11/26/2019

Dear Veena ~
Thank you so much for your wonderful
support & friendship, especially when I was
struggling with cancer. You are such an
- angel! God bless you always!

with TONS of Love &
Gratitude, ♥
Amor

BEEN THERE, DONE THAT

PRACTICAL TIPS & WISDOM
FROM CANCER SURVIVORS FOR CANCER PATIENTS

Amor Y. Traceski

gatekeeper press

Columbus, Ohio

Been There, Done That: Practical Tips & Wisdom from Cancer Survivors for Cancer Patients

Published by Gatekeeper Press
2167 Stringtown Rd, Suite 109
Columbus, OH 43123-2989
www.GatekeeperPress.com

ISBN (paperback): 9781619848375
eISBN: 9781619848368

Printed in the United States of America

Dedications

To my mother, Angela, now in Heaven, who ingrained in me
the critical importance of unconditional love, forgiveness, kindness
and sharing what I can
to be a channel of peace and to create a positive impact for others.

*

To my beautiful Catarina, who has always been
and will always be my inspiration and song.

Table of Contents

I always admire people who can look at any situation and see the positive. I met Amor almost two years before her ovarian cancer diagnosis, when she came in for group training at my fitness studio, My Core Balance. I was immediately impressed by her warmth, care, and authenticity. She struck me as one of those rare people who can reach out to a stranger with no context whatsoever, no introduction and, within minutes, become friends. She took some good time off for cancer treatment and returned with renewed determination to regain her health and physical strength.

I observed, firsthand, the care that Amor put into writing this book. As her personal trainer, she kept me updated on developments and I have been inspired by her excitement in sharing her stories Amor leads by example. No lectures, no judgment. She's a straight shooter, and she shoots from the heart. Rest assured that every word in this book was written out of a love and respect for you and what you are experiencing.

Not only is Amor caring and compassionate, she is also a powerful woman who follows through on her promises. Beginning her post-cancer treatment training with me just weeks after her last chemotherapy session, Amor walked in with a chemo cap on her bald head and a big smile on her face. She was ready to get down to the business of getting in shape.

As you can imagine, after the intense physical ordeal of fighting cancer, Amor's body was in a weakened state. The worst thing a beginner exerciser can do is be critical of themselves. At that delicate point in the process, the most important thing is consistency, even if the workouts are not very intense. Amor was disciplined, consistent, and determined. Gradually, with positivity and dedication, Amor strengthened her body. As her hair grew, so did her muscles. And so did her confidence in herself and what she can do. During a recent session, she completed a vigorous workout, alongside two other clients (who she encouraged every step of the way). She is all about sharing and helping. This book is a logical progression of that character. It is no accident that her name means LOVE.

I wish you all the best in your journey. You have a wonderful guide in Amor Traceski. She is truly here to support you.

Best of luck and God bless.

In health,
Chris Janke-Bueno

Owner/Personal Trainer, My Core Balance

Acknowledgments

Well, I must say that producing this very special book took a lot more time than I first thought. But then, from the idea, everything happened organically, which was actually a wonderful experience, despite the "hiccups." The combining of a ton of input together with the act of creating the material to, ultimately, publishing this book was, no doubt, a daunting task and I could not have done it without the support and generosity of some extraordinary people.

I am deeply grateful to all of the featured survivors in this book who I've come to know as my survivor sisters and brothers. **Aaron Cross, Bob Goodwin, Cindy Lewis, Cindy Reading, Glenn Mooty, Hilda Kurtovich, Jacki Spiteri, Joan Smith, John Bernard "JB" Ocampo, Rev. Linda Siddall, Rachel Salinas, Rick Sanders, Scott Michelsen, Sondra Williams, Susan Merport, Tet "Mesky" Mescallado, Vida Bonus Anderson and Yesi Lechuga:** Your courage, strength, graciousness, wit, intelligence, and willingness to share your individual vulnerabilities and wisdom borne from experience has really been awe-inspiring. I truly could not have written this precious book without you!

To my incredible partner in life, **Bill Stone.** From the very beginning, you supported me, taking precious time to proofread my manuscript, providing honest feedback and encouraging me along the way. Most of all, you gave me your love and guidance, especially in making sure I took care of myself and my health. You are my rock.

When I first told my family about this project, they believed in me from the get go. When I hit snags along the way and things painfully slowed down, they only gave me their understanding, lovingly and gently lifting me up to move forward one step at a time. I cannot thank you enough my beautiful daughter **Catherine** and my everloving siblings **Roman, Joy, Melody and JunJun.** Your unconditional love through the years, no matter the physical distance that separates us, is so overwhelmingly beautiful! I love you all so much!

What a blessing it has been to have the love of special friends who selflessly came to my rescue when I needed help with the seemingly mind-numbing task of proofreading and editing my manuscript. Thank you so much for all you've done to help me, my awesome BFF **Valerie Klazura** and my wonderful "big sis" **Linda Lepley!**

To those who generously provided motivation and financial support to help me get this book done and also to help me with my medical bills, words are not enough to truly convey my immense gratitude. Thank you so much **Joy Yamsuan Sanchez, Roman Yamsuan, Sidonie Sansom, Marsha Kliewer, Marty & Sam Lucky, Macy Tan, Lucy Tan, Mercy Yamsuan, JunJun Yamsuan, Amy Tanner, Ditas Malapitan, Pedro Angulo, Red Reyes, Silvana Garetz, Val & James Klazura, Beth Dugan, Joan Smith, Glenn Mooty, Martha & Steve Sandy, Jim Traceski, Art & Janis Kiesel, Sam Lerner, Sharon Lee, Susan Merport, Myse Salonga, Mary True, Rich & Connie Lee, Ray & Christine Rosenthal, Ilan Rosenthal, Karen Abolt, Barbara Bergero, Roger Chin, Carolyn Cox, Hazel Reyes, Steve & Phyllis Moore, Beatrice & Rama Ramachandran, Tess delos Reyes, George Menzoian, Kathy Carag, Dra. Joan delos Santos, Misa & Ed Flank, Doug Crom, Matt Corm, Jody Johnson, Veena Kallingal, Ambassador Ted Osius, Alma Avanzado, Joni Martin, Kim & Bob Shriver, Arnel Megino, Rebecca Palisoc, Judy Tsai, Sim Su, MCV and Pamela Jones.** Each of you are God-sent. Thank you so much!

During my health challenges throughout the years, I've met exceptional medical professionals and complementary health practitioners and would like to take this opportunity to personally thank them for their dedication to healing me and everyone whose lives they've touched.

Dr. Susan Marks, as my radiologist at Peninsula Diagnostic Imaging in San Mateo, CA, your dogged determination to identify suspicious shadows in my mammogram led to finding my breast cancer early. Thank you so much for taking the time to show me the images and explaining your findings and my options.

Dr. Pamela Lewis, as my breast surgeon in San Mateo, CA, your kindness in patiently making sure I understood everything about the mastectomy I was to undergo was invaluable. In your capable hands, my fears disappeared. Thank you for your awesomeness!

Dr. John Griffin, not only did you masterfully recreate my breasts as my plastic surgeon in San Mateo, CA, you also provided me with awesome care, reassuring me that I would be happy with the results ... and I have been ever since. Thank you for your expertise and for being there for me!

Dr. Jennifer Brown, as my breast cancer medical oncologist at California Cancer Care in San Mateo, CA, you made me feel valued as a patient. You also amazed me with how you answered my many questions before I asked them. Thank you so much for your insight and your caring!

Dr. Tae Noh, as my gynecologist in Santa Clara, CA, you identified the tumor in my ovaries and took immediate action. No doubt, the cancer would've advanced if not for your genuine concern for my health, which led to the finding of my ovarian cancer in its early stages. I am forever grateful!

Dr. Jeff Lin, I truly appreciate your surgical work, as my gynecologic oncologist, in performing my total abdominal hysterectomy, salpingo-oophorectomy, lymphadenectomy, enterolysis and the other procedures to remove my cancer.

Dr. Shane Dormady, how truly blessed I am to have had you as my ovarian cancer medical oncologist at the El Camino Hospital in Mountain View, CA, managing my chemotherapy and other treatments. You constantly inspired hope and gave me so many reasons to trust you with my health. You are a truly remarkable human being!

Charis Spielman, oncology nutrition specialist at the El Camino Hospital in Mountain View, CA. Your genuine care for me and my fellow cancer patients there was so evident. When you noticed our physical struggles, you didn't wait for us to come to you, you came to us. And you guided us with the right nutritional information to help us regain our health and strength. We have been so blessed with you!

Dr. Heather Lucas-Ross, as my current primary care physician at Western Sierra Medical Clinic in Penn Valley, CA, I've found, not only the best doctor for my care, but also a beautiful human being. Thank you for your selfless devotion to healing others and for giving me so many reasons to trust you. You are such a blessing to me!

Dr. David Campbell, I have been blessed with you as my current medical oncologist at the Sierra Nevada Memorial Hospital in Grass Valley, CA. Not only have you treated me with dignity and respect, you've also shown me kindness and patience, sharing insights about my cancer care that have been so enlightening. Thank you for helping me grow stronger in body, mind and spirit.

Dr. Justine Corbett, my integrative health doctor at Sierra Nevada Memorial Hospital in Grass Valley, CA, how wonderful it has been to learn from you about the amazing world of complementary medicine and the many opportunities available there for me to grow stronger in all ways. Thank you for being there for me!

Chris Janke-Bueno, my totally awesome personal trainer and friend who has guided me through my healing path towards strength and health. Both Bill & I are so grateful for all you do that truly makes a difference in our lives!

Anya Devi of Sacred Shakti Healing Arts in Grass Valley, CA, your skillful application of the Chi Nei Tsang massage to help me with my abdominal concerns, has opened up a whole new world of possibilities for me. Because of your amazing massages, I feel more energized. Thank you!

Lisa Swanson of Dharma Acupuncture in Grass Valley, CA, your expert acupuncture treatments have helped me in so many ways. I am truly grateful for your healing ways and look forward to more healing visits with you!

The oncology nurses and staff at the El Camino Hospital Cancer Center in Mountain View, CA are particularly special to me, because they helped to make all of my visits to the Cancer Center comfortable and pleasant. It was really a unique experience to feel the love and kindness they freely gave me and all of their patients. My heartfelt gratitude to nurse practitioner **Katie Kuhl**, business manager **Jaimee Chow**, my oncology nurses **Shelly, KB, Tamara, Major, Larisa, Lori, Sarah, Sharon, Theresa** and **Smita** and appointment coordinator **Maisie Tai**. Thank you so much for being the angels on earth that you have been (and continue to be) for all those you care for!

I am filled with deep gratitude and love for my many friends and relatives who lifted me up in prayer, sent me their positive thoughts, shared their time and energy with me, brought me food, cooked for me, cleaned my house, tended to my wounds, drove me to appointments, brought me flowers, balloons or gifts, sent me get-well cards ... So many wonderful acts of kindness and love for me, I am forever thankful!

To my wonderful extended family **Mom & Sam, Kelley & Dave, Wendy & Dave** and **Sean & Cory,** thank you so much for your continued love and support. It means so much to me!.

To my truly beautiful, awesome fellow Lions of the Foster City Lions Club who cheered me on through both my breast and ovarian cancers: **Karen Abolt, Wood Andrews, Barbara Bergero, Roger Chin, Chris Colgin, Carolyn Cox, Doug Crom, Matt Corm, Kateryna Davydova, Lori Eubanks, John Ficarra, Ed Flank, Jon Froomin, Jeanne Gallagher, Bob Goodwin, Shikha Hamilton, Don Isaacs, Jody Johnson, Veena Kallingal, Art & Janis Kiesel, Marsha Kliewer, Rich Lee, Sam Lerner, Terry McIntosh, Steve Moore, Phyllis McArthur, Pierre Morrison, Joe Pierucci, Chris & Kris Powell, Beatrice & Rama Ramachandra, Sandi Rocco, Danielle Rosenthal, Ilan Rosenthal, Ray Rosenthal, Martha Sandy, Joan Smith, Patrick Sullivan, Masako & Takao Suzuki, Willie Swan, Lucy Tan, Macy Tan, Spike Traceski, Mary True, Maria Vorobiev** and **Wing Yu.**

To my fabulous girlfriends through the years **Hilda Kurtovich, Janet Reyes, Dora Navales, Ria Nelson, Ellen Chao & Therese Williams**. Though our times together are few and far between, our "sisterhood" is so special to me! Thank you for your awesome love and support!

How blessed I've been to have my **Reyes** and **Yamsuan** relatives around the world cheering me on. Thank you all for your continued love and prayers during my health challenges. And **Sherry Wang**, my special neighbor who called 911 and accompanied me to the emergency room, you really were my God-sent angel! I especially would like to thank cousin **Amy Reyes Tanner** for being like a wonderful sister, caring for me on behalf of my family in Manila.

I've been so blessed with my classmates from College of the Holy Spirit in Manila, Philippines who showered me with positive thoughts and prayers from afar, namely: **Julie Famorca, Alma Avanzado, Susan Lim, Maggie Tipoe, Cathy Ledesma, Mabel Chua, Tina Medrana, Malou Tejada, Mica Calica, Mari de leon Hautea, Colette Marcos, Lia Torralba, Ma-i Matias, Angie Villegas, Anabel Macalinao, Jocelyn de Leon, Monique Cuenco, Joy Basuil, Claire Zarate, Angie Villegas, Leah Lazo, Lucy Sy, Ruby Melo, Cita Dee, Nela Sulit, Nimfa Trias, Angelica San Mateo, Bett Esposo** and, most especially, **Tet "Mesky" Mescallado** and **Vida Bonus Anderson.**

Most of all, I am grateful beyond words to my God who has blessed me with so much and has guided me throughout my writing of this book. Without my God, there would be no book; there would be no me.

Thank you, Lord, for unconditionally loving me!

~♥~

Introduction

"You gain strength, courage, and confidence by every
experience in which you really stop to look fear in the face.
You are able to say to yourself, 'I lived through this horror.
I can take the next thing that comes along.'
You must do the thing you think you cannot do."

~ *Eleanor Roosevelt*

WHAT'S DIFFERENT ABOUT THIS BOOK.

First and foremost, this is a down-to-earth, honest book that contains detailed information about my battles with breast and ovarian cancers, as well as, first-hand, actual experiences of nineteen of my brave amazing cancer survivor sisters and brothers ranging from 21 to 92 years of age. The cancers that they fought include adrenal gland, blood & bone marrow (chronic lymphocytic leukemia), breast (including triple negative & triple positive), colon, kidney, liver, lung, ovaries, pancreas, prostate, rectum, salivary gland, skin, soft tissue and stomach.

It is a no-nonsense, no-regrets book written to provide you with realistic accounts of what transpired during our cancer journeys. Although some of the content may be considered upsetting because of graphic details, we all believe it necessary to share the facts - both the good and the bad. Basically, anything caused by cancer is bad and anything that relates to beating cancer is good. As cancer survivors, we experienced highs and lows in our journeys, so it would be too for cancer patients. That is reality.

We share our stories, tips and advice, so that you can learn and, hopefully, benefit from the wisdom we've gained through our experiences, amidst the difficulties. Knowledge is power. Knowledge is strength. It is up to you to determine for yourself what story or practical advice is applicable to you.

NECESSARY REPETITIONS.

The accounts shared in this book describe our experiences characterized by a variety of physical and emotional factors. Due to the fact that some of these experiences happened simultaneously, you will find various accounts repeated throughout the book. This repetition is necessary to ensure that the topic or topics you are interested in can be quickly referenced, based on each symptom or circumstance, and nothing is missed.

PRACTICAL ADVICE, NOT MEDICAL ADVICE.

The purpose of this book is to convey information. It is not meant to be interpreted as medical advice, nor is it intended to diagnose, treat or cure your condition, or to be a substitute for advice from your doctor or other healthcare professional. The practical methods and advice provided here are personal to each of the cancer survivors featured in this book. They are intended to give you ideas on how to cope and live with your cancer.

HOW THIS BOOK CAME ABOUT.

When I first learned that I had cancer, I remember having to search for answers to my many questions on the Internet, at the library, in magazines, from documentaries, or from cancer survivors. It was not an easy task. It was sometimes confusing and definitely overwhelming. When I experienced my second cancer, I was still at a loss and wished that there was one central book that contained what I needed to know about my cancer, how to cope, what options I have, what the various medical terms mean, what I could expect, etc. I searched everywhere, but couldn't find what I needed; what, I believe, anyone experiencing cancer needs. And so, I created <u>Been There. Done That: Practical Tips & Wisdom from Cancer Survivors for Cancer Patients.</u>

HOW TO USE THIS BOOK.

This is not a regular book. I wrote it to serve three main purposes:

1. to be a "one-stop-shop" reference for cancer patients, survivors, caregivers, or anyone experiencing symptoms and conditions similar to those described here, whether it be first-hand or second-hand. It is not only for those suffering from the cancers the featured survivors in this book experienced;
2. to provide a deeper insight into how people experience cancer, from diagnosis to treatment to survival, and
3. to share practical tips and wisdom borne from experience from everyone featured in this book in hopes that it will benefit the readers and help them cope with their challenges.

Listed below is a brief description of each part of the book. Feel free to go directly to the part or parts that interest you.

- PART ONE is a compilation of profiles for each of our featured brave and awesome cancer survivors
- PART TWO is a special message from an extraordinary breast cancer patient
- PART THREE of the book will read like a guidebook or reference for patients or caregivers needing to find realistic and practical ways to deal with the cancer diagnoses, including:

  - how to share news with your family and friends
  - how to cope with possible treatment side effects
  - how to deal with medical treatments & procedures
  - how to get a handle on scans, biopsies, blood tests and similar processes
  - how to adapt to personal cancer treatment devices & accessories
  - how to wrestle with your natural negative emotions
  - how to carry on with daily life activities
  - how to relate to your medical team
  - how to organize your medical records

- PART FOUR contains various other ways to cope with cancer and treatment including:

  - good stuff to help you get through
  - how integrative healthcare coordinates conventional and complementary approaches to healing
  - cancer-fighting nutrition
  - effective cancer-fighting workouts

- PART FIVE addresses the subject of survivorship:

  - facing survivorship
  - the new "normal" and ways to move on
  - ways to create your own cancer survivor network

- APPENDICES is where other resources you can use are contained, e.g.

  - information to help you understand the major types of cancer, cancer stages & grades, and the general types of cancer treatments
  - cancer support resources, e.g. American Cancer Society, Cancer Horizons, Cancer.net, WhatNext.com and other sites where you can find information about cancer, treatments, programs, guidelines, options, active cancer communities you can join, etc.
  - tips for caregivers and how to support someone with cancer

- GLOSSARY OF TERMS. I gathered a great number of terms that you may come across in communicating with your medical team and health insurance team. I also provided their definitions to help you understand what those terms mean, so you can make better decisions.

IT'S ABOUT HOPE AND TRIUMPH.

Been There. Done That: Practical Tips & Wisdom from Cancer Survivors for Cancer Patients was written to prove that we can overcome our adversities and somehow find the strength from within to rise above our circumstances. Yes, it is a book about survival. However, it is mostly a book about hope and triumph over cancer. As you go through your cancer journey, we hope that you will find this book a source of comfort, strength, peace, hope, and love.

Fellow breast cancer survivor and multi-talented singer-songwriter Sheryl Crow stated, "More than 10 million Americans are living with cancer, and they demonstrate the ever-increasing possibility of living beyond cancer." All survivors featured in this very special book are included in the more than 10 million cancer survivors that Sheryl is referring to. We've been there and done that. We are proof that you can live beyond cancer. Here's hoping and looking forward to you being included in that growing number too!

Amor

"What lies behind us and what lies before us
are small matters compared to what lies
within us. And when we bring what is within
us out into the world, miracles happen."

~ *Ralph Waldo Emerson*

PART ONE

Chapter 1

ABOUT OUR FEATURED AMAZING CANCER SURVIVORS

This chapter contains the profiles of each of the brave, amazing
cancer survivors and warriors featured in this book.
Where, before cancer, we were individuals living separate lives,
we are now survivor sisters and brothers working together here towards a common goal:
To make a positive difference for you on your cancer journey.

"You never know how strong you are
until being strong is your only choice."

~ *Bob Marley*

"We cannot change what happened.
But we can change how we relate to it."

~ *Eva Mozes Kor*
Holocaust survivor

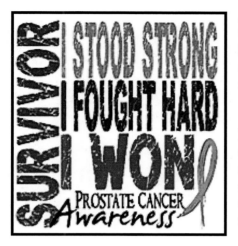

Aaron is a dashing, energetic, charismatic, smart and big-hearted 55-year old Caucasian male. He is divorced and lives in a multi-level house in the suburbs of Southern California. He has two beautiful daughters, eleven and fourteen years of age, who he's very proud of. He enjoys spending time with them and his girlfriend, who has been there for him through thick and thin.

He and his half-brother, 19 years his senior, grew up in different households. His father had no cancer issues, and his mother had no known cancer issues other than possible skin cancer, but Aaron is not sure. His brother, who had a different father, had prostate cancer in his mid-60s and is a survivor who used radiation treatment for his stage III prostate cancer diagnosis. Their mother lived until she was 95½ years of age, a testimony to their family's history of longevity. They follow the Catholic faith.

Aaron was a law enforcement officer for more than 20 years and retired more than five years ago. Despite being retired, he still keeps himself very busy as a consultant in a similar field of work. Aside from relishing precious time with his daughters and girlfriend, Aaron likes playing the drums. He was a cool drummer for a rock band a long time ago and still carries his "coolness" with him wherever he goes. In 1998, Aaron learned he had skin cancer (basal cell carcinoma) and in March of 2016, he was informed he had prostate cancer stage II. Here is Aaron's story.

When I first learned I had skin cancer in the lower eyelid of my left eye, I was shocked and upset. The doctor I had seen the year before told me that I just had a stye in my eye. His misdiagnosis cost me unnecessary pain and anger. Fortunately, the MOHS surgery I went through to remove the cancerous skin tissue was relatively "simple" and effective.

News of my prostate cancer diagnosis in 2016 hit me like a ton of bricks. It was hard to believe because I didn't exhibit any physical symptoms, whatsoever, e.g. pressure, pain, lumps on my prostate, etc. I was shocked also because the odds were like one-in-fifty that men under the age of 55 get prostate cancer! This all began when, after some time of getting my PSAs (prostate Specific Antigen) checked every few years, I noticed that the number was starting to rise. My doctor recommended prostate biopsy, but I didn't want one because my PSA was 3.6 ng/ml and the PSA threshold for biopsy is 4.0 ng/ml. So, three years later, I had my PSA checked again; the number increased to 3.9 ng/ml. That's when I agreed to get my prostate biopsied.

Before I had the prostate biopsy, I told my doctor, "I want to be unconscious for this." He said, "Sure." You see, just the thought of them inserting the biopsy device with needles up my rectum made me cringe, so I didn't want to be awake for it. Results of the initial biopsy revealed stage I cancer, i.e. about 5% cancer cells contained within the prostate. But, the pathology of my prostate after its removal during surgery revealed stage II and 20% cancer, with a few cancer cells close to the bladder. Luckily, I had a low Gleason score, which meant a non-aggressive cancer type.

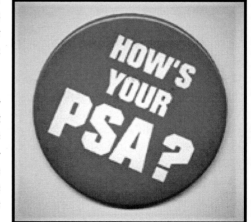

For treatment, I had the option of radiation, but I didn't like the downside. You see, with surgery, the side effects are immediate. But then, you get better and the side effects go away. Whereas, with radiation, you don't get the immediate effects. They happen later. So, I figured that I would be out of commission for a year and a half. In the big scheme of things, I'll (hopefully) have 30 more years of life and this episode will be a blip. I've got two kids; I can't be dead by the time I'm 70 years old! If you have children, you've got to live for your kids. At least, be around for a while and enjoy them.

My girlfriend was with me when I got the call. So she knew right away. As for my daughters, I just told them. Of course, they were worried that I was going to die. I said, "No, I'm not going to die. I'm going to have surgery." Then I said, "I'm going to be a little bit out-of-commission for a while, but your dad's going to be fine." I have a healthy relationship with my daughters, and I'm very honest with them. When they came over to be with me, there were a few things I couldn't do, like run and chase them around the house, like I used to. For ten days I had to wear a catheter and one day, they saw the

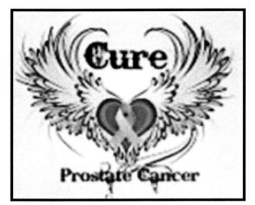

drain bag attached to my leg. So, I had to explain to them that I had to urinate into the bag. Then, I told them, "I need you to help me do this and that..." At first, they got grossed out by it. But after, they were totally cool with it, because they wanted to help me. You know, help their daddy.

I was really fortunate to get the best surgeon to operate the Da Vinci Robotic Surgical System during my radical prostatectomy, the surgery to remove my prostate gland. My doctor decided to remove a couple dozen lymph nodes from my groin region, since they were inflamed when he was doing surgery. Luckily, there was no cancer located in my lymph nodes. From the surgery, I experienced a few side effects, like constipation, pain, fatigue, bladder problems, lymphedema, and weight loss. I'm glad I didn't have to go through radiation or chemotherapy. However, I did have to wear a catheter for ten days, which was miserable, because of all the stuff that was connected to me.

Now that my cancer is passed me, I'm very grateful that I survived when some of the men I knew, sadly, did not. I strongly advise men to get their PSAs checked on a regular basis. The doctors don't usually like to check men's PSAs until they're 65 years old,but I would not wait that long. Start in your late 40s. My doctor said that the fact that I was proactive and had it checked early was the reason the cancer was caught early. That's what you've got to do because it can spread all of a sudden and kill you if you ignore it. It's unusual for someone under 55 to have prostate cancer, but it does occur.

Like I said earlier, when I learned I had cancer (both times), I was in shock. It's natural, given the fact that the news just seemed to come out of nowhere and went against the odds. I also had to deal with anxiety and irritation, something that is expected with the various adjustments I had to make in my activities, especially the limitations. I didn't let those limitations get the better of me though. I was determined to beat this cancer and get on with my life. I researched a lot about the disease and my options, so that I could be smart about what I needed to do and how. I asked the doctors and medical staff questions when I had questions and asked for their help when I needed their help. I was continuously engaged when it came to my treatment, because I really believed that it was critical to my recovery. I kept my focus on healing and regaining by strength. As soon as I could, I worked out at the gym and returned to my regular life activities. Of course, I had to start slow, but at least, I was able to return to living my life again. All throughout my cancer experience, I kept thinking about how I had to keep on fighting, so that I could be around for my kids and enjoy them. Now that it's behind me, I'm really thankful. I'm looking forward to spending time with them and watching them grow up.

Although it has been more than two years since my surgery, I am still not 100% recovered. My bladder still leaks and my erections are not as they were prior to surgery. If I consume too much salt, my left ankle will swell up. My doctor says that once my body adapts to the loss of lymph nodes, the swelling will subside. My only frustration, as a man, is still not having 100% normal function as I did prior to surgery. My recommendation to men, in my similar situation, is to buy and use the Tena Pads for men, and exercise your Kegel muscles regularly to help regain your bladder control more quickly – but have patience as it takes time. I have realized that this is a long, slow recovery process. But, I am hopeful to completely recover in the not-so-distant future. ~ *Aaron*

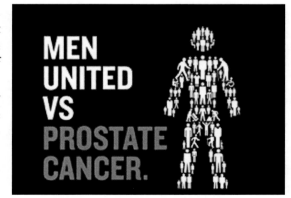

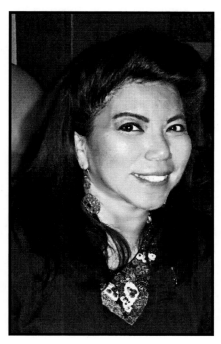

Hello Everyone! Since I put this book together, I thought I'd just share with you candidly about myself and my cancer journeys. As of this writing, I'm 58 years old and live in Penn Valley, CA with my amazing life partner Bill. I have one child, my beautiful daughter Catherine, who has been my joy and inspiration throughout my health challenges.

I am of Filipino-Spanish-Chinese ancestry, the second oldest of five siblings: Roman, Joy, Melody and Romy, Jr. We were born and raised in Taiwan where our father, Romulo, was a jazz band leader. Our mother, Angela, who was an English teacher, died of cervical cancer at the age of 73. Two cousins on my mother's side also had breast cancer, as did two of my paternal grandmother's sisters. No one in my family's history had ovarian cancer.

Before my cancer experiences, I was a human resources executive in the corporate world. I was a career-centered workaholic and kept myself constantly on-the-go, foregoing sleep a lot. Yes, it did make for a stressful lifestyle, but at the time, I focused on being successful and climbing the corporate ladder as high as I could. Outside of work, I was an active board member of the Foster City Lions Club. I enjoyed volunteering and being in the company of like-hearted friends there, working on fundraising and service activities for our community. Even though being able to share is fulfilling for me, my enjoyment in being with others led to my tendency to put myself last, and I didn't know then how to change. I remember telling myself, "I'll balance my life later." Unfortunately, I was too deep in the rat race, I just couldn't find my way out. And so, I learned … the hard way … that my health also should be a priority.

In 2013, I was given the formal diagnosis of multifocal stage I, HER2/neu negative, hormone receptors strongly positive cancer breast cancer. My treatment included a modified radical mastectomy of the left breast with sentinel lymph node biopsy and unilateral microvascular DIEP breast reconstruction. Since I was not in menopause yet, I was given hormone therapy of Tamoxifen to take for five years following the surgery.

After a week's stay at the hospital, I was sent home only to return to the hospital's emergency room the next day via ambulance due to a staph infection (cellulitis and sepsis). I stayed an additional week in the hospital, the only viable veins in my right arm pummeled with strong antibiotics, sulfa drugs and vancomycin. Although it was a really scary experience, I found strength in God and somehow knew I would survive. The love and support that was showered upon me also gave me a boost. Even though my daughter Catherine was away at college and couldn't physically be with me, she arranged for us to spend time together via Skype video chats, which was truly precious and comforting.

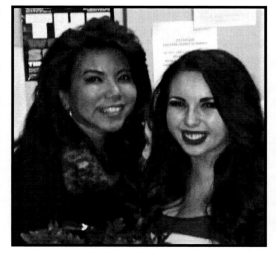

In January 2016, my gynecologist noted a large abdominal mass after my annual pap smear. Results of an ultrasound and biopsy showed that I had ovarian epithelial cancer. Thank God, it was detected early, and I was told that I should need only three chemo infusions. Unfortunately, after the three chemo sessions, my CA125 cancer marker was still high at 361.5 (normal is 35). Also, at that time, I observed strange gurgling sounds when I breathed. Results of a CT scan showed a "large" pleural effusion (fluid buildup) in my right lung, multiple enlarged nodes in the space between both lungs (mediastinum) and around my left breast/armpit area and a 7 cm soft tissue mass at the vaginal cuff. My oncologist was "highly suspicious for progression of one or both" of my cancers and my heart sank.

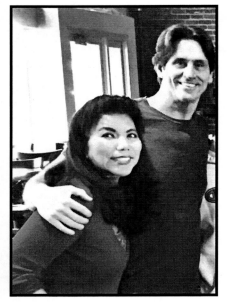

Nevertheless, I was determined to continue my fight. I went through a thoracentesis (pleural tap) where over three quarts of fluid was removed from my right lung. Biopsies of the nodes and the soft tissue mass were taken and I had a PET scan to identify where cancer had "spread" in my body. Bill and I braced ourselves for the bad news that the cancer had spread. When we met with my oncologist, he hesitantly said, "I don't know what to say ... The PET scan was clear ... There is no evidence of cancer!" Bill & I were stunned and cried tears of joy! I thanked God because I truly felt that it was a miracle! My oncologist agreed and said that everything pointed to recurrence or progression of cancer. He couldn't explain the results. Unfortunately, my CA 125 cancer marker was still high at 115.1 and cancer cells can still hide in our body undetected. On my trying to get out of more chemo infusions, my oncologist sternly warned me, "This is a matter of life and death. Don't play with your life." With that, I completed the rest of my chemotherapy treatments.

Between both my cancers (breast & ovarian), I went through a multitude of treatments and procedures, including chemotherapy, breast reconstruction (diep flap) surgery, hormone therapy, mastectomy, medical port implant and removal surgeries, MRIs, CT scans, biopsies, thoracentesis, catheterizations and x-rays. My experiences ran the gamut of side effects, including abdominal adhesions, allergic reactions, alopecia, anemia, arthralgia (bone & joint pain and weakness), chemo brain, constipation, delayed wound healing, diarrhea, dizziness, eye/vision problems, fat necrosis, fatigue, feet changes, fever, gas, hearing problems, hot flashes, hypothermia, a staph infection, itchiness, kidney/bladder problems, leg, foot and toe cramps, leukopenia, loss of appetite, lung problems, lymphedema, mouth & tongue changes, muscle cramps & pain, nausea, neuropathy, numbness, osteopenia, pain, poor sleep, poor veins, stiffness/rigidity, swelling, taste and smell changes, weakness, weight loss and a a really bad yeast infection. Although I always tried to keep an attitude of gratitude, there were times when my emotions were a bit wobbly, and I gave in naturally to negative emotions, like anxiety, confusion, depression, fear, frustration, sadness, loneliness, feeling overwhelmed, resignation, self-pity, shock and uncertainty.

Sure, going through cancer twice was really tough. However, looking back, I appreciate the experiences because I grew so much from them. Being surrounded by so much love from Catherine, Bill, my siblings, Roman, Joy, Melody and JunJun and my awesome, loving friends everywhere truly lifted me up. My faith in God kept me strong in ways I could never have imagined otherwise. It taught me a depth of happiness and peace that I never knew could exist, especially under very challenging and painful circumstances. Yes, there were times I thought God would take me and I was ready to go. However, I also felt enlightened and knew that I would be okay. There is a beautiful reason why I am still here. I am on a mission to spread hope and peace and joy and, most of all, love. ~ *Amor*

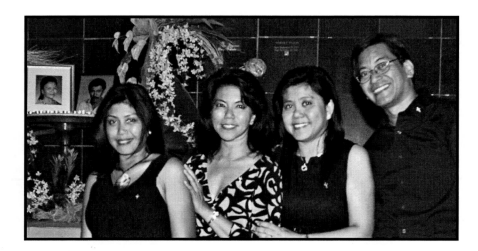

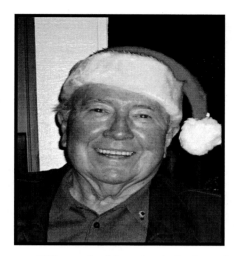

Bob is a fascinating and charismatic nonagenarian widower; a gentleman with a great sense of humor who embraces life with his positivity and wisdom! At 92-years young, he keeps fit by swimming regularly. His favorite role is great grandfather to his great grandchildren.

He and his wife Elizabeth raised three beautiful daughters: Vicky, Leslie and Kathleen. Sadly, Elizabeth passed away 12 years ago. On family history of cancer, Bob's mother died of stomach cancer and his sister died of skin cancer (melanoma). Not only does Bob's family have a history of cancer, they also have Lynch Syndrome, a type of inherited cancer syndrome associated with a genetic predisposition to different cancer types. This means that all of his family members have a higher risk of certain types of cancer. His family is aware of the gene that they carry. Two of his daughters are also cancer survivors.

When asked how he feels about having Lynch Syndrome, Bob says, "Well, what can we do? It's all a matter of having the right attitude." And Bob has loads of that! Bob is the youngest of four children and almost died before his other three siblings. His oldest brother died 20 days short of turning 94. Bob remarked, "He was nine years older than me, so I have a ways to go to beat him. But, who cares?"

He remembers how he and his siblings had to work newspaper routes growing up and how they learned to be practical and frugal. He recalled a time with his mother, "When I graduated junior high school, my mother bought me a new suit, new socks, new underwear....the whole works! Then she said, 'I want you to be sure to pick out something you will use again because from now on, you buy your own clothes.' I was 14 at the time, so for Christmas, instead of asking for toys, I asked for clothes!"

Starting out, Bob chose to see the world and become a merchant seaman. He was commissioned as a Merchant Marine Ensign with the U.S. Maritime Service (USMS). After the service, he worked selling appliances by pounding the pavements, going door-to-door and driving a truck for the grocery chains Safeway and Best Foods. Although he did not stay long in those jobs, he recalled those tough times fondly. Eventually, he landed in real-estate. While Bob bought and sold property, he asked his wife Elizabeth to handle the paperwork aspect of the business because he was "the world's worst bookkeeper". She was very methodical and with his success in real-estate, they "never had to worry about a nickel" since.

When asked about his favorite hobby, Bob – without hesitation, with a twinkle in his eyes and in a loud booming voice – said, "Chasing the females!" Laughter then followed. Just one of the many wonderful qualities about Bob is how he brings with him joy, wit and laughter that can brighten up the gloomiest room!

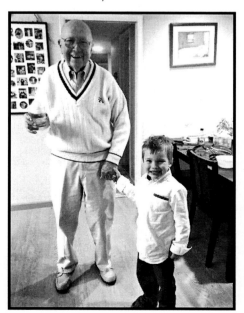

Bob has always kept active and believes it has contributed to his health through the years. He didn't stop swimming and dancing, even during treatment. He said, "I can't swim in the sun because of my skin. I still swim, but not as often and not as long. Now, I'm back up to swimming my half-hour time. I'm slower, but I figure that I'm the only 91-year old man still swimming!"

He is a member-at-large of the Foster City Lions Club (a service organization), which he has been active in for over 50 years. Aside from being a Lion, Bob has also been a member of The Elk's Lodge for over 20 years. As a valued member of the Lions Club in Foster City, Lion Bob is known for his outstanding work promoting one of the projects of Lions Clubs International: the Peace

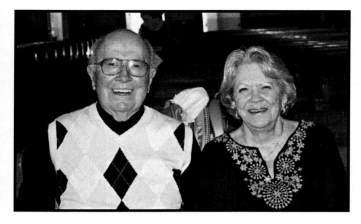

Poster contest. This is a contest for children that encourages them to express their visions of peace. Lion Bob was recognized for his commitment to this project, engaging various Lions Clubs with the youth in their community to sponsor their Peace Posters.

When Bob was 63 years old, he survived his first cancer: soft tissue sarcoma, which is a rare cancer in adults (representing only 1% of all adult cancers). He has since survived several cancers and the multiple surgeries associated with them. He's had surgery to remove his spleen and surrounding tissues and, after radiation, radical surgery to remove his left kidney, 50% of his colon, one to two back ribs, some muscle and more tissue. He has gone through more than 25 surgeries through the years to remove skin cancer found in his body, many of which he's found himself through proactive self-examination of his skin.

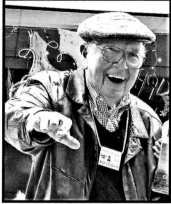

One of Bob's coping strategies is to keep life in perspective and go with the flow. Don't let your circumstances get you down he says. He also believes that it is important to communicate your needs and stand your ground if your situation calls for it.

Bob is constantly aware of how fortunate he has been and how much life there is still to live. So, what if he's 91! He enjoys time with his family and his wonderful partner Connie. Aside from having an abundance of stories and jokes, he keeps a plethora of original quotes that he likes to share. Here are a couple of great ones: "I may never ever work again, but I will NEVER RETIRE!" And, one to really keep in mind. "If it rains, you have to enjoy the rain. If it's foggy, you have to enjoy the fog. Because we don't have time to wait for the future!" ~ *Bob*

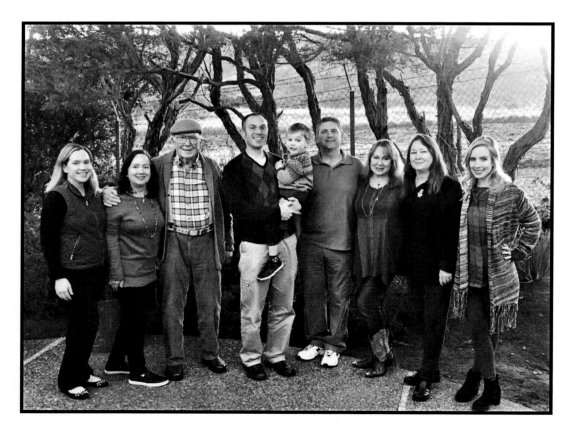

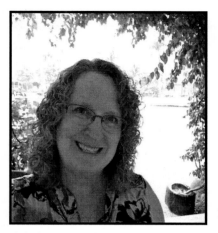

Cindy is a wonderful, remarkable 50+ year old woman with a heart of gold. She and her husband of 36 years, Ed, have four children: Brennan (32), Ali (31), Harrison (28) and Katy (25). They have lived in their one-story family home in Navarre, Florida for the past 15 years.

Of German-English-Irish-Scottish heritage, Cindy is the middle child and only daughter in her family. She and her two brothers were raised by their parents, Jack and Barbara Riddle in Columbus, Ohio. Their family has a history of cancer: Cindy's maternal grandmother had endometrial cancer; her maternal grandfather had bladder and skin (basal) cancer on his hand; her mother had basal cell cancer on her face, squamous cell on her leg, and her father had squamous cancer cells on his arm. According to Cindy, "No one in the family had kidney cancer, which was odd because both my brothers had frequent problems with kidney stones, but not cancer, and I didn't have kidney stones, but I was the one who had cancer."

Being a nurturer by nature, it was hard for Cindy to accept nurturing from others. Aside raising her four children, she volunteered in their schools, was PTA (Parent-Teacher Association) president for many years, visited schools throughout the San Francisco Bay Area to guide them on disaster preparedness, earthquake drills and even wrote the disaster preparedness plans that are currently being used in those districts. After motherhood and volunteerism throughout California, she went on to her second career as a registered nurse and a birth doula in Florida. Cindy is a people person and always wants to make a positive difference for others.

Cindy loves photography and enjoys writing her blog called, "The Midlife Express" where she hopes to be able to continue helping women and men alike on issues that approach them during midlife, such as health concerns, elder parent care, dementia, etc. On October 27, 2016, Cindy had surgery to remove her left kidney and received word that she had kidney cancer (clear cell renal carcinoma). Here is Cindy's story:

In December of 2014, I was placed on Prometrium (the female hormone progesterone) and took it daily as instructed. In July of 2015, I started itching in my hands, my feet and the back of my legs (calves). It was very strange. When I had it checked, the doctor had blood work done. When the results came in, she told me that my bilirubin was high, I was jaundiced, my triglycerides had tripled, my cholesterol levels were fine and we should just wait until next year to see if anything more develops. Well, that didn't sound right to me at all. So I just said to her, "No, I don't think so" and found another doctor.

As a nurse, I figured that my strange itchiness was a reaction to the Prometrium that was causing my liver to struggle. And so, I went off of that. At that point, a lot of things started happening really fast. I went on a very low carb diet, quit sugar and started losing weight at an alarming rate of speed, i.e. 48 pounds in a very short period of time. In December of 2015, my doctor called for an abdominal ultrasound and he said, "There's a cyst on your left kidney. Don't worry about it. These things are usually benign." Well, something in the back of my mind said, "No, we are going to worry about this." We agreed to follow-up in six months. In August, 2016, I had another ultrasound. Two hours later, he called to tell me that he found something suspicious. Since I have a heart issue and take beta blockers, we agreed that I was to get an MRI vs a CT due to the contrast dye. After a review of the results, he referred me to a urologist and said that there was a 95% chance I had cancer. Looking back, a

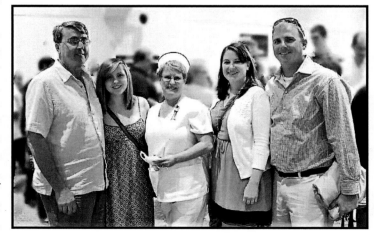

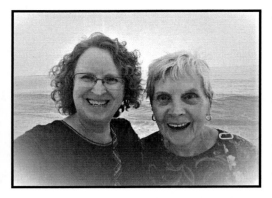

whole year had passed and the cyst in my kidney grew. When it was removed at the end of October, the urology oncologist stated it had probably been there 6+ years. The fact it was misclassified by radiology and, therefore, dismissed as benign by my primary doctor goes to show that even though medical professionals are trained and they care, it's important to still question them.

For treatment, I had a radical nephrectomy to remove my left kidney and all the surrounding tissue. Fortunately, I didn't have to go through chemotherapy or radiation. I did, however, go through so many changes in my body from the surgery that led to side effects like fatigue, gas (flatulence), low blood pressure, hot flashes, hypothermia, bladder problems, foot cramps, loss of appetite, nausea, pain, poor sleep/insomnia and weight loss.

During recovery, I also suffered negative emotions, like anger, anxiety, fear, frustration, grief, guilt, loneliness, feeling overwhelmed, resignation, self-pity, shame, shock, stress and uncertainty. I struggled with having to live life functioning with only one kidney versus two. Even after my physical body healed, many of the negative emotions persisted. I was still stressed, anxious, overwhelmed and at a loss. Those negative emotions were paralyzing me, so I sought professional help from a psychologist. I learned so many lessons that I've shared with my family and friends. And, I continue to share those lessons when and where I can, so that others may benefit. I learned that it's important to validate our humanity and know that feeling those negative emotions are natural, given our circumstances. I learned that we can't be happy 24/7, so when we feel unhappy, we should feel it, own it and then move on. Just don't unpack and live there!

I also learned to create my new "normal" and realize that as I've been trying to adjust, my wonderful husband Ed, my amazing children and all of my supporters have also been trying to adjust. I cannot thank them enough for their patience and love and support. Life continues and things can get better. I am inspired by Bob Marley's quote: "You never know how strong you are, until being strong is your only choice." I definitely grew from this experience. I am strong! ~ *Cindy*

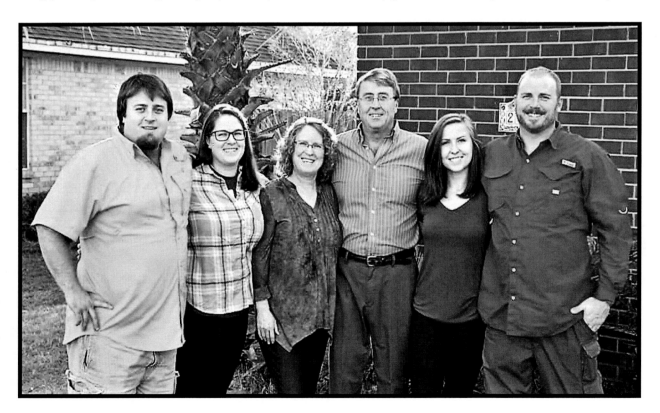

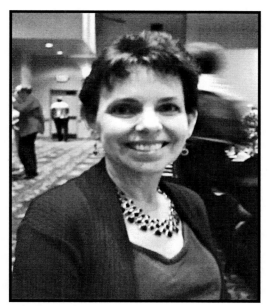

Cindy is an amazing 54 year old woman with a beautiful, kind and adventurous spirit. She lives in single story home in Valley Springs, CA with her loving dogs Harley and Shelby, who are her constant companions.

Cindy is of European descent and has two younger sisters, Karen and Lynette. Her close-knit family has a history of cancer; her father had prostate cancer. Just three months after Cindy's diagnosis, her younger sister, Karen, learned she had breast cancer and two years after, her mom learned that she, too, had breast cancer.

Before Cindy's bouts with cancer, she worked as an underwriter with a mortgage company. She led an active lifestyle, going to concerts and festivals, attending football games rooting for the Oakland Raiders, going horseback riding, camping, training and walking her dogs and traveling. She enjoys arts and crafts (e.g. jewelry making) and loves to dance, cook and bake, among many other activities. Cindy prides herself in having a good read for people and has found inspiration in her favorite book: Lance Armstrong's "It's Not About the Bike: My Journey Back to Life."

In 2004, Cindy learned she had stage III breast cancer. After she completed her treatment and went into remission, she was, unfortunately, involved in a head-on collision, which left her permanently disabled. She suffered broken ribs, a concussion and her back, one leg and an arm were broken. Then, in 2014, ten years after Cindy completed treatment for breast cancer, she found out that she had stomach cancer. Only, that was a misdiagnosis. Two years after faring poorly in the treatment of her stomach cancer, they realized that Cindy's stomach cancer was actually a metastasis of her breast cancer from ten years prior. So they drastically adjusted her treatment, which she finally responded to quite well. Here is Cindy's story:

I was 39 years old when I first noticed an inversion in my right breast, I kept looking at it and thinking, "Well, it's nothing." Still, I paid attention and noticed that it kept growing. Naturally, I got nervous. When my doctor said that it was nothing, I was not convinced and insisted on having it examined. The CT scan revealed that I had a lump in my breast the size of a golf ball. I had stage III breast cancer. My family and I were shocked, because there was no history of anyone in my family ever having breast cancer. Still, I kept positive throughout the entire treatment, focusing on what I could learn and how I could adjust to changes I had to make in my life. I enjoy keeping things light and I love to laugh. So, that's what I did as much I could, which I know helped me to heal faster.

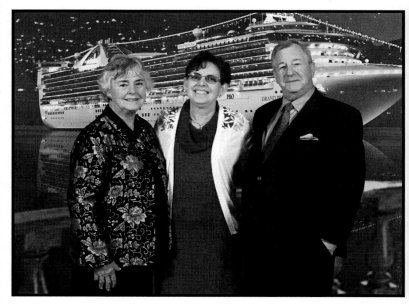

Not long after completion of my treatment, I got into a really serious, head-on collision car accident where the other driver, unfortunately, died, and I lived. But I'm permanently disabled. I broke my leg, my arm, my ribs and my back and had a concussion. Before the accident, everything was healing and I was able to get mobility back. Then with injuries from the accident, I've been in constant pain since. I realized,

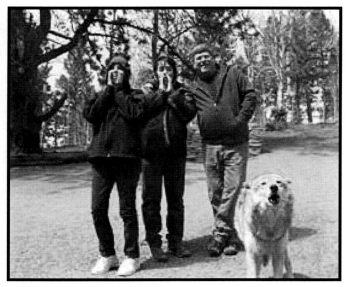

though, how fortunate I am to still be alive. So, I thanked God and told myself, "Okay, I'm going to fight this disability by being strong in my spirit and attitude and not worry about other things." It's really just a matter of doing what you can.

Around the 10th year anniversary of my breast cancer diagnosis, I noticed that my appetite was decreasing. I didn't feel any pain, just something like a cramping sensation. Results of a biopsy done on my stomach revealed that I had stomach cancer. I was completely shocked. I didn't understand at all and I was angry and afraid at the same time. After two years of treatment, I just wasn't getting any better. I was so sick; it was really awful. My doctors realized that my stomach cancer wasn't a separate cancer; it was actually a metastasis of my breast cancer from ten years back. So, they immediately changed my treatment plan, which has finally been working wonders!

It has been quite a ride dealing with both my cancers. I went through multiple rounds of chemotherapy, several hormone therapy treatments, a hysterectomy, a double mastectomy, double breast reconstruction, radiation and targeted therapy. I experienced numerous side effects, including alopecia, anemia, chemo brain, constipation, bone & joint pain, diarrhea, dizziness, fatigue, flatulence, hot flashes, infections, leukopenia, lymphedema, nail changes, nausea, neuropathy, pain, poor sleep and taste & smell changes. Although I was able to keep a positive attitude most of the time, I still went through some anger, anxiety, fear and uncertainty. Those emotions didn't last long because I willed myself to always look at the bright side and be thankful, no matter what.

I've been so blessed to have my wonderful family (especially my mom and sisters) and so many friends supported me throughout both my cancers, as well as all those people all over the world who prayed for me. I believe that everyone's prayers really helped. I just love my family so much and feel so very blessed to know that they love me too!

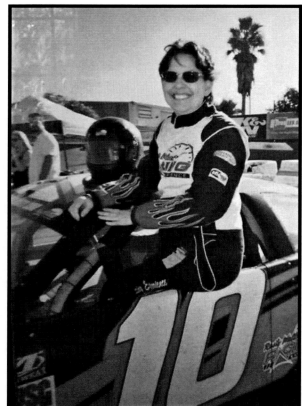

Even though I went through feelings of uncertainty that were crazy because they actually gave me an "expiration date" saying, "You have three months to live," I knew that it wasn't 100% guaranteed either. So, I kept telling myself, "Okay wait, I only have today really. Whether or not I have cancer, I have today. So, what I'm going to do is make it good for me and to make it good for others too, as much as I can." I was determined to change the situation for myself and went for one of my dreams, i.e. to drive a NASCAR race car! It was insane and it scared me, but I did it, and I had the best time! I feel that even though we go through all this painful experience, we can still have fun and be into things we enjoy. Sure, I was tired and not feeling good at all, but life is short. It is. However, we can also make it just a BLAST! ~ *Cindy*

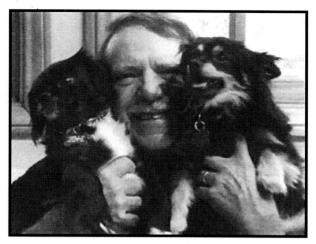

Glenn is an extraordinary human being; a kind and gentle man who loves to share his jokes, poems and many, many, many stories. He is 68 years old and just sold his business, ready to finally focus on his health and enjoy life in his retirement. Earlier this year, Glenn's wife of 47 years, Barbara, sadly succumbed to breast cancer. They have four children, three grandchildren and six great-grandchildren. He lives in a quiet, rural neighborhood where he is surrounded by nature and animals, an inspiration to him whenever he feels like getting some peace and writing his poems. When Glenn owned his business, he was passionate about getting the projects done right; he prided himself in the stellar reputation of his business. Once he learned he had cancer, he knew it was time to focus on his health and, thus, sold his business.

Glenn has a wonderful talent that he enjoys, i.e. writing stories and poems. Putting rhyming thought to paper (or computer) comes naturally for him, as long as he's inspired. He has composed many thoughtful stories and poems for his doctors, nurses and those he loves, as a way of expressing heartfelt gratitude, admiration and affection. His creative work also covers the abundance of wildlife around his home, email in Heaven, great-grandparenthood, the importance of twist-off bottle caps, a soldier's going home, his wife's conception and a poem of gratitude to his mother-in-law, among many others. His most powerful and meaningful poem was for his wife. According to Glenn, when Barbara had to get a mastectomy and told him how worried she was that he wouldn't want to look at her anymore after the surgery, Glenn wrote her a beautiful, love-filled poem entitled "Molecules," which read: *"You should know by the way I look at you, touch you, by the way I sing to you, that I love every molecule that is You. If someday there are less of them, it will only make the remaining ones more precious."* ♥

Of course, because Glenn loves to make people smile, he reaches out and shares his thoughts, time and even gifts. Sharing is such a big part of him that he gives generously, even to complete strangers in Costco and other public places, such things like backscratchers, toothbrushes and stylus/flashlight pens that he custom- orders. He makes friends easily and protects those he loves.

Despite living with cancer, Glenn finds humor in everyday life and uses his wit to see situations in clever and unique ways. At a recent function celebrating the Cancer Center's anniversary, Glenn eyed a large cake there that had "Happy 10th Anniversary, Cancer Center" written on it. He cut out the part with "cancer" written on it, placed it on a plate and then opened his mouth wide, striking a pose as if he was going to take a big bite out of cancer! Everyone who saw Glenn with the cake laughed and was truly amazed by his demonstration of wit. One of the oncologists there remarked, "No one, but Glenn, could come up with that idea!"

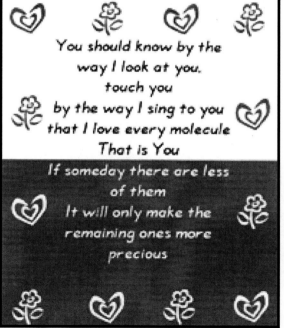

Glenn believes in actively engaging with the medical team when it comes to his treatment. He doesn't hesitate to ask questions and even give his opinions. He's quite tech-savvy and researches what he can about his cancer, the procedures, medications and everything associated with his treatment.

A flat polyp missed in his 2010 colonoscopy was discovered in Glenn's 2014 colonoscopy. Unfortunately, it was too late. Glenn had stage IV colon cancer. The tumor was missed because it was outside the colon, so the cancer had already metastasized to his liver. Here is Glenn's story:

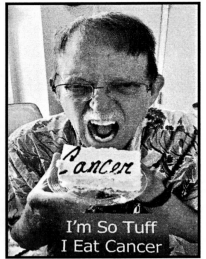

I'm So Tuff
I Eat Cancer

When I was told I had stage IV colon cancer, I was shocked and kept saying, "Sh*t! Sh*t! Shi*t!" I didn't know what I was going to do and sort of panicked. Fortunately, my wife Barbara was there to take care of me. So, I just toughed it out, with her support. It was good that, even though she too had cancer, we didn't go through treatment at the same time. Otherwise, we'd be in trouble.

I went through ten 2½2 hour cyberknife treatments, six months of chemotherapy, two radioembolization treatments, TURP surgery for my prostate, a colectomy and other surgeries to kill the cancer that had started on my colon and spread to my liver, adrenal gland and one of my lungs. I experienced multiple side effects, including brittle nail syndrome, chemo brain, constipation, delayed wound healing, diarrhea, dry mouth, fatigue, feet changes, gas, hearing problems, hyperthyroidism, nausea, neuropathy, pain, poor sleep, restless legs, skin changes, taste and smell changes, weakness and weight loss.

Looking back, it felt as if my emotions were on a roller coaster! I'm a fairly positive person; I try to look at things with optimism. Of course, when my health was down, especially when Barb, who was suffering from breast cancer, wasn't doing well, I couldn't help but feel anxiety, confusion, depression, fear, frustration and impatience. Those negative feelings, however, were temporary. I didn't want to dwell on them. I knew they didn't do me or Barb any good, and I wanted to be strong for her too.

Barb loved me and knew me inside out. She supported me through my cancer battles, even when she was the one who needed support with her cancer battles. After one of my "train-wreck" moments when my heart hurt so much seeing her suffer, and I tried hard not to soak my pillow with tears, she quietly said to me, "You're going to be okay." There she was on her deathbed and she was worried about me! We have loved each other for so long and continue to do so, even though she is no longer on earth. I know she's happy in Heaven, without pain, rooting for me to go on. I know there's still so much to do and experience in life, and I want to do it all!

Of course, I couldn't do it without my family, my grandchildren (especially Heather), my great grandchildren and my friends who have supported me...AND my dogs Maggie and Molly who definitely comfort me, but also annoy the heck out of me! I still love them though. Life is temporary and we'll all get to the end; that's reality. For me though, "When I get to the Pearly Gates, I'll just go in. I don't need an appointment!" ~ *Glenn*

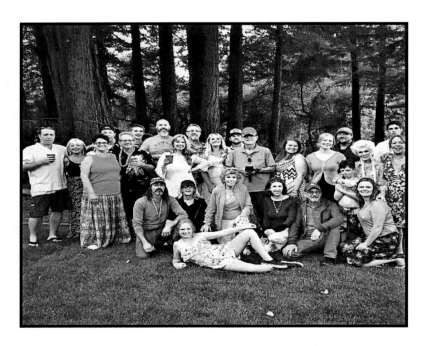

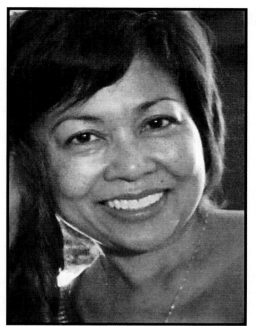

Hilda is a strong, incredible and gorgeous 50+ year old woman with a huge heart and a warm soul. She and her husband Tony have two beautiful daughters, Jessica and Adri, who were 20 and 10 years old, respectively, when Hilda was diagnosed with stage III colon cancer. They reside in a single family home in the city of Belmont, California.

Hilda is of Filipino descent and speaks fluent English and Tagalog (Filipino). She is Catholic and one of six children. She has three older sisters, an older brother and a younger brother. Her family does have a history of cancer. One of her sisters, Frieda, survived cervical cancer the year before Hilda was diagnosed and her other sister, Nida, had lymph node cancer 25 years ago. While Nida was treated with radiation and chemotherapy, Frieda's treatment required only surgery and nothing further.

Hilda has worked in local government service as a Human Resources Manager for many years. For her leisure time, she enjoys watching movies, shopping, reading murder mysteries and novels. She also enjoys traveling with her family and friends.

Before Hilda learned she had cancer, she scheduled herself for her first colonoscopy because she was approaching her milestone 50th birthday. The results of the procedure were shocking: She had stage III colon cancer! What followed was a whirlwind. Here is Hilda's story.

Since I was about to turn 50 years old in October 2011, I scheduled myself for a Colonoscopy, a four-hour procedure. I took the day off from work and my oldest daughter, Jessica, dropped me off at the hospital and picked me up after they released me. When I woke up after the procedure, my doctor came in and informed me that they did find something and would need me back for a reevaluation; but nothing to worry about, at this point. So, I just went home and chilled.

Returning to work the next day seemed normal; nothing new, until I received a voicemail message from my doctor saying that they had actually found something, and he needed to talk with me as soon as possible. I returned his call and when we talked, I learned that it was very serious. I said "Oh, SH*T!" Of course, I was shocked. Fortunately, no one was with me during the telephone conversation. I have a tendency to deal with bad news better when I'm on my own, because it gives me time to compose myself and think clearly about my situation and my options.

Having a very, very positive attitude and being as objective as possible is how I've been taking care of myself. I never think of the worst that could happen. Instead, I think of how things could get better. I think that it's very important to have a positive attitude because it makes you stronger. Otherwise, you'll just make yourself weaker. Anyway, that's how I handled the news of my cancer. I kept my attitude in check, so I could get the best possible outcome. And it worked!

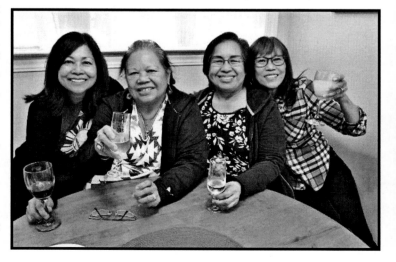

Treatment to remove my cancer included a laparoscopic colectomy and chemotherapy. Because the laparoscopic colectomy involves only little incisions in my abdomen for the camera and surgical tools to go through, it was minimally invasive and I was left with only five small scars on my abdomen. A large part of my colon, however, was removed during the surgery.

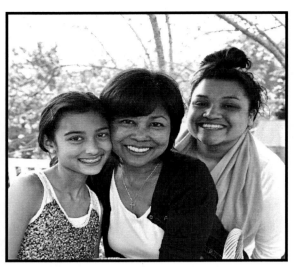

During the surgery, they also implanted a medical port (mediport) on the top left side of my chest. Treatment continued with chemotherapy (chemo) infusions at the cancer center every two weeks for six months. Before the infusion, however, they had to wait for my blood levels to be good before I could start my chemotherapy "chemo" infusions. After every infusion, I was sent home with a "chemo bag", which was definitely an interesting experience.

I did encounter several side effects from my chemotherapy treatment, which were thinning of my hair, constipation, dizziness, hypothermia, mouth and gum changes, nail changes, neuropathy, numbness and pain. During my treatment period, I also went through some naturally negative emotions, like anxiety, panic, fear and uncertainty. In spite of it all, I believe I coped well with the challenges. At one time, I thought that I was doing well enough to travel to Europe for a week. Well, when my oncologist found out, I had to change plans. That's okay, because I understood, and I still was able to travel to Europe. I just had to go later when my immune system was strong enough and I got clearance from my doctor.

My medical team was awesome! I couldn't have asked for a better team of doctors and nurses. The head nurse and my oncologist who I especially trusted, were such a blessing to me! They helped me maneuver through the process and were so full of heart. I also believe that my faith in God and my trust that He would guide and strengthen me, helped me conquer my fears.

From the very beginning, I was really determined to beat this cancer and put it behind me. I maintained a really positive attitude, worked out to strengthen my body and made sure I didn't stress. I did what I could to keep my daily activities as "normal" as possible and listened to my body. I allowed my friends and family to take care of me when I needed help and I also allowed myself time to relax and heal. Through the whole ordeal, my family gave me so much love and support; I know I am so blessed!

Experiencing cancer and going through treatment was definitely a challenge. I know God heard my prayers and gave me strength to help me cope. I am moving forward with more gratitude and a much brighter outlook in life. Yes, even with my attitude before cancer already being positive, I've learned ways to be even more positive! ~ *Hilda*

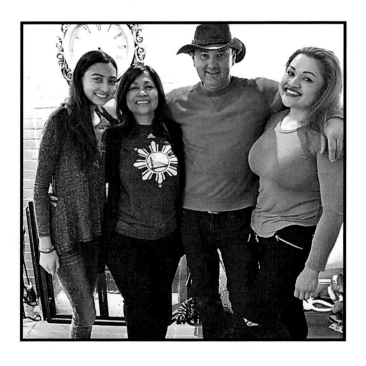

Amor Y. Traceski

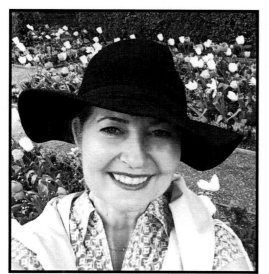

Jacki is an amazing, energetic and effervescent 50+ year old lady who was diagnosed with breast cancer in 2006. She is an ice skating coach, and her husband George is in the ice skating business. Their daughter Jenise, who was 12 or 13 years old when Jacki was diagnosed, is passionately into snowboarding as well as ice skating. They are devout Episcopalians and live in a beautiful house in the suburbs where Jacki also works part-time at her daughter's former elementary school as a yard supervisor and chaperone.

Since her husband George's family is from Malta., Their daughter Jenise (now 25 and a college graduate), will represent the country of Malta at the Winter Olympics. She is definitely a great source of pride for proud mama Jacki!

Unabashedly a Disney fan, Jacki really enjoys everything about Disneyland, i.e. dressing up, the shows, the parades, the songs, the characters, the costumes...everything! Around the time Jacki learned she had cancer, she was scheduled to chaperone her daughter's band and choir on a trip to Disneyland where they were going to perform. When she informed their choir director, he told her that the choice was hers to make. Jacki then told him, "I have loved Disneyland from the time I was six years old. I would love to go to Disneyland and won't even think about my cancer the whole time I'm there. Who thinks about cancer when you're in Disneyland?" Yes, Jacki is a very positive, lively and colorful lady who embraces life!

Jacki's family does <u>not</u> have a history of cancer, thus, the shock when they received her diagnosis. Still, she stayed positive and chose to keep the faith, living one day at a time. Here is Jacki's story.

When I learned I had breast cancer, I didn't really have any information going in. I didn't know anybody who had cancer. So, I just learned on my own because I guess I didn't personally know of anyone having a bad time with it. There was no history of cancer in my family at all. I was shocked and a bit scared. It was surreal. The only time I was very upset and sad and questioning was the day I found out it was cancer. Since I initially didn't have much information to go by, I didn't know what to do or how to cope with it. Still, I said, "Life goes on." And, of course, I looked at everything positive, which is just my nature. I woke up the next morning and continued to do whatever I do every day. I certainly didn't think it was the end of the world. It was just part of life.

I followed whatever my doctor advised me to do and talked with cancer survivors to learn more about their experience and what I could expect. Once I gathered more information from the doctor and the cancer survivors about what breast cancer is, what my options were and how I was going to deal with it, I just lived each day, planning on making a full recovery.

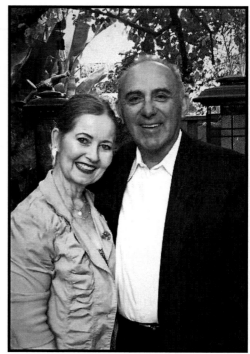

My family was always checking up on me. My mom had passed away, so I didn't have my best support there. I received my cancer diagnosis six months after my mom passed away. I believe the stress of her passing probably may have brought on the cancer. The other thing I was thinking about that could've given me this cancer was the fact that I am an ice skater. I was always a competitor. I was brought up in ice arenas. Always out on the ice and after the machines ~ the Zambonis ~which would make some new ice, I'd have to go back on the ice again and train. So, whatever fumes were left on the rink

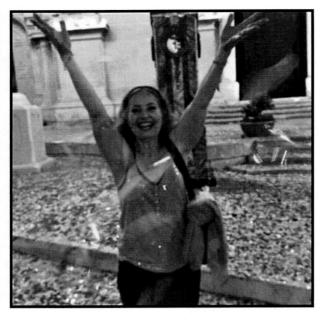

from the Zambonis is what I would breath in. Therefore, I have a feeling that could've been a little bit of what I was just breathing ... those toxins going into my body from the machine. Again, we had no family history of cancer.

To fight my cancer, I had a lumpectomy, nine rounds of chemotherapy, and 36 weeks of radiation. I'm fortunate that I didn't experience a lot of treatment side effects, only alopecia, some nausea and some chemo brain. Although I did feel the negative emotions of shock and fear, I felt them only in the beginning when I initially didn't know what was happening and if there was anything I could do about it. Once I got more direction and more information, I tried to work with what I did have and stayed positive. Except for my days at the hospital and a couple days of recovery after surgery, I continued my regular activities at work and with my family. I went out and enjoyed time with my friends and family, shopping, traveling ... basically, I continued living my life, even though it started out at a slower pace.

Going into all my chemo treatments, I had a friend who is also one of the ice skaters I coach. She had other friends who also went through cancer and so she knew that to help out was a very positive thing for a cancer patient. So, she did something special for me. Before I went to each of my nine chemo sessions, she would hang a little gift bag containing five to seven fun pink things on my front door. There was every little pink thing you could think of, e.g.: A pink ribbon for my hair. A pink pen. A pink notebook. A pink pair of socks. A pink nail file, etc. So, before each chemo, I would open up my front door and there would be my pink goody bag! ⬜ That a wonderful kind gesture that definitely helped me feel better as a cancer patient and helped me cope with my chemo sessions. After I was done with the chemo treatment, and I stopped receiving the goody bags, I found that I wanted to continue my own support for breast cancer prevention and breast cancer patients. I've been buying pink things from stores and donating them to companies that support breast cancer Awareness. Since October is breast cancer Awareness month, I wear pink clothes and pink jewelry every day in October, except for the week of Halloween when I wear my Halloween costume.

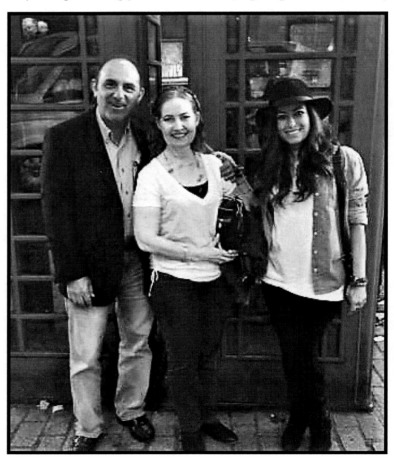

I started out in shock and fear, not knowing what to do. Now, I've grown from this experience and feel so blessed to have the support of my loving family, my wonderful husband George and my beautiful daughter Jenise. I thank God for them every day! ~ *Jacki*

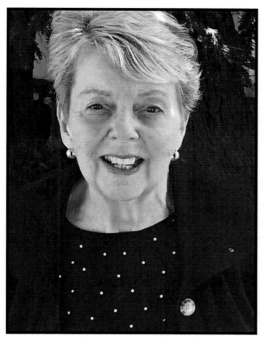

Joan is a wonderful, kind-hearted and inspiring 74-year old widow who is socially engaged in her community in Foster City, California where she lives in a two-story townhome. She has two beautiful daughters, Lori and Shelley, with whom she shares a very strong bond of love. Together, as a family, they're quite close-knit.

Of Irish, Scottish and Norwegian heritage, Joan is the younger of two children in a Catholic household. There is no history of cancer in her family.

Joan worked almost all her life (over 40 years), and before retirement, was an Office Manager, responsible for accounts receivable, accounts payable, payroll, etc. She has gone through many chapters in her life and is now very happily retired. Joan feels truly blessed with her family, her new friends as well as her old friends.

She enjoys being active, especially going to the theater, restaurants and shopping. She also enjoys playing games among other fun activities like bingo, cards and bunco. Since Joan belongs to two theater societies, she goes to twelve to fourteen plays a year with her friends. She also belongs to a sorority and is a very active member of the Foster City Lions Club where she participates in fundraising and service activities for the community. As a matter of fact, Joan was awarded "Lion of the Year", an honor given only to those who exemplify excellence in Lionism with their selflessness, hard work and outstanding service to their communities. Joan serves as a role model and an inspiration for those facing difficulties because despite it all, Joan feels passionately blessed and wants to continue sharing what she can with others. Here is Joan's story:

After my 2014 colonoscopy, I was informed by the specialist that I had stage III rectal cancer. When I heard the news, I was so upset, I felt like all my brain was floating way! Then, I looked at my daughter and she had tears rolling down her cheeks. It was such an awful feeling. But reality soon set in, and I prayed for acceptance.

After I settled down, I realized that I'm over 70 years old and never had a serious illness. I thought of all the ill children and gave thanks to the good Lord for the 71 healthy years I was able to live. When one of my friends told me, "You didn't deserve this" I told her, "I'm 71 years old. How many children have cancer?"

In all honesty, I know people who are living to be 90 or 100 and I don't know what the good Lord has in store for me. But when you reach 71 and you haven't had any health issues, it's a blessing! That reality and being able to appreciate what I have been blessed with is what has really helped me cope with my challenges.

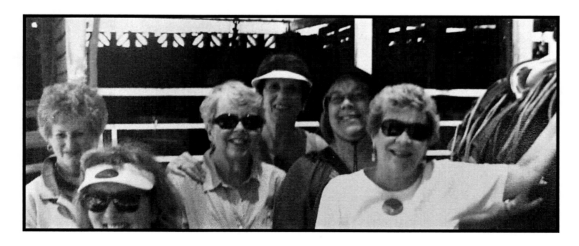

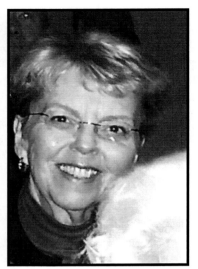

For my treatment, I went through 25 rounds of radiation (five days a week for five weeks), LAR (Low Anterior Resection) Surgery to remove my rectal cancer and surrounding tissues and lymph nodes, chemotherapy infusions and chemotherapy pills twice a day. In between my chemotherapy sessions, I suffered several complications that landed me in the hospital seven times. I did experience multiple side effects, like diarrhea, incontinence, fatigue, hypokalemia (very low potassium levels), loss of appetite, lymphedema (intense swelling), nausea and weight loss. I also went through negative emotions, like fear, shock, guilt, impatience and irritation. A permanent byproduct of my treatment is having a colostomy bag, something that I honestly dislike immensely, but have accepted because it is a fact of life and now a part of me. Instead of focusing on what I cannot control here, I choose to focus on all the wonderful things that I've been so very blessed with, especially my loving family and my wonderful friends.

Before cancer, my life had been difficult. My mother and my husband passed away just before my diagnosis. When I was told I had rectal cancer, I knew I had another huge battle to overcome. Sure, it was scary. I was afraid of the unknown and what could happen. It wasn't easy. What helped me was prayer, keeping positive, and being thankful. Prayer helped me feel calm. Keeping positive made me feel better about my situation, however difficult; it gave me hope. And, being thankful, just reminded me of how blessed I am. Again, there are ill children, who have it far worse than me.

I learned a lot from my experience, which I am sharing with you here. However, one of the most important messages I have is for those who are 50 years old and above: Make sure to get your colonoscopy and then follow the schedule for your next colonoscopy. Having a colonoscopy could mean the difference in whether your cancer is found in its early stage or late stage and what treatment you will need. Don't procrastinate or drag your feet. The rest of your life depends on it!

Even though everything that I went through is part of the past, I know I'm not out of the woods yet, health-wise. Still, why get myself all anxious about possible future challenges? I am very optimistic and always hopeful that things will turn out good for everyone. Right now, I'm having a lot of fun with the many activities I enjoy!

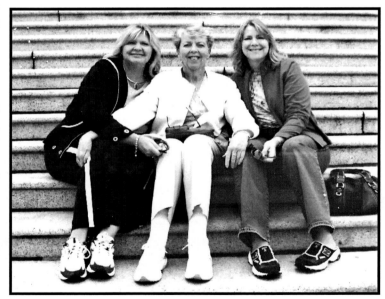

I just can't tell you how important my family and friends are to me. Life can be difficult at times, but as the Bible says, "This too shall pass". I always look forward to being with my girls (Lori and Shelley), my grandchildren (Tiffany, Victoria, Morgan and Grace) and my sons-in-law (Doug and Charlie). I am so thankful for their unconditional love and support! "We've got your back!" is what my girls would always tell me. I also want to express my gratitude to the many wonderful friends who showered me with their get-well wishes, prayers, comfort food, their energy and their time, especially Carolyn, Mary, Janis, Jody, Barbara, Sandy and Susan.

I live with the knowledge that God is in charge. It gives me joy, and I am so thankful for all the blessings He has given me throughout my life. That's why it just makes sense to stay positive. God is in charge! ~ *Joan*

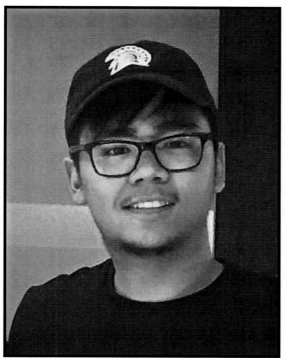

John Bernard aka "JB" is an exceptional young man who, at 21 years old learned he had a very rare form of cancer: salivary gland cancer. He is a junior at San Jose State University, majoring in Business Administration with a concentration in Accounting. He is the younger of two boys in his family.

JB lives with his family in a two-story home in the San Jose, CA and attends services with his girlfriend, Melody, at the United Methodist Church every Sunday where he accompanies the choir with his guitar.

He enjoys sports and playing video games. But, the activity he most looks most forward to is working out at the boxing gym. This is actually the same gym that the great boxing champion, Manny Pacquiao, trained at. As a matter of fact, JB is so passionate about boxing that, a month after his surgery, he returned to working out at the boxing gym. Of course, he was cautious and made sure he didn't hurt himself. Now, JB is feeling really strong and looking forward to competing in his first boxing match.

JB is level-headed and has a good head on his shoulders. He's the kind of young man who keeps calm in the face of crisis. His character shone true when he learned he had cancer.

Here is JB's story:

My cancer journey began in mid-November of 2016. I had an unusual growth on the right side of my cheek and went to the doctor to check it out. He had it biopsied and then he called me. At the time, aside from college, I was working part-time as an office assistant at a small machine shop in the San Jose. I was on the road, driving my boss's high-school aged son home when I got the call from my doctor. He asked if I had a moment. Because I knew it was important, I pulled to the side, parked the car and got out, so that I could talk to my doctor in private. What he told me definitely stunned me. He said that it was the worst possible case and used the word "malignant". He explained that I would require further testing. The whole thing was kind of surreal, and I felt confused. When I returned to my boss's son in the car, I didn't say anything. I just continued on my way. The first person I told was my dad and then my mother and girlfriend, Melody. Everyone was shocked.

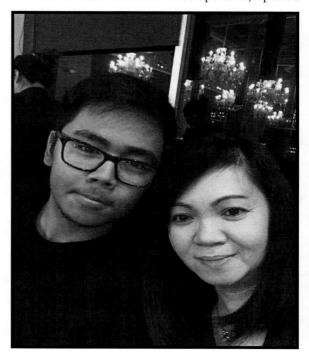

When my doctor confirmed my cancer and informed me that I would have to go through treatment and therapy, I resigned from my job, but continued my college studies.

For treatment, I had a Parotidectomy (surgical incision or removal of the parotid gland, the major and largest of the salivary glands) and radiation treatment five days a week for seven weeks. I did experience side effects from treatment (fatigue, loss of appetite, teeth changes, skin changes and taste and smell changes). Also, because salivary cancer is very rare, I initially experienced anxieties that led to poor sleep

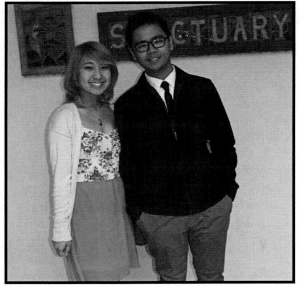

habits. It was interesting to experience the emotions that came with the diagnosis.

My last treatment was about a year ago, and I feel relief. Before my radiation treatment, my case went before the Tumor Board. Because radiation therapy actually adds risk for me developing a separate type of cancer, this group of oncologists had to discuss whether radiation treatment would benefit me in both the short term and the long run.

Since I'm so young, they determined that the radiation therapy would be the best option for me. Psychologically, I have to worry about recurrence, but I was told my odds are good, considering my age and health. If my cancer were to recur, then it may happen in 10 or 20 years. This possible recurrence causes me anxiety. However, I'm learning everyday how to cope with it.

I learned a lot about myself during my cancer journey, and I believe that I grew in strength and wisdom. There's nothing I can't do when I put my mind to it. Although the side effects of treatment are inevitable, I learned that there are ways to work around them. For example, scheduling activities that require focus and energy outside of the times fatigue would hit my body.

Although I would be inclined to not eat due to loss of appetite, I learned to force myself to eat foods high in protein to keep my weight up, so that my health didn't weaken and my body had the fuel it needed to recover.

Although my body would be inclined to stay inactive due to fatigue, I learned that I could be creative in my physical activities, like walking, to make sure I kept moving.

Although my nature is to spend lengthy periods of time researching answers to my many questions, I've learned that doing so to the extreme will only increase my anxiety and cause confusion. Moderation is key and the proper amount of sleep is important to health and healing.

Although I have a tendency to isolate myself when faced with personal challenges, I learned how wonderful it feels to open up and have the support of my girlfriend and my family who love me.

That last lesson was my favorite. ~ *John Bernard "JB"*

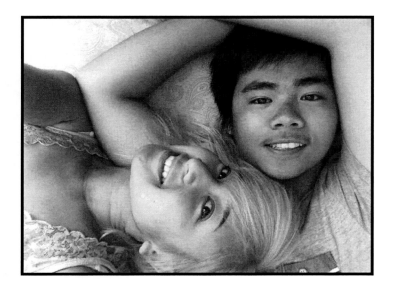

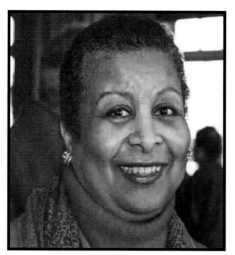

Rev. Linda is a beautiful spirit and a wise soul who retired after nobly working for the community as Director of Spiritual Care at Mission Hospice and Home Care in San Mateo, California. She is 71-years old and, despite living with cancer, still serves as a Minister and Chaplain where she lives in Illinois. Rev. Linda's personal theology: mystical Christianity, the teachings of Jesus, the immutable laws of science, and Buddhism. She relies on it to live her life in blissful and challenging times.

The older of two children, Rev. Linda was raised by her mother and step-father. Their family has a history of cancer, but none pancreatic. She lives in a wonderful single-story house in the city where she relishes time with her playful and handsome black mini schnauzer Murphy. She enjoys cooking, coloring, reading, word games, laughing with friends and family, going to church services and watching her favorite TV shows.

Rev. Linda was first diagnosed with stage II pancreatic cancer in 2016. After completing treatment, she went into remission. Unfortunately, less than a year later, her cancer returned … and returned a third time the following year. Here is Rev. Linda's story:

When I was diagnosed with stage II pancreatic cancer in July 2016, I was quite upset. I had just bought a house, retired and moved to Illinois from California two months prior. I was looking forward to enjoying retired life with my family and friends, especially my mother, Ma Mere, who has Alzheimer's. Having cancer and going through treatment was the exact opposite of what I had envisioned. So, I was really shocked and angry when I received the diagnosis. I had suspected cancer, but not pancreatic cancer. Thankfully, I had good friends there with me; they saved me from hysteria. When I finally calmed down, I mobilized myself to address it – physically, emotionally, mentally, and spiritually. I informed my immediate family and closest friends, because I wanted them to know the truth.

Learning that my cancer returned less than a year from my first diagnosis and yet again, the following year, despite surgery and over twenty chemotherapy sessions, really shook me. I knew I had no choice, but to accept and move on. To this day, I continue my attempts to normalize my life and stay in the present moment, while my subconscious continues to work on my concerns. Still, I go on. Again, I have no choice. I go out with my mother (Ma Mere) who has Alzheimer's, attend church on Sundays and meet and chat with friends. Every so often, there are times I don't feel well and would prefer to remain at home rather than go to church. But that still, small voice urges me to go and when I do, the Sunday lesson turns out to be what I just needed to hear.

For years, I erroneously believed I was one of the most conscious people on the planet. I was empathetic, compassionate and spiritual. I took professional development classes to expand my thinking, my views, and my heart. Never would I have imagined that I was just a novice in this thing called "Life", until I was diagnosed with a deadly form of pancreatic cancer.

I've gone through a lot of emotions and soul-searching since I was first diagnosed. Behind the wheel, on the road driving a total of six hours round-trip to and from my appointments to St Louis, MO for 30-45 minute appointments definitely afforded me time to ponder. Yes, consolidation of appointments would've been great, but it is what it is and I just do what I can. I have gone through so much

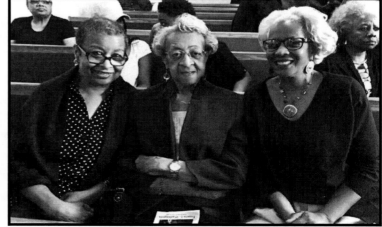

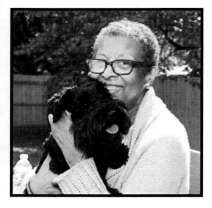

waiting; my patience truly has been tested. Waiting to get to my appointments ... waiting to take tests ... waiting for results.... waiting for the doctor to interpret the results ... waiting to see what's next... I'm not so great at waiting, but I am being reminded constantly that I control nothing about this process. Nada.

Treatment for my first bout with pancreatic cancer was surgery (the RAMPS procedure to remove the pancreatic tail, tumor and spleen) and eighteen chemotherapy sessions. I experienced a wide range of side effects, namely: alopecia, bone and joint weakness, chemo brain, constipation, diarrhea, fatigue, flatulence, loss of appetite, low white blood cell count, myalgia, nausea, pain and weight loss (I lost 44 lbs.). Treatment for my recurrence included more aggressive treatments, starting with radiation, followed by more chemotherapy. The success rate for these options is 20%. I see myself being in that 20%. I've already experienced the side effects I went through earlier, plus new side effects not yet experienced, like thickened tongue, higher-pitched voice, perplexing sensitivities to cold due to my neuropathy and vision problems. Continuing treatment for my third round with pancreatic cancer has been even more intense and draining. Even though this round of chemo won't end until the tumor markers normalize, I am living my life as if I am cancer-free.

My cancer is my cancer and side effects are side effects. I have high-energy days and I have low-energy days. For the former, I enjoy what I can. I have Girls Night Out with girlfriends I've known since we were kids. We laugh often and hard. I'm just trying to stay alive. I have no time for, nor interest, in nonsense these days. None. Nada. Zilch.

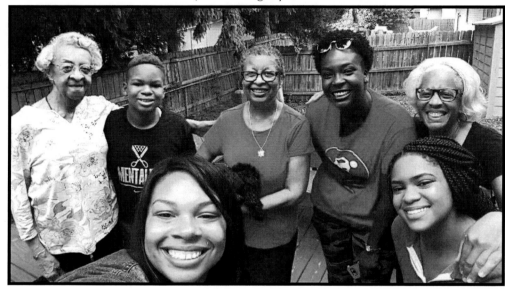

Being told that a high risk factor for pancreatic cancer is a sedentary lifestyle is driving me to tell everyone, "If you aren't doing so, get off your tushes and MOVE for at least 30 minutes a day." I try to move and be active, even while I'm going through treatment. Nevertheless, there are days when my body is fatigued and tells me to rest... and I listen.

It's been amazing to feel all the love and support I've received from friends and relatives, and even strangers. My sister Sam put her life in San Diego on hold to be here for as long as she needs to be; she dropped everything and rushed over for me. How blessed I am to have such an amazing loving sister in Sam! If words alone could cure and heal me, I would be completely well today from all the caring posts, messages, and emails I've received. The love showered upon me daily washes over me like a cleansing rain. I am completely and humbly overwhelmed by the companionship and support I've received on my cancer journey. And I am deeply grateful! As my dear friend Rosella Sims, said, "This cancer experience stretches me. It stretches me in ways I could never have imagined or grown from without actually having the cancer. Yes, I would have preferred to learn in a less lethal way, but this is the experience I have." I have wasted so much time on the petty nonsense that consumes far too many of us, time that we won't get back. Today that stops. No more. I am more awake and aware now than ever, and I hope you wake up, too, and begin living fully while you can. ~ *Rev. Linda*

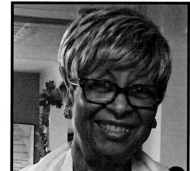

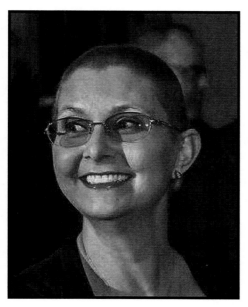

Rachel is an amazing and spirited 42-year old woman; a wife and mother of two wonderful sons, now five and 15 years of age, and a beautiful 22-year old daughter. She is speaks mainly English and simple conversational Spanish. She and her family live in a single-story family home in Manteca, a city in the Central Valley of California. Aside from her children's many activities, Rachel works in the medical field for a manufacturing company and also volunteers her time and energy in helping others. During treatment, she did what she could to continue daily life activities, like taking care of the kids, doing dishes, laundry, etc. She said, "I had to move forward. I couldn't stop because of my children. I just tried to keep things as normal as possible for them."

Rachel is a fighter, who continuously exhibits the strength to battle adversity, knowing it also serves as a model and a legacy for her young children. Here is Rachel's story:

I was diagnosed on May 27th 2016 with stage III triple negative breast cancer. The news stunned my husband and me because there was no real history of cancer in my family, except for cancer of the mouth. Since everything I do is for my family, especially my kids, I knew they would be directly affected. So, I knew I had to be strong and fight with all my might to beat cancer!

I first knew that something was wrong when I felt kind of achy just in my breast on and off for a couple of weeks. I didn't really think anything of it because my youngest was a baby, only 1½ years old at the time and I had just weaned him from nursing. I knew it would take several months to dry up, so I didn't think anything of it. On a Sunday morning, my little one came and laid up against me and it hurt so bad, I had to move him away. That's when I felt the lump.

I was scared and went into the hospital to be checked. Unfortunately, I was given vague, inconclusive information by the clinical nurse there, who basically said that although they found a lump, "it's probably just a cyst" because "cancer doesn't hurt." I went in for an ultrasound, followed by a mammogram, which I never experienced because I had not yet reached my 40th birthday. After the mammogram, the doctor came in and said that my lump needed to be biopsied immediately <u>and</u> my lymph nodes as well. I broke down crying because, in my head, I believed that once cancer hits the lymph nodes, my life is "done." I know now that is not true. The doctor called himself to inform me that my biopsies were positive; I had stage III triple negative breast cancer. Hearing the news, I pretty much fell to the floor and called my

husband, Eusebio. I have no idea what I told him. I don't even think he understood me between my non-stop sobbing. My sister and my best friend came over to comfort me, and, they both stayed until my husband got home.

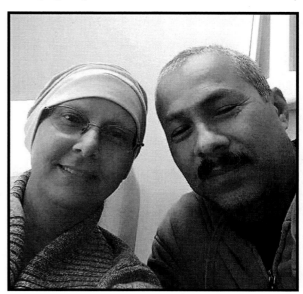

My husband and I researched what we could about my cancer, and I decided to get a double mastectomy. All the doctors (my oncologist, the surgeon...everybody) tried to talk me into just doing a single mastectomy, not a double. Thankfully, I made the right decision because during the surgery, they found two lymph nodes on my left side that were abnormal and not yet cancer, but would've developed into cancer had I not made that choice. Multiple times, they said I had triple negative breast cancer. That means, "it's not IF the cancer comes back, it's WHEN it comes back!"

Before my double mastectomy, the biggest fear I had was about what people were going to think. I was between a C and D cup

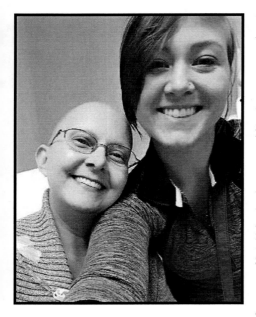

before my surgery. The plastic surgeon told me, "When you do reconstruction, you're mostly going to be an A." I said, "I don't care. I'll be alive to be an A. How's that?" I then asked my husband, "Do you care if I'm going to be an A?" He said, "Nope. You'll be here with me. That's all I care about!" Before, I cared a lot about what others thought of me. Now, it doesn't matter to me. If people don't like the way I look, then don't look at me. I didn't have hair, and I've got no chi-chis. So what? It really doesn't matter. I didn't have this confidence before. I do now!

After my surgery, I had three months of chemotherapy and five weeks of radiation. I experienced many side effects from the treatment drugs, like losing my hair. Since I used to have my long hair cut and then donated to cancer patients, I didn't have a problem with it. However, a couple of the side effects hit me really hard like the hot flashes, lymphedema and painful skin changes. Still, I toughed it out. My coping mechanism was my family.

I had my children and my family to motivate me. I fought knowing that, even though I couldn't control this disease, I could control my attitude. There's a lot to be said about attitude. When I was down, I turned on music, danced and laughed with them. They made me stronger. When I was sick, I told myself that it meant the treatment was working, and that it would not last. I would repeat to myself, "This is only temporary." During the nights I felt horrible and literally thought I was going to die, I just kept repeating to myself, "It's temporary!" And, this IS just temporary. I have the rest of my life!" That got me through a lot.

I also made an early decision that I was not going to let cancer eat me alive; I was going to make life as good for my kids as I possibly can because God forbid if I don't survive this, they will have good memories; not bad memories. I was determined that I was <u>not</u> going to leave this world and have them think of me as always being upset. I want them to think, "My mom was very positive and my mom was happy".

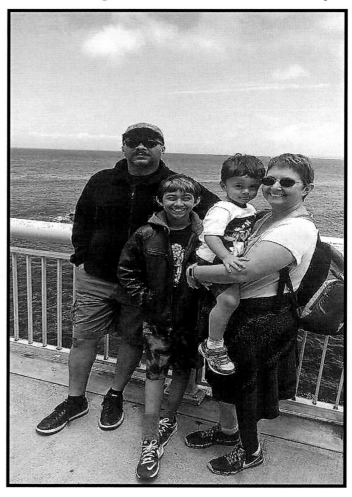

When I asked "why me?" I would remind myself of others who have it worse and then would stop feeling sorry for myself. I began to want to help others. I began to thrive on the idea of helping others. I began to live for it. This made me stronger.

"People who go through cancer become part of a club no one ever wants to belong to. But, when they get into that club, they're met with nothing but love and compassion."

Learn to be comfortable with the "New You." Life will never be the same as it was before. And that's OKAY. You will come out stronger than you ever knew was possible! ~ *Rachel*

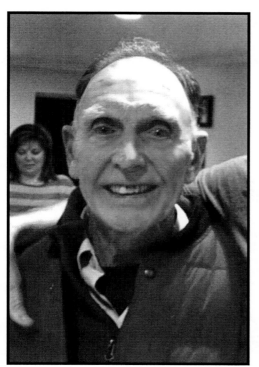

Rick is a remarkable and extraordinary 75 year old man who has experienced much in life. He has two daughters and lives in a retirement community in an urban neighborhood in the city of Santa Clara, CA. His family (he has two siblings) has a history of cancer. Both his parents are deceased; his mother passed away from colon cancer.

Rick grew up and has lived with faith since he was a little boy. He said, "The Bible and I grew up together because I had cerebral palsy." When he was small, Rick couldn't walk. He was in a wheelchair for years, and he was also in braces for years. But then, he learned how to walk and then, he learned how to run and then, he learned how to climb mountains. So, he said, "It was all tied in. The Bible gave me strength."

He worked as a Civil Rights Advisor Community Officer at Moffett Naval Air Station in Mountain View and as a Civil Engineer in the U.S. Air Force. Rick enjoys running, being physically active, engaging with children and weightlifting. You can find him working out at the Senior Fitness Center for hours lifting weights that those half his age would struggle with. He uses weightlifting as a way to combat the muscle weakness from his condition. He's also found it to be quite therapeutic.

Rick belongs to the Assembly of God and participates in the services of two churches in his community: First Presbyterian Church and Garden City Church in Santa Clara. He is an active church-goer, serving as a Greeter and serving in Children's Ministry, supporting Sunday school workers. He has been such a role model for Ministry work that Garden City Church produced a special video of him for the congregation, entitled "Rick's Story". It's a must-see and can be found in the Garden City Church's Facebook site. Here is Rick's cancer survival story:

On September 27, 2009 when I was 65 years old, I was diagnosed with chronic lymphocytic leukemia (CLL), which is cancer of the blood and bone marrow. It was discovered by accident when I was rushed to the hospital on emergency because I had double pneumonia. I was shocked at the news that I had leukemia because I had always taken care of myself. I informed my daughter that I had CLL, but I just briefly told her because I didn't want her to worry about it.

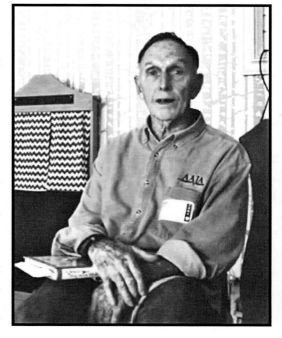

For treatment, I had chemotherapy for four months. Around the same time, I became ill with BPH (benign prostatic hyperplasia) aka an enlarged prostate and my primary doctor scheduled me for TURP (transurethral resection of the prostate) surgery. When my oncologist found out, just three days before my scheduled surgery, he put a stop to it. With my chemo drug also being a blood thinner, any surgery on me would cause serious problems for me. I learned a very important lesson there. If you have more than one condition that needs treatment, always make sure that your doctors communicate with each other. It's mind-blowing to think what would've happened if my oncologist hadn't found out. I did have my TURP surgery three weeks later and then resumed my chemotherapy treatment.

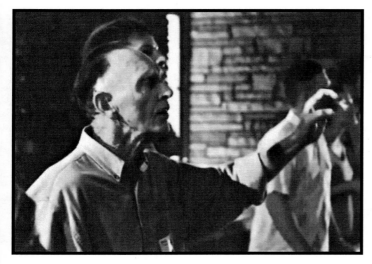

I didn't experience many physical side effects from my treatment~ Just fatigue, itchiness, loss of appetite and a bit of weight loss. I did experience emotional side effects, but I learned from them as well.

I went through anxiety about what was going to happen to me. But nothing ever happened. They were just negative thoughts that I just built up in my own mind. I learned to cope with my anxiety by getting out, going for a walk, talking with people, etc. I learned to not be alone, which is the same advice I would give for coping with depression, sadness, frustration, self-pity...all that. Sitting in the chair or laying in the bed for hours not doing anything is a waste of time and does not help you. It just makes matters worse. Instead, fight your anxiety, depression, sadness or frustration by going for a walk or talking with someone or exercising or doing some activity you enjoy. When you talk with someone, they can't change the feelings you have inside; nobody can do that. But, you can talk, and you can get your mind off what you're going through and make yourself feel better.

I've always been pretty independent ever since I was a little boy with cerebral palsy. I worked really hard to be strong and not let my condition get in the way of my daily activities. It was the same with having my cancer CLL. Even though I was shocked and experienced negative thoughts, I still learned to fight what I had and keep active because I understand how important it was to my health. Whenever I felt bad, I'd try to walk around the block. And if I felt really bad, then I'd walk around the block TWICE, just to show my body that, "I ain't gonna give up!"

I keep on moving and keep active. I volunteer where I can, whether at the churches I go to or at my retirement community where I help set up and move our big band's instruments. My favorite activity, of course, is working out at the gym, which has been my go-to activity for years whenever I was down. When I feel my muscles getting stronger, I feel really good.

I am grateful for all the people from my church who accompanied me to my chemo sessions and supported me there. I am grateful to my doctors and the nurses who did everything they could to make sure I was comfortable with my treatments, as much as possible. I am grateful to those of my friends who helped me cope in many ways. I am grateful for the opportunity to serve in Ministry at my church, especially the Children's Ministry. The more I got involved, the more I felt the caring of my church family.

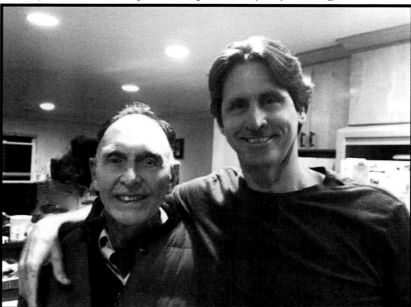

To that point: "If you have somebody you care about, go ahead and care about them more than anything in the world. It'll help you get your mind off of yourself. You take good care of them, and you make sure they're okay. You love them, and that helps you lose yourself in them. When they're not there, then you're happy you sent them off feeling loved and doing well." I am grateful for my family, especially my granddaughter, Ethel. ~ *Rick*

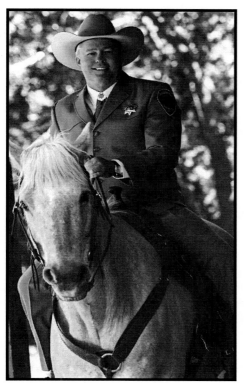

Scott is an exceptionally tough and remarkable 59-year old retired U.S. Air Force combat rescue and special operations pilot. He is a survivor of metastatic stage IV colon cancer, which means that his cancer spread from his colon to his liver, pancreas and prostate. According to Scott, "I was as far-gone as you possibly could be." Scott lives in an urban suburb, which he also considers rural, given their four dogs, seven cats, five chickens and two horses, all on over an acre of land. He has a 23-year old son and a 20-year old daughter, both of whom were in high school when he was diagnosed with cancer.

He is half Norwegian and a quarter Scot and belongs to a non-denominational, ecumenical Christian church. He and his older sister were raised by both their parents. Their family has a history of cancer, i.e. his mother died of leukemia at the age of 78 and his grandmother died of colon cancer in 1965 at the age of 68.

After retiring from the U.S. Air Force, Scott worked with a Palo Alto startup selling medical equipment to the Veterans Administration. The start-up was later acquired by the giant products and services company Bosch. When Scott was diagnosed with cancer, he retired a second time.

Scott is one of a very small percentage of metastatic cancer survivors who beat the odds. It's been almost seven years since his diagnosis and he looks great! When a friend of his asked, "So Scott, what do you think about having only a 5% chance of living?" Scott looked at him and said, "Is that what it is? Well, ok. Somebody's gotta be on the top 1%... and it's gonna be me!" Scott is re-writing the statistics. His message to others is: "Do not believe what you see on the Internet. Don't even go there. Don't let it worry you. You fight your own battle. There are people at both ends of the spectrum, and you want to be the one at the winning end. Have faith in yourself. I'm tough and resilient and I'm not taking "NO" for an answer. "I'm fighting this with everything I've got!" Here is Scott's story:

When I found out that I had stage IV colon cancer on April 27, 2011, I was kind of numb, but I was also really angry, because I was misdiagnosed the year before. I was told by the doctor then that I only had bleeding hemorrhoids and needed surgery, which I put off for a year, given a major government contract I was working on at the time. I also had not had my baseline colonoscopy and I was 52 years old. I wondered what that delay of one year cost me. If I had done a colonoscopy a year earlier, would I have been a stage III as opposed to a stage IV and improved my chances of survival? So I went through that anger. But, at the same time, I'm a fighter and am very disciplined, with 23 years in the military. For me, failure was not an option. So, I had the strength and fortitude to mentally say I'm going to beat this!

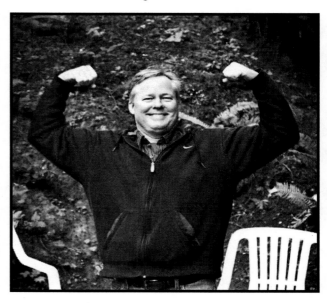

For treatment, I had a colon resection, six months of chemotherapy, two chemoembolization treatments, 43 days of radiation, a cholecystectomy, two cyberknife radiosurgeries and many endoscopies. From the numerous treatments I received, as well as the many medications I was given, my experience with side effects basically ran the gamut, from easy to very difficult, with some temporary and some permanent. They included: chemo brain, constipation, delayed wound healing, fatigue, hot flashes, infections, itchiness, mouth ulcers/dry mouth, loss of appetite, nail

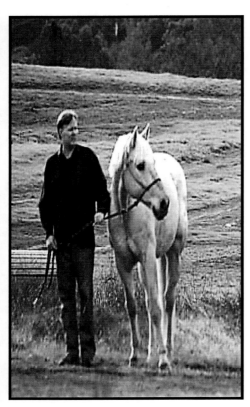

changes, neuropathy, pain, pancreatitis, poor sleep, skin changes, severe weight loss and vision problems. Naturally, I went through emotional roller coasters too. Despite it all, no matter how tough it got, I fought hard to keep positive and keep the focus on my strength, will power, and desire to continue living.

There was a time when I rapidly lost 70 lbs. due to my pancreas being inflamed and everybody thought I was going to die. Good thing they didn't tell me because that thought never crossed my mind. There was also the time when my body's response to the first part of the chemoembolization for my liver was so horrific that my doctors did not want to perform the second part. They both told me, "We don't think we should do the second half." And I said, "Hey guys, what was the plan?" And they said, "To do both halves". And I said, "Well, I'm going to survive the second one. It may be tough, but we're doing it." So, we did it and sure enough, I was again in the hospital for a week, sicker than a dog, and it again knocked me on my butt for two months ... but, I DID IT!

I realize that things could've been worse. I'm very grateful for what I have and I try to find the good in everything. So what if my feet hurt. I can get some medication to lessen the pain. It's still a beautiful day, and I'm enjoying the blue skies with the gentle breeze. You just have to find the good in life and move on.

Life is too valuable. It's too precious. I just can't imagine giving up on it, no matter how tough. There are days when I think, "Oh, I can't do this anymore". But then I remind myself that I can. I just have to. That's where meditation and mindfulness comes in. I spend ten to fifteen minutes per day meditating; just having nothing on my mind; letting it go blank. If a thought comes to me, I acknowledge it, then I push it aside. Same with mindfulness.

Mindfulness. I'll sit and I'll think how I want it to be.....think positive reinforcements; those kinds of things. You are your primary thought. If I think that I don't have cancer, then I don't "have" it. I read something where it said, "Every cell in your body eavesdrops on your mind every moment." If you say you're sick, all your body cells are going to say, "Hey guys. We're supposed to be sick, so ..." But, if you say, "Oh, I'm perfectly healthy," then all your body cells will say, "Okay, guys, we're all supposed to be really healthy. So, if any of you are not healthy right now, let's get you fixed. Immune system, kick in over here." That kind of thing. That's why I envision it. I'm the same way. Try and stay positive and no stress. I walk away from stress. If something gets stressful, I just say, "Sorry, not for me," and I walk away. It's not worth it. I've got more important things to do.

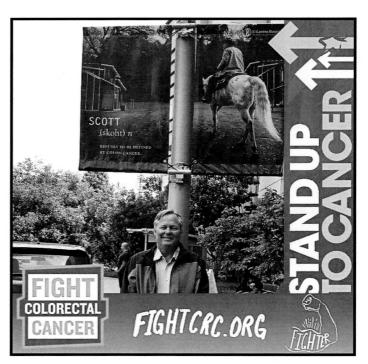

"I think everyone, at the end of the day, should be completely happy, at peace, completely satisfied, have the complete feeling of fulfillment, be loved and in love, and then you've had a great day. Then, tomorrow, repeat." ~ Scott

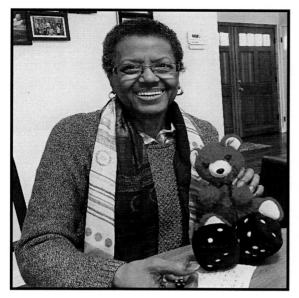

Sondra is a beautiful, gracious and extraordinary 75-year-old retired career woman who has a lot of soul and wisdom. She has been married for over 45 years to her husband Kenneth. Together they have their daughter Dawn, and their granddaughter Kayla. They belong to a non-denominational Protestant church in Mountain View, CA where they lived for over 35 years. When Sondra was diagnosed, they moved to a condominium to be closer to her doctors.

Sondra is the eldest of two brothers and one sister, raised by both parents in separate households. Ethnically, they are a mixture of African, Irish and Native American. Sondra's family does have a history of cancer. From her grandparents down to her aunts and uncles, there was stomach cancer and pancreatic cancer. Then, looking at her generation, for example, her cousins, there were several with breast cancer, stomach cancer and prostate cancer. But, no history at all of anyone in the family with ovarian cancer. "It's interesting how cancer showing up more in the cousins than the other generations" said Sondra.

Before Sondra retired, she was an organizational development consultant. Her favorite pastimes include going to museums and the beach, photography shows, and movies. The beach is BIG for her and her family. For personal time, Sondra delights in music, pen and ink drawing and working on her adult coloring book. She would like to also learn to play the piano. Throughout the physical and emotional challenges Sondra has had to battle, she exemplified grace and faith-based strength. Despite difficulties, she still shares love, joy, and peace with everyone. Here is Sondra's story.

When I went in for my annual physical exam in December of 2014, I told my doctor that I noticed thickening in the ovaries; I felt it when I moved around and knew something was different. I had put my hand down there and felt tightening and knew that it didn't feel like it did before. You know your body more than anyone. Results of an ultrasound in January 2015 were clear. Fives month later (June), I felt something was just not right. So, I contacted my gastroenterologist. Around the same time, I also had an appointment to see my urologist about my kidney. Both specialists noted fluid in my abdomen, which is not normal. So they ran some tests. Since I've been diabetic for about six years prior, my gastroenterologist initially thought that either my liver or my pancreas was causing the problem. So, more tests were run.

Negative. Then, it hit me! I realized that I had been describing my abdominal discomfort as "fullness" and for years, I had paid attention to the symptoms of ovarian cancer because they miss it so often. I remembered that one of the symptoms for ovarian cancer is "fullness." So, I thought to myself, "Whoa! I'm seeing fullness. This is not good." When I told my doctor, she did a cancer marker test on me, which came back positive for cancer. Shocked, I said to her, "No, this can't be. I just had an ultrasound in January." She replied, "That was then. This is now." That was my first reality check.

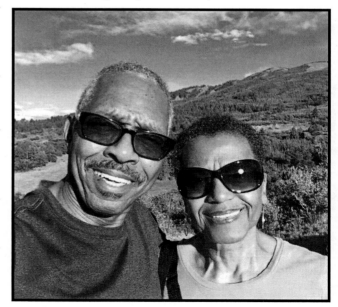

During that time, I had also been caregiving for my 95-year-old mother who was wheelchair-bound. Making arrangements for her to move into a facility in Ohio where my brother was, while also getting myself scheduled for my radical hysterectomy and subsequent treatment was very stressful, to say the least. Still, I made it through.

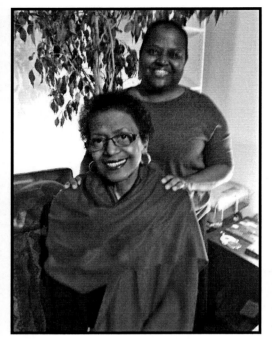

It was in July of 2015 when I found out that I had stage III ovarian cancer. I went through four months of treatment and went into remission. In January of 2016, my PET scan showed that I had spots in my lungs. Results of my lung biopsy revealed that it was just "chemo junk" lodged in my lungs' lymph nodes ... Whew! Unfortunately, my cancer returned and disseminated throughout my abdomen. So, I went through a second round of treatment, followed by maintenance chemo to keep me in remission..

Throughout my cancer journeys, I experienced many side effects, including alopecia (hair loss) twice, anemia, bladder problems, chemo brain, diarrhea, vision problems, fatigue, feet changes, gas, high blood pressure, hypothermia, kidney/bladder issues, low white blood cell count (leukopenia/neutropenia), mouth changes, nail changes, neuropathy, pain, poor sleep habits, taste and smell changes, poor veins, skin changes, swelling/edema and weight loss. For treatment, I went through a radical hysterectomy, chemotherapy twice, immunotherapy and targeted therapy. There were challenges in my treatment, because my body had adverse reactions to so many of the drugs. Still, my oncologists were really amazing in working with my sensitivities.

Naturally, I experienced a lot of negative emotions, namely anxiety, confusion, fear, frustration, sadness, impatience, irritation, loneliness, night fears, stress and feeling overwhelmed, shock and loss. Looking back, I can easily say that all of my experiences with ovarian cancer taught me so much. Stress does contribute to cancer. So I learned that it's really important to not take on too much and to set some boundaries in order to be able to take care of myself.

When my family and friends got angry because I was initially misdiagnosed, I knew that I couldn't get caught up in the anger because it would just be detrimental to my health. So, I decided to let go of that. Like my doctor said, "That was then. This is now." A huge lesson I also learned and that I want to make sure to pass on to every woman is this: "If you think that you may possibly have cancer, then you need to have the CA 125 blood marker test for ovarian cancer done. If necessary, insist on it. Also, get an ultrasound done too."

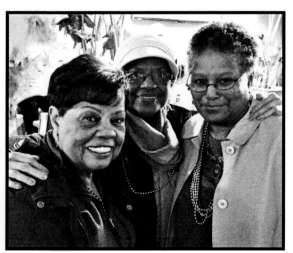

However difficult my experience, I did find peace and comfort in my God. My faith enabled me the grace to feel His Presence, and it was beautiful! I knew that there was much more life for me to live. That's why I worked really hard to beat cancer ... and won!

Words cannot adequately express the love and gratitude I feel for my husband Kenneth, and my daughter Dawn, for being my rocks of strength, sacrificing time, energy and more to take care of my needs. I am so very grateful for my siblings, my granddaughter Kayla, supportive pastors, my amazing church families, and my wonderful friends for their prayers and all they did to lift my spirits and give me their support. Feeling the outpouring of love and prayers for me was beautiful beyond words. It only goes to show that there is no place for cancer where God and love are present. ~ *Sondra*

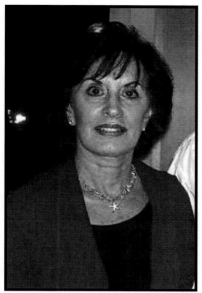

Susan is an amazing, strong and very determined 72-year old woman who is a devoted wife to her husband, Ken, and a loving mother to her beautiful daughter Stephanie, who has been by her side through thick and thin.

She is the older of two sisters raised by both their parents who are of Italian heritage. Her family did have a history of cancer. Her mother had ovarian cancer, and her sister had Lung cancer. Susan speaks English, is Catholic and lives in a single-family home in the suburbs with her family.

When Susan was 37 years old, she was diagnosed with stage II ovarian cancer; her daughter Stephanie then was only eighteen months old. Thirty-three years later and two weeks after Susan retired as a college, career and financial aid advisor, she was diagnosed with stage II pancreatic cancer. Two years later, cancer was found in her right lung, a metastasis of the pancreatic cancer. Nevertheless, Susan is fierce in fighting the disease with treatment and a healthy lifestyle which, fortunately, has kept cancer at bay.

Currently in remission, Susan is embracing a healthy lifestyle, which includes meditation, yoga, working out at the gym, eating organic food, using GMO-free products in her home, avoiding negativity in all its forms (e.g. negative news, negative people) and joining RANN (Roseville Area Newcomers and Neighbors), an active non-profit social organization. She is a picture of strength and determination; a role model and inspiration to many. Here is Susan's story:

It was December 1984 when I was diagnosed with stage II ovarian cancer, after my hysterectomy. Although I was somewhat surprised, I knew it was hereditary because my mom had it. The worst part was the gripping fear I felt thinking I would never see my then eighteen-month old baby grow up. However horrible I felt, I knew that I had to really focus on recovery for my family's sake.

In January of 2016, I was rushed to the ER because I was quite jaundiced and felt pain in my abdomen. Tests showed that my liver blood count was very high also, so they ran a CT scan. From the results, I was given a diagnosis of stage II pancreatic cancer. Fortunately, my daughter, Stephanie (now all grown up), was with me and immediately started researching the disease. In July 2018, a follow-up CT scan and biopsy showed cancer present in my right lung. Despite feeling great, I decided to be proactive and go through another round of chemotherapy.

Both cancers presented their difficulties and challenges; some similar, some not. Both brought me back to my faith and prayer. The Serenity Prayer: "God grant me the Serenity to accept the things I cannot change...the Courage to change the things I can... and the Wisdom to know the difference" resonated throughout my journey. When I had ovarian cancer, I prayed to God for the miracle of a cure and I was healed. When I had pancreatic cancer, I again prayed for the miracle of a cure, and I am currently in remission. I truly believe in miracles and am so grateful to be able to continue living, especially for my family.

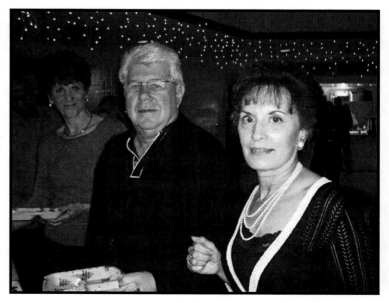

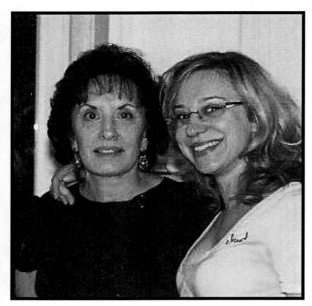

Between both cancers, my treatments included a total hysterectomy, a seven-hour surgery called the Whipple procedure aka pancreaticoduodenectomy, hormone therapy and a total of thirty-six chemotherapy sessions on top of several medical procedures and tests. I experienced physical side effects, like alopecia, chemo brain, diarrhea, fatigue, loss of appetite, nausea, pain, poor veins and weight loss. I also struggled to cope with the natural negative emotions of anger, anxiety, fear, hopeless, sadness and loneliness.

Having cancer is life-altering. It turns your life upside-down. It is okay to have anxiety, to be scared or to cry. This is normal. But, remember FIRST to take care of yourself ... before family and friends. The best way to heal is to put yourself FIRST. Of course, it will help to communicate this mindset with your family and friends, so they are aware. You can't take care of others if you are not well. So, if people offer to help, i.e. cook a meal, drive you to the doctor or appointments, visit you, take you out, well then...take it!

I kept my illness quiet for a long time-my way of coping with the huge challenge I was presented with. As I mentioned earlier, I am thankful for having survived both cancers. Yes, I fought hard and won, but I know I couldn't have done it without the unconditional love and support of my family and friends who knew of my illness. I realize that their taking on the role of caregiver, especially for my second cancer, was difficult for some.

I definitely have a stronger appreciation for life and for all those who have been with me through thick and thin. Having survived cancer twice, I am, without doubt, wiser from my experiences. Survivorship, however, is something I believe I have to continuously work on. That means actively do everything I can, physically and mentally, to prevent another recurrence. I'm proud to say that I'm making headway and feeling such a positive difference. I am very determined, not only for myself, but for my daughter Stephanie and my husband Ken. I continue to do weekly yoga classes and walk, eat healthy, take daily vitamins, and keep my faith in God. I am fortunate that I feel great and the time off from chemo is giving my immune system a chance to become stronger.

The reality also is that some days are great, and there are also days that are a little sad. I try not to dwell on the sad- things that are not within my control, and to keep life in perspective, appreciating what I do have. Aside from my family, I am so grateful for my true friends who were there for me when I needed support, namely, Mary, Susan W., Barbara, Laura B., Laura C, Robert and Amor.

I continue living with faith and trusting God to guide me through the rest of my life. I'm blessed every day to be here and pray for many more healthy years. I just have too many things left on my bucket list to do! This is my prayer: "Today, I just want to thank God for the gift of life. No requests, no complaints; I'm just thankful to be alive."

~ *Susan*

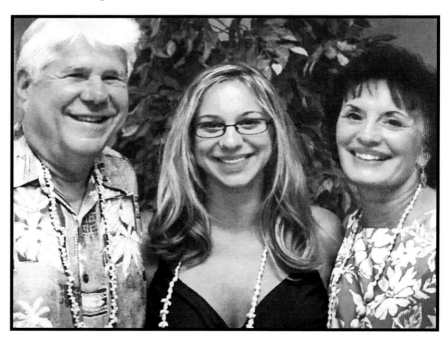

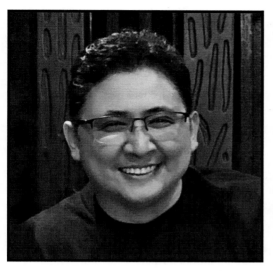

Teresa, Tet, or "Mesky" (as she was fondly called in college) is a kind-hearted, effervescent and wonderful 54-year old soul with a remarkable spirit. She lives with her family in Toronto, Canada.

Her heritage is mixed — Filipino, Spanish and Chinese. There is a history of cancer in her family, such as. lymphoma cancer on her father's side and liver cancer on her mother's side. She is Catholic and, aside from English, she speaks fluent Filipino (Tagalog) and some Spanish.

Tet enjoys reading, writing, traveling and social media. She was a graphic designer who's known for her humor, good nature and positivity. She is also known for her creative writing, especially the fun and witty stories she shares of her continuing experiences at Costco Wholesale, where she works as a member services associate, a jester and a "Happy Face Producer" for the kiddies. Here is her story:

When I turned 50, it made me mull over what has been a heck of a ride so far. People I care about deeply have come and gone, while others, thankfully, continue to ride the wave with me. One of the people whose passing affected me immensely was my grandmother. She had saved me from choking to death when I was a baby. If it weren't for her, I wouldn't be here to talk about my life.

Fast forward from infancy to decades later. I was a graphic designer for a publishing house in Toronto and fighting a perpetual battle against my weight. I was ecstatic when co-workers started paying me compliments on how I was looking good in my jeans. Weeks later, I started getting abdominal cramps. Ahhh, eating too much sashimi was doing a number on my tummy. I told myself, "It'll pass." When it didn't, I finally went to see my physician. He suspected it was gas and gave me a prescription to ease the cramps. No sweat. *Or so, I thought.* Days later, the cramping didn't stop and I found blood in my stool. Tests were performed and showed that I had a malignant tumor in my colon, a blockage measuring 9 cm long. This was right before Christmas in 1991, and I had just turned 27 at the time. But at least colon cancer helped me lose some weight. Where there's bad news, there must be good news in exchange, right? Right. Always. And it has been quite a journey since.

Fortunately, my dad, my brother, and my best friend were there to support me when I got the news. I couldn't believe what I was hearing; it felt surreal. In January 1992, I had my first colectomy (the surgical removal of all or part of the colon) performed in the Philippines. The surgeons here in Toronto wanted the entire colon removed. There would have been a drastic lifestyle change if I had opted to have it done here.

Eight years later in 2000, my colon started growing polyps at an alarming rate. The cancer was threatening to return. Instead of another colectomy, I combated it by completely eliminating red meat and cured food like bacon from my diet, taking megadoses of Vitamins A, C, E, Beta Carotene and Selenium. My next colonoscopy revealed that about half of the polyps disappeared. My gastrointestinal doctor told me, "Whatever it is that you're doing, keep

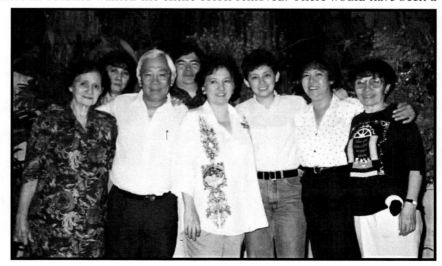

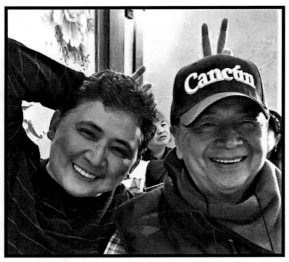

it up because it's working." This went on for a few years. However, the threat of cancer recurring hadn't stopped.

In 2005, I had to undergo a second colectomy as a pre-emptive strike against colon cancer because I was again growing polyps at an alarming rate. Since they also found three large fibroids in my uterus ranging from 3 cm to 9 cm, I decided to have a hysterectomy as well. We did leave one ovary behind, so that I wouldn't go into menopause. The added bonus was, menstruation ceased right after the procedure. To women reading this, I ask you: "Just how awesome is that?

When cancer became a part of my life at a young age, it forced me to grow overnight. It transformed me into a stronger person. It put a lot of things in perspective, and I've learned to pick my battles to let little things slide and lock horns with bigger issues. During the darkest times, there's always hope to pull you through. You'll realize that you have inner strength that you didn't know you had until your back is shoved against the wall. I was extremely lucky to have my family and friends around who have showered me with unconditional love and support. I may not be bulletproof, but they have become my bulletproof vests. There's no price tag for that. It made me realize how blessed I am. Now don't get me wrong...many positive things happened in the course of half a century. But today, I want to focus on adversities, challenges, and all the good that comes out of it. Heaven forbid, if you should face life-altering challenges, know that you are surrounded by people who care about you. Know that you can pull through. Just hang on to faith, hope, love and you'll make it. In the event you don't make it, you can at least say that you gave it your damned best, and that's all your loved ones would want you to do. Don't you ever forget to laugh through it all because it can work wonders.

As of this writing, life has once more taken me to the crossroads. My recent colonoscopy revealed the rapid growth of two 2 cm polyps, one polyp measuring 1 cm and approximately 50 smaller ones having an average size of 5 mm. The doctor removed everything he could within safe parameters. Should I finally go for the third and final surgery the doctors have been wanting for me all along and end up with a colostomy? Or should I keep fighting the way I have for decades and try to live a relatively normal life?

Thankfully, the results of my biopsy taken from the specimens removed during my recent colonoscopy tested negative for cancer. I have escaped the much dreaded colostomy yet again. Whatever the case may have been, I am grateful for all the amazing support I've been receiving from my amazing family and friends.

It's been a good run so far — 27 years of battling colon cancer and counting. I won some and I lost...no, I *learned* some. The thought of having a colostomy scares me, but as with anything in life, I would get used to it if it came to that. I will eventually make jokes about it. I'll be saying goodbye to unscheduled runs to the bathroom. I'll say *adios* to colonoscopies. And the best part? I'll say "So long, colon cancer! It's been a slice!" (Literally and figuratively...and yes, pun was intended.) I can tell you this much: Whichever path I choose, I WILL WIN THIS WAR. Watch me.
~ *Tet, aka Mesky*

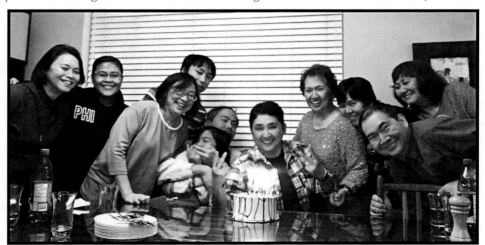

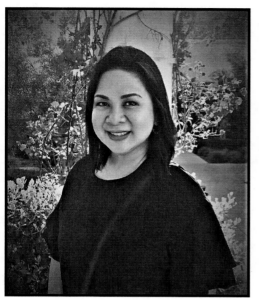

Vida is an amazing and spirited 50+ year old woman whose breast cancer journey started in 2015. She lives in the Philippines and has two daughters Michelle (29) and Monica "Nikki" (27), both of whom reside in California.

Of Filipino ethnicity, Vida is the fifth of six children (four sisters and two brothers). She speaks both English and Tagalog (Filipino) fluently. She lives in a multi-story townhouse in Quezon City, Philippines that has three floors, plus a basement and an attic. Vida and her family are close-knit. Despite the physical distance that separates them, they're in constant communication, thanks to technology. The only family member she knows who has had cancer is her sister who had uterine cancer. Fortunately, it was found in its early stages.

Vida is an artist who designs glass art which is therapeutic for her. At the time of her diagnosis, she owned a glass art and interiors business. When treatment was completed, she decided to sell her business and pursue another venture; this time, designing fancy, elegant head wraps for formal or celebratory occasions. Her favorite pastimes include playing badminton, mahjong, shopping and spending time with her family and friends.

When Vida suspected she had breast cancer, she chose to seek counsel from various sources, including alternative medicine practitioners to better decide what her options were. Here is Vida's story:

The first time I suspected something was wrong was when I was being massaged. I felt pain on my left breast and felt a big lump there. I was 50 years old at the time and never had a mammogram. Of course, my discovery was a big reason for me to finally get a mammogram. When I received a copy of the results, it indicated that I was a "BI-RAD 5." A good friend, who's both an oncology nurse as well as a breast cancer survivor herself, explained the term to mean that the chances of my having cancer were very strong. When I met with my cousin, who's a doctor, he told me that the results of my mammogram were "bad" and I needed a biopsy done, as soon as possible. That was difficult for me to accept, because with everything I had heard about cancer treatments, I was already of the mindset that I would never get chemotherapy, if I ever got cancer.

To learn more about my options outside of chemotherapy and radiation, I went to see a couple of famous herbal doctors. The first herbalist, Apo, without any physical examination, told me that I had a large lump on my left breast. He then strongly cautioned me to not get a biopsy because if I did, "it will poke the mass and the mass will spread." He instructed me to drink a special tea that consisted of a variety of herbs he grew. I still drink it to this day. When I met with the second famous herbalist, he looked at me and, pointing to my left breast, said, "You have a lump right there and it's big. Don't get a biopsy." That was exactly what Apo said! When I heard that, I felt so lost and confused, I couldn't sleep for days. So, I prayed really hard for God to guide me on what He wanted me to do.

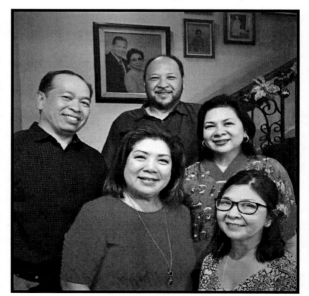

When I felt God telling me to get the biopsy, I finally had it done. My wonderful friend, Masa, was in the room with me, holding my hand. When my doctor cousin told me that my biopsy results tested positive for breast cancer, my sister was with me. Being there with me as I went through my shock and my fears meant so much to me!

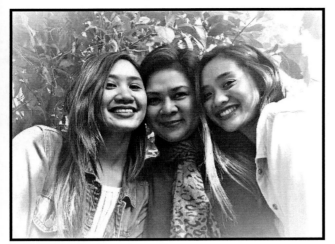

To remove the cancer in my body, I went through a mastectomy of my left breast, chemotherapy, and radiation. I also decided to get reconstruction of my left breast. Throughout my journey, my faith kept me strong and positive. Of course, I did go through some negative emotions, like depression, impatience, irritation and numbness, all of which didn't last long because of my faith and my loving family and friends.

I suffered many side effects, like allergic reactions to medications, loss of my hair, anemia, bone and joint pain, chemo brain, cold sweats, diarrhea, vision problems, lightheadedness, fatigue, fever, gas, hot flashes, itchiness, bladder problems, loss of appetite, low white blood cell count (leukopenia), swelling of my left arm (lymphedema), dry mouth with difficulty swallowing, muscle cramps, nail changes, nerve pain (neuropathy), osteopenia, pain as a side effect from some of the medication and pain from my mastectomy, collapsed veins, shingles, skin changes, taste changes and weight loss.

During the course of my experience, I learned so much about myself and what is truly important in life. The number one lesson I learned is that we are never alone, even though we are by ourselves physically. God is with us through everything. He is there to guide us and to help us. God is always there for us to talk to anytime. All we have to do is ask God for help and He will heal us inside and strengthen us. So, yes, my faith in God was strengthened because of my cancer experience. That's why prayer and faith is so important.

During my cancer journey, I learned two other important lessons that made such a difference also. One was a deeper understanding of love and the other was a beautiful lesson on forgiveness. Love makes everything more colorful. When I was at the lowest point in my life when everything looked black and white, love added so much color! Love made me so happy that my sickness became secondary. If we emphasize love, instead of taking it for granted, we will actually feel the love of those who support us and appreciate them. I have never felt so much love before! It was so amazing! And then there's the power of forgiveness when I let go of everything negative from my system ~ all the anger, the stress; everything that made me cry or lose sleep. Those negatives led to my cancer and they're not worth it. So, the lesson is to take away the negativity and focus on the positive, which includes forgiveness. Just keep all the good thoughts and the good energy.

I'm a new person now. I enjoy how beautiful the world is...the clouds, the trees, everything in nature. I now enjoy life with renewed appreciation of my family and friends and enjoy sharing love with them. I thank God for gifting me with life. I am so grateful. and I want to share my joy with everyone! ~ *Vida*

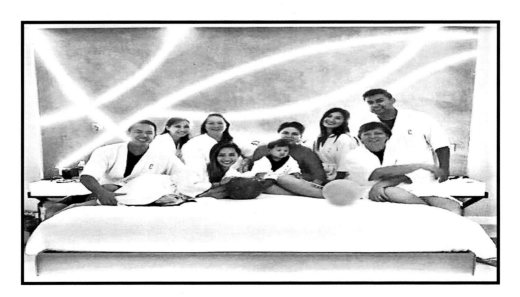

Amor Y. Traceski

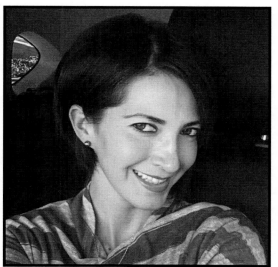

Yesi is a stunning and vibrant 35-year old, happily-married wife to her husband Ryan and mother of her beautiful eight-year old daughter Zoe. She came from a family of three children and was born in Mexico.

When Yesi was nine, she immigrated to the United States. She speaks English and Spanish fluently and is eager to learn yet another language; perhaps Portuguese or Italian. Yesi lives with her family in the wonderful city of Sunnyvale, CA where she works in hotel sales. She is a California girl, at heart! For her leisure time, she enjoys gardening, cooking and absolutely adores nature, greenery and water. She says, "It's definitely what keeps me going. It just gives me energy. I love spending time with my family and I just enjoy every day like it's the last." Yesi fervently believes there is a higher power and that "God is with me every day"! Here is Yesi's story:

I was diagnosed with cancer at the age of 32 and am the first in my entire family to have cancer. My mother who has nine siblings and my father, who is one of five siblings, informed me that there is absolutely no cancer on either side of the family. So, of course, the news of my cancer was devastating to all of us.

My story began in the summer of 2014, when I discovered a marble-sized lump in my right breast as I was doing a self-examination. The first doctor I saw, learning that I had absolutely no history of cancer in my family and seeing my young age (32), said, "It seems like it's just a fibrocystic breast. Just give it a couple of cycles and it should go away. Check back with me after a cycle or two." I was relieved. The following month, however, the marble-sized lump in my breast had doubled in size; like the size of a bubble gum ball, and it was definitely growing! So, I knew something was wrong. The next doctor I saw was my regular doctor. She saw me right away and said the same thing the first doctor said, after examining me. She said, "Honey, you have fibrocystic breast. Don't worry about it. You're young and healthy. You should be fine."

I really felt that I was not being taken seriously, so I insisted that there was something seriously wrong, and I begged her to have more tests done. Because of my persistence, I was referred to the most amazing team of professionals at the Cancer Center in Mountain View. I tried to remain positive even though I was scared.

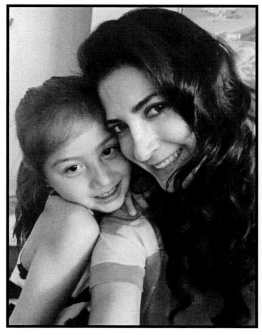

After a series of tests and procedures, I was given the shocking news that I had stage III (almost stage IV) carcinoma in situ triple positive breast cancer. Upon hearing the news, I didn't cry. All I could think of was my daughter Zoe, who was then four years old. Although we asked about what the next months, the next year was going to look like, I really didn't remember a thing. I had gone into a different world. All I wanted to do was feel peace, so I told my husband that I didn't want to talk to anybody. All I wanted to do was process the news and be with nature. So, we went for the longest hike in Rancho San Antonio, and I just lost myself there. I know it sounds weird, but I actually felt peace and was not afraid. I knew I was going to be fine.

Since we knew our 4 ½ year old daughter Zoe was going to witness changes in me, we carefully shared the news with her. She then referred to my tumors, not as cancer, but as "bubble gums" and even told me that she had a dream that "the doctor took all the bubble gums out and you are going to be fine!"

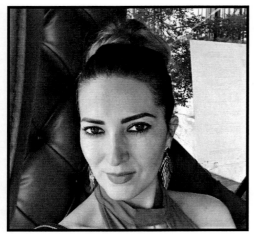

Yes, I accepted my diagnosis. But, at the same time, I declared war against cancer! I said, "My daughter needs me, and I need her. I am going to fight with everything I have. I have an amazing support team of doctors, family, friends, and I'm going to fight! This is a battle, and I am going to win!" That was my approach.

So, I went through several rounds of chemotherapy every other week for eight weeks, two rounds of targeted therapy weekly for 12 weeks, a total of 24 rounds of radiation, a bilateral mastectomy, and a series of tests and procedures to beat my cancer.

For treatment, my body had to process a lot of toxic drugs in my system. I experienced a lot of physical side-effects, like alopecia (hair loss), anemia, bone & joint pain, brittle nails, chemo brain, constipation, delayed wound healing, diarrhea, fatigue, fever, hot flashes, infections, kidney problems, cramps, low white blood cell count, lymphedema, mouth sores, neuropathy, pain, poor veins, taste & smell changes, weakness and weight loss. Still, I remained positive. The amazing support of my wonderful family and friends kept me going!

I also experienced a lot of emotional pain, like anger, bitterness, anxiety, depression, fear, frustration, grief, impatience, irritation, loneliness, moodiness, passiveness, feeling overwhelmed and shock. However, because of my family and friends' support, especially, my husband, mother and daughter and best friend, I remained emotionally strong.

The only time I lost control of my emotions was <u>after</u> my treatment was complete. I was supposed to feel happiness in having survived cancer, but I didn't feel happiness or a sense of accomplishment at all. Instead, for over a year, I felt negatively about my past experience and my situation. I wasn't aware of how my behavior was affecting everyone around me. After a very serious discussion with my husband that knocked some sense into me, I finally met with a psychological therapist who explained to me how various cancer treatments can affect the brain. In my case, my treatments sucked my brain dry of serotonin, a chemical responsible for maintaining mood balance. She gave me a prescription of antidepressants, which have been a lifesaver for me, and guided me through my survivorship issues.

Now, I definitely understand that I beat cancer's ass and was given a second chance in life! That experience is behind me. I am very happy, and it's one of the most amazing feelings! I am also very grateful to be able to continue living life with my wonderful family, especially my beautiful daughter Zoe! ~ *Yesi*

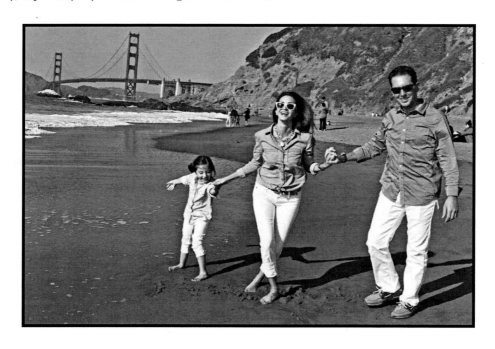

PART TWO

BARBARA MOOTY'S MESSAGE THROUGH HER CANCER SURVIVOR HUSBAND GLENN

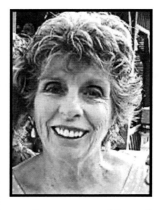

Barbara Mooty was the wife of stage IV colon cancer survivor, Glenn Mooty. They were married for 47 years and have four children, three grandchildren and six great-grandchildren. Together, they created a special love story that transcends time and space. On February 21, 2017, Barbara passed away from breast cancer.

Known to be loving and straightforward, Barbara did not mince words, especially when it came to providing insight she believed would benefit others. Here are some tips and insights that Barbara shared through her husband, Glenn.

1. Consider being Aggressive.

"Making the decision about how aggressive you should be in your cancer battle is something that must be discussed with your own doctor, of course. In my case, it wasn't a very difficult decision. With the pleasure of watching great grandkids grow up, I decided that I wanted to live as long as possible and that treatments with their side effects were the price I had to pay. I was bothered by the nearly constant anxiety and worry of not having an effective plan to fight it.

So in January of 2000, I had a double mastectomy, even though I had not yet been diagnosed with cancer. After the mastectomy, lab findings of the tissue that was removed confirmed that I had cancer. So, I made the right decision, even though it was made without input from the doctors."

Glenn's account of how it happened:

During the first half of 2000, Barb was agonizing about the risk of getting breast cancer. She had a series of "suspicious mammograms" and "pre-cancerous needle biopsies". She was already having so much anxiety, she couldn't sleep. This worry wasn't helpful.

Barb was pretty aggressive for someone who wasn't even diagnosed with cancer. She wanted to have a double mastectomy as a preventative measure. But, as she talked about it with friends, she found out that one friend (her co-worker at the Unicorn where she worked) had had a mastectomy 20 years prior. After the surgery, her friend told her that her husband refused to look at her body naked. Naturally, this woman was very hurt and disturbed by how her husband treated her.

This concerned Barb very much. She came home that day and asked me if we could talk. "How is it going to affect you if I have this surgery and possibly not have breast reconstruction? I will have a flat chest and be scarred. I need to know how you're going to handle it." So I asked her, "Can I give you my answer later today?" "Yes, that's fine" she said.

I have never liked "free verse poetry (where no attempt is made to rhyme). I agree with Robert Frost when he said, "Writing free-verse is like playing tennis without a net." But in this case, I decided it was worth a try.

I needed something simple, quick and straight from the heart. So, I wrote "Molecules", made a card out of it and recited it for her before I gave her the card. It turned out to be the most important and powerful poem I had ever written, because the next morning, she called her doctor and asked him to schedule her for the surgery.

Only after her breast tissue was sent to the lab did they confirm Barb had cancer. "Lobular carcinoma in situ (LCIS)". In converting the metric, it was .17 inches; exactly the size of a BB. We thought that was more than a sufficient margin and that we didn't have to worry about her with breast cancer any longer. That was not the case. It came back and Barb sadly passed away seventeen years later.

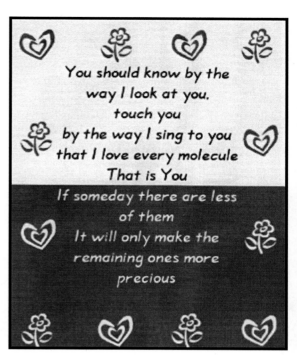

You should know by the way I look at you,
touch you
by the way I sing to you
that I love every molecule
That is You

If someday there are less
of them
It will only make the
remaining ones more
precious

2. Barbara says, "Be Sincerely Supportive."

If you are a partner of a cancer survivor, it is critically important that you be supportive of him or her. There is no need at all to share that you are repulsed.

Glenn agreed and continued...

The emotional damage caused by the husband of Barbara's friend, although no doubt unintentionally done, was very hurtful, as well as, damaging to the healing process. So the point is, IF you want your partner to survive and thrive, then do your part and be **sincerely** supportive. If you have a problem with that, then you might need a different kind of treatment yourself.

3) See Doctors Who See Other Doctors.

Doctors need medical treatment themselves from time to time, just like the rest of us. Where do they go? Generally, they see top medical specialists who have a very good reputation in their chosen field. That's what you should do as well. And, it's not always easy. Even if you have to make an appointment that you have to pay for out-of-pocket just to get a referral, do it! We did just that.

Glenn agreed and continued...

Unless you have known a doctor for years, don't expect him or her to give you a referral for free. We had a favorite doctor who was in his late 80's and had been practicing general medicine for 60 years. He knew he was going to need cataract surgery when he kept losing the golf ball after hitting it during his games. So, of course, he went to the top ophthalmologist and got a great result with no problems.

When I needed cataract surgery, I did not see the top doctor. I saw the ophthalmologist I had gone to for years for my glasses. Consequently, because of my ophthalmologist, I had halos around the oncoming car headlights in night traffic, after my cataract surgery, and I couldn't drive at night again for the rest of my life.

4) Cough It Up!

For some, this advice may seem too disgusting a subject to talk about. But, the truth is, it's really important that people know about this. It's a fact of life that the body has a natural response to removing infectious material through the action of coughing it up and spitting it out. Being able to remove these infectious material could make the difference in your treatment or recovery from an illness.

Glenn expounded on Barb's thoughts...

> The slang phrase I use is "hocking up a loogie". The definition of "hock" is to clear the throat of phlegm. The definition of "loogie" is a large wad of spit or phlegm, sometimes mixed with nose snot or nasal mucus that has accumulated in your throat.
>
> Make sure that you and the young people you know learn the importance of being able to cough up a "loogie". Children should learn this skill before they become teenagers, as much as possible. Typically, women or girls have more of an aversion to coughing up this material than men or boys, because it is considered "gross" and not "ladylike". However, when your body tells you to get rid of something, it's critical that you listen to your body. By the way, we knew a mature, seasoned oncology nurse who could easily be brought to the brink of vomiting, just from the sound of someone coughing up a "loogie". So, for some people, this could require some training or coaching ... from boys or men.

5) Dealing with a Gag Reflex. Taking Oral Medications and Pills.

Make sure that the young people you are exposed to, are able to down fairly large pills without throwing up. People with mild to severe gag reflex may have a very difficult time getting down some or all pills. In my case, I grew up practicing Christian Science, which doesn't believe in using medicine to heal the body. I was raised, instead, to believe that God will take care of us when we get sick. So as a young person, I did not learn how to cough up and spit out anything. I would gag just brushing my teeth. Inevitably, capsules, especially sticky ones like Ibrance, were nearly impossible for me to get down. After the more common estrogen blocker medications stopped working, I was basically left without medical treatment. Then, the cancer took over.

Glenn agreed and continued...

> Women or girls may likely have more problems learning the important skill of taking oral medications and pills. Nevertheless, it is critical that they learn this ability. Maybe some of the nice men or boys out there can help with that.

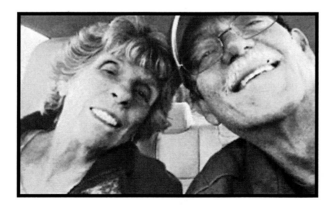

Good luck with your fight,
Barbara & Glenn

PART THREE

Chapter 2

FINDING OUT YOU HAVE CANCER

When we learn that we have a serious illness, our emotions come into play. When we learn we have a serious illness that could lead to the end of our life, stronger, deeper emotions like disbelief, shock, anger, panic, etc. come into play. No one can tell you how you're going to react or how you should react. In this chapter, cancer survivors share how they learned they had cancer, and they give you a glimpse of how they handled the news, given the circumstances.

♥ **Aaron** (*Prostate cancer, Skin cancer.*)

Skin cancer: I noticed a small, red lump in the lower eyelid of my left eye. When I went to the hospital, the doctor there said that it was just a stye. A year went by and it got worse. Only then did they realize that it wasn't just a stye; it was skin cancer. The dermatologist I saw told me that the doctor I saw a year back misdiagnosed me and should have known that I had was skin cancer, not a stye. So then, I had to have special surgery to remove the cancer. Of course, I was upset and really irritated.

Prostate cancer: After some time of getting my PSA's (Prostate Specific Antigen) checked every few years, I noticed that the number was starting to rise. In 2013, when my PSA was 3.6 ng/ml (normal is considered 4.0 ng/ml), my doctor recommended a biopsy. But, I didn't want one at the time. I said, "No" because, as a rule, they become concerned when it's about 4.0 ng/ml. So then, in 2016, when it increased to 3.9 ng/ml, they again recommended a biopsy, which I got. I didn't have any lumps or anything on my prostate, but then the results came back.

My doctor called me to give me the results. I had stage I prostate cancer. The cancer showed in 5% of my prostate. I was shocked! Immediately, I asked him, "Are you serious?" Then, I said, "Go figure, I would get it.." My girlfriend was with me when I got the call.

I remember that my mom figured I would get cancer of the prostate because statistics have shown that one in seven men get it. Also, when I was a motorcycle cop, I was exposed to a lot of chemicals. I had to work in a carcinogenic environment, breathe in benzene found in gasoline and be exposed to the ultraviolet rays of the sun, both of which are known to cause cancer. So, I believe that was part of the reason I got cancer at an early age. Still, I was shocked because the odds were, one in fifty men get prostate cancer under the age of 55.

At first, I didn't even want to have the surgery. I said, "Screw it!" But my doctor said, "If you don't do anything about it, it'll kill you in ten to fifteen years. You have a long life ahead of you. Your mother lived a long time (she died when she was 95 ½ years old). Your brother's still around; he's 74. So, you're better off getting it done now. Get through the process. Then, you'll be able to live the rest of your life normally."

I also had the option of radiation. But I didn't like the downside. You see, with surgery, the side effects are immediate. But then, you get better and the side effects go away. Whereas, with radiation, you don't have immediate side effects. They happen later. So, I figured that I would be out of commission for a year and a half. In the big scheme of things, I'll (hopefully) have 30 more years of life and this episode will just be a blip. I've got two kids. I can't be dead by the time I'm 70 years old. If I had stage IV cancer at the age of 70, I'd be dead! That's how I had to look at my situation.

So, I progressively did all my research, talked to other people and then decided that surgery was my best option. I also interviewed a few doctors who could perform my surgery. Fortunately, I found the very best surgeon at the hospital I go to. He had the most skill and experience with the specific surgery I needed (robotic surgery) and even had trained the other doctors that I had interviewed before him.

ADVICE #1: Even though the doctors don't usually like to check people's PSAs until they're around 65 years old, I would not wait that long. Start having your PSA checked when you're in your late 40s! My doctor told me that the reason they caught the cancer early was due to the fact that I was proactive and had it checked early. So, that's what you have to do because it can spread all of a sudden and kill you if you ignore it. It is unusual for a man, under 55 years of age, to have prostate cancer. But it does occur, obviously. So, that would be my first recommendation.

ADVICE #2: Do the research. I did a lot of research to help me determine if it was better for me to do radiation or surgery. The difference is: If you do radiation, the doctors can't go back and re-radiate the area if they don't get it all. So, you don't have a back-up option there. Now, radiation would be good if you're 75 years old or towards the end of your lifespan because, most likely, you are going to die of other causes before the prostate cancer gets you. If you're younger, like me, and you have a family history of longevity, surgery is probably the best bet. Although it is a slower recovery process, they can always go back and radiate if they're not able to get all the cancer out. So, with surgery, you have a backup option.

That's why I eventually chose to have robotic surgery, which is the most advanced, least invasive method of surgery. Then, I interviewed about four or five doctors and, fortunately, found one who actually taught robotic surgery techniques to all the doctors I had interviewed before him.

♥ Amor (Breast cancer, Ovarian cancer)

Breast cancer: After my annual mammogram, my radiologist informed me that she saw something highly suspicious, but needed to run more tests. I have dense breast tissue, so this was expected. Well, I went through more than one test, i.e. an ultrasound guided core biopsy, a stereotactic core biopsy, an MRI and then a final ultrasound before they called me at home and told me that I have cancer in my left breast. I was alone and stunned. Although I took the news calmly, it sounded like a death knell. After the call, I told myself, "Well, garbage in, garbage out" and immediately searched the Internet for whatever information I could find about Breast cancer, treatments and their outcomes, including death. I even looked at really graphic pictures because I wanted to be prepared for the worst. I felt that arming myself with knowledge would help keep me strong.

I had the BEST radiologist. She really took time to provide me with information, so that I could make the right decision for myself. One day, she brought me into her office, which was lit only by two images on her computer screens. One was of my diseased left breast where the breast tissue looked like a mesh of lightning & thunderstorms, and the other was of my healthy right breast where my breast tissue looked silky smooth. It was obvious that my left breast looked like "garbage" and it had to go!

Ovarian Cancer: During the manual examination of the pap smear process, my gynecologist said that he felt something different; a firm tissue mass. He then asked me if my previous gynecologist had mentioned anything about it. I told him that results of my last pap smear were clear and nothing else was mentioned. He scheduled me for an ultrasound, explaining that we definitely need to have the mass tested. My boyfriend Bill, thankfully, accompanied me. During the ultrasound, my gynecologist and the ultrasound technician quietly had a discussion between themselves while looking at the images. When I asked what was going on, they just gave me vague responses, e.g. we're still reviewing, or we don't know yet.

When Bill and I later met with my gynecologist to discuss results of the ultrasound and the biopsy that he had done of the "firm tissue" in my abdomen, he stated that I have a malignant tumor, which tested positive for Ovarian cancer. Fortunately, he said, it was only in stage II, meaning it was caught early and my chances of a full recovery were pretty high. He then proceeded to explain the next steps, which included a total abdominal hysterectomy, oophorectomy, omentectomy and other procedures to make sure they remove any sign of cancer from my body. I took it quietly, as I had gotten bad news like this in the past. Again, my thought was "garbage in, garbage out." However, as this was Bill's first time to receive such news, he was quite upset.

I researched everything I could about ovarian cancer and my options. Most of all, I prayed continuously to God for strength and direction, trusting God to be with me and show me the way. In my surrender to God, I felt safe. I felt strong, and I also felt peace.

<u>ADVICE</u>: Everyone's individual reaction and way of handling challenges is different, and I totally respect that. I would, however, like to impart some thoughts that hopefully will help those who feel "lost in the darkness and confusion."

- First, take good time to acknowledge your fears and emotions: honor your humanity. Cry if you need to; don't hold back your tears. Vent your emotions to release your negative energy. When the dust settles, when your emotional balloon has somewhat deflated, you'll be able to think more clearly on the steps you'll need to take.
- Next, put aside your emotions and think of the facts. Write them down if that helps. <u>Fact #1:</u> You have cancer. <u>Fact #2:</u> You have options.
- Next, look at your options. What are they? Ask your doctor and research information. Get a second or even third opinion if you need to. Write these down. I've found that the activity of writing down my questions and the facts helped me cope. When I actively asked my doctors questions and discussed my options with them, I felt like I had more control. I didn't want to just follow everything they told me to do. I wanted to be fully informed and understand what I was up against and what I had to go through.
- <u>Fact #3:</u> Your emotions do have an effect on our overall well-being and recovery. For me, "happy cells = healthy cells". Yes, honor your humanity and emotions and give yourself a time limit to vent. However, don't wallow in misery and stay in the "darkness"; you'll just spiral downward. It just makes matters worse and doesn't help your situation. I gave myself 10 minutes, tops, to cry my heart and head out. Afterwards, my head was clear and I was able to breath. Of course, I had many, many crying episodes. They were all part of my human experience.

When you are able to breathe and be calm, try to look objectively at your situation. Try to put your emotions to the side and focus on the facts. Get organized. A cancer diagnosis can make you feel out of control. Putting together a binder or notebook that will house any information related to you diagnosis and care, e.g. medications, tests, procedures, images, lab results, etc. will help you focus on what you need to do. Learn as much as you can about your cancer, the stage, and your treatment options. Then identify what you can do and what you'll need help with.

Have someone who supports you accompany you to your medical appointments. List questions to ask your doctor, and take notes of your meeting with him or her. Many times, just learning of your diagnosis is overwhelming. Your companion can be your extra set of ears, speak on your behalf or help you digest important information, like tests and appointment dates.

Find the best care you can. Research the background of doctors and surgeons, including experience, special skills and reviews given by other patients. Being with doctors or surgeons you trust is critical to your overall treatment and recovery. If necessary, get a second opinion. Seek outside advice, but don't get too many opinions because that will only create confusion.

Find support. This is an emotionally difficult time for you, so it is important to find family or friends you can lean on for support. You'd be surprised at how many people want to help. Of course, it's best not to set expectations on anyone. People like to give freely, without expectation.

Questions to ask your treating physician:
- What are the treatment options for my cancer? - Treatment paths differ from patient to patient, depending on cancer type, stage and other health issues present. Some patients have surgery and then chemo and radiation. Others have chemo and then surgery, followed by radiation. Treatment is not a one-size-fits-all.
- What stage is my cancer? - From the answer to this question, you'll know how big your cancer is and if or where it has spread. Staging your cancer enables your doctor to determine the right treatment for you.
- How long will my treatment take? - Find out when you'll complete treatment, so you can gauge when you can return to work or make post-treatment plans for yourself. Knowing that will help you plan your future.
- Are there any markers that define my cancer? - Markers are substances that cancer tumors produce that are found in your blood or other fluids. Doctors use these markers to fine-tune diagnoses and treatments.

♥ Bob (*Soft Tissue Sarcoma, Skin Cancer*)

Soft Tissue Sarcoma: It definitely started in the tissue. Then, when it latched on to the spleen, it reacted, which is my good fortune. I was driving up to Reno with my wife and I got sick up there. When I saw the surgeon, I could tell something was wrong. By the look in his eyes, I could tell that I wasn't out of it; but something was still wrong. But he and the other doctors weren't telling me. Nobody ever told me that I had cancer. But the way they described what they were going to do, I had a strong feeling that it was cancer. One day, going to the hospital, I told my wife, "They haven't told me what it is, but I'm going to have surgery, and I just want you all to be prepared because it's really bad...very bad." When we got to the hospital, they took out my spleen, but the doctors then never officially told me. I guess everyone thought that someone else told me. Note: I moved a little of the copy because the paragraph was confusing otherwise.

ADVICE: If you think something is wrong, ask your doctor, so you know for sure.

♥ Cindy L. (*Kidney cancer*)

In December 2014, I was instructed by my doctor to take Prometrium (a female hormone progesterone) daily. Seven months later, in July 2015, I started itching for no apparent reason. It was a very strange itching; just in certain parts of my body, i.e. my ears, hands, feet and calves (back of my legs). Since the doctor I had been seeing just retired, I went to see a new doctor. She ordered blood work for me. When she got the results, she told me, "Oh, your bilirubin is high. That means you're jaundiced." I asked her, "So, that's what's causing my itching?" She answered, "Well, your triglycerides are tripled, but your cholesterol levels were fine. Let's just wait until next year." I said, "No, I don't think so."

I found another doctor and he jumped on the problem. Because I am a nurse, I figured that my strange itching was a reaction to the Prometrium that was causing my liver to struggle, and so I went off of that medication. At that point, a lot of things started happening really fast. I went on a very low carb diet and started losing weight at an alarming speed, i.e. 48 pounds in a very short period of time. Yes, it was on purpose; I quit sugar. My diet wasn't horrible before that; I just quit sugar. That alone was enough to get my body to dump the weight when I went off the Prometrium, which was keeping me heavy. My doctor ordered an abdominal ultrasound and checked my liver. I was diagnosed with fatty liver. Then he said, "Oh, by the way, there's a cyst on your left kidney. Don't worry about it. These things are usually benign."

Well, something in the back of my mind said, "No, we ARE going to worry about this." So, I said, "I'm going to wait six months, and then we're going to look at it again." This was in December of 2015. So in August of 2016, I went back to my doctor and requested the ultrasound. Within two hours of that ultrasound, he was on the phone and said, "We need to see what this is." After meeting with him again, we decided that I would get an MRI of my kidney versus a CT scan. That's because I have a heart issue that could cause me to have problems with the particular contrast that they use with the CT scan; we felt the contrast with the MRI would be better handled by my heart. Within a couple of hours of the MRI, I got word from him that they were referring me out to a urologist because there was about a 95% possibility that I had cancer in my kidney. My husband, thankfully, was with me from the very beginning; whether I was on the phone with my doctors, or when I met with them.

When I learned that I had kidney cancer, I got mad. Yes, I was crying, but I got mad. My daughter was having problems in UCF Orlando. She was having serious medical issues; kept fainting and we didn't know why. She was taken to the emergency room three times in an ambulance when she would faint. We didn't know if was her heart, her brain, or what. And, I was headed down the very next day to see her. So, yes. When I found out I had cancer, in the middle of everything that was going on, I got pretty upset and more angry at what I was about to go through instead of having a lot of fear.

ADVICE: It's never easy to learn you have cancer, especially when you have other matters you have to deal with. It's natural to get upset and cry, so allow yourself to vent. I was fortunate to have my husband by my side to support me. Hopefully, you do too.

♥ Cindy R. (*Metastatic Breast cancer to the Stomach*)

Breast cancer: It was in 2004 when I initially noticed that there was an inversion in my right breast. I kept looking at it and thinking, "Well, it's nothing." I was 39 years old at the time. Still, I paid attention and noticed that it kept growing.

Naturally, I got nervous. When I went to my doctor, he said, "Oh, yeah, it's nothing." He didn't even think a mammogram was necessary because I was too young. But I insisted and said, "No. No really. We've got to figure this out. Something's wrong." So, they did a CT scan and found out that there was a lump there. Then I went in for the biopsy and sure enough, it was cancer; stage three Breast cancer. The cancer had gone into my lymph nodes too. I was shocked!

There was no history at all of breast cancer in my family, of breast cancer ever. I was like, "What?!" My dad had prostate cancer, but no one in my parents' generation, nor any one of cousins had had Breast cancer, ever. So, it was very shocking. My mom and my sister, who were with me, were shocked too.

It sounds weird but, thankfully, I insisted that my breast be checked, which led to finding my cancer, because three months later, when my sister noticed something was not right with her breast and insisted it be checked, they found that she had stage one Breast cancer.

A few years later, my aunt found her breast cancer early (stage one). And, the following year, my mom also found out that she had stage one Breast cancer. So, they all realized how important it was to regularly examine their breasts and pay attention to anything that was off. And, if there was something there that was questionable or not right, then they knew to have it checked right away.

ADVICE: Learn how to perform breast self-exams and do it regularly. Pay attention to anything that's off. Know your body, because if something doesn't feel right or if there is something questionable, then you'll know to get it checked right away. The sooner you get yourself checked, the better.

Stomach Cancer: Around the 10th year anniversary of my breast cancer diagnosis, I started noticing that my appetite was decreasing. I wasn't a huge eater, but I got to a point where I thought, "If I ate another bite, I would just throw up." I didn't feel any pain. What I felt was like a cramping sensation. I just knew something wasn't right. I thought I had IBS (irritable bowel syndrome) or something like that. It was weird. So, I told my oncologist, and he had a biopsy done on my stomach. Well, it turned out that I had stomach cancer. At first, I was like, "Ugh, that wasn't what I thought it would be, but okay." But then after, it hit me and I said, "What? Wait a second! Why is this happening now?"

It just didn't make any sense because I had already passed the five-year remission period when I was "released" by my oncologist and told, "Okay, you can just go to your primary care doctor now." So yeah, I was shocked when I was told I had stomach cancer. I was also angry and afraid.

The fear mainly came from my primary care doctor telling me, "Well, I know one other person that had this happen and I haven't seen him since." I said, "Oh my God!" He's pretty straight forward, which is kind of good and kind of not so good. Still, it was crazy finding out. Again, my mother was with me and our mouths dropped open in shock. We both said, "What? Wow, what the crap!"

After my first diagnosis (breast cancer), I thought, "Okay, I'm dying. That's it. It's over." At that time, I didn't know what else to think. Ten years later, after my mom and I learned that I had stomach cancer, I said, "You know what? No. This is not right. First of all, I want ice cream. So, let's go get that. Second of all, I am fighting this thing. I don't care what they say. I don't care what they do. This is not happening. This is not right. This is not happening." Yeah, it really took me for a loop because the likelihood of getting cancer again after 10 years is pretty low.

After several treatments for my stomach cancer, which didn't seem to work at all, my doctor looked deeper at the pathology and realized that the cancer in my stomach was actually a metastasis of my breast cancer from 10 years prior; not a separate cancer.

ADVICE: Always be aware of changes in your body, including your appetite. When you observe that something is off, even if it's just a feeling of something that's not right, let your doctor know right away, so that you can have it checked.

It is natural to be shocked or angry when you receive bad news. However, instead of feeling like a victim and feeling sorry for yourself, focus your energy on fighting the disease. Even if your body is weak, you have to take on the attitude that you're not going to let it control you.

♥ Glenn (Metastatic Colon cancer to the Liver, Lungs & Adrenal Glands)

A flat polyp missed in my 2010 colonoscopy was discovered in my 2014 colonoscopy. Unfortunately, it was too late. I had stage IV Colon cancer. The tumor was missed because it was outside the colon, so the cancer had metastasized to my liver.

I actually learned the news through my granddaughter Heather because the doctor couldn't reach me when I was on the job. So, they called her since she is my backup contact. When I was told I had stage IV colon cancer, I was shocked and kept saying, "Sh*t!...Sh*t!..." I didn't know what I was going to do and sort of panicked. Fortunately, my wife Barbara was there to take care of me. With her support, I was able to tough it out.

<u>ADVICE:</u> As much as possible, have someone you trust with you when you receive the news. That way, they can help you up and get see straight when you get the news that basically knocks you down.

♥ Hilda (Colon cancer)

Since I was about to turn 50 years old in October 2011, I scheduled myself for a colonoscopy. Given that it's a four-hour procedure, I took the day off from work and asked my daughter Jessica to drop me off at the hospital. I told her that I would call her to pick me up once they released me.

My doctor and his nurse prepared me for the procedure and told me that when I woke up, the colonoscopy would be done. Then, they had me count backwards, and I went under not too long after. When I woke up, they put me in Recovery and, basically, waited for me to have a good sense of my surroundings before releasing me. However, before I was released, my doctor came in and informed me that they did find something, and they'll need me back for a reevaluation; but nothing to worry about at this point. So, that was cool and I felt better. When Jessica picked me up, she asked, "How did it go, Mom?" I said to her, "Everything sounds good, but they have to check again because they did see something, so I'll probably go back later." Being such a positive person, my daughter said, "Ok, Mom, I'm sure it's going to be fine." "Yeah, I think so too," I said. Since I took the whole day off from work, I just went home and chilled.

When I went back to work the following day, everything was like it was before; nothing new. When my doctor called, I was unable to take his call, because I was at work, so he left me a message. When I retrieved it later that day, my doctor said in his message, "We found something. I need to talk with you as soon as possible." I said "Oh, sh*t!". His message prepared me for something. Knowing that I had to make that call, I took a break and I went outside because I didn't want to be in the office. I remember walking around. I was still in the Dublin, Pleasanton office at that time. It was a hot day in October, right before my birthday. I remember walking around the parking lot, just trying to make that call. And then, I called and talked to him.

My doctor told me that they did find something and that they needed to schedule an appointment with me immediately because it looked pretty aggressive. I was saying to myself, "Sh*t!" and I was, of course, shocked, but I was alone and I tend to deal better with challenges on my own. So, it was actually a "good" time. If I had been in the office or at home taking that call, it would've been a bit hairier. But I dealt with it and I composed myself. I had to think clearly as a mom, what the best thing was for me to do next. After giving my situation some good thought, I called my doctor back. He informed me that he would make the necessary calls and get me scheduled with a team of doctors for me to meet. I was to expect a call from someone with the details. I said, "Okay, that's fine. Go ahead and do that."

When I went to the Cancer Center for my meetings, I remember the young man at reception. He was very upbeat and familiarized me with the steps. He told me that the first person I was going to meet was going to be the head nurse who was going to explain everything to me. When the head nurse came out, I immediately recognized her as Marie, the mother of my daughter's classmate. I was so happy, because I felt relief knowing her personally and knowing she was there for me. And in her profession, she understood confidentiality. Nobody knew about my condition, except her and me.

I told Marie, "I'm really glad it's you because I can talk to you more openly." Marie told me what to expect, who I'm going to see, who my surgeon was going to be, who my oncologist was, etc. She said they didn't think it was necessary to assign me a radiation oncologist. They wanted to evaluate first how I did with the initial treatments. When Marie told me to be prepared for my meetings with the doctors, I remember asking her, "What should I say to them? Do you have anything to tell me?" She said, "Tell them that you are healthy and you want them to be aggressive. Tell them you want them to take your situation seriously."

I first met with my surgeon, who was a young, upbeat kind of guy. He told me that I have colon cancer and explained how he was going to remove the cancerous tumor from my colon. He reassured me and said, "Don't worry about it." He described the "twirled up" position the colon is normally in and, when stretched, it would be like so long that having half of it taken out wouldn't be a big deal. He reassured me, "Don't worry. We're just going to do it." He also explained about the four stages of cancer and, and as far as they could tell, I was at stage III. However, they would confirm the stage of my colon cancer after the surgery. I told my surgeon, "All I can say is please be aggressive. Don't hesitate to take extra because

I don't want it to come back. Take out as much as you want and, if you find it spread to other parts of my body, then while you're in there, please take them out too! Take out the uterus...whatever you have to take out. Take it out because I want to live!" I added that I wanted to live and see my children get old. He was really nice. I felt a good connection with him.

Afterwards, I met with my oncologist who was also very nice. She was going to take care of my chemotherapy treatment. I was given the opportunity to have a second opinion if I wanted it, but I chose not to because I felt good about both doctors. My surgeon even told me, "I do want to move this along as quickly as possible because of the stage; it's urgent, so I'm going to make an opening for you. Thursday morning is the first appointment I could have. I'm going to come early and take care of it." I met my doctors on Tuesday, and my surgery was scheduled for that Thursday, just two days later! It all went very fast, so I knew it was time to tell my husband because now I knew all I needed to know.

ADVICE: If your doctor wants to speak with you about the results of your test, find a place where you can speak with him or her without interruption or background noise. Whether you have someone there with you or not is your choice. For me, I wanted to process the news on my own.

When you meet with your doctors and you are otherwise healthy, don't hesitate to let them know that you want them to take your situation seriously and be aggressive in treating the disease. Because you want to live, you would want any possible threat to be removed too.

♥ Jacki (Breast cancer)

When I learned I had Breast cancer, I didn't really have any information going in. I didn't know anybody who had cancer, so I just learned on my own because I didn't personally know of anyone having a bad time with it. There was no history of cancer in my family at all. I was shocked and a bit scared. It was surreal. The only time I was very upset and sad and questioning was the day I found out it was cancer. Since I initially didn't have much information to go by, I didn't know what to do or how to cope with it. Still, I said, "Life goes on." And, of course, I looked at everything positive, which is just my nature. I woke up the next morning and continued to do whatever I do every day. I certainly didn't think it was the end of the world. It was just part of life.

ADVICE: Breathe and learn about your cancer. It also helps to talk with cancer survivors to understand the experience and what you can expect.

♥ Joan (Rectal cancer)

After my colonoscopy, I was told to see a specialist. So, I went with my daughter Lori to see the specialist and was told that I had stage III rectal cancer. When I heard the news, I was so upset, I felt like my entire brain was floating away! Then, I looked at my daughter, and she had tears rolling down her cheeks. It was such an awful feeling. Reality soon set in, and I prayed for acceptance.

After I settled down, I realized that I'm over 70 years old and never had a serious illness. I thought of all the ill children and gave thanks to the good Lord for the 70 healthy years I was able to live.

ADVICE: Learning you have cancer is not easy. After you settle down from being upset, it helps to think of those who have it far worse than you and move forward to doing what you need to do to get better.

♥ John Bernard "JB" (Salivary Gland cancer)

My cancer journey began in mid-November of 2016. I had an unusual growth on the side of my right cheek and went to the doctor to check it out. He had it biopsied, and then he called me. At the time, aside from college, I was working part-time as an office assistant at a small machine shop in the San Jose. I was on the road, driving my boss's high school-aged son home when I got the call from my doctor. He asked if I had a moment. Because I knew it was important, I pulled to the side, parked the car and got out, so that I could talk to my doctor in private. What he told me definitely stunned me. He said that it was the worst possible case and used the word "malignant." He explained that I would require further testing. The whole thing was surreal, and I felt kind of confused. When I returned to my boss's son in the car, I didn't say anything. I just continued with my day.

♥ Rev. Linda *(Pancreatic cancer – 3x)*

When I was diagnosed with stage II pancreatic cancer in July 2016, after completing a series of tests prompted by lab results, I was quite upset. I had just bought a house, retired, and moved to Illinois from California two months prior. I was looking forward to enjoying retired life with my family and friends, especially my mother, Ma Mere, who has Alzheimer's. Having cancer and going through treatment was the exact opposite of what I had envisioned, so I was really shocked and angry when I received the diagnosis. I had suspected cancer, but not pancreatic cancer. When I finally calmed down, I mobilized myself to do what I needed to do to address it – physically, emotionally, mentally, and spiritually. I informed my immediate family and closest friends because I wanted them to know the truth.

Learning that my cancer had returned less than a year from my first diagnosis and, despite surgery and 18 chemotherapy sessions, really shook me. I knew I had no choice but to accept and move on. To this day, I continue my attempts to normalize my life and stay in the present moment while my subconscious continues to work on my concerns. Still, I go on.

> **ADVICE:** I advise patients to follow up on negative results QUICKLY if there's any suspicion of cancer. Delaying can be the difference between early and late stages. Also, for cancer patients, be fearless about saying what you need, and what you do not need, about what is helpful, and what is not.

♥ Rachel *(Breast cancer: triple negative)*

I was diagnosed on May 27, 2016 with stage III triple negative breast cancer. The news stunned my husband and me since there was no history of cancer in my family, except for cancer of the mouth. Since everything I do is for my family, especially my kids, I knew they would be directly affected. So, I knew I had to be strong and fight with all my might to beat cancer!

I first knew that something was wrong when I felt kind of achy just in my breast on and off for a couple of weeks. I didn't really think anything of it because my youngest was a baby, only 1½ years old at the time, and I had just weaned him from nursing. I knew it would take several months to dry up, so I didn't think anything of it. On a Sunday morning, my little one came and laid up against me and it hurt so bad, I had to move him away. That's when I felt the lump.

I went into the hospital the following morning where they confirmed that they found the lump. But they told me "cancer doesn't hurt". So, there should be no worries; it's not cancer. "It's probably just a cyst". Since they saw how scared I was, they said, "We'll go ahead and do an ultrasound anyway. But you shouldn't worry about it because "cancer doesn't hurt." Two days later, I went in for an ultrasound. My sister was with me and stayed out in the lobby. When they decided that I needed to be biopsied, I asked to have my sister with me, but they refused! That was the most lonesome time! I was standing at the corner of the room waiting for the doctor to start the procedure...and I have never felt so alone in my life. Ever!

The ultrasound was followed by a mammogram. Since this all happened a month before my 40th birthday, I had never experienced a mammogram before. As soon as the mammogram was done, the doctor came in and said I needed a biopsy of my lump immediately. Then he said that he also needed to biopsy my lymph nodes as well. I broke down crying because, in my head, I believed that once cancer hits the lymph nodes, my life is "done"! Less than a week later, I got a call from a clinical nurse there who deals with scheduling for cancer patients. She said, "We don't have the results yet, but I'm pretty sure it's cancer...but, the results aren't in yet." I was at work when I got this phone call.

At 4:00pm the next day (Friday), the doctor himself called me and confirmed that my biopsies were positive; I had stage III breast cancer. I was home with my then 1½ year old son who was in the living room watching TV and my older son was in school. Hearing the news, I pretty much fell to the floor and called my husband, Eusebio...I have no idea what I told him. I don't even think he understood me, between my non-stop sobbing. Then, I called my sister who left her camping trip to be with me. My best friend also came over to comfort me. They both stayed with me until my husband got home.

I met with the clinical nurse the following Tuesday, since Monday was a holiday. She told me that my breast cancer "wasn't stage III. It was stage 1, possibly stage II, because of the lymph nodes." She further stated that they made a mistake. They had gotten my results mixed up with someone else's when they initially told me stage III." So, I left there feeling a little better. However, that clinical nurse also told me that they couldn't confirm the stage, until after my surgery.

I researched what I could about my cancer and decided to get a double mastectomy. A couple of days later, I met with all the doctors: my oncologist, the surgeon ... everybody. They kept trying to talk me into just doing a single mastectomy, not a double. Thankfully, I made the right decision because during the surgery, they found two lymph nodes on my left side that were abnormal and not yet cancer, but would've developed into cancer had I not made that choice. Multiple times, they said I had triple negative breast cancer. That means, "it's not IF the cancer comes back, it's WHEN it comes back!"

ADVICE: Get as much support around you, as quickly as possible, if you can. When you get that initial call, saying, "Yes, it is cancer", you do not want to be by yourself. So, make those phone calls to family and friends for support. They will drop whatever they're doing to come and be with you because the aloneness you feel can really be overwhelming.

Also, research your cancer, so you have information to make decisions for yourself. If I had followed the doctors' decision and just had a single mastectomy, the abnormal lymph nodes that were about to develop into cancer, would not have been found until much later.

♥ Rick (*Chronic Lymphocytic Leukemia, CLL – blood & bone marrow cancer*)

On September 27, 2009 when I was 65 years old, I was diagnosed with Chronic Lymphocytic Leukemia (CLL), which is cancer of the blood and bone marrow. It was discovered by accident when I was rushed to the hospital on emergency because I had double pneumonia. I was shocked at the news because I had always taken care of myself.

♥ Scott (*Metastatic Colon cancer to the Prostate & Pancreas*)

A year before my colonoscopy, I was misdiagnosed by an internal medicine doctor and surgeon who both told me that I had bleeding hemorrhoids. Since I was doing a major contract with the government at that time, I put off doing the hemorrhoid surgery for a year. When I was finally ready for the hemorrhoid surgery a year later, I told them, "Oh, by the way, I'm 52 and I haven't had my baseline colonoscopy yet. Can you give me that?" They referred me to a gastroenterologist. After my colonoscopy, she came out saying "Good news, bad news. The good news is you don't even have a hemorrhoid. The bad news is that you have a 3½" malignant tumor." I looked at her and said, "Are you sure it's malignant?" And she said, "Oh, yes. I've already called the surgeon. He's expecting you to call to do the colon resection." The date was April 27, 2011.

When I went in for the surgery, the surgeon saw on my x-ray a little bit of shading on my liver that he didn't like. So, when they did the colon resection, he sliced me open a little bit higher than he normally would. And, he went ahead and biopsied that shaded area. Since they did the pathology in the operating room, they were able to determine immediately how far my cancer had gone. I started right off the bat with stage IV Colon cancer.

The way I reacted to the news, I was kind of numb, and I also was really angry because I was misdiagnosed. I wondered what that delay of one year cost me. If I had done a colonoscopy a year earlier, would I have been a stage III as opposed to a stage IV and improve my chances of survival? So, I went through that anger. I even sought the advice of a medical attorney to see if I had a medical malpractice claim. But, for the state of California, it's a "he said-she said or he said-he said" kind of thing. At the place where I was diagnosed, they had "canned verbiage", like a boilerplate kind of verbiage that said that they had advised me to do the colonoscopy when, in fact, they hadn't advised me of anything. So, I was pretty angry.

But, at the same time, I'm a fighter. I was 23 years in the military; very disciplined. Failure is not an option, so I had the strength and fortitude mentally to say we're going to beat this.

ADVICE: I have not been shy. I tell everyone I know, especially those around my age, "If you haven't had a colonoscopy by the time you're 50, then you're overdue. You get your butt in, literally, and get it done." I don't want anybody to go through what I went through. I got lucky; I'm surviving it. I had one friend who went in, was told he had bleeding hemorrhoids and he told the doctor, "No, no, no. I've heard this story before" (Because that's what I was told one year before my diagnosis). Well, my friend went in the next day, got his colonoscopy and found out that he had stage II colon cancer!

When you're given bad news, process it, but then get over it and focus on what you're going to do to beat it. Think: "Failure is not an option".

♥ Sondra (*Ovarian cancer - 2x*)

In December of 2014, I went for my annual exam with my gynecologist and told her that I noticed thickening in my ovaries, which I felt when I moved around. When I placed my hand on the area, I felt tightening that was never there before. She checked, but could not feel anything. She examined me standing up and lying on the table. Because she believed that I know my body better than anybody else, she said, "Let's send you for an ultrasound." I had the ultrasound in January of 2015, and when the results came back, everything was "beautiful. As a matter of fact, before I left the imaging center, they told me that everything was fine, and they sent my doctor the report. They also said that my ovaries looked great, my uterus was great and there were no problems, whatsoever, that they could see. So when I went back to see my doctor, she confirmed that good news, and I breathed a sigh of relief.

In June, I began to have some symptoms and I knew something was not right in my abdomen. So I called my gastroenterologist because I thought it was some type of digestive issue going on. Her office gave me an appointment about three weeks out. Four days later, I felt that things just weren't right; they were actually getting worse, so I called them up again and said, "I need to see her sooner." They asked, "Oh, because you're having bloating?" And I said, "No, it's not bloating." I said, "It's more like a fullness."

Coincidentally, it was also about the time I was due a routine x-ray of my kidney area because the year before I had a kidney stone. That prompted me to get my kidneys checked once a year to make sure nothing is happening there. So, the lady at my gastroenterologist's office pushed up my appointment. In the meantime, the report came back about the kidney area, and I noticed that it said there was some fluid in my belly.

It was good that I already had an appointment to see my urologist about my kidney. He works in partnership with my gastroenterologist. When I told him that I was going to have my gastroenterologist see me sooner because I felt something was wrong, he said, "Yes, you should see her." So I said, "Send her the report that was given to you, so she can see it."

Now, that's the report that indicated there was some fluid in my abdomen. My gastroenterologist received my report that day. Soon, my home phone was ringing, my cell phone was ringing... everything was going off. As soon as I answered the phone, my gastroenterologist very excitedly said, "There's fluid in your belly. I want you to come in." When I came in later that day, she told me, "That's not normal. We're going to do some tests. Something is going on somewhere."

Since I've been diabetic for about six years prior to this, my gastroenterologist initially thought that it was either my liver or my pancreas causing the problem. She immediately scheduled me for tests on my liver, pancreas and colon, all of which came back negative. So, I thought, "Okay, this is a good thing." But then I realized that I had been describing my abdominal discomfort as "fullness." And for years, I had paid attention to the symptoms of ovarian cancer because they miss it so often. I remembered that one of the symptoms for ovarian cancer is "fullness." So, I thought to myself, "Whoa! I'm noticing fullness in my abdomen. This is not good."

I experienced bloating once and remember that it was from my lower abdomen. The fullness I felt was high up my abdomen, like almost to my chest, but starting from my abdomen.

My gastroenterologist then said, "Okay. There's another test. I'm going to do a cancer marker test." I had that right away. Afterwards, she said, "We're going to draw out some fluid from your belly and test that." In the meantime, my abdominal area was extending, beginning to really stick out. Before she drew out the fluid from my belly, she had received the results of the cancer marker test. She informed me that the test came back positive for Ovarian cancer. I was puzzled and said to her, "No, this can't be. I just had an ultrasound in January."

When she replied, she said something to me that has been impactful ever since. She said, "That was then. This is now." And, that was the way she got the reality through to me that we're dealing with a different situation from the last time they told me "everything was fine." That was the first reality check I received about my situation.

When they drew the fluid from my belly (known as a paracentesis or abdominal tap), they removed a gallon, which seemed like a huge amount to me. But then they told me that they remove two and, even, three gallons from other patients. I was like, "Oh wow!" because that seemed a like a lot to me. Then, my gastroenterologist told me that she wanted me to see two excellent doctors she knew. One was a gynecologic cancer surgeon and the other was a medical oncologist.

When I met with the surgeon, he asked, "Why are we here at this point?" He knew that I had felt something in December and he knew that the cancer had been missed on the ultrasound. So, he was a little bit perturbed that it hadn't been caught sooner. The surgeon was really good. He went over everything, explaining exactly the situation that I was in, what they were going to do about it and what the surgery would be like. He informed me that I had to decide whether to have chemo first and then surgery to remove everything (hysterectomy) or have surgery first and then do the chemo.

During the time I was informed I had cancer, I had been caregiving for my 95-year old mother who was wheelchair-bound. I had to make arrangements to send her to my brother in Ohio, so she could be placed in a facility there. When I told my doctor that I was going to be gone for two weeks to take care of family matters, he said, "You do need to get your mother taken care of by other family members, because you will not be able to do anything for her care." He continued, "But, you only have one week. You need to be back here in a week because we need to be doing the surgery." That stepped me up a little bit more into the urgency. First, I had the reality. Then, I had the urgency.

Fortunately, my daughter was able to take off from work and go with me to Ohio because we had to deal with my mother being wheelchair-bound. On the flight, everything went smoothly. However, things did not go smoothly getting her into the facility. It was very stressful. Eventually, I felt the tiredness and the stress of all that I had to do before I could even go in for my surgery. I was there for a week.

In the meantime, my doctor scheduled the surgery. I felt like I was in a whirlwind. Things were just happening left and right. We were busy with my mother, and then the surgery was scheduled. I flew back to California on my birthday, of all days. And then, I had to get ready and get some tests done immediately the very next day. It was just a whirlwind of activity, I didn't even have time to really take it in!

Reacting to the news, I was stunned because I had mentioned that I thought something was wrong and they had assured me that nothing was wrong. With that, I felt relief. But then, Boom! Something was definitely wrong.

ADVICE: Keep in mind my doctor's statement: "That was then. This is now." It helped me to face the reality of my situation and not go back to what could have or should have been. When you have cancer, you have cancer. Thinking of how or why it happened doesn't make it go away. So just think of your present situation and how you'll move forward.

For those of you who are taking care of others (children, parents, etc.), you'll need to make arrangements to have someone else take care of them because you will not be able to: physically, emotionally and mentally. This is the time you have to focus on yourself. Communicate your needs with your family, your doctor and all those who support you. Most of all, take care of yourself.

♥ Susan *(Ovarian cancer. Metastatic Pancreatic cancer to the Lungs)*

Ovarian cancer: In December of 1984 when I had my hysterectomy, they performed a pathology on the tumor that was found in my ovary. My gynecologist informed me that the pathology revealed that I had stage II Ovarian cancer. No one was with me when I received the news, and I cried after the doctor left. I was somewhat surprised, but I knew it was hereditary because my mom had it. The worst part was the gripping fear I felt thinking I would never see my then eighteen-month old baby grow up. However horrible I felt, I knew that I had to really concentrate on recovery for my family's sake.

Pancreatic cancer: In February of 2016, I was rushed to the emergency room because I was quite jaundiced and felt pain in my abdomen. Tests showed that my liver blood count was very high also, so they ran a CT scan. From the results, I was given a diagnosis of stage II pancreatic cancer. Fortunately, my daughter Stephanie was with me and immediately comforted me. After we talked it over, she started researching the disease.

Lung cancer: In July 2018, my follow-up CT scan showed two small nodules (6 mm in my left lung and 1 cm in my right lung). A biopsy was performed, which showed the 1 cm nodule in my right lung had cancer cells. This news did upset me, but my determination to fight the cancer gave me the strength to choose four months of aggressive chemotherapy treatment. Fortunately, I feel great and I am thankful.

ADVICE: If you can, have someone with you when your doctor gives you the news. It is natural to get upset, even if you had the experience before. After you calm down, make sure to get yourself refocused on what you need to do to move forward. Then do it.

♥ Tet "Mesky" *(Colon cancer – 3x)*

Before Christmas 1991, I experienced abdominal cramps, which my physician at the time thought was gas pain. I mean, really, when you have cramps, you wouldn't automatically assume it's cancer, right? After a few days, I found blood in my stool. That was the alarming sign that something was seriously off. The next step was to do a barium enema. It was then the X-ray showed a blockage in my colon. Later on, I learned that I had stage III Colon cancer. The presence of my dad, my brother and my best friend certainly alleviated some of the stress dealt to me as I was being told of the test results. A surgeon dropped by the recovery room where I was at and recommended complete removal of my colon. This was during Christmas time and finding a doctor who wasn't on vacation was quite a feat. He seemed exhausted, thus lacked some bedside manners. We then sought a second opinion and the second surgeon we saw said the same thing. That's when my family (most of whom were in the Philippines at the time) stepped in and insisted that I fly home and get the surgery done there. This I did and our family doctor, who performed the surgery, upon his insistence, did a phenomenal job at extending my life with minimal "aftershocks", if any.

> **ADVICE: Allow time for the news to sink in. Take your time and lean on family and friends who are there to support you and are capable of being objective. Don't rush into any decisions that need to be made because decisions made when we're emotional, more often than not, may turn out to be erroneous.**

♥ Vida (*Breast cancer*)

After playing badminton with friends for about four hours straight, I felt so exhausted; I needed a massage, so, I went home and called for a home-service massage. During the first half of the session, while my back was being massaged, I felt pain on my left breast and wondered what it was. During the second half, when I had to lay on my back, I touched my left breast to see if there was a lump. And there was ... a big lump! I realize that if I had not played badminton and needed a massage afterward, I wouldn't have found the lump on my breast, so I am very grateful that I found it.

At that time, my cousin who is a doctor and the Breast cancer Director at a large hospital here was out of the country. When he returned, I told him about what I found. He told me that I should get a mammogram immediately. When he asked me if I ever had one, I said, "No, I never had one." I was 50 years old then.

I was so afraid. However, I tried to be positive. I kept telling myself, "Maybe this is nothing." But then, I remembered the stress I had been feeling earlier from the really serious argument that I had with my best friend. I thought that the stress of that argument, together with all the stress that built up from my past (my ex-husband, the business and our two daughters, finding ways to pay for their education, etc.) must've contributed to my cancer. Then, I thought, "We don't have any cancer in the family, except for my sister who had uterine cancer." My emotions were just going back and forth.

After my mammogram, I was anxious and afraid. Not too long after the mammogram, my doctor cousin called. He got the results and wanted to see me. I was anxious and afraid. Since I also received a copy of the results and read that I was a BI-RAD 5, I called a good friend of mine to ask her about it. She is an oncology nurse who, at that time, was also going through the same thing; only she was diagnosed earlier. She said that it meant the chances of my having cancer are very strong. However, I had to get a biopsy to confirm the findings. After that, I decided to finally see my doctor cousin and had my sister accompany me for support. My cousin doctor told me that the results of my mammogram were "bad" and that I needed a biopsy done as soon as possible. That was really difficult for me to accept because of all the things I had heard about cancer and chemotherapy. I was already of the mindset that I would never get chemotherapy if I ever got cancer.

To learn more about my options outside of chemotherapy and radiation, I went to see a couple of famous herbal doctors. One was a Chinese herbalist and the other was a farmer in the province of Pampanga who was believed to be "gifted." When I met with the gifted herbalist farmer (he was called "Apo"), he cracked open an egg and dropped it into a half glass of water. He observed it for a while and then the egg yolk suddenly had a lump with a dark spot in it. I was stunned and said, "Oh my gosh! What is this?" He said, "You have a mass on your breast" and he pointed to the left breast where my lump was. And he said, "It's big and it's right there". In the air, he drew a circle the size of my lump with his finger. Then he said, "Don't do the biopsy, because if you do that, it will poke the mass and the mass will spread." I said, "Oh no!" Then, he gave me a list of herbs, which he actually grows because he's a farmer. They were not expensive at all, so l bought 30 kinds, like branches of a cactus, roots, parts of flowers, parts of leaves and parts of the coconut, including coconut flowers. I was told to boil them to make a special herbal tea. To this day, I still drink it every day. Apo also gave me a list of what I could and couldn't eat. For example, I could eat eggs, beef and pork. However, I couldn't eat grilled foods, radish or fish without scales. In following his instructions, I lost a lot of weight.

The famous Chinese herbalist was the one who my friend's mother insisted, cured her. She had a massive cancerous tumor on her neck 30 years ago, which disappeared after following instructions from this Chinese herbalist. When I met with him, she said that he looked at me and, pointing to my left breast, said, "You have a lump right there and it's big.

Don't get a biopsy." That was exactly what Apo (the other herbalist) said! Yes, it was the second time I heard that, and I felt so confused, I couldn't sleep for nights.

After some time had passed, my sister said, "Why don't you have your biopsy already? You should get your biopsy done." I knew my doctor cousin was waiting and I didn't want him to feel bad. Yet, I just felt so lost and confused. So, I prayed really hard. I said, "Dear God, please tell me what to do. You be my boss. Just please take care of me. I don't know what to do. Please tell me what to do." When I felt God telling me to get the biopsy, I finally had it done. My wonderful friend, Masa, was in the room with me, holding my hand.

I had a core needle biopsy to remove the suspicious tissues from my breast. During the procedure, I couldn't look at my own breast. I just kept looking at the monitor of the biopsy machine where I was able to see the mass. It looked really big because they enlarged the focus on the tumor. I was able to see when they pulled a trigger and the core needle removed the tissue samples they needed. It wasn't painful at all because of the anesthesia.

When my doctor cousin called and asked me to come in to discuss the results of the biopsy, my sister accompanied me. When he said that my biopsy tested positive for Breast cancer, my sister cried. I didn't cry. I guess, somewhere along the way, I kind of accepted it. Yes, I was shocked, but that wasn't evident until after the fact; after we left the doctor's office. My sister hugged me so tight and cried so much; I realized the gravity of my situation, and I began to cry too. What made it harder was the fact that my best friend and I just had a very serious argument and weren't in speaking terms. I felt so very sad.

ADVICE: If you suspect you have cancer, do what you can to learn about your options. If necessary, get second or third opinions from other sources, even those who practice alternative medicine. It's important to get as much information as you can, so that you can make the best decision for yourself. As much as possible, have someone you trust with you when you receive the results from your doctor, whether it be in person or over the phone. No matter how strong you are, having someone support you when you receive the news goes a long way.

Most of all, you need God to guide you. You can talk to God and lean on Him and trust Him. When you experience dark times and feel lost, having faith and believing that God is there to guide and comfort you will definitely give you the inner strength to cope. In truly believing, you won't feel alone. You'll feel Him there with you all the way.

♥ Yesi (*Breast cancer: triple positive*)

My story begins in the summer of 2014 at age 32. I discovered a lump on my right breast as I was doing a self-examination. I had always been very curious about how our body developed and even considered breast augmentation. When I felt a marble-sized lump, I screamed in fear. I'm a very positive person and for some odd reason that day, I wasn't. I screamed and told my then husband, "Please come! I have a lump, and it's cancer!" The words slipped out of my mouth. He came to my rescue and tried to calm me down, saying, "Don't get ahead of yourself. It's nothing. You're going to be fine." Of course, I was in a real panic. So, I immediately called my doctor. When I was told that she was on vacation, I went ahead to the medical office and saw a doctor that was available. (Note: At that time, I had taken a much-needed and much-deserved year off from work, so I was unemployed. Since I was unemployed, I had no insurance. So, I was forced to go under the state-sponsored MediCal.). The doctor performed a manual exam and checked the lump on my breast. When he learned that I had absolutely no background of cancer in my family and considering my young age, he said, "It seems like it's just a fibrocystic breast. Just give it a couple of cycles and it should go away. Check back with me after a cycle or two." So, hearing from a professional, I went about my life and gave it some time. I saw him in June. In July, I felt this marble-sized thing in my breast doubling in size; like a bubble gum! It was definitely growing, so I knew something was wrong.

When my original doctor returned from vacation a month later, I called her and made an appointment. She saw me right away. I had the same experience with her as I had with the doctor I saw earlier. After a manual examination, she said, "Honey, you have fibrocystic breast. Don't worry about it. You're young and healthy. You should be fine."

I don't know if it was because of politics with MediCal and the cost of diagnostic testing, but I really felt that I was not being taken seriously, so I begged her and insisted that there was something definitely wrong. Bless her heart; she heard me and made a phone call to the most amazing team of medical professionals. I came in only for an ultrasound and walked out of there with an ultrasound and a mammogram.

A week later, I was scheduled for a biopsy. I knew something was definitely wrong. When I asked what was found in the mammogram and the ultrasound, they told that they found not one mass, but two masses and suspicious cells. Not being familiar with medical terms like masses and suspicious cells, I tried to remain positive. I came in for a biopsy the next week accompanied by my husband. I was scared. Although I didn't know what the outcome was going to be, I tried to prepare myself.

The biopsy was definitely painful and uncomfortable. I felt a pressure, but it was bearable. Within four days, the hospital called and asked, "Can you come in?" I said, "Sure, let's get an appointment." But then, they asked, "Can you come in today?" I knew the news was not going to be pleasant. So, my then husband and I went into the office and were introduced to the Nurse Navigator. It was then that we were given the shocking news: I had stage III (almost stage IV) carcinoma in situ triple positive Breast cancer. Still in denial, I didn't cry. All I could think of was my daughter Zoe, who was then four years old. Although we asked about what the next months, the next year was going to look like, I really didn't remember a thing.

I had gone into a different world. All I wanted to do was feel peace. And all the things that make me feel peaceful are in nature, so I told my husband that I didn't want to talk to anybody. All I wanted to do was process the news. I wanted to go for a hiking trip. So, we went to Rancho San Antonio.

We went for the longest hike, and I just lost myself in nature. That's how I was able to process my news. I know it sounds weird, but I actually felt peace and was not afraid. I knew I was going to be fine.

~ 0 ~

Chapter 3

SHARING NEWS OF YOUR ILLNESS

Deciding on whether or not to share news of your illness is entirely up to you. It truly is an individual thing. Some people are very private and some are very open to sharing everything. There is no right or wrong to this. Although you are strongly encouraged to share your news with others, doing so is still your prerogative alone; no one else's. The only exception to sharing news of your illness is to make sure that you share ~ if not with family or friends – with your medical team. In this chapter, cancer survivors reveal who they shared the news with; some also provide their reasons why.

♥ Aaron (*Prostate cancer, Skin cancer*)

My girlfriend was with me when I got the call, so she knew right away. As for my daughters, I just told them. Of course, they were worried that I was going to die. I said, "No, I'm not going to die. I'm going to have surgery." Then I said, "I'm going to be a little bit out-of-commission for a while, but your dad's going to be fine."

ADVICE: It's your choice on who you want to share the news with. For me, it was important to share it with my daughters and my girlfriend.

♥ Amor (*Breast cancer, Ovarian cancer*)

Breast cancer: I initially didn't want to tell anyone, including my daughter, Catherine, and my siblings. I didn't think it was necessary, because I believed I could do it on my own. I also didn't want to be a burden to anyone. I prayed really hard to God for guidance, and then it dawned on me ... I needed to let Catherine and my siblings know. I realized that not telling them would be unfair because if the tables were turned and my loved ones were in a health crisis, I would definitely want to know. I would want to be there for them and know how they're doing. If they kept me in the dark, I would be so hurt. I certainly didn't want to do anything to hurt them, so, I informed Catherine and my siblings Roman, Joy and Melody first. Then, I shared the news with my close friends, as well as my wonderful fellow Foster City Lions.

When I informed them, I made sure that I was objective and took as much emotion out of the conversation as possible. I assured them that I would be fine, and this matter would pass. When it looked like someone was going to get emotional, I let them know that I needed only positive thoughts and energy. Though it was not a good situation to be in, negative thoughts of sadness or worry would just not benefit me at all. I knew I had to just focus on the facts, not the hypothetical "what if this or what if that?" Negative scenarios in our thoughts are fear-based. Positivity, objectivity, and of course, prayers and faith were what I needed.

Using Facebook, I posted pictures of me in the hospital after surgery and also during my unexpected stay following my staph infection. Every time a picture was taken of me at the hospital, no matter how I was feeling, I put on a BIG smile. I wanted to show everyone that I was happy that the cancer was removed from my body and that I going to be fine. My body may be weak, but my spirit was strong.

After treatment, I shared my breast cancer experience with anyone who expressed interest, either for themselves or for those they knew. I showed them pictures of me in the different phases of treatment and healing, including my body's wounds, bruises and swellings. I did this to show them that the difficulties experienced were temporary and the wounds, however unsightly then, healed nicely in the end. They all appreciated that. To this day, I share my breast cancer experience with those who express interest.

Ovarian cancer: My boyfriend Bill was the first to know that I had Ovarian cancer. He was with me when my gynecologist gave me the diagnosis. I then proceeded to calmly inform my daughter Catherine and my siblings in the Philippines and Taiwan. I shared the news with my close friends and my wonderful Foster City Lions Club friends, and Bill relayed the news to his family (my extended family).

I had no qualms about letting others know that I had Ovarian cancer. As a matter of fact, I used Facebook to post pictures of me after my hysterectomy, me during my chemo sessions, me with my falling hair out, me dressing up my bald head with my wig ,or the many colorful scarves and caps I had collected, as well as pictures and videos of the head-shaving party I organized for my family and friends to shave my head bald..

As with my breast cancer experience, I continue to share information about my ovarian cancer journey with anyone who wants to know. I really believe that knowledge is power. The more a person knows about their ailment, their options, along with wisdom borne from experience shared by those who went through the process, the better and more prepared they would be for their own experience.

ADVICE: How you share news of your illness is up to you. Do what you're comfortable with. However, please don't keep the news to yourself. It would hurt those who love you. When you share your humanity in informing others of your cancer diagnosis, do it for yourself. It will free you from worrying about trying to hide your sickness. If you're concerned about what others may say then, for your own peace of mind, ignore them. They're not going through what you're going through.

If you have children, it is critical for you to be honest and open with them. It lets them know that you trust them and it gives them permission to talk with you. Describing it objectively as a sickness that you're being treated for will help them cope with seeing you sick. If they don't know what's happening, then they'll worry about the unknown, which is often worse than the reality of the situation. Most of all, your children and loved ones should hear about your cancer diagnosis from you, not your neighbor, friend or even another family member. Telling your loved ones directly lets them know that you trust them. Let them know that it's ok to tell you what they're feeling or thinking. If someone asks a question that you don't feel like answering right away, just let them know that you need to think about it and will get back to them.

♥ Cindy L. (*Kidney cancer*)

It was difficult to share the news with my family because my children are all over the place. My oldest daughter Ali lives in Royal Oak, Michigan. My oldest son Brennan lives in Tampa, Florida, and my Katie and Harrison both live here. Harrison is married and has four little girls. He's a busy dad and I'm a busy grandma.

It was especially tough telling my Ali, because she was going through such a difficult time. When I got there and saw her, I called my husband and said, "I'm bringing her home. We have to deal with this." Ed drove over to meet us, we pulled her out of school, and she was placed on medical leave. Unbeknownst to me at that time, we would be driving back on the caravan with her and all of her stuff. We brought her back, so that we could all be able to discuss things together, as a family with everybody in one town.

ADVICE: Having your loved ones together in one location is ideal, so you can share and discuss things together. However, if your loved ones live in different states or are far away, you'll have to carefully consider each individual's situations. Be honest. That way, everything is out in the open and you can all better support each other.

♥ Cindy R. (*Metastatic Breast cancer to the Stomach*)

I was working at the time. I was in the mortgage industry. When I left the office, I called my boss and said, "I've got cancer." After talking to my oncologist, she said, "You know, what? You're taking the time off. You're gonna go on disability. You're gonna take care of yourself." That was the best news I could think of, cause you just don't know day in and day out how you're gonna feel. Especially a stressful business like I was in. You know, you just can't even think about that. You gotta think, "Okay, it's for me now, I gotta do this for me."

> **ADVICE:** You gotta take care of yourself. It's respecting yourself. It's like "Wait a second. This is a whole new world and I gotta do all these other things and I gotta do it for me."

♥ Glenn (*Metastatic Colon cancer to the Liver, Lungs & Adrenal Glands*)

Of course, my granddaughter was the first to learn of my cancer since they had to call her to reach me, because it was hard to get a hold of me when I was on the job. I don't remember how I communicated my illness to my children, who are all grown now. It was a long time ago.

♥ Hilda (*Colon cancer*)

After I met with my doctors and got the information I needed, I was already tripping. Like, how was I going to tell my husband? How was I going to tell my kids? And, when I tell my husband, I know he's going to freak out because I know that he's sensitive and emotional when it comes to anything medical. I knew I had to accept the news myself first. I had to be strong for myself and for my family. So, I decided not to say anything to them after the first conversation with my doctor over the phone. That's because I needed to find out exactly what was happening before I could share the news with anyone.

When I told my husband Tony, who is not openly emotional, he was shocked. But the fact that I already accepted it, helped provide some sort of calm to the news. For me, I did this all by myself, so there's no reason for anyone to be uncertain. There's no need for panic or to think of a "death sentence." This was really happening. I was going to have my surgery and go to chemotherapy treatments and go through the whole ordeal of it all. I really felt that I took the best approach, and that helped me. I really felt that I wasn't going to die, and I was going to be fine. Everything was going to be okay because I was going to take care of it. Again, it helped that the head nurse Marie was there if I needed her further. I knew I could count on her.

After my husband Tony processed the news, we told our family. And, as expected, he treated me like I was convalescent; that's how his natural reaction is. He treated me like I was helpless. I insisted that I was going to be fine. He then told my family, i.e. my sisters, my mom and, eventually, everybody. I actually didn't want to tell everyone because I didn't want to go over it again and again. When I was with my close girlfriends, I remember trying to tell them about my cancer. But, when we got together, we were all having so much fun, I just didn't want to deal with it and bring everyone down. Anyway, I told myself that I was already getting better.

My ten-year old daughter didn't know the severity of it. I didn't think it was necessary for her to know; I didn't want her to worry. For me to know the severity is okay because I was already prepared to do everything I could to beat this cancer. Although some may not agree with how I communicated my illness, what I did was my way to prepare myself and family for what was to come.

I eventually told my office that I was going to be out on medical leave, and that I was going to take all the vacation and sick time that I had accrued., There really was no reason for me to rush back to work. However, I did keep them up-to-date on developments.

> **ADVICE:** How you share news of your illness and who you share it with is up to you. You may want to make the decision on your own or with others input. It's up to you. It's an individual thing. You are the one going through the experience, so those who love you should understand and support your decision.

♥ Jacki (*Breast cancer*)

I first informed my husband George and my daughter Jenise. I later informed the rest of the family. I didn't want to give it too much attention, so I didn't really talk about it much to others outside of my family.

ADVICE: **Tell those you are closest to first.**

♥ Joan (*Rectal cancer*)

My daughter Lori was with me. After our meeting with my doctor, we contacted my other daughter Shelley to inform her of my diagnosis. It was important to me that my family knew first. Then, Lori put an itinerary together of my stage III rectal cancer diagnosis and what was going to happen to me before surgery. She emailed it one of my close friends (and fellow Foster City Lion) Carolyn who told everyone at the Foster City Lions Club, as well as our sorority. That took care of that. I also informed my soul sister Bev and friends I've known since junior high. They also spread the news of my illness to my other friends.

I wasn't afraid to share the news with others. In fact, sharing my diagnosis helped me in so many ways, especially when everyone supported me through the many challenges and helped me back on my feet. I couldn't have done it without them, especially my family.

I remember a time when I went to the cancer center for another infusion. I met a woman who brought her father there. This man was just starting his first chemo infusion and his daughter said to me, "My father can't keep anything down." I told her, "That's where I'm at too." I told her about the one power protein drink (Premier Protein) I found that was the only thing I could keep down, and I recommended he try it.

ADVICE: **When you share the news that you have cancer, you learn you're not alone. Those who love you will do what they can to support you. It really helps in the healing process to feel their love and caring and support. Also, when you share your cancer coping tips with those who are experiencing similar challenges, it makes you feel good.**

♥ JB (*Salivary gland cancer*)

After I gave myself a chance to settle, the first person I told was my dad, then my mom and, eventually, my girlfriend, Melody. They were all shocked.

♥ Rev. Linda (*Pancreatic cancer 3x*)

When I first learned I had cancer, and then when I learned of its return both times, I informed my immediate family and closest friends because I wanted them to know the truth and I wanted to prevent rumors from running rampant in the community.

ADVICE: **I advise cancer patients to do what they feel comfortable doing at the time.**

I've also come across times when I would be asked or I would be moved to share my cancer experiences with other patients. For example, one day while I was at the Oncology/Hematology Infusion Center in Champaign, IL, I was pleasantly surprised to see that God had been using me as a teacher and comforter all day. My first assignment was with "Mike" and "Sue" (not their real names, of course). It is Mike's first time here. Only a few days ago, he received a diagnosis of inoperable pancreatic cancer. Ten years ago, his wife, Sue, was treated successfully for colorectal cancer. We now have the same oncologist. We chatted a long time and more briefly throughout the day. I hope we can continue to support each other.

For my second assignment, my oncology nurse brought by a tearful woman who was debating having a port catheter implanted. My nurse asked me to speak with "Brenda" about the benefits of having one. I did and Brenda changed her mind. She was quite scared. I get it. So, I gave her my business card to call for extra support when she needed it.

My nurse told Brenda that I was a retired hospice chaplain with first-hand personal experience with cancer. Actually, I felt most useful again and taken out of my own sadness and occasional misery.

♥ Rachel (*Breast cancer: triple negative*)

When I got the phone call, I pretty much fell to the floor, called my husband...I have no idea what I told him. I don't even think he understood me, between my sobbing. And then I called my sister who came back from her camping trip to be with me. I called my best friend too and she also came over. And they both stayed with me until my husband got there.

My children knew what was going on. The first day I found out, I had my neighbor pick up my then 12-year old son from school. Once his dad got home, his dad & I talked to him together. I never hid anything from my children, and I also never hid from them the severity of it. The only thing I did hide from them – not from my 20-year old, but from my 12-year old – is the fact the cancer will come back. He knows there's a risk of it coming back. He just doesn't know how high.

Everything else from the surgery, the lymphedema to the medications I took...the cannabis...my family knows all of it. I didn't hide anything from them. My 12-year old didn't ask too many questions. I think because I answered them before he had a chance to ask most of the time. He started kind of – not shutting down – but he was turning a lot to music and gaming as a coping mechanism, which was fine. I don't have an issue with it. He was still doing karate. One day, his sensei came to me and said, "I'm starting to get worried about him. He had a breakdown in class the other day." I said, "Ok". So, when we got home, I sat my 12-year old down and told him exactly what his sensei told me. He broke down crying. His question was, "How do you know the treatments are going to work?" I said, "They will". He said, "HOW do you know?" And I said, "I don't". I'm very honest with him. We have to have faith that it'll work. And so, a lot of it is based around that.

That's another thing I got criticized for, believe it or not~ People telling me I give too much information; I shouldn't be sharing everything with my kids. But, how can I expect them to cope and come out with a good outcome in their attitudes and their lives if they know I'm lying to them about everything. It doesn't work that way.

Something else that people need to be aware of. I think that when you get a diagnosis, all of a sudden EVERYbody becomes an expert. I got advice from everywhere, even if I didn't want it. I kept in mind that everybody was doing it because they care and they have good intentions, and there's no ill will, one way or another, even if I didn't agree with them. I listened to them, but didn't necessarily follow everyone's advice. In the end, I knew I had to do what's right for me.

♥ Rick (*Chronic Lymphocytic Leukemia: blood & bone marrow cancer*)

I informed my daughter Julie Ann that I had CLL. But I just told her quickly without giving too much information because I didn't want her to worry about me.

♥ Scott (*Metastatic Colon cancer to the Prostate & Pancreas*)

My two kids were in their mid to late teens when I received my diagnosis. I sat them down in a family meeting one evening, and told them that I had cancer. we don't know the extent of it yet, but by the size of the tumor, it might be bad. I wanted to prepare them and asked them if they had any questions, and, of course, they said, "No. Are you going to die?" I replied, "I don't know." They were scared. Then, as time went by, I kept them fully informed. As I would get information from the doctors, I would pass it along to them.

As far as work goes, the night I was diagnosed with the three-and-a-half-inch tumor, I called my right-hand guy at work, Eric. I said, "Eric, I'm not going to be in tomorrow, and I don't know if I'll ever come back because I've got a cancerous tumor in my colon, and I'm going to be out of commission for quite a while." As it turned out, that was the day I retired. Going through the colon resection and the chemo for six months and the healing and a couple of emergency surgeries after that, it just took me out of the picture for too long. And then with chemo brain, I couldn't see myself going back to work. So, I just kept it that I was retired. As far as coworkers and friends were concerned, I kept them fully informed too.

Another way I share the news. Here at the cancer center sometimes, the nurses will ask me to go introduce myself to a patient that's in one of the other chairs because they're here on day one. I'll go up and I'll introduce myself, and I just tell them my story. I don't ask them their story. I just say, "Hi, I'm Scott. I'm a stage IV colon cancer patient.. I've been here six years. I'm going into my seventh year." I do not look sick. In fact, I look very, very healthy, so it's easy for me to hide the fact that I do have cancer. Well, I don't have cancer per se. I'm three years no evidence of disease right now. They see me. I'm healthy, and it gives them hope. it gives them faith, and I feel really good about myself for helping that person in that way.

Some people are really, really bad off, and hope really, really helps them. Oftentimes, I counsel patients. If they're new to the process, they'll ask me, "Well, what was that like for you?" I'll tell them my story. I don't hold back. I tell them exactly what happened, so people might be prepared if it were to happen to them.

ADVICE: I think it's really important to be honest and open about your illness. That's so people understand your situation and will even work to support you.

♥ Sonda (*Ovarian cancer 3x*)

Aside from my husband Kenneth, I told my brothers because we were working on placing my mother in an assisted-living facility in Ohio. So, they needed to know. We held telephone conferences because one was in Charlotte, North Carolina and the other was in Solon, Ohio. I informed my 50-year old daughter, Lucy, and my 24-year old granddaughter too. Aside from my family, I also told my close friends.

My daughter and granddaughter took the news hard. What I saw was how they keyed off of my reaction and how they wanted to protect me. I told them, sort of calmly, what they wanted to know. After they got over the shock and sadness, they started listening to what we were going to do. They wanted to know how they could help and all that; they kind of "kicked in" that way.

I realized that when some people learn they were misdiagnosed, they get angry. They think of how the cancer was missed or how the hospital messed up and how they ought to sue them. Well, what I knew for sure was how I just couldn't get caught up in anger because it would just be detrimental to my health. I just needed to focus myself and save my energy on what we were going to do remove my cancer and recover my health. And so, I decided I would let go of that. I also told others of my decision, so that they could settle down and know what I wanted and didn't want. I told them that suing anyone wasn't what I wanted or needed to do. I said, "I know they missed a lot and, yeah, it is devastating to me. But I have to let go of that and be fine. It is what it is now and that's what I have to deal with."

ADVICE: A misdiagnosis is no small error, especially when it could've been prevented. However, fighting legal battles is not the priority when your life is on the line. You need to save every bit of energy you have to be positive and focused on your return to health and full recovery. Don't get caught up in the anger, because it would just be detrimental to your health. Focus on the positive. Focus on healing. After your battle with cancer is won, you can then determine if you want to address legal issues. No matter what, keep counting the blessings along the way ... there are many!

After speaking with others, I learned that there are two different reactions when people receive the news that they have cancer. Some people get busy, meaning they try to find out as much as they can, learn as much as they can about the disease, the treatment and so forth and so on. Now, I kind of fall in that camp because I had to make decisions. I knew that it would help to be more informed, so I could make better decisions. Also, having my faith was really important and it came in a lot during this time.

And then, other people who learn they have cancer don't seem to be interested or want to know anything about it. I came in contact with a person who had cancer the same time I did. Same thing: Ovarian cancer. I met her only by phone. Now, she didn't want to know anything, including her chemo medicine. She said that she asked them (the medical team) to tell her what they were going to do and she would do it. It seemed hard for her to learn more about it. She just didn't want to know.

Me? I want to learn everything. It's a journey. What I learned is that, as I shared with my friends, they were really appreciative to hear the details of what I had learned. And particularly, I wanted them to know about the CA 125 blood test because, actually, if I had had the CA 125 blood test at the same time I had the ultrasound, the doctors would have caught it.

So, wanting to learn everything about my cancer is what helped me through the experience. And I just learned so much! In November 2016, I attended a Cancer Connection conference and heard different speakers. From that, I learned some more and passed the information on to anybody who was interested. I wanted to share and be a light to others.

> ADVICE: As I've said to every woman I know and continue to say here: Look, if you even think you may have cancer ... and I know the doctors don't want to do it, because it gives a false positive ... If you're thinking something is wrong, you need to have the CA 125 test done. And if they say you need an ultrasound, you definitely need to get that done too.

♥ Susan (*Ovarian cancer, Metastatic Pancreatic cancer to the Lungs*)

Ovarian cancer: I first informed my husband, my dad and my baby daughter's godfather. Later, I told my girlfriends and my employer.

Pancreatic cancer: My daughter was with me when the doctor told me I had stage II pancreatic cancer. I then immediately called my husband and one girlfriend. Eventually, I told several close friends and a few family members. I did not tell everyone until after I had surgery and was home from the hospital. I chose to keep my illness quiet for a long time. I just felt it was better for my healing.

> ADVICE: I think it's important to share news of your illness with your family and close friends. You don't necessarily have to share it with everyone immediately. It's your choice. Do what is comfortable for you.

♥ Tet "Mesky" (*Colon cancer 3x*)

After I was able to process the news, I informed the rest of the family in the Philippines.

> ADVICE: It's very important to share the news gently and in person if possible. Try to soften the impact by offering positive thoughts and ideas on how they can support you. Assure them that things will be fine. Believe it or not, it may be equally difficult for our loved ones to deal with such news.

♥ Vida (*Breast cancer*)

I didn't have any qualms about sharing news of my cancer. My sister was with me when I was given the diagnosis, and I informed my children and my other siblings about it right away, and they immediately showed me their support.

I also told my close friends and my very best friend who, herself, had experienced breast cancer and a mastectomy several years back. She knew how it felt and wanted to be with me and support me through my journey. I have shared everything with her, and she has supported me, unconditionally, from the very beginning.

> ADVICE: #1. Having cancer is not something you should be embarrassed or ashamed about. When you inform your family and friends who love you, you'll enable them to support you, and you'll all benefit from the experience. #2. Love makes everything more colorful. At the lowest point in your life when everything looks black and white, love will add color to your life. If you emphasize love, it will make you so happy that your sickness will become secondary. The love you feel from those who care for you, support you and pray for you; that's love that is so strong and powerful. So, open yourself more to loving and being loved. #3. Forgive your past and those who hurt you. You have to get out of your system everything that is negative because they just cause you stress, which is what contributes to cancer. Just be positive and forgive, as much as you can. If you cannot forgive a person, just don't think about them at all. Just keep all the good thoughts, good energy and positivity.

♥ Yesi (*Breast cancer: triple positive*)

About sharing the news with my beautiful Zoe, who back then was four-and-a-half, almost five. We actually didn't share the news with her the day we found out. We waited for a couple of days to process it ourselves. After, we felt it best to be very open with her and not hide anything from her because I was going to go through a lot of transformations that she was definitely going to see. And, children are very intelligent at that age. We also decided it best that we just tell her how it is; of course, in a way that her little mind can process.

So, we told her that Mommy had a lump. Since we didn't know how to describe it, we just told her that Mommy had this lump that the doctor was going to take care of. We explained that I was going to be taking some very strong medicine and that the medicine was going to make me lose my hair. We also told her that I probably wouldn't be able to pick her up anymore because I was going to be very tired. But, no matter what, I still love her with all my heart, and we were going to get through it.

The next day, Zoe had a dream. When I went to check on her, she told me, "Mama, I had a dream last night. I dreamed that the doctors took your bubble gums out". She named them! My then fiancé and I couldn't come up with a name for the tumors and she, with her innocent little mind, called them bubble gums! Zoe added, "Yeah, and the doctor took the bubble gums out, and you are fine!" I said, "You are absolutely right! And, guess what? I think they're gone already!" So, basically, from that day on, we referred to my tumors, not as tumors or as cancer, but as bubble gums.

As far as sharing the news with family … Again, we were very open. It is what it is. It was definitely shocking for the entire family, because being the middle child, the one with a very positive attitude and the strong one out of the whole family, for me to be facing something like this was quite shocking. Of course, my mother thought the worse. How could she not? Just the simple thought of losing her daughter ….

Yes, I accepted the diagnosis. But, at the same time, I declared war against cancer! I said, "My daughter needs me, and I need her. And, I am going to fight with everything I have. I have amazing support of doctors, family, friends and I'm going to fight!" That was my approach.

~ 0 ~

Chapter 4

COPING WITH POSSIBLE TREATMENT SIDE EFFECTS

Anytime medication is administered, there is always a possibility of a reaction or side effect. And then, because every individual is different, reactions or side effects vary.

In this chapter, we share our personal experiences with treatment side effects and what we did to cope. We were honest with our descriptions, so that you can prepare yourselves for what <u>may</u> happen. Again, side effects and individual experiences vary from patient-to-patient. Whatever the case may be, there are lessons we survivors have learned from our experiences, which we have provided in the form of advice, given at the end of most of the accounts here. It is our hope that, if you are to encounter treatment side effects, you will find the information and advice we provided here, useful.

<u>AUTHOR'S NOTE:</u>

Given the fact that some side effects may happen simultaneously and the descriptions of our experiences can be characterized by a variety of both physical and emotional factors, you will find various accounts repeated across this chapter and even throughout this book. This repetition is necessary to ensure that the topic or topics you are interested in can be quickly referenced, based on each symptom or circumstance, and nothing is missed.

ADHESIONS & INTERNAL SCARS (FROM SURGERY)

After surgery, attention is usually given to external scars and steps are sometimes taken to remove visibility of those scars through ointments, creams and even surgery. However, surgery can also create scars on the inside. These inner scars are basically tough tissue bands that form between the abdominal tissues and organs. They make our normally slippery internal tissues and organs stick together. They can also twist and pull our small or large intestines, causing obstructions, which sometimes leads to pain. They're considered a normal surgical outcome and 93% of people who have abdominal surgery develop an adhesion; most having no problems. It's impossible to predict how much scar tissue you'll have, though. It varies from person to person.

* ***Amor T.*** *(Breast cancer, Ovarian cancer)*

During my radical hysterectomy to treat my ovarian cancer, my surgeons had to deal with a lot of adhesions found in my abdomen. They performed a procedure called a lysis of adhesions (enterolysis) to release the tough tissue bands that had formed in one area of my bowels, causing an obstruction. Those adhesions were actually internal scars from my past surgeries, mainly the caesarean section birth of my daughter 22 years prior and my diep flap breast reconstruction surgery from three years back, where a large portion of skin, fat and blood vessels were taken from the lower half of my belly and moved up to my chest to form my new left breast.

After recovering from my hysterectomy, I noticed a difference in movement in my abdomen. At first, it seemed like a tightening of part of my abdominal muscles. As time went by, that tightening developed into cramp-like movements, which were especially painful when I did abdominal exercises, like crunches. So, I either stopped the abdominal exercises or adjusted my positioning. Unfortunately, the constrictions increased in frequency and I found there were times when I had to drop whatever I was doing, lay flat somewhere to stretch my abdomen (if I could) and relax/breathe calmly while I gently pressed my hands down on the really firm tissue that popped out from under my left rib cage and jutting up against my skin (yes, something like an alien...ugh!). It felt like a tumor too. If I were someplace where I couldn't lay flat (like at Sunday mass), I would stay seated and just press down firmly on the tissue until it slid back under my left rib cage.

I discussed my concern with my doctor and re-created the appearance of the firm tissue by doing an ab crunch. She thought that it looked like a hernia, but wasn't sure. So, she sent me to get an abdominal ultrasound. To make sure the radiologist could pinpoint the area of concern, re-created the appearance of the firm tissue for her, which helped her see it. She explained that the firm tissue was not a hernia nor was it a tumor (whew!). It was actually an abdominal muscle that was being pushed upwards by abdominal adhesions. With that, I asked my doctor if she could have the adhesions removed, because they were causing me pain. Unfortunately, she said that unless the adhesions were obstructing my bodily functions, my insurance would not cover their removal. Besides, whenever the adhesions are removed during a laparoscopic procedure, they eventually return.

So, I continue having to deal with the adhesions and learning how work with them. Initially, whenever I experienced the constrictions, I would say, "My innards want to come outwards." Now, I refer to those innards as "Ingrid." When others witness my having constrictions, I just explain to them that, "Ingrid wants to come out."

I'm very conscious of how I move and twist my upper torso, especially in a seated or half-seated position when my abdominal muscles have to work. My physical trainer Chris, owner of My Core Balance, suggested that I try keeping my spine in alignment with my legs to avoid twisting my upper torso & abdominal muscles unnecessarily. That means, to get into the driver's seat of my car, I go in backwards, butt first, then swing my legs together with my upper body into the car. That advice has helped a lot. Thanks, Chris!

Another helpful solution to my adhesions problem was Chi Nei Tsang, which is a centuries-old healing touch therapy from China that focuses on deep, gentle abdominal massage in order to "train" the internal abdominal organs to work more efficiently, which in turn is said to improve physical and emotional health. I was fortunate to have found a wonderful Chi Nei Tsang practitioner, through my Integrative Health doctor, to work on my abdomen. Not only did she perform Chi Nei Tsang to remove the complex adhesions that have been developing in my abdomen for years, she did it also to work on my liver that was found to have several fluid-filled cysts (the largest being 10.5 cm, as of this writing.) From the very beginning, I have seen a marked difference in my movement, my breathing, my digestion and my sleeping. I continue to perform Chi Nei Tsang on my abdomen every morning.

ADVICE: Adhesions or internal scar tissue, form to help the body heal from surgery. After healing, they can create strong glue-like bonds that last a lifetime. Abdominal adhesions can pull the body forward, making it difficult to stand straight. That's why I didn't use a walker when recovering from my diep flap breast reconstruction where my abdomen was slice from one end of my hip to the other.

When your abdominal wounds have healed, gently massage your abdomen while you're lying down. Start by placing the fingers of both hands together to move in a circular motion around your navel in a clockwise direction. You're working to soften the adhesions that are forming in your small intestines. Then, gradually move to the areas where you any organ or tissues were removed. Focus on gently softening the adhesions below the surface. Remember, adhesions or internal scars are much like the outer scars we have on our skin when we get a cut or a wound. When those bands develop in our abdomen, they attach themselves to our organs, intestines, muscles or tissues and keep them from functioning like they should. It really is important to try and eliminate them.

If you those abdominal constrictions caused by the adhesions, first relax and then try to find a place to lay down. Breathe calmly and with both your hands, press your fingertips on the firm tissue that's protruding and gently push down until that adhesion slips back down and you no longer feel the constriction.

Avoid movements that involve you twisting your upper torso to the side, even if done slowly. Crunching your abdomen will most likely get the adhesions to surface too. When you get into a car to take your seat, go in backwards where you can plant your butt on the seat first without twisting. Then, swing your legs around together with your butt to the front of your body, without twisting your torso.

There are three ways I know of to remove the adhesions, i.e.:

1. A surgical procedure called Lysis of Adhesions (Adhesiolysis and Enterolysis). It involves cutting or burning the adhesions, which actually creates more adhesions (scars) to heal from the very surgery designed to remove them;

2. A manual therapy regimen called the WURN Technique. Here, pressure and "shearing" is applied to the adhesions to detach the crosslinks that the adhesions are made of. Focus is treating adhesions affecting the soft tissues of the entire body, i.e. fascia (connective tissue), muscles, organs, nerves, ligaments and tendons. It feels like a deep tissue massage, but it aims at finding and detaching internal scar tissue (adhesions) that wrap around abdominal or pelvic organs and cause constricting pain. Ask your doctor if they know of a WURN technique practitioner, and last but certain not least,

3. A centuries-old healing touch therapy from China called Chi Nei Tsang (CNT). It focuses on deep, gentle abdominal massage in order to "train" the internal abdominal organs to move and work more efficiently, which in turn is said to improve physical and emotional health. It also supports digestion, metabolism, detoxification, lymphatic/immune function, respiration and much more. This is the natural method that I highly recommend.

* Rachel S. (Breast cancer: triple negative)

Before I was diagnosed with cancer, two years after the caesarean section (c-section) birth of my son, I felt this excruciating pain. I knew that scar tissue from my c-section surgery had formed in my abdomen and was pulling all of my internal organs into one central location. Basically, it was like, my bladder, which was supposed to be in front and below my stomach, was actually in my back!

When I saw my doctor, I tried to get him to do a laparoscopy to get rid of the scar tissue. Unfortunately, he told me that they won't do laparoscopies to get rid of scar tissue anymore, because even if the laparoscopy removes the scar tissue, they will just come back.

I knew he was right, because I had laparoscopic surgery done twice to remove scar. The first one was done 8 years ago. At that time, I was in so much pain; doubling over. I would move slightly and it was excruciating! When I went to the hospital, they found that scar tissue from my first c-section had formed and all my organs were pulled downward. After my second c-section, I felt excruciating pain again and they found scar tissue had pulled all my organs inward and my bladder was in my back.

When I insisted that I had laparoscopic surgery to remove scar tissue twice before, he just stated that it is no longer common practice. He did say that the only time they'll perform the laparoscopy, is if the scar tissue impedes the patient's ability to go to the bathroom.

ADVICE: If you are feeling excruciating pain in your abdomen and, especially, if you are not able to go to the bathroom because of it, let your doctor know immediately. Ask for laparoscopy to remove the scar tissue that is pulling your organs together and giving you intense pain.

ALLERGIC REACTION(S)

An allergy is a damaging immune response by the body to a substance to which it has become hypersensitive. During treatment, we may respond to certain medications or materials used, which cause symptoms such as itching or inflammation or tissue injury.

* Amor T. (Breast cancer, Ovarian cancer)

After the thoracentesis procedure, where the doctor aspirated excess fluid from the lining of my right lung, they used adhesive bandage to cover my wound. When I got home, the part of my skin where the adhesive bandage was attached to was really itchy and red. I first thought that I should just clean the area and replace the adhesive bandage. Unfortunately, the itching and redness continued, this time accompanied by tiny blisters where the adhesive bandage was. So, I decided to just not have any covering over the wound. I had to wear tube or tank tops or camisoles that did not touch the affected part of my skin, especially since the blisters were seeping. When I showed the wound to my doctor, he realized that I had an allergic reaction to the adhesive bandage, so he cleaned my skin and used paper tape bandage to affix the gauze over my wound.

When my mediport was first implanted below my right collarbone, they initially placed a gauze over it with a bandage to secure it in place. I did not notice that it was an adhesive bandage, the kind I was found to be allergic to earlier, until I started itching in that area. When I realized it, I got some paper tape bandage to replace the adhesive ones. And, the itching ended.

> **ADVICE:** Two things to remember: (1) Alert your doctors and nurses about any allergies you have and make sure they properly note it in their records. (2) Even if you alerted them about your allergies, before a procedure, reiterate your allergies to them and don't be shy about it, because it's you who will suffer the consequences, not them. I say this, because my allergy to the adhesive bandages was already recorded, but someone, apparently didn't check the records. Looking back, I would reiterate to my doctors and nurses before the procedure, just to make doubly sure they understand.

* *Bob G*. (Soft Tissue Sarcoma, Skin cancer)

During the second stage of my treatment, I reacted to the radiation.

* *Vida B.A*. (Breast cancer)

During my first chemo infusion, I experienced an allergic reaction to one of the two chemo drugs I was given. I felt shooting and sharp pains on the nerves of my big toes and my tailbone. The nurses stopped the treatment for 30 minutes and made some adjustments. I don't know exactly what they did, but when we resumed, the pains weren't there anymore.

I remember falling asleep through half of the session. My best friend was with me throughout my experience, which was so comforting. She told me that while I was sleeping, I was also moaning and groaning. Well, I also had a really unexplainable pain that was "emotional"; like my body didn't know how to react to how I was feeling during the chemo infusion. Since I was half asleep, I can't explain it. Nevertheless, I was able to take it. The rest of the chemo sessions, for me, were uncomfortable. It felt like my body didn't know how to react to the drugs and I kept feeling pain. It could've been an allergic reaction or psychological; I don't know for sure. I'm just glad it's done and over with.

> **ADVICE:** Receiving chemotherapy is something your body is forced to adjust to. Observe how you're feeling during the infusion process. If you feel any discomfort, especially shooting or stabbing pains, let your doctor and nurses know immediately. You may be allergic to the chemo drugs. Your dosage may be adjusted or the chemo drugs removed altogether.

ALOPECIA (TOTAL OR PARTIAL HAIR LOSS)

Alopecia or the lack or loss of hair from areas of our body where hair is usually found is a known side effect of some cancer treatments, such as chemotherapy, targeted therapy, radiation therapy or bone marrow/stem cell transplants. Certain drugs from these treatments cause hair loss by harming the cells that help hair grow. The amount of hair loss varies from person to person. Hair loss may occur completely or partially. It may fall slowly or quickly, or it may just become thinner, duller or dryer. It usually begins to fall out after several weeks or cycles of treatment. Most of the time, new hair will grow back in one to three months after treatment. And when it does, you may notice a difference in color, texture or volume.

* *Amor T*. (Breast cancer, Ovarian cancer)

Falling Hair. My first chemo treatment was on May 13, 2016 and I noticed my long hair starting to thin and fall out three weeks after. It did not all fall out immediately; it happened gradually and, as time passed, I noticed more and more of my hair on my pillow, the sink, the floor, my clothes ... everywhere. So, I had my hair cut really short and styled like a pixie. Once clumps of my hair fell off, I knew it was time to shave it all.

Shaving my Head. Funny thing, I was actually excited to shave it all off, because my falling hair had become so annoying to deal with. I so wanted freedom from the mess that it created. And, I was also excited to start wearing my new wig and the various colorful head covers I had collected. So, I organized my own head shaving party, calling my family and friends to help me shave off all my hair. It was such a gorgeous day, so we held it in my backyard. During the head shaving, each person was asked to use the electric shaver and shave the remaining hair off my head any which way, e.g. zigzag, stripes, polka dots, train tracks, etc. I really wanted it to be a fun and positively memorable event for everyone to remember with smiles & laughter, not sadness nor tears. After I was shaved completely bald, I went in to get my wig and donned it for the first time for everyone to see. (applause... applause...) We all look back to that event with positive memories. It really was a lot of fun!

Fun with Head Covers. Initially, I thought that I would use my wig all the time, but discovered that I actually didn't need to. I wore my wig when I had to go to social functions, e.g. church, movies, meetings or dining out. Other occasions, like visiting family and friends, grocery shopping, going to the hospital, etc. I didn't feel were necessary for me to wear my wig. Collecting a bunch of head covers was fun. I got a lot of chemo caps made of different materials. Some were plain colored and some had designs. I had the basic neutral colors of black, white and tan. Sometimes I wore them as is and sometimes I used them as a base, placing on top of them a designed cap that was complimentary. For me, it added to my look, especially when I coordinated my clothes with my head covers. I also collected a lot of scarves - I mean, a LOT of scarves! There were so many ways to twist and tie them; I really enjoyed finding creative ways to cover my head.

Loss of Facial Hair. Alopecia is a condition in which hair is lost, not just from the head, but from other areas, if not all areas of the body. I also lost my eyebrows, eyelashes and pubic hair from my armpits and private areas. I felt like I looked super clean, like a baby, in a way. I also didn't have to shave any more (for that period in time, anyway).

When it came to my face without eyebrows or eyelashes, I knew I had to draw them in. I thought of celebrities who had gone bald at one time or another, like Sinead O'Connor, Demi Moore and Natalie Portman. Even though they had no hair, they had make-up that accentuated their features. So, I learned how to draw my eyebrows on to look natural and accentuated my facial features with makeup, e.g. eyeliner, eye makeup, blush on and lipstick. Because I'm a great believer that a smile can make a positive difference, I chose to keep my smile on. Turns out, our smile is our face's best feature!

Nightcaps. Being bald caused me to get cold easily, especially at night when I slept. So, I wore a nightcap; something I never thought I had to wear. And no, I'm not referring to the alcoholic drink some people have before going to bed.

Hair Growth after Chemo. After my last chemo session my final chemo session, it took a couple of weeks before I noticed my hair starting to grow. My head looked like a peach fuzz. To my horror, the fuzz looked like it was all white! As it grew longer, however, the black hair started showing. Then, my hair came out kinky, then curly. As it grew longer, it started to straighten out. I noticed that the volume of my hair increased a lot. My hair was really full, very healthy and shiny. It was and is really beautiful; more beautiful than it was before treatment. I've been calling my hair my "second baby hair."

Wigs and their Accessories. My wonderful sister Joy generously bought me a beautiful, quality wig that looked like my original long hair. Along with it came the necessary accessories, like a mesh wig cap liner, a wig band, wig shampoo, wig conditioner, wig comb, wig stand, etc. The ladies at the wig salon referred me to a stylist who was skilled at cutting and styling wigs. When I met with her, I described exactly how I wanted my wig to look like my original hair and she did a great job!

When I was bald, I used the mesh wig cap liner that covered my entire head, to secure the wig onto my head. When my hair started growing, the wig cap liner couldn't grip my head, because my growing hair was creating a "slippery" surface. That's when the wig band came into the picture. It had a very wide band with velcro fasteners at each end and it did the trick of securing my wig to my head.

Not wasting energy on what people think. I knew that people would look at me and know that I lost my hair to chemo, but I just smiled at them. For me, my hair or lack of, didn't define me. Sometimes, while visiting family or friends, I would remove whatever head cover I was wearing (scarf, wig, cap or hat) and show them my bald head. I always did that with a big smile. Sure, I didn't have hair. But, I was still me and removing my head cover was just me without hair... nothing more to it ... just that.

One windy day while walking from our car towards a restaurant, my daughter Catherine noted that my wig was about to slip off my head. I laughed and said, "Well, that would've been funny!" and that's the truth. It really didn't matter to me if people made fun of me with or without my hair or wig or head wear. I've learned that, no matter what I do or look like, people will judge, for whatever reason. Their judgments or opinions don't matter to me. I like and respect myself, so why should I care what they say? I'm just happy to be alive and I'm so thankful for my many blessings!

ADVICE: Ask your doctor or nurse practitioner if your treatment will cause you to lose your hair. If so, ask them around when you can expect it to happen. Do some pre-planning so you're prepared for the inevitable. Shop for wigs (You can get a free one at numerous cancer support organizations like the American Cancer Society) and take a friend with you. It can be fun when you have someone to share the experience with.

If your hair is long, have it cut short and consider donating it to charity organizations that provide wigs for disadvantaged children like Locks of Love (www.locksoflove.org), Hair We Share (https://hairweshare.org/), Wigs for Kids (https://www.wigsforkids.org/) and the like. When you notice your hair falling out more, it's best to have your head shaved. Having head-shaving events with a friend, family member or a bunch of both can be fun and memorable. Try not to see your falling hair or getting bald as a "loss." Think instead of how you will GAIN life, because of treatment, and how you will ROCK you new look, starting with your smile and a positive attitude!

If you lose your eyelashes and eyebrows, no worries. There are a lot of good tutorials on how to create eyebrows and eyelashes for those who are suffering from alopecia on YouTube.com. Just search for "Eyebrow makeup for alopecia." YouTube.com also has tutorials on how to apply makeup in general.

Our body's heat escapes mostly through our head, because it's exposed. You'll notice getting colder going through treatment. So, wear a cap at night when you're sleeping. During the day, you can keep your head warm with caps, hats, scarves, etc. and your wig, if you did decide to purchase one.

Try not to think of what people are saying about your being bald. Ignore them. What they think doesn't benefit you, so it's not worth your time or energy. Keep your head up high and stay positive.

* *Cindy R.* (Metastatic Breast cancer to Stomach)

Breast cancer: I lost my hair completely when I was going through chemotherapy to treat my Breast cancer. Every follicle of hair on my body, I lost. I had super long hair before chemo. Since I knew my hair would fall out eventually, I got it cut really short, at first, because I didn't know if I just wanted to shave it all off yet. Then when it started falling out, I thought, "Well, I should just shave it now."

I did use a wig, but I did not like it at all. It just was the most uncomfortable thing, so I just wore a scarf. I also wore chemo caps at night or whenever it got cold. And I was always so cold. I wore a lot of caps and scarves to cover my head because I didn't like to wear the wig I had. I only wore my wig on occasion, like the time my sister got married, and we went to Hawaii. I was part of the wedding party and I wanted to, at least, look halfway normal. It was so uncomfortable for me, so, I took it off whenever I could and put it back on only when I really needed to. I was more comfortable wearing bandanas, caps and those kinds of things.

My sister and I actually had some fun making our own little hats too. They were almost like babushka hats that you can tie around. We sewed them from different materials and got to be creative. I just wanted to have fun with it.

Stomach Cancer: This time with chemotherapy, I lost some hair, but not all of it, like I did the last time when I was being treated for breast cancer.

By the way, the American Cancer Society has a program that's called "The Look Good, Feel Better" program that helps women with cancer, manage the appearance-related side effects of treatment. Their, trained volunteer beauty professionals teach cancer patients simple techniques on skin care, makeup and nail care and give practical tips on hair loss wigs and head coverings (scarves, caps, turbans, etc.). Workshop participants receive a free cosmetic kit and style tips. The workshops are free to women undergoing chemotherapy, radiation or other forms of treatment. I also got a free wig from them.

The program is a great resource, especially for those patients who learn that treatment will cause them to lose their hair, and they won't know what to do and where to go when that happens. It's really helpful.

* Hilda K. *(Colon cancer)*

At the Cancer Center where I was treated, they had a program to help patients deal with physical changes, like a dermatologist, a cosmetologist to teach you how to put on makeup or someone to teach you how to tie scarves. I was prepared to have a "shave day" and a "scarf day" with some of my family members, but I ended up not having alopecia per se or losing all of my hair. That's because the way they administered my chemotherapy wasn't hard-hitting or aggressive; the dosage was dispensed gradually. I learned that each cancer has different levels of treatment. So, with my Colon Cancer, I did lose hair, but as soon as I lost some hair, new hair was also growing back. So, I never went completely bald.

Although I still had hair, it was thin. That, along with my chemotherapy treatment, made me feel cold a lot. So, I did wear hats or caps. At my oncologist's office, there was a basket of gloves, hats and scarves that were knitted and donated by someone. If I forgot my hat, I didn't have to worry, because I could get a knitted hat there. And, every time I went there, I got a different color.

* Jacki S. *(Breast cancer)*

Before I lost all my hair, well that was a little tricky. It was after about the third or fourth chemo session, I noticed my hair starting to fall out. And I knew it was going to fall off little portions at a time. It wasn't a lot until one day, I got into the shower and just lightly massaged my head to get a little shampoo in because I still had hair. I noticed that it started falling out more in clumps. It was really coming out. Then I had my one and only panic in the shower. My husband came to my aid and I realized that I had filled up the drain with my hair, so that was pretty hard. He helped me get out of the shower and he took care of all the hair in the drain. It wasn't one of those things you could turn around and look at. I didn't want to see all my hair laying there. I didn't really miss my hair when it was all gone. But at the same time, it was one of those kind of things you have to think about other people looking at you.

I did opt for a wig versus wearing head scarves. For me, head scarves are very noticeable on cancer patients and they would draw more attention to me than if I wore a wig. So then, after that one shower when I realized I lost a lot of hair, I let my daughter cut the rest of my hair off. She loved that because she got to style-cut my hair in whatever way she wanted. That was a fun little episode we had out in the garage. I put a hefty garbage bag over my head (I cut a little hole in it, of course) and sat on the chair. My arms weren't available. So, I just let my daughter have the scissors, and she cut as much as she wanted. She styled it first and then cut the rest off. She really enjoyed that, and it put a smile on my face because it made her happy. And in a way, your daughter (or son or other family member) is having to deal with this just like you are. And sometimes, it's harder on the kids than it is on the adult going through it. I knew my daughter was also a very strong individual trying to help me out, so our beauty session in the garage was a fun, humorous time for us. After that, I went to Supercuts and let them do the buzz cut all the way ... cut all the rest of it ... Gone!

Another aspect of having alopecia, which is probably very common, is that you also lose all the hair on your body. The pubic hair is gone, underarm hair is gone. You don't have to shave your legs anymore. It's all gone! Therefore, you feel like you've gone back to being a young girl again, which is quite interesting. Since I also lost my facial hair (eyebrows, eyelashes), I ran with a group of cancer patients and survivors at the hospital in a program called "Color Me Beautiful." In that program, we were shown how to apply makeup, how to make our eyebrows again, how to put the eyeliner on (because we didn't have eyelashes), how to put blush on our face and how to give ourselves a little more of a bright lipstick because it can enhance our face a little bit more. After the program, we all got a box of our own cosmetics to take home. That was a special treat.

Something fun that I experienced when I had no hair was getting the free hats when I went in for radiation. Because there are so many patients that go in for radiation and don't have their hair yet, there's a special group of women (I don't know who they are; they're just angels) who make hats for patients who need them. What they do is they put these hats in a basket right inside the office. Before you go in for your radiation and, if you feel like you need a new hat or you would like to have a hat for another occasion, the hats are in the basket for you to take, free of charge! So, that was very nice. I did have a bunch of them. But then, I brought some back to the radiation department and some I took to the Salvation Army because there is always someone who could use them.

Everybody has to make their own decision about what to do when they lose their hair. I bought wigs and my husband was so supportive. In fact, he liked the way I looked when I lost my hair from the chemo. I did buy a wig that was pretty expensive, and then I had some fun cheap ones as well. But my husband liked me without the wig and he liked me to make kind of wild makeup because he said I looked like Cleopatra. I had a good looking head without hair on it, which I guess doesn't happen for everybody. So, my family was very supportive, and he gave me compliments on how I looked.

ADVICE: Do whatever makes you comfortable. It's your decision whether to wear wigs or scarves or caps or hats. It's your decision to make, no matter what anybody says. You have options and whatever you decide to do, just do it for you and do it your way.

* Rev. Linda S. (Pancreatic cancer 3x)

I went through chemotherapy after my initial diagnosis and then again, after the return of my cancer. The first time, chemo straightened and then thinned my hair. Since my chemo began in September and ended in March, I wore scarves and hats to keep my head warm. For spring and warmer weather, I wore a wig for social occasions or church services. I chose not to shave my head because of the cold weather. For my second round with chemo, I decided to shave my head after I noticed small strands of my hair on my iPad screen. The weather is warmer too. As with my previous experience, I wore scarves and hats and a wig for social occasions or church services.

ADVICE: Again, I advise patients to do what feels right for them.

* Rachel S. (Breast cancer: triple negative)

When I was told that I would lose my hair as a side effect of the treatment drugs I would receive, I made the decision ahead of time to just chop off all my hair. When it started, I asked my husband to take me to go get my haircut. When he asked, "Why?" I explained, "Because I want to save it and make a wig of it. And, I need to do it before chemo hits it." I felt that this was the one thing I could control. At that time, I felt I couldn't control anything else. This, I could control.

My hair was always very long. I've grown it out many times and donated it to cancer patients in the past. And, around the time of my diagnosis, I was actually about ready to do it again. And so, I went and chopped off all 12 inches of my hair and I saved it. About a week after my chemo started and I was at work, I just scratched my head and a handful of hair came out.

The week after, we went down to see my dad and visit *Disneyland. He and I went together to his barber and had both our heads shaved at the same time! Actually, it wasn't as difficult as I thought it would be. My dad kept it light-hearted! It was just what I needed, because if I had shaved my head at home where a lot of people knew me, it would've been more emotional for me. My twelve-year old son was also with me when we did it and we cried together. He himself has donated his hair several times, growing out a tail to be donated. So, he cut his tail and gave it to me. My husband, my best friend, two brothers-in-law and my best friend's husband all shaved their heads for me. So, we were all in this together! [*Note: My doctor gave me his blessings to go to Disneyland during my treatment period, because my dad got me an electric wheel-chair for the trip!]

I originally was going to have a wig made, but I did some research and I found out how they feel so heavy and can also feel itchy. Also, I learned that they're hard to take care of. So, I just came to the realization that, you know what, I don't care what people say right now. I'm going to do this; I'm going to be comfortable. So, I didn't wear a wig; I went around bald. I really didn't care. I did wear scarves and chemo caps, but not all the time.

ADVICE: If you were told you'll lose your hair, the best way to deal with it is to accept it. First of all, it's temporary and will grow back after treatment. And, second, you really don't need hair. So, don't care what others think. They're not going through what you're going through; they're not you. No matter what you have covering your head, your smile can be the main feature. Your positive attitude also can be your main feature. Besides, you can be creative and try on different scarves or caps. Or, you can get fashionable wigs, if you want.

If your hair is long, you can have it cut and donate it to cancer patients. One important note: If you do, make sure to have your hair cut before chemo. This is so that the hair you donate will still be healthy, without the chemo toxins in them. That way, you hair can be strong in its use by those with cancer.

* Sondra W. (Ovarian cancer 3x)

I did lose my hair. And oddly enough, that didn't bother me. It was interesting that prior to my chemo infusions, my nurse practitioner gave me the chemo treatment calendar and encircled the date I was going to lose my hair. And that's exactly when I lost it. I was like, "Wow! They got this down." Since she had informed me beforehand and even pinpointed the date, for some reason, it [losing my hair] didn't bother me.

My hair loss happened within a couple of weeks after my first chemo infusion. At first, some hair came out in small clumps. But then, I believe, on the third week, I put my comb in my hair, and then big, BIG chunks came out. I was like, "Well, she had that right." Then I thought, "Okay. Well, I'll just have some fun with this. I'll get different scarves and hats and wigs and just have a little fun with it." Since I couldn't get wigs made of real hair, I got the synthetic ones. Unfortunately, they made me perspire so much that I would get drenched. Even when I wore it for only five minutes, I would be wet. I had two wigs that I was not able to wear. It was winter, and it was cold. So, I thought the wigs would help me stay warm. Well, they didn't work that way because they made me perspire, and I just got wet. So, I gave up on the wigs and, instead, used carves and different caps.

Now, the chemo caps were something I could be fashionable with too. I wore them all the time, even in the house because I was so cold. My head was so cold. I know some people thought, "Oh, it's okay for you to be without your hair. You can leave your cap off." And I would explain, "No, no. It's not that. My head is freezing, and I'm really cold." I think it was hard for people to understand. Well, heat does leave through the head and the extremities, our fingers and toes too.

When I went into remission, my hair grew long and straight, which is different from how it was before cancer. Now, I have to cut it down really, really low. Every time they change my medication, my hair changes texture. It's interesting.

ADVICE: Ask your doctor if your treatment will cause you to lose your hair. If it will, then ask for an estimated date your hair will start to fall out. Since treatments and schedules vary by individual, then hair loss will too. When you lose hair, just think of it as temporary. It will grow back. In the meantime, have some fun with it. Get some wigs, hats, scarves and caps. You can be fashionable and change colors every now and then. The main thing is to keep yourself warm by keeping your head covered.

* Susan M. (Ovarian cancer. Metastatic Pancreatic cancer to the Lung)

Ovarian Cancer: After all my hair fell out, I bought some scarves and two wigs to wear. I just did not feel comfortable without them.

Pancreatic Cancer: For my first round of chemo, I didn't lose hair, but it did thin out. Fortunately, it wasn't necessary to wear a wig. For my second round, however, the chemo drug Gemzar caused my hair to really thin out, so I had to get a wig.

ADVICE: Do what makes you feel comfortable. You don't have to follow anyone. It's your experience, so it's your preference.

* Vida B.A. *(Breast cancer)*

When I got up one morning and saw that a lot of my hair had fallen on my pillow, I immediately decided to have my hair shaved off. I didn't want to go through the depressing experience of seeing clumps of my hair on the ground or just patches of hair on my head. To me, it just wouldn't look good, so I thought it best to just accept it and go for the head shave.

Since it's usually hot and humid here in the Philippines, I didn't wear anything to cover my bald head, if I wasn't going anywhere. At home, my head was bare. However, when I had to go out, like when I had to attend a wedding and other social functions, I had a variety of head wraps and wigs to choose from to cover my head.

I decided to enjoy wearing head wraps and wigs and collected different ones in a wide variety of colors. It was my way of coping, because sometimes my self-esteem was low and I felt ugly. With my collection of headwraps and wigs, I could put makeup on, try to look nice and not look sick. Being able to do that made me happy. I chose to make the best of what was happening to me.

ADVICE: Of course, it's hard to lose your hair when you're going through treatment. However, you don't have to look sick or depressed and feel bad about your situation. You can do something to control how you look and, therefore, feel good about yourself. To cover your head, there are so many different kinds of head wraps and wigs ... so many designs, colors, lengths you can choose to wear when you go out. You can put on makeup to help you look good too. Taking some control over how you look with head wraps and/or wigs and makeup will help you cope better with your situation and make you feel good. Focusing on what you can do is much better than focusing on your sickness and your hair loss.

* Yesi L. *(Breast cancer: triple positive)*

Losing my hair was definitely the first major side effect I had to deal with. From my research, I read that it would happen 14 days after treatment and that was absolutely right. Before all that happened, however, I already told myself that I was not going to let cancer take my hair. I was going to proactively take my own hair away. Before treatment, my hair was down to my waist: long, beautiful, healthy hair. I definitely did not want it to be a sad thing. I wanted it to be something that wasn't frightening for me or for my daughter, Zoe. I wanted her to be part of my choice, so, we had a "Hair Party." It was very intimate~ just my husband, my daughter, my best friend and my hairstylist, who is a good friend.

Because I wanted to donate my hair, it was braided. Zoe had the pleasure of cutting off the first braid. She was excited and saw that I wasn't sad. Internally, I was sad; I just didn't show it. I knew my beautiful hair had to go, but I was glad that I was being proactive and in control. Well, at least for the time being. I had my hair cut very short, like a boy's haircut. I loved it and I rocked that hair for about a week.

Around that time, the Avon 2K Walk in San Francisco was happening. I felt so weak from the treatment side effects, but I really wanted to go, so I still walked it. And on that day, as I styled my hair with gel, I knew that it would be the last time I was going to be able to style my hair for a long time. I did the run and enjoyed it. I was very exhausted when I got home and took a shower. I knew that the gel was holding my hair together, so, when my daughter asked to join me in the shower, I allowed her. However, when I started to shampoo my hair, it came off in chunks! That's when I realized it's finally happening and now, I'm no longer in control. When my daughter saw me, I told her, "Mama needs some mommy time." She understood and got out of the bathroom right away.

I didn't even want to touch my hair. I finished showering and wrapped my head with a towel. When my husband came into the bathroom, he shaved my head. It was definitely very emotional, but I was going to fight through it. I was really grateful to have had hair, but that's it. It was just hair. I knew there are things in life that are far more important.

ADVICE: If you know you'll be going through hair loss, try to rock it. Whatever comes your way, just rock it. So, for me, it was a time to wear colorful scarves. I didn't bother with buying expensive, fancy wigs. I found them extremely uncomfortable. If you are considering a wig for yourself, there are a lot of places that donate them like Cancer CAREpoint and Bay Area Cancer Connections.

There may be those times when you have to go to a special event and you do not want to wear a scarf. I had those times and so I did wear, what I called, my "party wig". The wig was itchy, but it was just for partying. Other than that, around the house, I would have absolutely nothing on my head. For cold weather, I would have just a beanie or a scarf.

Bald, Brave, Strong & Beautiful Survivors

Rachel S. *(Triple Negative Breast cancer)*

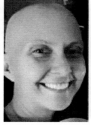
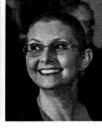
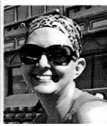
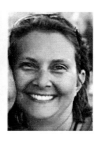

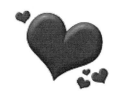

Rev. Linda S. *(Pancreatic cancer 3x)*

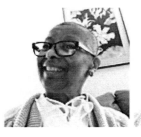
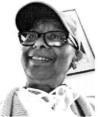
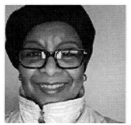
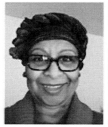
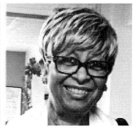

Yesi L. *(Triple Positive Breast cancer)*

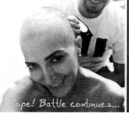
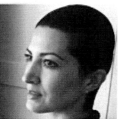
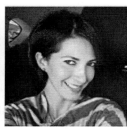
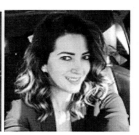

Amor T. *(Breast cancer. Ovarian cancer)*

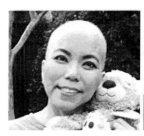
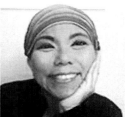
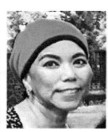
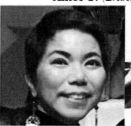
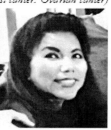

Sondra W. *(Ovarian cancer 3x)*

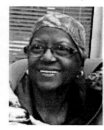
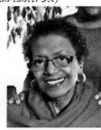
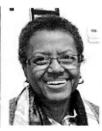
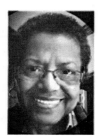

Vida B.A *(Breast cancer)*

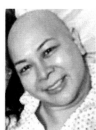
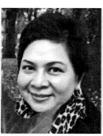
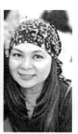
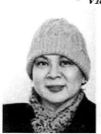
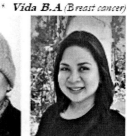

Amor Y. Traceski

Anemia is a condition in which our body does not have enough red blood cells to carry oxygen from the lungs throughout the body to help it work properly. If we are anemic, we can feel very tired, short of breath, and lightheaded. Other signs of anemia may include feeling dizzy or faint, having headaches, a fast heartbeat, and/or pale skin.

* Amor T. (Breast cancer, Ovarian cancer)

After my week's stay in the hospital for my mastectomy and breast reconstruction, I was sent home only to return the next day on emergency due to a high fever that was climbing (101.5F to 103.5F+). It was later diagnosed as a staph infection (cellulitis and sepsis). About a week later, my doctor told me that he was sending me home early. I was confused and told him that I was still didn't feel right. I was still very tired and a bit dizzy. He acknowledged that my red blood cell count was low (anemia), but with the iron medications he'll be sending home with me, I'll feel better. He added that it would be best for me to leave the hospital environment and continue my recuperation at home. "Huh?", I asked. He explained that even though the hospital is supposed to be a sterile environment, it's still a haven for bacteria to grow and spread. He didn't want to risk me getting another staph infection there; I'm much better off at home. So, despite my having anemia, I was sent home. The iron supplements he prescribed did the trick and my red blood count level was back to normal when I saw him again at my follow-up appointment.

ADVICE: Aside from taking your prescription iron medication as directed, eat foods rich in iron, like spinach, liver, beef, sardines, tuna, beans, tofu, turkey, ham, oysters, cereals rich in iron, etc.

* Cindy R. (Metastatic Breast cancer to Stomach)

During an appointment with my primary care doctor, he found that my red blood cell count was pretty low. So he put me on iron tablets. They helped some, but I still needed to really be careful. I found that if I turned around too fast, I would get dizzy and go down. So, I just had to be really careful. I didn't climb ladders or do any crazy movements that would cause me to lose my balance.

ADVICE: When you're going through treatment, it's really important to pay attention to your red blood cell count. If it's low, be careful with how you move. Don't turn around too fast or else you'll go down. Let your doctor know if you're getting faint or having dizzy spells, so that he or she can help you.

* Rachel S. (Breast cancer: triple negative)

They told me to eat more red meat and take vitamins. Originally, they told me to stop eating red meat, but then they told me to bring it back. Correct way? I think it just depends. I don't know. I just did what they told me to do.

* Sondra W. (Ovarian cancer 3x)

During my first round of treatment, there were times when my I was so deficient in red blood cells (anemia) that I needed blood transfusions. The transfusions helped because I was just worn out. I had extra pain and then the diarrhea. Everything was really wearing on my body, so those transfusions really helped.

During my second round of treatment with chemotherapy, I experienced more trouble with my red blood cells going down. Carboplatin, the stronger chemo drug, knocked down the red blood cells harder this time. Usually, blood transfusions were given six weeks apart. So, when I needed another transfusion two weeks later, that was unusual. At first, they started with the booster shots, but they didn't work. Once I got on the Carboplatin, I needed the transfusion.

My symptoms were shortness of breath, "strange" fatigue and hypothermia; I was freezing! They kept asking me how I was feeling because they were testing the dosage, and they were watching the numbers. Each and every time, I communicated how I was feeling.

* Vida B.A. *(Breast cancer)*

Sometime after my third or fourth chemo session, I was craving a Japanese noodle soup (ramen). Since I was getting used to the chemo side effects, like fatigue, I thought that I could eat out with my girlfriends. So I asked them to accompany me. At that time, my red blood cell count was low.

At the restaurant, we ordered a big bowl of ramen that the three of us shared; I had a small portion. After I ate it, I felt like my blood sugar or something went down really quickly, because I felt like I was going to pass out. I was also having cold sweats and laid my head on the dining table in the restaurant, so my blood would go down and not up to my head. I knew to do this, because when I was younger, I was anemic and had similar episodes of lightheadedness. My friends were panicking and called the restaurant's security guard for help. He got me a wheelchair and they wheeled me to our car to take me home. I rested at home and recovered not too long after. Looking back, I think my body reacted to the MSG (monosodium glutamate) in the food.

ADVICE: When going through chemotherapy, it's really important to be careful about what you eat, because your body is going through so many serious changes with the chemo drugs. This is especially true when you go to restaurants where you don't have control over the ingredients they have in the dishes they serve. If you get cold sweats or feel like passing out, immediately let your companions know, so that they're aware and can support you. Lightheadedness and cold sweats are symptoms of anemia.

* Yesi L. *(Breast cancer: triple positive)*

I was anemic and so, I had a diet that had a lot of iron, such as beans, lentils, etc. I'm so blessed that my mother lives right next door to me. She cooked a lot for me. I am so very fortunate.

ARTHRALGIA AND BONE PAIN

Arthralgia is defined as aching, stiffness or pain in the joints (without swelling). We may experience arthralgia in different joints in the body, including hands, knees, and ankles. Bone pain is the experience of discomfort in the bones. Both Arthralgia and bone pain can occur as a side effect of cancer treatment.

* Amor T. *(Breast cancer, Ovarian cancer)*

Before receiving chemotherapy treatments, my bones were fine and strong. Unfortunately, that changed while I was going through chemo. And, the changes to my bones and joints are much more apparent now post-chemo. During treatment, I experienced strange jolts in my bones that would just come out of nowhere. They were like lightning bolts directly hitting my bones. All of a sudden, no matter what I was doing, I would get the jolts. Sometimes they happened in quick succession, I would feel drained in the end. Thee jolts weren't seriously painly; just really unnerving and even annoying. Imagine being quickly pricked everywhere. Yes, really annoying.

I also felt awful aches deep inside my bones that felt like the aches I got when I was a little girl growing in height. The pain was dull and, fortunately, did not last that long. I dealt with the aches by talking with someone, distracting myself with things that would take my mind away from it, e.g. watching TV; basically.

After treatment, I went through a DEXA scan to measure my bone density. Results showed that I had osteopenia. So, my doctor arranged for me to get Prolia injections twice a year. By the time I received my second injection, I also received a bill for $6,000. Big Ouch! I asked my doctor to switch my prescription to a bone medication that wasn't so expensive. So he prescribed Fosomax, which I was fine with ... initially.

After some time had passed, I started feeling stiffness in my arms, hips and legs. I thought that it was due to my osteopenia. Then, after more time passed, the stiffness spread to my shoulder and neck and I could barely lift my arms up. It was painful and I started to get really worried. So, I did some research on the internet about Fosomax and also talked with some people about it. One lady told me that after taking Fosomax for a year, her femur actually broke and she sued the company. When I researched the drug on the internet, I was aghast to find there was a class action lawsuit filed by hundreds of users who suffered from severe bone diseases, femur fractures, osteonecrosis of the jaw (ONJ), heart rhythm problems, and other serious problems associated with the use of the drug. Of course, I immediately stopped taking Fosomax.

To strengthen my bones, I increased consumption of foods that are high in calcium and vitamin D, in addition to calcium and vitamin D supplements. Since weight bearing exercises also help to increase strength and bone density, I added that to my bone strengthening regimen.

ADVICE: Going through a DEXA scan is fairly easy and quick. I just laid on the exam table, the technician position my legs, the scan passed over me quickly and then I was done. Quick, simple and painless.

Review the scan results. A "T-score" is a comparison of a person's bone density with that of a healthy 30-year person of the same gender. A T score of 2.5 or lower qualifies as osteoporosis and a T score of -1.0 to 2.5 signifies osteopenia, meaning below normal bone density without full osteoporosis.

Prescription medication for bones can do you more harm than good. Always discuss potential harmful side effects with your doctor and check the literature too. Beware of drugs like Fosomax. If you must take it, pay close attention to how your body is reacting to it.

Two natural ways to increase bone strength are:
1. Increase consumption of foods that are high in calcium, vitamin D and increase bone health, like salmon and fatty fish, dark leafy green vegetables (e.g. kale, collard greens), milk, tofu, molasses, prunes, grapefruit, etc.
2. Take calcium and vitamin D supplements
3. Do weight bearing exercises to increase strength and bone density, like planks, "inchworms", "bear crawls", "donkey kicks", dancing, hiking, using the elliptical machine

* Cindy R. (Metastatic Breast cancer to Stomach)

The bone and joint pains hit me like a day or two after the chemo infusions. I pretty much just tried to relax and take it easy. Every once in awhile, I took Tylenol. Other than that, I don't remember taking anything else. My bone and joint pains were just always there, and I just had to deal with them.

ADVICE: The bone and joint pains from chemotherapy treatments are common. Aside from taking the occasional Tylenol to deal with the pain, the best thing to do is just try to relax and focus your attention on something else. Doing that helps to keep your mind off the pain in your bone and joints.

* Rev. Linda S. (Pancreatic cancer 3x)

When I first began my chemo treatments, I would have bone and joint aching around the 12th of the scheduled eighteen chemo treatments for which I took Tylenol and rested. Now on my third round of chemo, I'm experiencing the worst bone and joint pain, which happens the third day after chemo.

My oncology nurse said the bone pain is from the Neupogen (white blood cell booster) "digging deeply" into my bone marrow to stimulate white blood cell growth. Tylenol for Arthritis helps, as well as rest, which is essential to recovery in my view..

ADVICE: Take Tylenol for Arthritis or whatever painkiller you have and rest. Rest is essential for recovery.

* Rachel S. (Breast cancer: triple negative)

Yes, I got bone and joint pains from my treatment. Unfortunately, I still suffer from them.

* Vida B.A. *(Breast cancer)*

During treatment and sometime after, my hands were really painful in the morning. The pain seemed to come from the bones and the nerves. They felt like cramps in my hands, even though they weren't cramps. The pain seemed to come from my bones. After several rounds of chemotherapy, I had a bone density scan. My doctor told me that my bones were getting very brittle and that I was a candidate for osteoporosis. I still have bone and joint pain. When I wake up in the morning, get up from bed or when I stand up, I can't walk immediately, like before. I feel a lot of pain on the soles of my feet; I feel like a very old woman. The only thing I know to do is to take calcium supplements twice a day.

ADVICE: If you're feeling pain in your bones and joints, let your doctor know that you would like a bone density scan. This will test the strength of your bones and can diagnose osteoporosis before a broken bone occurs. Also, take calcium supplements (and vitamin D for better absorption), which help to increase bone density and strength

* Yesi L. *(Breast cancer: triple positive)*

I definitely experienced bone and joint pain and weakness too from my treatment.. I now have Osteopenia, which is a less severe bone loss than Osteoporosis. I have the "junior". But then again, it's a diagnosis; it doesn't define who I am.

For treatment, I got injected every six months in my abdomen (stomach) with Prolia, which helps prevent bone fractures. I used to hurt for days, even weeks after being given that shot. The one side effect I felt with the Prolia was sore muscles; I was sensitive to touch. Nobody could touch me because I felt so much pain in my bones. I just let those around me know that I was sensitive to touch.

I have a very high tolerance for pain, so I just took the pain and those around me knew not to touch me. My daughter knew I could not carry her and my husband knew that when he touched me, he had to be very, very gentle.

ADVICE: Whenever you're in pain, just make those around you aware of what you're going through and be very open about it.

CHEMO BRAIN / "CHEMO FOG"

Chemo brain *aka* chemo fog describes the cognitive impairment that can result from chemotherapy treatment. Approximately 20–30% of people who undergo chemotherapy experience some level of post-chemotherapy cognitive impairment. The phenomenon first came to light because of the large number of cancer survivors who complained of changes in memory, fluency, and other cognitive abilities that impeded their ability to function as they had pre-chemotherapy. How long chemo brain lasts can vary from person to person. Unfortunately, there is no definitive answer.

* Amor T. *(Breast cancer, Ovarian cancer)*

I didn't know what "chemo brain" was about until I saw a flyer at the Cancer Center for "Introduction to Chemo Brain and What to Do About It." I was curious, so I went. The speaker, a psychologist, explained that those being treated with chemotherapy may experience difficulty with short-term memory, multi-tasking, new learning, reading comprehension, working with numbers and a decrease in concentration ability. She then showed us pictures comparing a brain before and after chemo, as well as parts of the brain affected by chemotherapy. Two of the coping strategies I remember her giving us were: (1) to keep a notebook and pen/pencil handy to take notes, and (2) to give those with us a head's up that we may forget their names or what they just said. She ended her presentation with the saying, "If you treat your brain as a mental muscle and exercise it, your mental functions will improve."

At that time, I didn't notice any change in my cognitive abilities. Ah but, soon after, it became apparent. I found myself having problems focusing, multitasking, remembering things, learning new things and finding words. So I did some research of my own to learn more about chemo brain and what I can do make the best of it. I learned that chemo brain is temporary and the symptoms of chemo brain are similar to those of dementia, i.e. memory problems, increasing confusion and reduced concentration. Dementia, however, has the added symptoms of loss of ability to do everyday tasks, personality or behavior changes and signs of depression or withdrawal. I had none of the final three symptoms, so that was a relief ... Whew!

Nutrition was a subject that wasn't covered at the Chemo Talk. So, I did some research on my own to learn how nutrition could boost my brain's performance and found the following foods for brain health: fatty fish, broccoli, tofu, turmeric, dark chocolate, blueberries, nuts, oranges, pumpkin seeds, eggs, green tea and coffee.

I've never let my having chemo brain get me down. The way I see it, it is what it is. Sure, I sometimes get forgetful, uncoordinated or overwhelmed, like when multiple people are talking at the same time. However, I remember to be kind to myself. Toxic chemo chemicals have affected my brain and there's only so much I can do to cope. As of this writing - two and a half years after my last chemo infusion - I still have chemo brain. Fortunately, it's not as prominent.

ADVICE: Simplify your life, by doing one thing at a time. Carry a personal calendar or notebook for notes and lists. Relax, meditate. Work with puzzles to exercise your brain. To improve brain function, eat the following foods: fatty fish, broccoli, tofu, turmeric, dark chocolate, blueberries, nuts, oranges, pumpkin seeds, eggs, green tea and coffee.

Also, forewarn those around you that you may forget what they just said or you may forget certain details. It's really nothing to be embarrassed about, because chemo brain is chemo brain ... No ands, ifs or buts. It is what it is. Besides, when you communicate what you're having to work with, there's better understanding for everyone involved.

* Cindy R. (Metastatic Breast cancer to Stomach)

Yes, I have chemo brain. And, you know what's funny? I was never into technology that much, but decided to buy a smartphone (iPhone) and learn how to use it for everything because I needed help remembering things and keeping things organized. I keep all kinds of notes in the Notes app and I use the Calendar app a lot too. I also play "Words with Friends" on my smartphone because it helps to exercise my brain cells. Boy, if I ever lost my smartphone, I'd be in real trouble.

ADVICE: If you go through chemotherapy treatments, you may experience thinking and memory problems after. Writing down things to do and remember helps. So, keep a pen or pencil and a notebook handy. Or, if you have a smartphone, you can use the "Notes" app to write down things you need to remember, and you can use the "Calendar" app to note appointments you need to keep. Now, if you don't have a smartphone, it may be time to get one because it's a really useful tool when you have chemo brain.

* Glenn M. (Metastatic Colon cancer to the Liver, Lungs & Adrenal Glands)

For me, chemo brain or chemo fog, as it's called, was the worst of my treatment side effects. I would get embarrassed about forgetting what I talked about mid-sentence. There were times I told someone a joke, only to be reminded that I had already told them the same joke a couple of days before. It's kind of frustrating, but I'm trying to learn to live with it. That's hard because it does bother me. But then, it's a fact of my life now, so, I'm working on not letting it bother me.

ADVICE: I write things down more to remind myself, and I try not to let my chemo brain bother me.

* Jacki S. (Breast cancer)

Yes, I had brain fog or chemo brain. I just dealt with it however I could; one day at a time. I also tried to be positive.

ADVICE: Deal with our chemo brain however you can. Be positive and just take one day at a time.

* Rev. Linda S. (Pancreatic cancer 3x)

Having chemo brain was especially inconvenient since I manage two households – my own and my mother's because she has dementia. Some days I felt as if I had it [dementia], too.

I also notice that I've been forgetting important tasks and responsibilities and worse, breaking my word because of this forgetfulness. I sent out a blanket apology to ask for forgiveness from my family and friends. With chemo brain, you're not your "usual self." Concentration is hard.

ADVICE: Just do what you can. Communicate with your family and friends; send them a blanket apology, so they can understand and support you.

* Rachel S. (Breast cancer: triple negative)

I did chemotherapy treatment for five months and noticed that I didn't remember conversations, like I used to and I didn't remember seeing people, like I used to. So, I tried to take notes. But, after three months of trying to work while going through chemo, I had to stop working, because I just couldn't function at all. I couldn't focus, look at the computer or anything like that.

When I returned to work after treatment, I still had chemo brain, but I found ways to do my job and do it well. I learned to adapt, like take notes and create a schedule for myself. I learned that it was important to rest my brain, so I napped in the car during my breaks. To help my memory and build muscle, I started taking martial arts classes last summer. I also did that to pass the test for abdominal muscle and blood flow, which was a requirement for me to able to have my diep flap breast reconstruction surgery. the following January and it worked; I passed!

ADVICE: If you feel your thinking is fuzzy when it used to be clear, then you may have chemo brain. Try taking notes on a little notepad you can carry around with you, if need be. If you're in a job and find that you can't focus or work like you used to be able to, then take time off from work. Talk with your manager or human resources. If you take time off from work, you may be able to get disability benefits from the state.

There are many ways to adapt to chemo brain. Aside from taking notes, you can create a schedule to help you keep track of things. Rest is critical for your brain, so take breaks to relax and calm your thoughts. To strengthen your memory, learn a new skill, like taking martial arts classes.

Be kind and patient with yourself. Yes, some things will take longer than others for you to grasp and it can be overwhelming at times. But, remember, your entire body (including your brain) went through chemotherapy, which is a brutal, toxic treatment for your body. And you are alive because of it. So, instead of being hard on yourself for not having the same brain function as you did before chemo, be kind and patient with yourself. You deserve it!

* Scott M. (Metastatic Colon cancer to the Prostate & Pancreas)

I have pretty advanced chemo brain where I am very, very forgetful. That's just the way I am. I just accepted it. I tell people I'm going to forget things. I tell people I've known my whole life, that there will be times I come up to them and say, "I'm sorry, but I forgot your name." It's the drugs messing with my mind. And, I just try and accept it.

ADVICE: chemo brain is a fact of life; a side effect of treatment that you have no choice but to accept. The best way to deal with chemo brain is to first accept it, and then communicate that fact to people. That way, they can adjust and know what to expect.

* Sondra W. (Ovarian cancer 3x)

Oh yes, I had chemo brain. I learned to write things down. Unfortunately, my chemo brain affected my handwriting as well. For a while, no one could hardly read what I was writing, including me! That shocked me a little bit because when I saw that I wrote so badly, something about that made it seem like I was sick. Other things about having cancer didn't bother me. But, for some unknown reason, that did. Nevertheless, I got over it in time. It just was the way it was.

ADVICE: The way to cope with chemo brain is to expect it, accept it and adjust to it. If you can't remember things like you used to, that's just the way it is. If your handwriting gets really bad, then just accept that it's gotten really bad. Complaining about it is not going to make your memory or your handwriting better. As a matter of fact, it may even make them worse. So, don't expect too much of yourself. Cancer treatment is serious and there are side effects to take into consideration. Think of all you've been blessed with and focus your energies on recovering. Negative thinking doesn't help at all.

* Susan M. *(Ovarian cancer. Metastatic Pancreatic cancer to the Lungs)*

I experienced chemo brain or brain fog with the chemo treatments I received for both my Ovarian and Pancreatic Cancers. Both times, my mind would just go blank sometimes.

ADVICE: You need to just be patient and focus as best you can. Don't worry too much about it because your memory does come back. Of course, you can also adjust by taking notes or repeating several times what you need to remember. The main thing is to not stress about it.

* Vida B.A. *(Breast cancer)*

I noticed that my brain was not functioning like it used to before my chemo. Some of my friends suggested that I make a journal, but I was too tired to do that. I wanted to just rest. Resting my body and healing was my priority. I tried to take notes, but it was hard too. My brain was just not up to it. Although, at the time, I did go on Facebook a lot to post updates and comments.

ADVICE: Rest is really important for your body (and your brain) to heal, so that takes priority. Since your brain also needs activity, going on Facebook would be a fun activity where you exchange thoughts, ideas, pictures, updates, etc. with your family and friends. When an activity is fun, it easier to do; it won't seem like work.

* Yesi L. *(Breast cancer: triple positive)*

When I first experienced chemo brain in 2014, I gave myself a hard time because I didn't know what was going on, and I didn't know about chemo brain. After I learned about it, I told myself to be gentle and kind to myself. Now, three years later, I still have chemo brain.

One of the ways I cope with it is to just make fun of it. It is what it is! I also take notes; lots of notes, especially at work. If I used post-it notes before, I do so now more than ever. Post-it notes are everywhere, even if the subject is very fresh in my mind. I still write it down because I know that there is a big possibility I can forget it.

My chemo brain also happens when I'm dealing with clients. When it happens, I'm not ashamed. I simply tell them that I'm having a "brain fart" or "chemo fog". And they'll actually look at me and ask, "Like chemo brain?" And I'll reply "Yes". This definitely starts a conversation. And, there is an opportunity to create awareness.

CONSTIPATION

Constipation is a condition in which our stool becomes hard, dry, and difficult to pass, and bowel movements don't happen very often. Other symptoms may include painful bowel movements, and feeling bloated, uncomfortable, and sluggish.

* Aaron C. *(Prostate cancer, Skin cancer)*

I experienced a bit of constipation after my surgery which, I was told, is normal. I just took the prescription stool softener they prescribed to me and that was it.

ADVICE: If you're constipated, just let your doctor know, so that he or she can prescribe to you the stool softener you need to take care of the problem.

* Amor T. (Breast cancer, Ovarian cancer)

After my radical hysterectomy, I suffered serious constipation. Since I experienced constipation before, I initially thought nothing of it. Well, I was in for a HUGE surprise. The constipation I experienced was so painful, I didn't know what to with myself. When I informed my surgical oncologist, he suggested I take fiber supplements, like Metamucil and Benefiber, together with stool softeners. Well, I did and my constipation worsened! I got so bloated, I couldn't eat. Not only did I not feel like eating, I was afraid that anything I ate would just get stuck in my bowels and not come out. I was so uncomfortable, frustrated and in pain. My doctor suggested that I get Fleet Enema at the drug store and try to see if it worked to relieve my constipation. I used it several times. Unfortunately, it didn't work either. I was at my wit's end!

When I first met my medical oncologist to discuss my chemotherapy treatments, I informed him of how much I was suffering from constipation. He suggested I take MiraLAX; it would definitely take care of my constipation. He explained that with my constipation, I didn't need to produce more fiber, which the fiber supplements Metamucil and Benefiber did. Instead, my body needed help releasing hardened stool from my digestive tract. Miralax is not a fiber-based supplement. It functions by coating the colon and pulling water into the stool to help relieve constipation. Since my constipation was severe, he had me initially take more than the recommended dose of Miralax. When I followed his instructions, I was finally relieved ~ thank God! I wished I had met with him sooner!

> **ADVICE:** Take MiraLAX! It was such a godsend to me when I suffered serious constipation. Also, it helps to drink plenty of liquids, especially hot liquids (coffee, tea, soup). I also took a stool softener, but really, MiraLAX was the one that saved me.

* Cindy R. (Metastatic Breast cancer to Stomach)

Since I was really, really sick, I wasn't eating well at all. So when I had constipation, I had to use stool softeners, and I tried to drink as much water as I could. You know how important that is. I also drank tea and used suppositories when it was necessary to keep things moving. I tried all kinds of crazy things to keep it going.

> **ADVICE:** You have to let your doctor know if you're experiencing constipation, so he or she can prescribe something to help you. Prescription suppositories really help. Also drinking liquids (especially water) help to keep things moving.

* Glenn M. (Metastatic Colon cancer to the Liver, Lungs & Adrenal Glands)

I had both constipation and diarrhea at the same time, which is interesting. I never thought it would be possible!

* Hilda K. (Colon cancer)

I try not to take medications unless I really have to. Because chemotherapy made me constipated, I just took some stool softeners. I didn't change too much of what I ate, except for the fact that I ate less red meat because red meat can cause constipation. I also ate more soups because I like my food to be warm. I still drank coffee, but I didn't drink as much wine as I used to. Although I wasn't a big smoker to start with, I stopped smoking altogether because I knew it wasn't good for me. I was trying to be good to myself.

> **ADVICE:** Get an over-the-counter stool softener or get a prescription for stool softener from your doctor. Avoid red meat and alcohol because they cause constipation.

* Rev. Linda S. (Pancreatic cancer 3x)

I suffered severe constipation and laxatives were ineffective. When I realized that my sister, a retired nurse, knew how to "disimpact bowels" I called her and she came over to help. I was really elated. I'm also grateful for small miracles. Bowel impaction is part of the "daily indignities of cancer", which I am experiencing. Nothing to be ashamed of.

* *Rachel S. (Breast cancer: triple negative)*

Yes, I experienced constipation and had to take Miralax and a stool softener pretty much every day.

* *Scott M. (Metastatic Colon cancer to the Prostate & Pancreas)*

When I get constipated, I take MiralAX. A couple of times, I've had to use suppositories and stool softeners. I even had to use a fleet enema, at one time.

* *Yesi L. (Breast cancer: triple positive)*

I have to say that constipation was probably one of the most painful, hardest things that I had to deal with during my treatment. Similar to all of those mothers that experienced internal hemorrhoids after giving birth (which is very common), going through chemo treatments affects your most sensitive, private areas more than ever. And so, when you're constipated, those visits to the bathroom are almost like giving birth.

DELAYED WOUND HEALING

Delayed wound healing occurs when it takes longer for a wound to heal than normal. Chemotherapy and radiation therapy can slow wound healing. In cancer patients, normal body processes, such as cellular replication, inflammatory reactions and tissue repair, are impacted by cancer treatments.

* *Amor T. (Breast cancer, Ovarian cancer)*

The diep flap breast reconstruction procedure that I went through entailed the surgeon making a 20" incision across my abdomen from one extreme side of my hip to the other. A surgical drain bulb hung out from both sides of my hip where the incision started and ended. When I got home from the hospital, I noticed that I was getting a little itchy in the immediate area where both surgical drains were coming out of, but it didn't concern me at all. Later that day, I developed a fever, which I thought was due to an allergic reaction to medication I was taking. Unfortunately, my fever climbed to 101.5F and I was shivering uncontrollably. My neighbor called 911 and I was rushed to the hospital that night.

In the emergency room, my fever had gone up to greater than 103F, which is considered dangerous. My doctor informed me that I had a staph infection; a cellulitis infection, followed by sepsis, to be exact. The staphylococcus bacteria had entered my body through my surgical wounds and my body responded by releasing chemicals that were out-of-balance into the bloodstream to fight the infection. My treatment included some really heavy antibiotics that were being continuously coursed through the veins on my right arm. [Note: Since lymph nodes were removed from my left side during my mastectomy, the veins in my left arm can no longer be used for medical tests or procedures.] At the end of a week's stay, my doctor came in to let me know that they will be discharging me and sending me home, even though my red blood cell count is still low. He explained that with a staph infection, I definitely did not want to get infected again, and with the hospital being a haven for bacterial growth, it would be much safer for me to recover at home than there. I went home with the antibiotic Keflex and did finally heal from the staph infection.

> ADVICE: Always observe how your surgical wounds are healing. That way, you can see the progress or notice if anything is wrong. Itching, redness and swelling are the usual warning signs. Developing a fever is a HUGE warning sign. Inform your doctor immediately. In the meantime, keep the area clean and covered until you get treatment.

* Glenn M. (Metastatic Colon cancer to the Liver, Lungs & Adrenal Glands)

My "wound" was actually my skin that kept breaking, because it was thinning, ,so I wore gloves. Wearing gloves helped to protect my skin and also keep it moisturized. When I wore gloves, I was able to stick my hands under hot water or grab a hot pan if necessary.

> ADVICE: If the skin on your hands has a tendency to break because it's thinning, wear gloves to protect them and keep them moisturized.

* Scott M. (Metastatic Colon cancer to the Prostate & Pancreas)

I had to deal with a little bit of delayed wound healing. The scars from my surgery didn't heal like they probably should've. I think that it's because I started chemo six weeks after the surgery, which was a major operation. So, the Avastin from my chemo treatment caused the wounds to heal slower.

> ADVICE: If you're scheduled for chemo treatment after major surgery, expect your wounds to heal slower. Your wounds may take a longer time to heal, but they should heal, eventually. Just be patient.

* Yesi L. (Breast cancer: triple positive)

Even after three years, I'm still dealing with delayed wound healing. Because everyone was so worried about saving my life during treatment, I went through as many rounds of radiation as possible. What I wasn't aware of (and what you should be aware of) is that radiation seriously damages the skin. And, as far as wound healing goes, after so much radiation, the skin is basically left with no blood vessels, no cells to be able to regenerate. It makes it very difficult for wounds to heal.

After four surgeries on my breast, I was trying to heal. But there was one little area (like a pore) that kept opening up; it was definitely infected. The doctors then had me go through Hyperbaric Oxygen Therapy (HBOT). Yes, I was placed inside a hyperbaric chamber, like the one Michael Jackson used. In that chamber, I was able to breathe pure oxygen in a way that allowed my body to fight the infection I had and allow my wound to finally heal.

DIARRHEA

Diarrhea is the passage of loose or watery stools three or more times a day with or without discomfort. It happens when water in the intestine isn't being absorbed back into the body for some reason. It can be caused by various cancer treatments, including chemotherapy, radiation therapy to the belly, treatment drugs, liquid food supplements and the like. It can also be caused by infections or the cancer itself.

* Amor T. (Breast cancer. ovarian cancer)

Fortunately, I only experienced a couple of diarrhea episodes and they were brief. When I got them, I immediately knew to follow the BRAT (bananas, rice, applesauce and toast) diet. Even though I had to eat my rice and toast plain, I still enjoyed them, as well as bananas and applesauce. So, the fix was easy.

I avoided dairy (cheese, milk, ice cream, etc.), gas-producing veggies, like beans, broccoli, cabbage, cauliflower and onions (a favorite), gas-producing fruits, like raisins, prunes, plums, and also fatty and greasy foods. Because of the latter,

I unfortunately, had to stay away from my favorite Filipino and Chinese dishes when I had diarrhea. Coffee has always been my go- to comfort drink. Unfortunately, I learned that coffee irritates the GI tract. So, I had to avoid it too. Oh yes, I had to stay away from spicy foods too, because they trigger diarrhea. Again, I didn't have many diarrhea episodes during treatment. So, I'm lucky there.

ADVICE: Stay away from dairy (cheese, milk, ice cream, etc.), gas-producing veggies, like beans, broccoli, cabbage, cauliflower and onions, gas-producing fruits, like raisins, prunes, plum

* Cindy R. *(Metastatic Breast cancer to Stomach)*

To deal with my diarrhea, I ate a lot of bananas because I knew that they "bind you up." I didn't eat tons to where I got constipated; I just tried to eat enough. Even though my doctor told me to take Imodium, I tried to take care of my diarrhea as naturally as possible. Rice is binding too,. so that was good to eat. If I had the real bad bouts, I avoided eating fruits and other foods that would trigger them, like oily or spicy foods.

ADVICE: Foods that are bland and "bind you up" are those that will help firm up your stool when you have diarrhea. Bananas and plain white rice are ideal, because they're bland and easy to digest. Bananas have a bonus in that they are high in potassium, which is needed to replace electrolytes lost when you have diarrhea. Try to take care of your diarrhea naturally first before you go for the imodium or whatever medicine your doctor prescribes.

* Glenn M. *(Metastatic Colon cancer to the Liver, Lungs & Adrenal Glands)*

Yes, I experienced diarrhea, but I was able to get a prescription medication from my doctor to help take care of the problem.

ADVICE: You can use over-the-counter (OTC) meds to help with your diarrhea; there are a lot out there. However, if it's pretty bad, then ask your doctor if he or she can give you a prescription for Lomotil. It's a very, very tiny pill. One of my doctors said they look like very tiny corks, and they do.

* Joan S. *(Rectal cancer)*

I did experience diarrhea and took anti-diarrhea pills that I bought at Costco, which I took twice a day. I did not eat whole grains.

ADVICE: Don't expect your surgery to immediately heal you. It'll take at least a year. It does get better as time goes by. Don't be afraid of anti-diarrhea pills. Eat sourdough bread, potatoes, and white rice.

* Rev. Linda S. *(Pancreatic cancer 3x)*

When I initially experienced diarrhea, I was able to manage it with Kaopectate. When my cancer recurred and I had to go through stronger treatment, my diarrhea came back with a vengeance. Fortunately, I found that Lomotil, along with a daily serving of Greek yogurt helped tremendously.

ADVICE: If you have diarrhea, using Kaopectate or some other over-the-counter anti-diarrhea medication may help. If they do not help, try taking Lomotil along with a daily serving of Greek yogurt.

* Sondra W. *(Ovarian cancer 3x)*

It took me the full six weeks to recover from my hysterectomy. Unfortunately, from that I experienced a lot of diarrhea and lost a lot of weight; about 30 pounds. I just couldn't seem to get over that. My doctor kept testing me to make sure I didn't have some bacteria. But the results were always negative. Finally, weeks and weeks later, I took one test that had a positive result. Even though I was given antibiotics, I still had a lot of intestinal issues going on. I eventually got to the point where I was just up all night; in the bathroom all night, and I was exhausted! This went on night after night. I remember thinking to myself, "Wow! I'm not going to make it through this night!" I experienced so much diarrhea; I really believe that it kept me from healing at the time.

Our friend Peter, who is a member of Kenneth's men's group at church and who used to work at a hospital, told us about a concoction that helped give me relief for my diarrhea. It was a mix of coconut water, green bananas, yogurt, and Pedialyte. That mix helped me for a while because it coated my stomach. Unfortunately, as I continued with treatment and the cumulative effect of the chemo drugs in my body increased, the yogurt began to be a problem. That's why I couldn't use the nutrition drinks Boost or Ensure or anything that had any kind of dairy-milk base. So, I made Peter's concoction without the yogurt. Aside from that, I also used the anti-diarrhea medication Imodium A-D. Initially, I used it following the instructions in the package, which was basically, if you have loose stool then take it.

Well, eventually, I got so thin that the nutritionist at the Cancer Center stopped me one day in the hall and said, "You're not looking well. I think we need to talk." She told me to take the Imodium A-D diarrhea relief medication twenty minutes before I eat to slow everything in my system down. And that's when I began to feel better. At that time I was down to 108 lbs., and I was still losing. But now, following her directions by taking the Imodium A-D twenty minutes before I ate, being proactive versus reactive, I started to be able to keep the wholesome food down.

For a couple of months, I was off chemo, and all the diarrhea went away. I didn't have to take the Imodium A-D. But the moment I had to go back on chemo, the diarrhea started up again. So I use it now, in combination with Metamucil, which my surgeon and nutritionist both recently advised me to take. That and probiotics too.

Now, I had to fool around a little bit with the probiotics. For a while, I used the VSL#3 that my nutritionist recommended and that worked. Then I tried some different ones. For me, trying to understand probiotics, what I needed to take and finding the right one was the hardest thing to do. But they do help with the diarrhea.

I also had to be on a low-fiber diet. Before my diagnosis, green salad was a mainstay for me. So, that cut out a lot of nutritious vegetables because I wasn't able to digest them anymore. Now, I was limited to potatoes, carrots and eggs. Also, my system couldn't tolerate beans or grains. It was hard, really hard. I was trying to pick up weight and eat nutritious food, but then I couldn't have vegetable salad and foods that I liked. In time, gradually, I was able to add to the nutritious foods I could eat. Unfortunately, with the limited choice of nutritious foods to eat at that time, my energy level was affected.

ADVICE: If your doctor tells you to take Imodium A-D for your diarrhea, talk to your doctor about taking it twenty minutes before meals to slow your system down prior to eating. That way, you're being proactive versus reactive, which is just miserable.

Also, try "Peter's" Concoction. It is a mix of coconut water, green bananas, yogurt, and Pedialyte. I don't have the exact measurements, but just mix them together to your taste and start with a small amount. It'll help by coating your stomach. If it stops working, the yogurt may be the culprit. Just don't include it next time you make the concoction.

Make sure to add probiotics, which strengthen your digestive system and help to prevent and treat diarrhea. You may have to try different ones before you find the right one. Research or ask your doctor or nutritionist for guidance.

* Susan M. (Ovarian cancer. Metastatic Pancreatic cancer to the Lung)

About every few weeks, I experienced diarrhea, as a side effect of my chemo to treat pancreatic cancer. The doctors did not want me to take anti-diarrhea pills because at the time with my condition, taking them would've caused severe constipation. So, I ate rice and bananas instead.

ADVICE: If your doctors will not allow you to take anti-diarrhea pills, try eating rice and bananas. They are low in fiber and can help make your stools firmer.

* Vida B.A. (Breast cancer)

During treatment, I experienced diarrhea and, on top of that, I was dehydrated. Because I also had a high fever, I had to go to the emergency room. There, they rehydrated me. And, since my immune system was so weak, they put me on a neutropenic diet. The diet helped protect my weakened body from harmful bacteria. I also had to drink lots and lots of water. But, it was so hard to drink, because I had a tough time swallowing the water, which also, for some reason, tasted really bad. Nevertheless, I had to force myself to drink water. To give it a better taste, I put a little bit of Gatorade in my water. That definitely helped.

ADVICE: If you experience diarrhea, you need to make sure you hydrate. With diarrhea, you lose a lot of nutrients and minerals that your body needs, so drink lots and lots of water and liquids. If you find it difficult to drink the water because of the taste, then add some Gatorade. It'll be easier to drink. Getting a high fever along with diarrhea is really serious. Go to the nearest emergency room for immediate treatment.

* Yesi L. (*Breast cancer: triple positive*)

Diarrhea, definitely! It was like constipation. I went from one extreme (constipation) to the other (diarrhea). There were times, depending on the medication, that I had to deal with diarrhea. What worked for me was using Imodium. I used it in dealing with diarrhea symptoms and dealing with the diarrhea itself.

DIZZINESS / LIGHTHEADEDNESS

Dizziness or lightheadedness is an impairment in spatial perception and stability. We feel as though we are about to lose our balance or that the room is spinning around us. We might also feel like we are about to faint and, if we stand up, walk, climb the stairs or simply move our head, we may fall. Many types of chemotherapy and radiation therapy to part of the body related to the nervous system cause dizziness. Other possible causes of dizziness are high blood pressure, heart problems, low blood sugar, infection and dehydration.

* Amor T. (*Breast cancer. ovarian cancer*)

I had dizzy spells from my anemia, which I felt when I was in the hospital being treated for my staph infection. My doctor prescribed iron supplements, which helped bring up my red blood cell count. Anytime I felt dizzy, I just laid down, closed my eyes and stayed still. I found it also helped to stay calm and drink water.

ADVICE: When you feel dizzy, try to lie down, close your eyes and stay still. Drinking water and keeping calm will also help.

* Cindy R. (*Metastatic Breast cancer to Stomach*)

During an appointment with my primary care doctor, he found that I had anemia, i.e. my red blood cell count was pretty low, so he put me on iron tablets. They helped some, but I still needed to really be careful. I found that if I turned around too fast, I would get dizzy and go down, so I just had to be really careful. I didn't climb ladders or do any crazy movements that would cause me to lose my balance.

ADVICE: When you're going through treatment, it's really important to pay attention to your red blood cell count. If it's low, be careful with how you move. Don't turn around too fast or else you'll go down. Let your doctor know if you're getting faint or having dizzy spells, so that he or she can help you.

* Hilda K. (*Colon cancer*)

Sometimes I panicked while I was going through treatment. That's when I felt dizzy. I remember the nurse giving me medication to calm me down. Whenever I had to bring the chemo pump home, I remember also getting a bit dizzy. I realize that my anxiety or panic attacks caused my dizziness. Even though I was given medication for dizziness, I didn't take much of it.

* Vida B.A. *(Breast cancer)*

Sometime after my third or fourth chemo session, I was craving a Japanese noodle soup (ramen). Since I was getting used to the chemo side effects, like fatigue, I thought that I could eat out with my girlfriends. So I asked them to accompany me for some Japanese ramen. At that time, my red blood cell count was low.

At the restaurant, we ordered a big bowl of ramen that the three of us shared; I had a small portion. After I ate it, my blood sugar or something seemed to go down really quickly and I felt like I was going to pass out. I had cold sweats and laid my head on the dining table in the restaurant, so my blood would go down and not up to my head. I knew to do this, because when I was younger, I was anemic and had similar episodes of lightheadedness. My friends were panicking and called the restaurant's security guard for help. He got me a wheelchair and they wheeled me to our car to take me home. I rested at home and recovered not too long after. Looking back, I think my body reacted to the MSG (monosodium glutamate) in the food.

EYE / VISION PROBLEMS

Some cancer treatments, such as chemotherapy, biological therapies, long term steroid therapy and hormone therapy can cause eye or vision problems. These vision changes can vary and include blurred vision, irritated or dry eyes, tearing, redness and eye pain.

* Amor T. *(Breast cancer. ovarian cancer)*

During treatment, I noticed blurriness in my vision, which I expected as one of the side effects of chemo. Since I thought it would be temporary, I just ignored it. However, a month after treatment, I noticed a change in my vision that frightened me. I saw bright flashing lights on the sides of my eyes and I also saw floaters coming down fast on my right eye. When I drove, especially at night, the bright flashes were more evident. I thought that my retina was tearing. After running some tests, my optometrist explained that my retina was weak, a side effect of chemo. He said that he would monitor any developments and, in the meantime I should get new contacts and glasses. Fortunately, the flashes and the shower of floaters stopped. To this day I still get little floaters in both my eyes. Yes, they're distracting, but I'm used it to them now; no big deal.

It is recommended that people try to learn to see around their floaters. The floaters usually settle to the bottom of the eye like the snow in a snow globe and stop being as bothersome as time passes. The brain also gets tired of looking at a floater all of the time and starts to ignore it. You will always be able to see the floater again if you concentrate on it, or if you're looking into the sky or another very light background.

* Rev. Linda S. (*Pancreatic cancer 3x*)

My vision is slightly blurred, and it magnifies the pixels in online text, making all the letters look like small dots with tiny white spaces between them rather than a solid black outline.

* Rachel S. (*Breast cancer: triple negative*)

Yes, I had eye and vision problems like blurriness and not being able to focus. I also had eye strain, like my eyes just hurt. I just had to wait it out.

* Scott M. (*Metastatic Colon cancer to the Prostate & Pancreas*)

Yeah, I think I have little bit more blurry vision. I don't wear glasses, but I'm starting to wear glasses for reading.

ADVICE: If you notice your vision is blurry, get your eyes checked. Or you can get non-prescription reading glasses from the drug store, if your reading vision is blurry.

* Sondra W. (*Ovarian cancer 3x*)

During my initial treatment, I had an episode in my right eye. I experienced problems with brightness and pain. When I went in for an eye exam, the ophthalmologist saw some inflammation from my chemo treatment. He then prescribed around of medicated eye drops, warm compresses twice a day and lubricating drops during the day.

Later, we discovered that chemo-induced high blood pressure had been impacting my macular and retinal area. Once again, my ophthalmologist ordered the same prescription as she gave me earlier, i.e. medicated eye drops, warm compresses and lubricating drops. However, when I informed her of the chemo-induced high blood pressure I had been experiencing, which was impacting my vision, she then prescribed a beta blocker for me to take with my high blood pressure medication. The beta blocker would lower my blood pressure by lowering my heart rate, as well as, relieve the impact on my eyes. She explained that I had distorted "fishbowl" vision in my right eye, meaning it was like looking through fishbowl lens. The chemo not only impacted my eyes; the high blood pressure caused by my chemo treatment also affected my vision.

Recently, my ophthalmologist decided to not do anything to my eyes, because my body was in such a state of flux, she wanted to give it a rest. Despite my body being in remission, the toxic chemotherapy drugs are still in my system, so my body needs time to process it all out. Vision is one of those side effects. My ophthalmologist said that once my body stabilizes, the side effect of the vision problems will go away. That's the reason why no treatment, other than warm compresses and the eye drops as prescribed.

ADVICE: If you experience pain, brightness or notice a difference in your vision, have your eyes checked by an eye doctor (optometrist or ophthalmologist). That way they can examine your eyes to determine what can be done to give you relief or make your problem go away. Also, and this is very important, let ALL the doctors on your care team know what's going on. They all have to be on the same page, so they can determine the right treatment for you, within their respective specialties.

* Vida B.A. (*Breast cancer*)

My vision got blurry during my chemo treatment. Initially, I thought it was just a sign of me getting old. But then, I was told that it was a common side effect of chemotherapy. Fortunately, it didn't last long. So I didn't have to do anything.

ADVICE: Getting blurry vision is a common side effect of chemotherapy. If you get it, don't panic. You don't have to really do anything, unless it's really bad. Let your doctor know. It should go away after treatment.

Fat necrosis is a benign condition in which fat tissue in the breast or other organs is damaged by injury, surgery, or radiation therapy. The fat tissue in the breast may be replaced by a cyst or by scar tissue, which may feel like a round, firm lump. The skin around the lump may look red, bruised or dimpled.

* *Amor T.* (*Breast cancer. ovarian cancer*)

After reconstructive surgery was done on my left breast, I met with my plastic surgeon several times to check on how my reconstructed breast was healing. I noticed that the majority of breast tissue was softening except for a medium-sized lump located on the top portion of my reconstructed breast. My surgeon told me that it was fat necrosis, which is basically scar tissue that had formed where some of the fatty tissue, transferred to my reconstructed breast, died. He said that this is commonplace and that, in time, the firm tissue would soften up. To date, the fat necrosis has diminished in size and the rest of my reconstructed breast tissue has softened up to the point that it is almost as soft as my healthy right breast.

The only thing I did to try and soften up the firm tissue was massage it in such a way where I'm trying to separate the the tissues from each other. Whether that lead to its diminishing in size, I'm not sure. I am just happy that I don't feel it as much as I used to.

ADVICE: If you got a DIEP flap or tram fat breast reconstruction, ask your doctor about fat necrosis, so you'll understand developments of your surgery better and watch for it. If fat necrosis developed, then regularly massage the area, so it will soften up. The sooner and more consistently you massage it "down", the faster it will soften up or just disappear, altogether.

FATIGUE / WEAKNESS

Fatigue is a feeling of tiredness or exhaustion or a need to rest because of lack of energy or strength When you're fatigued, you have no motivation and no energy.

Weakness is a lack of physical or muscle strength and the feeling that extra effort is required to move your arms, legs, or other muscles.

* *Aaron C.* (*Prostate cancer, Skin cancer*)

After surgery, I lost a lot of strength. So, I couldn't lift any weights. I lost strength and muscle because I stopped working out. I also lost some weight, which didn't help. It took about six months to regain the strength and weight I had lost in just three months. I'm not completely back to full strength, but I continue to work at it and am determined.

ADVICE: Since your body takes a big hit from major surgery, expect your strength to decline. It's temporary. You can regain your strength, as long as you're determined and work at it.

* *Amor T.* (*Breast cancer. ovarian cancer*)

Breast cancer: I experienced a lot of fatigue and weakness while trying to recuperate from my mastectomy and breast reconstruction. It was really tough. Since the surgery, I was I was pretty sore and bruised and could barely move. It took the wind out of me, initially, to walk or move around, even at the slightest. I just wanted to lay down and sleep most of the time. Unfortunately, there were times when I could no longer lie down because my head would hurt, so I would just sleep sitting up, which then hurt my neck (*sigh...*).

Since I was afraid I would get addicted to the painkillers, I decided to hold off unless it was really necessary. I was instructed to take the oxycodone every six hours. Well, I refused to do that. So, what followed was my not moving around, in order to avoid any pain. I learned later that that was not a very smart thing to do. Since I refused to take my painkillers, which would have allowed me to move, I got sluggish and felt my energy waning, my body getting weaker; not stronger.

When I met with my doctor to follow up on my progress, I informed him that I was low on energy and I could barely move around. When he learned that I had avoided taking the Oxycodone painkillers he had prescribed, he gently scolded me. He said that, in order to heal, I have to move around and the painkillers would allow that. Besides, he continued, addiction would not set in until after many months of continuous use. I definitely was not on that path.

Ovarian cancer: After my hysterectomy, I was quite fatigued. I understood that my body just needed rest and was on its way to healing, so I just had to listen to what my body needed and rested when it signaled for me to do so.

Two months later, I started chemo treatments. Immediately after my first infusion, I felt fine, but then later on, fatigue hit me like a ton of bricks and I was down for the count. I felt like a wasted ragdoll. I couldn't lift my heads, my arms... my entire body. Walking was not an option. The only thing I could do was lay there and sleep. I did even have to try and sleep. I just did.

The days following were also hard; fatigue set in. Throughout my six cycles of chemo, I noticed that my first week would be the hardest and in my second week, I would also get fatigued, but not as much. And then finally, my third week was my happy week because that's when I would feel the most energy.

It is important to move I was told that it is important to move about, no matter how tired I felt. So, when I had even a little bit of energy, I tried to walk around, juts to get my blood circulation and immune system going.

> **ADVICE:** You will know when you are fatigued. You are just depleted of energy and want to just lay down and sleep. You should definitely follow your body's needs and lay down to rest. The thing is, moving about is also very important. So be aware of how much you have been sleeping and resting. If it has been for hours and you feel you have a bit of energy, first sit up, then stand up, and then take a couple of steps or walk slowly around ~ with the support of the wall o r nearby furniture) even if just for a short while or a short distance. Then, you can go back to lay down and rest.

* Cindy L. (Kidney cancer)

I still have fatigue. Every night, around 8:00 o'clock, I hit the wall. It has only ever gotten slightly better since my surgery and I think that is a physiological reaction of my body to only having one kidney. When I get fatigued, I don't feel guilty about getting some shuteye or a little nap in the afternoon. I don't sit back and read or type on the computer, or anything like that, because that doesn't help. I just need to actually shut my eyes and, at least, take a power nap. And then, in the evening, I just go to bed. That's all I can do when I feel fatigued.

> **ADVICE:** When you're fatigued, your body is telling you that it needs to rest. So, listen to your body and get your shuteye. Don't feel guilty, at all, about getting some shuteye. Things can be put on hold, so you can rest. If you need to stay up later in the evening, take a little nap. Try not to read anything or work on the computer, because that doesn't help with fatigue. Just shut your eyes and, at least, take a short power nap.

* Cindy R. (Metastatic Breast cancer to Stomach)

Breast cancer. During my breast cancer treatment, I experienced fatigue. I had regular blood tests done to see if my red blood cell count was too low to get the next chemo treatment and what we'd need to do if it dropped. It didn't get so low that I needed a blood transfusion or anything like that. However, they did monitor it.

To get my energy up, I did what I could to eat good, healthy foods. I also drank a lot of Starbucks coffee too, which my friend Leah went out and got for me. It helped to keep me going, even though I don't know that it was exactly a good thing to do. Still, I kind of took it easy and did what I could when I felt like it. I just relaxed and took care of myself.

Stomach cancer. This time around, when I felt fatigued, I rested when I could. But, I didn't want to just sit and mope away. So, I tried to get up and move a little. When I started to feel dizzy, I just told myself to wait a second and then sat down for about five minutes. Then, I'd get up and move a little again. I also tried to keep busy and keep my mind active by playing Words with Friends on my smartphone. .

I knew that I shouldn't be sedentary or inactive, because that is just not a good thing. I didn't go crazy either. I did what I felt comfortable with and listened to what my body was telling me, at the time.

ADVICE: Chemotherapy treatments are hard on the body and drain you of energy. So, when you feel fatigued, you should rest, relax and take it easy. However, it's really important to move around, as much as possible, even a little bit. It's what your body needs. Being sedentary or inactive does not help your body heal. Keeping your mind active is also important. If you have a smartphone, try playing "Words with Friends" or games like that to keep you busy. If you don't have a smartphone, you could still do a lot of things to keep you busy, like read, do puzzles, listen to music or chat with family or friends.

Have blood tests done to check your red blood cell count. Your doctor will monitor it. As for coffee, it's best to just take it in moderation.

* Glenn M. (Metastatic Colon cancer to the Liver, Lungs & Adrenal Glands)

During my radiation treatment, I got really low in energy; I was really fatigued. But, since I completed my radiation treatment, my energy returned.

ADVICE: I didn't do anything when I was fatigued, but sleep or rest when it hit me. If anything, I guess it's good to know ahead of time that radiation treatment can cause fatigue, so you're not surprised.

Yeah, hard to say the cause or causes of my weakness; a $64,000 question. I would guess the meds caused it, but then I also got out of my exercise habit. I like to ride my bike and walk my two dogs at the same time... safely ~ you know, with the helmet, elbow pads and knee pads – because my dogs conspire. They talk to each other. I can hear them thinking, "Okay, when we get to the pole, you charge left and I'll charge right and we'll SLAM him into the pole and then, we'll tie him up!"

To strengthen my muscles, I try to lift some weights and do some crunches with the bar. The bar has a pulley, a built-in pillow and padded handles. I do a set of 25 crunches with the bar, but I used to do three sets of 25. I do this in the living room with the dogs.

ADVICE: It's important to exercise even if you feel weak. Just exercise slowly and do what you can. Exercising helps you gain strength, which your body really needs when it's trying to heal.

* Joan S. (Rectal cancer)

During my chemo treatment, I got very, very tired. When I felt tired, I just took a nap and set a timer, so I didn't oversleep.

ADVICE: When you get tired from your chemo treatment, go ahead and take a nap. Set a timer, so that you don't oversleep.

* J.B. (Salivary gland cancer)

The biggest side effect I experienced was definitely fatigue. It just kind of hit me from out of nowhere when I was on my way to school. It happened about the third week into the radiotherapy. They did warn me that I would experience this. Since they knew I was in school, my nurses advised me to focus on intensive things like looking at assignments or studying earlier in the day because the fatigue tends to happen later in the night. I found it really hard to focus and study at night. So I organized my time and tried to do most of my work during the day. I was also advised to just keep moving and be active, like walk as much as I can throughout the day. That advice really did help me cope with my fatigue.

So, for the most part, I was able to continue with my hobbies and things that I enjoyed, although there were times I had to adjust. When I felt fatigued, it limited the amount of time I could do the things I enjoyed. As I mentioned, I did plan around the times fatigue would get to me.

* Rev. Linda S. *(Pancreatic cancer 3x)*

Fatigue always the day of and the day after chemo. So, I plan my activities around those days. On the days I feel fatigue, I nap, read or watch TV.

* Rachel S. *(Breast cancer: triple negative)*

I was constantly tired. Always tired. And the only thing I could really do was sleep as much as I can. It's hard when you have kids. A lot of the times, if my husband was at work, I had friends who came over and helped me out, as much as they could. I just lay on the couch and watched the kids. Unfortunately, I wasn't able to do a lot of things that I wanted to do with them. Like, I couldn't read to my son. We couldn't do things like that. They pretty much got away with a lot of things during that time too. But, they were safe; they were fed. My twelve-year old son did a lot of cooking for me. He would also go make his brother something to eat. And, he'd also go and make spaghetti. We ate a lot of Progresso soup or … just stuff like that to get through the time.

* Rick S. *(CLL: Blood & Bone Marrow cancer)*

I experienced fatigue, but not immediately. It happened around the third month into my chemotherapy treatment. Initially, I coped by spending a lot of time lying in bed, which I shouldn't have done. When I realized that I should try to keep on moving, I then started working out at the gym again. That really helped me feel better.

* Scott M. *(Metastatic Colon cancer to the Prostate & Pancreas)*

When I was on six months of the chemo drugs Oxaliplatin, Avastin and Xeloda, every day I still got up; I still showered; I still got dressed, and I still walked to the other end of the house. Then, because I was so fatigued, I laid on the couch, napped and watched TV. So, even if the only thing I did that whole day was walk to the other end of the house and lay on the couch and nap and watch TV, I wanted to show my kids that I was fighting through it. I was doing everything possible to have a normal day. It always started with a shower, which felt good, then getting dressed, which helped me feel normal and prevented me from getting depressed. I could've stayed in bed with my pajamas all day long, but I really think that would've just brought on more depression.

* Sondra W. *(Ovarian cancer 3x)*

Fatigue was HUGE for me, just huge! I felt I had a lot of things going against me. Not only did I have diarrhea, I also had all the extra pain. In the middle of all that, my husband and I had to pack up and move from a three-bedroom to a one-bedroom, so we had more than a lot to do. I also had to gather all my mother's belongings and send them back to her or get rid of them. And, that was the first year! Last year, we had to pack up again. That took a HUGE toll on my health and energy. I don't think I even recovered from our last move on October of 2016. That was a lot.

ADVICE: Trying to prepare for the unexpected is tough, especially when you're involved with a lot of things and have a lot of things going on. Finding out you have cancer in the middle of all that is exhausting, both physically and emotionally. You need to save as much energy as you can to cope with the fatigue you're experiencing. You need to make your health a priority, so you can beat cancer. List what needs to be done and request the assistance of your family, friends and other sources, e.g. church groups, volunteer organizations.

* Susan M. (Ovarian cancer. Metastatic Pancreatic cancer to the Lung)

Ovarian cancer: I really don't remember I had fatigue as a side effect of my treatment, because at the time, I also had a 20-month old baby and I was working full-time, as well.

Pancreatic cancer: I had a pancreaticoduodenectomy (Whipple Procedure), which was a seven-hour, major surgery where several of my organs were removed. Fatigue set in during my 22-day stay in the hospital and continued for several months. During my second round of chemo to treat the metastasis of the cancer to my right lung, I felt fatigue for a day or two after treatment and swelling in my throat a couple of times, but nothing major. Other than that, I've been doing well considering.

ADVICE: Listen to your body. If you are feeling tired or fatigued, REST. Sleep or just lay in bed or the couch and REST. Your body needs it to recoup from surgery and medication.

* Vida B.A. (Breast cancer)

After every chemo session and for the first two weeks after, I felt so weak. I remember just laying on my bed with no energy at all. Sometimes, I would get up to go outside my room. But then, when I reached the couch there, I would just lay there; again, with no energy whatsoever. Later, I would get up to go back to my bed, only to lay there, again with no energy. I couldn't even think. The TV would be on, but I wouldn't be listening; just staring at the TV. I was fatigued, for sure. My body and my brain just couldn't function. It just wanted to rest, so I just followed what my body wanted and rested.

ADVICE: Chemotherapy is a very serious treatment; the drugs are really strong, so when you have the chemo drugs in your body, your body is working with them to kill the cancer cells. The fatigue is your body's way of forcing you to rest, because it needs to conserve energy for the battle against cancer.

* Yesi L. (Breast cancer: triple positive)

I experienced a lot of weakness, especially after chemo treatments. During the first week after chemo infusion with Adriamycin and Cytoxan, I felt like I went from being a strong adult to pretty much a defenseless, little baby. Dealing with fatigue was one of the biggest side effects I had and something that, at times, I still experience.

ADVICE: My advice for those feeling weak during and after chemo treatments is to just let it be. Let it be. Do not give yourself a hard time. Do not punish yourself. If your body is tired, just simply listen to your body and give it rest. If you're feeling fatigued, take naps. Take naps throughout the day and you would feel absolutely amazing after! No judgment! Be kind to yourself and just allow your body to rest.

FEET CHANGES / "CHEMO FEET"

Certain types of chemotherapy affect the small sensory nerves in the feet and hands, causing symptoms such as numbness, tingling, and pain in fingers and toes. These symptoms are common after cancer treatment, but they may also have other underlying causes. Hand-foot syndrome causes redness, swelling, and pain on the palms of the hands and/or the soles of the feet. Sometimes blisters appear.

The feet can also experience peripheral neuropathy: pain, numbness, coldness, and cramping in the feet caused by nerve damage. (This condition can also result from uncontrolled diabetes.)

* *Amor T.* (*Breast cancer. ovarian cancer*)

Three things I remember from having neuropathy: my feet felt like they were walking on glass shards and/or they got numb and/ or they felt extremely dry and dirty. The times my feet felt extremely dry and dirty, I placed them in a basin full of warm water and scrubbed them hard to remove the "grime". One day, I felt I had to do that three consecutive times, because there was still "grime" on my feet. But, no matter how much I soaked and scrubbed, the "grime" was still there. That was really weird. Of course, I learned I was experiencing neuropathy.

Neuropathy affected my feet in other ways. They would feel numb, like I was walking on glass shards, which was a bit scary. I did not feel stable at all to walk, because it was not a constant feeling. It would just happen out of the blue; no warning. It discouraged me from walking outside. Fortunately, my boyfriend Bill was there to help me and encourage me. So, we walked around the neighborhood slowly, very slowly. In time, the neuropathy went away.

ADVICE: B vitamins are useful in treating neuropathy since they support healthy nervous system function. I recommend you take vitamins B6 and B12 separately versus one B complex vitamin.

* *Glenn M.* (*Metastatic Colon cancer to the Liver, Lungs & Adrenal Glands*)

Because my skin on the soles of my feet got so dry and tissue-paper thin, they cracked and opened up. You can't imagine how much it hurt every time I walked. I used Aquaphor on my feet to moisturize them. I also wore socks from CVS Pharmacy, which I prefer over others, because they have looser, gentler elastic bands that won't cut off my circulation when I wear them.

ADVICE: Use Aquaphor to moisturize your skin and wear socks to help keep the moisture in. I suggest getting socks that have looser elastic bands, so that circulation to feet won't get cut off. Now, before you get the socks, you have to consider how thick they are. Because, if they're too thick, then your shoes may be too tight to wear. Thin socks are great.

* *Sondra W.* (*Ovarian cancer 3x*)

Almost overnight, after my first chemo infusion, I started having pain and redness on my right foot, so I had it checked to make sure it wasn't an infection. I found out I had "Hand-and-Foot Syndrome" caused by one of the chemotherapy drugs, Doxil. The skin on my foot was crusty and leather-like, and turned black, like it had been burnt in a fire. Since my heel also became leathery, I had to cut some of the tough skin off with a pair of scissors. The friction of the skin of my feet rubbing against my shoes caused it to be discolored, inflamed and blistered. It was so painful that even if something soft (like a pillow) touched my feet, I had to take Norco to relieve the pain! I've been wearing post-surgical sandals since. We had hoped that when I went off the Doxil over a year ago, the problem would go away. Unfortunately, it's still here today.

When I felt the need to go to Urgent Care, at one time, the doctor there prescribed an antibiotic, which caused me a bleeding ulcer and landed me in the hospital. Apparently, he did not know how to work with strong chemo drugs like Doxil. Fortunately, my podiatrist was familiar with it and its side effects, and he helped me take care of my foot issues.

For the blisters, the doctors gave me Erythromycin gel, which has done a very good job of drying up the blisters.

While the blisters are running and open, I apply the Erythromycin and place a light gauze over them for protection against infection and also to give them air.

For my dry, leathery skin, I use Aquaphor. Before using it, however, I store the Aquaphor in the refrigerator, so that when I apply it to my skin, it will be cool and soothing. Ice packs are too cold for me, but the coldness of the refrigerated Aquaphor is perfect. I alternate it with Cetaphil lotion, which is also soothing, or a combination of the Cetaphil and coconut oil; they work really well together.

FEVER / NEUTROPENIC FEVER

A fever is a defined as any body temperature above 98.6°F, which is often due to an illness. Neutropenic fever is a single oral temperature of 101° F or a temperature of greater than 100.4° F. sustained for more than one hour.

Having a fever is a sign that something out of the ordinary is going on in your body. For an adult, a fever may be uncomfortable, but usually isn't a cause for concern unless it reaches 103 F (39.4 C) or higher.

* *Amor T.* (*Breast cancer. ovarian cancer*)

The day I returned from a week's stay at the hospital from my mastectomy & DIEP flap breast reconstruction surgery, I felt fine. That night, however, I started shivering, so I just covered myself with warm blankets and drank a lot of hot tea. Unfortunately, my shivering became uncontrollable. Since I was alone at home, I called my neighbor Sherry for help and she took my temperature - it was 101.5F degrees. When she said that I needed to go to the hospital, I told her that I was just there for a week and didn't feel the need to go back. My shivering increased and Sherry convinced me to go to the hospital and called 911.

The ambulance came and the paramedic firefighters, after checking my vitals, said that my fever was too high and that I needed to go to the hospital. I refused; I really didn't think my fever was a big deal. I could see that they were really concerned. When they tried to convince me again, I told them that I wanted to make a deal with them. I said that I would go to the hospital on one condition: that we get a group picture together. They looked at each other as if I just lost my mind! I explained that every time one of my girlfriends told me that handsome paramedics came to their rescue, they didn't have any proof. Well, this was my opportunity to get proof that handsome paramedics came to my rescue. With a lot of hesitation, but also a lot of smiles, they came around and had their picture taken with me. It was really amusing to watch their reaction! Thanks for obliging me, Gentlemen!

In the emergency room, my fever had gone up to greater than 103F, which is considered dangerous. My doctor informed me that I had a staph infection; a cellulitis infection, followed by sepsis, to be exact. The staphylococcus bacteria had entered my body through my surgical wounds and my body responded by releasing chemicals that were out-of-balance into the bloodstream to fight the infection. My treatment included some really heavy antibiotics that were being continuously coursed through the veins on my right arm. [Note: Since lymph nodes were removed from my left side during my mastectomy, the veins in my left arm can no longer be used for medical tests or procedures.] At the end of a week's stay, my doctor came in to let me know that they will be discharging me and sending me home, even though my red blood cell count is still low. He explained that with a staph infection, I definitely did not want to get infected again, and with the hospital being a haven for bacterial growth, it would be much safer for me to recover at home than there. I went home with the antibiotic Keflex and did finally heal from the staph infection.

* Vida B.A. (Breast cancer)

I experienced a high fever when I got diarrhea. I was also dehydrated, so I had to be taken to the emergency where they rehydrated me. Since my immune system was so weak, I was confined in the hospital for four days and they put me on a neutropenic diet. The diet helped protect my weakened body from harmful bacteria. I also had to drink lots and lots of water. But, it was so hard to drink, because I had a tough time swallowing the water, which also, for some reason, tasted really bad. Nevertheless, I had to force myself to drink water. To give it a better taste, I put a little bit of Gatorade in my water. That definitely helped.

For the neutropenic diet I had to follow, I was told that I couldn't eat anything raw or uncooked, like fruit or salad vegetables. Everything had to be cooked. My doctor advised me to avoid eating in restaurants. He said, "As much as possible, just eat at home, because then you know what's in your food. When you go to restaurants, you don't know what they put in it, like MSG and other unsafe ingredients."

* Yesi L. (Breast cancer: triple positive)

I was hospitalized twice with fever and at one time, I had a fever of 105. They called it Neutropenic Fever. That is a condition that puts you in a hospital. Since my white blood cell count was really, really low (Neutropenia), my having a high fever was really dangerous. So, I had to go to the emergency room twice.

GAS (FLATULENCE)

Gas (flatulence) is commonly known as farting, passing wind, or tooting. Flatulence is a medical term for releasing gas from the digestive system through the anus. It occurs when gas collects inside the digestive system, and is a normal process.

* Amor T. (Breast cancer. ovarian cancer)

Breast cancer. After my mastectomy and breast reconstruction surgery, it took me a while before I could pass gas. This was because my body had gone through major surgery and I was not eating solids yet. When my body healed a bit, I was allowed to eat solid foods again, and that's when I started passing gas... a good sign for recovery. Fortunately, it did not smell.

Ovarian cancer. Having radical hysterectomy was really intense. After my body healed and I was able to eat solids, I was able to pass gas, which was progress. One day, around the time I was still undergoing chemo, I felt excruciating pain around my body. So, the first thing I did was take my painkiller Oxycodone, which did not do anything for me. Since I also felt like I was on fire, I lay on several packs of ice. But, that did not do anything for me either. It felt like a pinched nerve all over my body. I remember being in a panic, crying, at a loss for what to do. Bill's son, Sean, ask me what he could do or how he could help. While I sat on a recliner with ice, I asked him to turn on the television. Going through the channels, I asked him to stop when we got to America's Funniest Videos. Fortunately, I enjoyed the show; it really helped to take my mind off of my intense pain.

After the show (still in pain), I went to look around our medicine cabinet. My eyes landed on GasX. Strangely, it seemed like it was the only thing I needed; all others just faded to the background. I took one and .... Lo and behold, my pains disappeared. With that, I understand that the excruciating pain I had experienced was due to gas going throughout my body. Who'd have thought?

> ADVICE: Gas trapped in your body can cause intense pain. If your pain medication doesn't relieve you of pain, then you may want to see if GasX or similar can help relieve the pressure of trapped gas you may hav

* Cindy L. (Kidney cancer)

After my nephrectomy, which was laparoscopic surgery, I had a lot of gas pain due to the carbon dioxide that they used during the surgery to work on my abdominal cavity. It went into my tissues and then got trapped in my intestines. The first night I had the surgery, my surgeon came in at about 11:30 at night to make me get out of bed. He said, "This is the only time that you're going to get a high-five for farting." So yeah, he made me laugh and I thought I was going to die because I was trying to get up and fart, at the same time!

> ADVICE: When it comes to gas, especially after laparoscopic surgery, you have to "let it rip!" It doesn't matter who's around. Just let it go, because it has to come out.

* Cindy R. (Metastatic Breast cancer to Stomach)

When I had gas, I tried to just deal with it the natural way by eating good and healthy foods. I tried to not get into meds unless I absolutely had to. Like, I didn't take Tums unless my gas was so bad that I just needed a little relief. I just tried to do everything as natural as possible. Of course, when I had to, I "let 'er rip!"

> ADVICE: Avoid foods known to cause gas, like beans, fruits, corn, asparagus, broccoli, cabbage, potatoes, onions, garlic, pasta and food and drinks that contain sugar. You can eat foods high in protein, like eggs, chicken, fish, beef and turkey. Good vegetables to eat are green beans, bok choy, cucumber, lettuce, tomatoes, zucchini, bell peppers and greens, such as kale or spinach.

* Glenn M. (Metastatic Colon cancer to the Liver, Lungs & Adrenal Glands)

Oh yeah, a few embarrassing moments there... I just "let 'er rip!" When I took Tums (an antacid), I threw up violently, which was odd, because I used to take it all the time before I had cancer. It helped back then, especially since it's supposed to calm the stomach down.

Since I had a lot of stomach acid, I took Prilosec and other over-the-counter things for gas. By the way, sometime ago (pre-cancer) when I had a thick cough, my ENT (Ear, Nose and Throat) doctor suggested I try Prilosec for a couple of weeks. I did and the cough went away. Go figure!

> ADVICE: If you have problems with gas, you can try taking over-the-counter antacids, like Prilosec or Tums. If it's not a big problem for you, then just let 'er rip, without being rude, of course.

* Rachel S. (Breast cancer: triple negative)

Yes, I definitely had gas. When I had them, I just "let 'em rip!" There's not much you can do about it.

* Sondra W. (Ovarian cancer 3x)

I experienced gas only during my second bout with ovarian cancer and only with the new chemo drugs Doxil and Avastin, which my oncologist said causes huge problems with the gastrointestinal system. It's the reason why I experienced diarrhea and had all kinds of issues. When I had gas, I had to sometimes just let it go. There's really no other choice. I did try different things, like drink water before meals, drink the "colorless" carbonated beverages (ginger ale and Sprite), which helped. Unfortunately, drinking them, after years of not having any carbonated drink, made my taste for them return and cause problems. So I turned to drinking tea using Arrowhead sparkling water and no sugar. When my stomach started hurting, my doctor informed me that my body cannot tolerate mint or ginger tea; they're too hard for my intestines. I'm now taking Protonix, an acid reducer. That has allowed me to have a little bit of chamomile tea. I'm still trying to experiment around, but don't have that down yet.

> **ADVICE:** Avoid foods that cause gas, like beans. Drink water before you eat. Try "colorless" carbonated beverage, like ginger ale or Sprite, but avoid Coke or any drink with caffeine. Also, there are over-the-counter gas relief medications you can get. Of course, there are times when you just have to "let it go" when you have gas. Experiment with different things to identify what works best for you. If nothing works, ask your doctor to prescribe an acid reducer, like Protonix.

* Vida B.A. (Breast cancer)

I had all kinds of stomach issues, some of which led to gas. I didn't take anything for it or try to stop it. I just let it happen. It wasn't a big deal.

> **ACTION:** If you have gas, just let it out. Don't try to stop it or keep it in, because doing that isn't good for you. Just let it out.

* Yesi L. (Breast cancer: triple positive)

I was hospitalized twice with fever and at one time, I had a fever of 105. They called it Neutropenic Fever. That is a condition that puts you in a hospital. Since my white blood cell count was really, really low (Neutropenia), my having a high fever was really dangerous. So, I had to go to the emergency room twice.

HEARING PROBLEMS / OTOTOXICITY

But many people are unaware that hearing loss is also a common side effect of cancer treatment, and it can impact patients years after treatment. Toxicities from chemotherapy and radiation can cause damage in the inner ear structures that leads to hearing loss. This is called ototoxicity.

* Amor T. (Breast cancer. ovarian cancer)

When I was going through chemo treatments, my hearing weakened. Bill and my other friends had to repeat what they were saying to me. Sometimes I had to ask them to speak a little louder, enunciate what they're saying and also speak slowly. What I did for my part was try to repeat back to them what they just said. That kind of helped me to not have to ask them again. I really appreciated their patience.

> **ADVICE:** If you find that you're having to ask others to repeat what they just said to you and you're having difficulty hearing what's being said, just ask them to speak clearly and a little louder (without yelling).

* Glenn M. (Metastatic Colon cancer to the Liver, Lungs & Adrenal Glands)

Before cancer, my hearing was already bad. Even so, my doctors had my hearing checked, because they were concerned some of the chemo meds could decrease my hearing ability. The chemo meds didn't seem to bother my hearing or make it worse. So, I quit getting the ear check-ups. I did spend over $10,000 on hearing aids already.

A blood pressure of 140/90 or higher. High blood pressure usually has no symptoms. It can harm the arteries and cause an increase in the risk of stroke, heart attack, kidney failure, and blindness. Also called hypertension

* Cindy L. *(Kidney cancer)*

High blood pressure runs in my family and I had high blood pressure before I lost 48 pounds. Although a bit lower it continued to run in the 130's/80's until my kidney was removed. Then it lowered to 115 or so over 70 or so. Looking back that was the ONLY indication anything was amiss but since high blood pressure runs in both sides of my family it didn't trigger a red flag.

One of the things that can blow up a kidney and cause permanent damage is high blood pressure. Unfortunately 2 years later I have gained back 20 pounds and so I have to work to lower my weight, which is done with exercising and eating healthier food. I'm still on my blood pressure medication and put myself on a pretty serious low carb diet, which consist of no adding of salt and keeping it at 2300mg a day of sodium.

For my diet, I also eat fruits and Ezekiel or sourdough bread, which have less sodium; a lot of Italian breads do too. Of course, I also try to skip the breads altogether. So, aside from exercise, that's just one of the ways I handle the high blood pressure. I'm within fifteen pounds of my normal weight, so not too bad.

ADVICE: High blood pressure is dangerous and can cause permanent damage. The two main ways to lower your blood pressure is to exercise and eat healthy. You should remove salt from your diet and drastically decrease your sodium intake, i.e. 2300mg per day. Keep in mind that about 1700 mg is required for body functions. When it comes to eating bread, choose the Ezekiel brand, especially the sprouted ones. They're low in sodium. I believe they're sold at Whole Foods, Trader Joe's and Publix supermarkets. Of course, skipping bread altogether is best if your goal is to lose weight in the effort to lower blood pressure.

* Sondra W. *(Ovarian cancer 3x)*

When I took Avastin as one of the chemo drugs during my second time round battling ovarian cancer, I developed high blood pressure. It was controlled with high blood pressure medication, which, unfortunately, also caused my feet to swell. My doctor kept a close watch on my condition to make sure my blood pressure was under control during treatment. However, the swelling continued, moving up my leg, causing discoloration and blisters.

I am now working with a kidney doctor, and with medication, have been able to get rid of 15 lbs. of excess fluid from my lower body. The focus on lowering the excess fluid and lowering my blood pressure continues.

ADVICE: If you get high blood pressure as a side effect to any of the chemo drugs, your doctor may give you medication to control it and monitor developments. Of course, treatment is on an individual, case-by-case basis.

Hot Flashes

Hot flashes are sudden feelings of warmth, which are usually most intense over the face, neck and chest. Your skin might redden, as if you're blushing. Hot flashes can also cause sweating, and if you lose too much body heat, you might feel chilled afterward.

* Amor T. *(Breast cancer. ovarian cancer)*

Before my breast cancer diagnosis in 2013, I was already experiencing hot flashes. However, after my radical hysterectomy to treat ovarian cancer, my hot flashes grew in frequency and intensity. Fortunately, those episodes are brief. What I do to cope is drink cold water or coconut water and just go on with whatever I'm doing. Sometimes, I wipe my face and neck with a really cold washcloth. I would also remove any outer layer of clothing I'm wearing or my blanket, if it happens when I'm sleeping. For me, hot flashes comes and then they go. They haven't been a big problem for me.

> **ADVICE:** Drink something cold. If you have an outer layer of clothing, juts remove that. Wiping your face and neck area with a cold washcloth also helps.

* Cindy L. (Kidney cancer)

I'm not sure what brought on my hot flashes; I'm not sure it was menopause. I had them before the surgery and then they stopped. Whether it's the adrenal gland or the physiological side effect having only one kidney, I don't know. When I did get hot flashes, they were just horrendous! It got to the point where I just felt like I was going to spontaneously combust! My face turned red. I'm a redhead. So, you can just imagine when my face turned red, everybody would ask, "Are you OK?" And, I'll respond, "Yes, just having a hot flash."

I could tell when my hot flash was about to come on. First, I got this odd sensation, which I can't describe. Then I got queasy. Then, I got real hot. Then, I got freezing cold for a while. Yes, it was very strange.

> **ADVICE:** When you get hot flashes, you just have to deal with it. Even though it's really uncomfortable, it comes and then it goes; it's temporary. It does help to be aware of how it comes on and any triggers such as hot beverages, an anxious moment. That way, you're prepared.

* Cindy R. (Metastatic Breast cancer to Stomach)

I was miserable with the hot flashes. They were awful! I tried everything under the sun to get away from them, like flip the covers off of me and that kind of thing. To deal with my hot flashes, I got something called the "Chillow Pillow." It definitely kept things cool for me while I slept.

The "Chillow Pillow" is a special cooling pad that I placed underneath my pillow case. I just laid on that and it cooled down the hot flashes that came at night; it allowed me to sleep at night. In the morning, I would place it back in the freezer to cool again and then place it on me whenever I was miserable from my hot flashes. The Chillow Pillow is like bluish in color and it's got some kind of pad in the middle that keeps everything cool. It's fabulous. I'm like, "Thank You!"

> **ADVICE:** Aside from drinking an ice-cold beverage or flipping the covers off of yourself, the best advice I can give you is to get the Chillow Pillow for yourself. You can get it online at Amazon or in stores like Walmart. It's reasonably priced and a real lifesaver!

* Rachel S. (Breast cancer: triple negative)

Oh, yes! The chemo sent me into menopause. The last time I had a period was over a year ago. I asked the doctor about that and she said that chemo can send you into menopause. And the hot flashes were horrible! There was nothing I could do because of the cancer and what I was going through. The typical hormone pills they give women to deal with it, I couldn't take them. I think one of the worse things about the hot flashes is that I could feel my mood changing really fast. Like, I would be totally fine one minute and then, suddenly, get a hot flash where I turn into the crankiest person in the world. I could feel it was about to happen, but couldn't stop it. I just tried to hold my tongue or, usually, I would just walk away to another room. Or, I'd stay really quiet, like really quiet. I wouldn't talk, because I knew if I did, I was just going to snap at someone that didn't deserve to be snapped at.

* Scott M. (Metastatic Colon cancer to the Prostate & Pancreas)

When I had the prostate cancer, because I was on chemo, I couldn't have any surgery. So, they gave me two injections (lasting three months each) of female hormones that was to bring my testosterone down to zero while I did 43 days of radiation for the prostate cancer. Well, in doing that, I got hot flashes. It was like I was going through menopause.

* Vida B.A. (Breast cancer)

Yes, I had to deal with hot flashes during chemo. I just dealt with them as they happened. And then, they just went away. All I could do was cool myself. Here, in the Philippines, it's very hot, so I've got the AC (air conditioners) on. But then, sometimes the ACs are not enough, so I also use the electric fans. Oh, I have a mini battery-powered electric fan that I use too.

When I slept, I felt the heat start in my neck and then spread all over my back, so I would remove the blanket I had on. After a minute, I would get cold again and put my blanket back on.

* Yesi L. (Breast cancer: triple positive)

Wow! Hot flashes at my age was something that was completely new to me. I thought I was having anxiety and panic attacks. What I felt was heat rushing from the top of my head down throughout my body and sometimes, back up. I also thought I was having a heart attack; I thought I was dying!

When I first realized that I was actually going through hot flashes, I immediately thought of my mother. I then went and asked her for forgiveness, because I remembered how my siblings and I would give her a hard time thinking she was exaggerating when she experienced hot flashes.

HYPERTHYROIDISM

Hyperthyroidism (overactive thyroid) occurs when your thyroid gland produces too much of the hormone thyroxine. Hyperthyroidism can accelerate your body's metabolism, causing unintentional weight loss and a rapid or irregular heartbeat.

* Glenn M. (Metastatic Colon cancer to the Liver, Lungs & Adrenal Glands)

Hyperthyroidism makes your metabolism work overtime and makes it very hard to hold weight. That's one of the reasons I'm still at 160 lbs. because I've only just recently, from the last scan or two gotten the TSH (Thyroid Stimulating Hormone) and the T-4 in range. So, if they're in range, I should be able to theoretically gain weight. However, they haven't been in range very long. I am taking medication called Methimazole and instead of my dosage being 10 mgs. per day, I got the script for 5 mgs, so I could avoid pill-splitting if I have to go lower. I have an organizer – the weekly pill box that has AM and PM every day. I put a 5 mg. pill on each side, so that it stays in my blood longer. I think that's maybe a good thing.

When it was discovered that I had hyperthyroidism, my endocrinologist treated me with Methimazole for two and a half years before he got me in remission. When my hyperthyroidism returned, the associate of my endocrinologist started me on 20mg of Methimazole, which resulted in my TSH going over eight. Since I was out of state when that happened, I was informed that the dosage could not be corrected over the phone, and the endocrinologist would have to see me in person. For that reason, I unfortunately, had to release him and have been treating myself since as I haven't been able to find a new endocrinologist.

Since I was getting blood draws every two weeks, it took me only 20 days to get the TSH back in range. However, even though my TSH has been in the desired range for the last month or so, I don't feel good about steering my own treatment and my oncologist is not comfortable treating my hyperthyroidism. At this time, I'm looking for a new endocrinologist to take care of my needs in this area.

> **ADVICE:** Learn about whatever condition you have, so you can ask the right questions that will provide you with the answers you need to take care of your health. Find a doctor you can trust, who will work with you and consider whatever unusual circumstances you may be in, like being physically out of the area, and unable to meet in person.

HYPOKALEMIA

Hypokalemia is when the blood's potassium levels are too low. Potassium is an important electrolyte for nerve and muscle cell functioning, especially for muscle cells in the heart. Your kidneys control your body's potassium levels, allowing for excess potassium to leave the body through urine or sweat.

* *Joan S.* (Rectal cancer)

There was another time when I got really sick. Everything hurt and my potassium levels dropped so much, I was close to having a heart attack! When I went into emergency, they gave me potassium through the IV, which was horrid because they gave it to me too fast. I felt like I was being electrocuted. Afterwards, they kept me overnight for observation because the low potassium levels was believed to have been excess anti-nausea pills.

> **ADVICE:** If you need to get an infusion of potassium to raise your levels, have them start at 40% and then gradually raise it. The higher they go, the faster the IV goes, which makes it really uncomfortable.

HYPOTHERMIA

Hypothermia is a medical emergency that occurs when your body loses heat faster than it can produce heat, causing a dangerously low body temperature. Normal body temperature is around 98.6 F. Hypothermia occurs as your body temperature falls below 95 F.

* *Amor T.* (Breast cancer. ovarian cancer)

Every time I went to get my chemo infusions, I got really cold, so I always wore warm socks and kept a very warm blanket or blankets on me. Losing my hair also added to my hypothermia. If I didn't have on my wig, I would wear one of my warmer (knitted) caps to cover my head. Interestingly, I easily got cold while I was sleeping. So, I always wore a night cap, which was one or two of my knitted beanies. I also drank hot or warm liquids only when I felt cold.

> **ADVICE:** This is a common side effect that is temporary. Keeping warm with extra clothes, socks, gloves or blankets to cover you and a warm cap or beanie to cover your head will do the trick. Hot or warm liquids will also help.

* *Cindy L.* (Kidney cancer)

I did experience hypothermia. I got it after my hot flashes. And then, I froze! My hands and feet got cold and my entire body shivered. So, I kept myself warm, as much as I could by drinking warm beverages and covering myself with a blanket or jacket. Even though these are side effects of having chemotherapy, which I didn't have go through, they're also the physiological effects of my body learning to live without a kidney. I am almost two years post surgery and still suffer from shivering cold at times. So, at this point, I don't know if the physiological effects will go away or not.

ADVICE: When you get hypothermia, it's important to do what you can to keep your body temperature up. Drink warm beverages and cover yourself with something warm, e.g. blanket, jacket, etc.

* Hilda K. (Colon cancer)

After each treatment, I would feel really cold. So, I basically lived in sweats and slept in sweatshirts, jackets and socks throughout the winter. Even when I had a comforter on top of me, I was still cold. For the six months I went through chemotherapy, no matter what I did, my body just would not warm up. Whatever the temperature was, my body was always really cold, so I just never exposed my skin. I always wore gloves whenever I went outside. I wrapped my whole head and face with a scarf because I didn't want cold air to touch me. I prepared myself for any situation that would cause my body to react to cold. I also used the scarf to cover my mouth, so that when I breathed in air, it didn't feel so cold in my throat.

I stopped drinking cold water because my body would react to anything that was cold. I kept thinking ahead; I kept preparing myself for possibilities, so it was easier to deal with. However, there was one incident when I forgot to drink warm water, and I drank cold water...I felt like I was suffocating because my throat was contracting, and I couldn't breathe! So, my husband called emergency. Once I calmed down, I was able to breathe normally again. It was one of those panic moments. That taught me a huge lesson, and I became even more aware of cold temperature and what I drank and ate.

ADVICE: Even if it's warm outside, always keep warm clothing with you or near you, just in case you unexpectedly feel cold. Cover your body, face, hands, head and feet...everything, to protect yourself from the cold. Be aware of the temperature of what you drink and eat because the experience of taking in cold food or beverages will cause your body to hurt, make you shiver uncontrollably and, in the case of drinking something cold, constrict your throat and breathing due to panic.

* Rachel S. (Breast cancer: triple negative)

There were times I was super, super cold. I just got blankets. It would happen just in the general day-to-day; no actual trigger. I want to say that it happened more right after chemo.

* Sondra W. (Ovarian cancer 3x)

Initially, I was cold all the time when I went through my first treatment. Aside from my hair loss contributing to my feeling cold all the time, I believe that my drastic weight loss caused by my problems with diarrhea during treatment was also a big factor. At that time, my weight went down to 108 lbs. After treatment, when I was in remission, I was able to increase my weight to 125 lbs., and did not feel cold all of the time. Unfortunately, on my second round battling cancer, I went back on chemo treatments and lost the weight I had gained. Back to 108 lbs., I also again started feeling cold all of the time. The journey continued.

At the Cancer Center, they gave me a mylar blanket and a mylar cap to keep me warm. We call it my "space suit," and they gave me the set to use at home.

One hour before each scheduled chemotherapy session, I had to have blood work done. Unfortunately, there were many times when the results of my blood tests were not good, and I had to get emergency blood transfusions. Since there was a lot of waiting involved, they gave me another "space suit" to keep me warm because the results of my blood test were not good, and there was a lot of waiting involved.

There were many occasions when my blood work would not allow me to get my chemo treatment. There were many times I had to wait for my blood test, and my blood work condition caused me to keep getting emergency blood transfusions.

ADVICE: Keep yourself warm by bundling up and, definitely, wear something to cover your head (e.g. cap, hat, scarf, etc.) if you don't have hair. Since there are various causes of hypothermia, make sure to let your doctor know you're experiencing cold all of the time. That way, he or she can look into your situation and find a solution.

Infection is the invasion and growth of germs in our body. The germs may be bacteria, viruses, yeast, fungi, or other microorganisms. Infections can begin anywhere in the body and may spread all through it. An infection can cause fever and other health problems, depending on where it occurs in the body. When the body's immune system is strong, it can often fight the germs and cure an infection. Some cancer treatments can weaken the immune system, which may lead to infection.

* *Amor T.* (*Breast cancer. ovarian cancer*)

The day I returned from a week's stay at the hospital from my mastectomy & diep flap breast reconstruction surgery, I felt fine. That night, however, I started shivering, so I just covered myself with warm blankets and drank a lot of hot tea. Unfortunately, my shivering became uncontrollable. Since I was alone at home, I called my neighbor Sherry for help and she took my temperature - it was 101.5F degrees. When she said that I needed to go to the hospital, I told her that I was just there for a week and didn't feel the need to go back. My shivering increased and Sherry convinced me to go to the hospital and called 911.

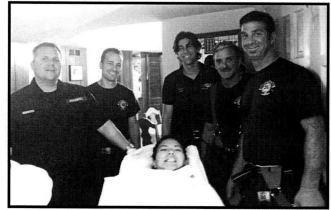

The ambulance came and the paramedic firefighters, after checking my vitals, said that my fever was too high and that I needed to go to the hospital. I refused; I really didn't think my fever was a big deal. I could see that they were really concerned. When they tried to convince me again, I told them that I wanted to make a deal with them. I said that I would go to the hospital on one condition: that we get a group picture together. They looked at each other as if I just lost my mind! I explained that every time one of my girlfriends told me that handsome paramedics came to their rescue, they didn't have any proof. Well, this was my opportunity to get proof that handsome paramedics came to my rescue. With a lot of hesitation, but also a lot of smiles, they came around and had their picture taken with me. It was really amusing to watch their reaction! Thanks for obliging me, Gentlemen!

In the emergency room, my fever had gone up to greater than 103F, which is considered dangerous. My doctor informed me that I had a staph infection; a cellulitis infection, followed by sepsis, to be exact. The staphylococcus bacteria had entered my body through my surgical wounds and my body responded by releasing chemicals that were out-of-balance into the bloodstream to fight the infection. My treatment included some really heavy antibiotics that were being continuously coursed through the veins on my right arm. [Note: Since lymph nodes were removed from my left side during my mastectomy, the veins in my left arm can no longer be used for medical tests or procedures.] At the end of a week's stay, my doctor came in to let me know that they will be discharging me and sending me home, even though my red blood cell count is still low. He explained that with a staph infection, I definitely did not want to get infected again, and with the hospital being a haven for bacterial growth, it would be much safer for me to recover at home than there. I went home with the antibiotic Keflex and did finally heal from the staph infection.

ADVICE: Always observe how your surgical wounds are healing. That way, you can see the progress or notice if anything is wrong. Itching, redness and swelling are the usual warning signs. Developing a fever, especially one that's climbing towards 103F, is a HUGE warning sign. Inform your doctor immediately. In the meantime, keep the area clean and covered until you get treatment.

* *Cindy R.* (*Metastatic Breast cancer to Stomach*)

After my double mastectomy, I decided to have breast reconstruction done. In the process, they inserted tissue expanders beneath my skin and chest muscles to stretch the area and make room for a future, more permanent implant. Then, I made several visits back for them to inject saline solution to gradually fill the expanders. Unfortunately, the right side kept getting infected. So I ended up going through a couple more surgeries where they removed the expander on my right side, cleaned it out, cleaned the area that it was in and then put it back to where it originally was. So, now I'm lopsided. I'm at the point where I'm like, "That's it. I don't even care. I can't take it anymore." It was crazy!

> **ADVICE:** If you decide to get silicone breast implants after your mastectomy, learn all you can about the process, especially the pros and cons. Have a good dialogue with your doctors, so you're all on the same page. My plastic surgeon knew exactly what to do when I got the infection. Sure, it was a painful and trying time. But you should do whatever you feel is right for you and your body. Whether you have breast reconstruction or not, it's your choice. If you choose to not have breast reconstruction, it's not the end of the world to have no breasts. If you do have reconstruction and come out lopsided, well, there are ways to solve that too.

* Scott M. (Metastatic Colon cancer to the Prostate & Pancreas)

There was a time I had a blood infection. We were over the hill in Santa Cruz driving home when it really kind of hit. I called the Cancer Center and said, "I'm coming in. I'm coming in whether you have space for me or not. You can put me in the closet, but I need treatment; I need help." The gal on the phone put me on hold a little and then said, "Are you the guy that always says this is your 'spa' day?" I said, "Yes". And she said, "Yes, come right on in." By the time we got there, they quickly and carefully "poured" me into a wheelchair and wheeled in. I was completely slumped over; white as a sheet of paper. The nurses took one look at me and said, "Over here!" and, immediately, I had a team of the Cancer Center's oncology nurses working on me. They knew exactly what to do to get me back to feeling good. It turns out my blood got infected from the single-access medical port (port) I had implanted. Since that port was used for my chemo infusions as well as to feed me, the sugars got in there, which led to bacteria growth that fed the blood infection. I realize now that I should've gotten a dual access port where the chemo cocktail goes in one and the food goes in the other.

[*I used to joke with the Cancer Center staff that my chemo sessions were my spa day because where else can a guy go, be welcomed by beautiful women, put in a recliner, have warm blankets put over you, be cared for and have a food cart wheeled up to you ... I mean it was a spa; it was great! And I'd get to nap, and they didn't bug me. So, I would always walk in and say, "I'm here for my spa day!" The staff got to know me that way.]

> **ADVICE:** If part of your treatment is getting food through your veins, alongside your chemo infusions, then make sure you get a dual-access port. That way, you'll avoid the infection I got caused by having only one port for both feeding and chemo purposes.

ITCHINESS

Itchy skin, also known as pruritus, is an irritating and uncontrollable sensation that makes you want to scratch to relieve the feeling. The possible causes for itchiness include internal illnesses and skin conditions.

* Amor T. (Breast cancer. ovarian cancer)

After the thoracentesis, where the doctor aspirated excess fluid from the lining of my right lung, they used adhesive bandage to cover my wound. When I got home, the part of my skin where the adhesive bandage was attached to was really itchy and red, so I just cleaned the area and replaced the adhesive bandage. Unfortunately, the itching and redness continued, this time accompanied by tiny blisters where the adhesive bandage was. So, I decided to just not have any covering over the wound and I had to wear tubes or camisoles that did not touch the affected part of my skin, especially since the blisters were seeping. It also helped to apply a cold pack; that helped keep the itching at bay. When I showed it to my doctor, he said that I was having an allergic reaction to the adhesive bandage. He cleaned the wound area and used paper tape bandage to affix the gauze over my wound.

ADVICE: First, make sure your medical team is aware of anything that you're allergic to. If your itching results in blisters, clean the area and apply a cold pack. Calamine lotion or an oatmeal bath could also help. Of course, you can also try to ignore it. Eventually, it will go away.

* Scott M. *(Metastatic Colon cancer to the Prostate & Pancreas)*

When I was in the hospital, I experienced itchiness from the Xeloda and morphine I was given. I needed 75 mg of Benadryl, but was initially given only 25 mg, by the hospital staff. That frustrated me, because they gave me 75 mg of Benadryl before to counter itching from the opioid drugs I was given. So, it didn't make sense to me. After discussing the issue directly with my oncologist, the issue was resolved.

ADVICE: When you experience itchiness, ask for enough medication (Benadryl) that should relieve you of your discomfort. If you do not receive enough medication, and you feel the hospital staff is not listening to you, then bring it to a higher authority, i.e. your oncologist.

* Vida B.A. *(Breast cancer)*

The breast implant procedure and recovery was painful. But I was able to tolerate it. One big problem was the itchiness on the skin surrounding my implants, which I believe, was an allergic reaction. My doctor said that it was psychological because the nerves were removed from that area. He told me to not scratch it and just put the topical steroid hydrocortisone on the area. He also said that if I wanted, he would give me a prescription for Gabapentin, a nerve pain medication also used to treat chronic itching. Since it comes in the form of a pill, and I'm the kind of person who doesn't like to take oral medication, I just applied the hydrocortisone and that helped.

ADVICE: If you're itching, let your doctor know, so that it can be checked. It may be an allergic reaction or not. Either way, your doctor may be able to give you something to relieve the itch. Try not to rely on pills, especially nerve pain medication because they're really strong and may cause side effects. Topical ointments or cream, hopefully, will do the trick.

* Yesi L. *(Breast cancer: triple positive)*

With my delayed wound healing on my breast, I experienced infection to the skin in that area. It was caused by bacteria entering the open wound. To treat it, I was given a lot of antibiotics. The caution with antibiotic treatments is that from curing one infection, a yeast infection can develop in a woman. And, it definitely developed in me.

ADVICE: If you are female and your doctor gives you antibiotics to treat an infection, be proactive and also ask your doctor to give you something to prevent a yeast infection.

KIDNEY / BLADDER PROBLEMS

- Some types of chemotherapy and immunotherapy can also affect or damage cells in the bladder and kidneys. Radiation therapy to the pelvis (including reproductive organs, the bladder, colon and rectum) can irritate the bladder and urinary tract. These problems often start several weeks after radiation therapy begins and go away several weeks after treatment has been completed.
- Surgery to remove the prostate (prostatectomy), bladder cancer surgery, and surgery to remove a woman's uterus, the tissue on the sides of the uterus, the cervix, and the top part of the vagina (radical hysterectomy) can also cause urinary problems. These types of surgery may also increase the risk of a urinary tract infection.

* Aaron C. (Prostate cancer, Skin cancer)

Incontinence was one of the side effects from surgery that I had to learn to cope with. It's a really slow process. I did a lot of Kegel exercises, but not as frequently as I should because I wasn't sure if they helped me, so I got sort of lazy about it.

I started at the gym again three months after surgery. But, it was around the fourth month mark when I started again with light weights, followed by walking around the block; that kind of stuff. I didn't swim at all because I couldn't control my bladder and I didn't want pool water rushing right up into my bladder.

When I first started lifting weights again, I strained and leaked urine because my bladder wasn't strong enough. My bladder is still not 100% at this point, but it's getting better and I don't leak as much. I noticed that my bladder's function improves more like on a month-to-month basis; not day-to-day or week-by-week.

It is funny how we take our bladder control for granted because we've been doing it all our lives. When we were toddlers, we learned how to control our bladders. We go 50 years without even thinking about our bladders; we take all that stuff for granted. And now with this situation, we think about it all the time! When it doesn't work, we're like "Holy sh*t!" But that's normal. It's expected.

It took me the first six to seven months to get my bladder functioning semi-normally. When I orgasmed after sex, I still leaked urine. At about the nine month mark, I started noticing a big difference. I had more control; my bladder was stronger. When the twelve month mark hit, my bladder was completely healed. I remember the first six months after surgery when losing control of my bladder was always on my mind. I'm finally at the stage now when I don't think about it all the time.

ADVICE: Do the Kegel exercises and don't be lazy about it. Although they may say that it will take at least nine months for your bladder to be reasonably healed, don't expect it to happen sooner. Be realistic about it when it comes to expectations about your healing. Regarding your bladder, it'll improve more on a month-to-month vs. day-to-day or week-by-week basis.

If you're a man, you can completely avoid wearing diaper pants. You don't even have to buy those things. Just buy the incontinence pads that are designed for men like Depend Incontinence Guards for Men (maximum absorbency). They're just pads; not the pants. That's all you need.

* Amor T. (Breast cancer. ovarian cancer)

Since I had multiple abdominal surgeries, I developed a web of abdominal adhesions that were keeping my internal organs from functioning smoothly. There were times I felt like urinating, but nothing would come out. It was the same feeling I had when I had urinary tract infections many years ago. However, I noticed that every time I had a bowel movement, that feeling of needing to urinate would go away. It dawned on me that with all my abdominal adhesions ~ like a rearrangement of my internal organs ~ scar tissue would press up against my bladder whenever I needed to have a bowel movement or just pass gas. So, if I had issues urinating, I would find relief in passing gas or having a bowel movement. To do that, drinking coffee or chocolate helps.

ADVICE: First, if you have problems with your kidney or bladder functions, let your doctor know. It may be a symptom of something more serious. If you're having difficulties urinating, sometimes simply drinking a lot of liquids helps.

* Cindy L. (Kidney cancer)

I had a nephrectomy to remove one of my two kidneys. So now I am functioning with only one kidney, and it's a struggle. I have to do everything I can to protect my one kidney, being the sole survivor in there.

I can no longer take any NSAIDs (non-steroidal anti-inflammatory drugs) for pain, like Motrin, Naproxen...any of that. However, I can take Tylenol and anything with acetaminophen in it. I also have to be careful about antibiotics, but I have a lot of antibiotic allergies anyway.

I don't take herbal supplements willy-nilly, because everything taken orally will go through my kidney. When I take oral medication, they'll first go through my liver and then will be excreted either by the liver or my kidney. Medications that are excreted by the kidney will put a strain on my kidney, so I need to avoid them, as much as possible.

Regularly, I am tested to determine my kidney's ability to handle creatinine. When the normal breakdown of muscle tissue occurs in the body, creatinine is produced, filtered through the kidneys and excreted in urine. The normal level of creatinine in the blood for women is 0.5 to 1.1mg/dL. We noticed that the level of creatinine in my blood at eight (8) weeks had gone back to its pre-surgery level of 0.8mg/dL. Post-surgery, it was 1.1mg/dL. Then, it went down to 1.0mg/dL. Now, it's back up to 1.13mg/dL. Levels are expected to fluctuate, but I'm trying to keep it low.

ADVICE: If you have kidney problems, be aware of your creatinine levels. That way, you can make whatever adjustments you need to keep your kidneys functioning properly. Avoid NSAIDs (e.g. Motrin, Naproxen, etc.), be careful about the antibiotics you take (always check with your doctor) and be wary of taking herbal supplements. Those medications and supplements can strain kidneys function. You don't want that. The number one piece of advice I can give is to drink a lot of water; even more than you think you need! It has helped keep my kidney within normal range.

I also experienced bladder spasms and I think that it was caused by tannins in the tea that I enjoy drinking. Teas have tannin and tannin is a bladder-irritating property. Some teas have more tannin than others. I used to love McDonald's unsweetened iced tea, but I don't anymore because drinking it irritated my bladder. I can drink the unsweetened tea at Panera, and it doesn't bother me. I try not to experiment too much because the bladder spasms are painful. Two years post surgery, I rarely have a bladder spasm, so it seems to have been a temporary issue. I still avoid drinking too much tea or coffee and stick to plenty of water.

ADVICE: For both bladder and kidney problems, drink lots of water. Also, you just have to be patient because it does take time. Try to flush out whatever irritation is in there. Usually, it will only last about a day and then it goes away. Avoid teas that have a lot of tannin in them; you may have to experiment. Just remember that teas have tannins that irritate the bladder. Do drink Cranberry juice. It's been proven to work for those with bladder or kidney problems

* *Joan S.* (*Rectal cancer*)

Because of all the surgeries I went through and also because of my age, I have to wear a pad because I leak. Many women and men have to wear pads too because of age.

ADVICE: It's a fact of life you have to live with. It's a good thing many stores carry a wide selection of pads you can choose from.

* *Sondra W.* (*Ovarian cancer 3x*)

I had the problems for sure during my first treatment, i.e. bladder bleeding and pain. No kidney problems; just bladder problems. I finally saw a urologist. He first examined me in a procedure called cystoscopy where he inserted a hollow tube (cystoscope), equipped with a lens, into my urethra and slowly advanced it into my bladder. After that, he conducted an intravesical bladder instillation where he injected medication directly into my bladder via a urethral catheter. It was a very painful procedure. But since I was already in so much pain from my bladder problems, the pain from the instillation was okay. And, boy, I tell you, I was thankful for my urologist!

Initially, the medication for my bladder lasted only three days, so I went through another dose of treatment and that lasted five days. After that, I returned for yet another round of medication, which then lasted a week. Finally, my bladder wall softened up and got better. Unfortunately and despite the several bladder instillations, we couldn't get rid of the bleeding. We got rid of the pain and the urinary tract infections, but we could never get rid of the bleeding.

Interestingly, when I went off of chemo, in two weeks all my bladder problems were gone; everything! They disappeared and never returned. That was definitely such a blessing because when I had it, it was really bad.

You see, my severe bladder problem was a reaction to one of the chemo drugs I was taking. And, I was told that my reaction was unusual. As a matter of fact, they even told me, "This is not part of the deal." But, that's also when they learned that I have a high sensitivity to different kinds of drugs. I actually have a whole page of medicines I cannot take because I react to them., so my doctors had to work with all that.

ADVICE: If you have bladder problems, you may be reacting to one of the medications, or you may not. Whatever it is, you need to see a specialist (urologist) to look into the source of the problem and the right treatment for you. If the urologist you see can't help you, find another one right away. Move on. If the urologist recommends a treatment, and that treatment doesn't work in about two weeks, you really should question it. If the urologist says that he is not sure what's happening or says that he hasn't "seen anything like it before", that is very unusual and the urologist is NOT helping you. Find another urologist who will.

* Vida B.A. *(Breast cancer)*

During treatment, I experienced a UTI (urinary tract infection) aka bladder infection problem once. It wasn't really that bad. I just drank cranberry juice and it went away.

ADVICE: If you get a bladder infection or UTI, drinking cranberry juice can help. If not, you should consult your doctor. Drinking lots of fluids can help too.

* Yesi L. *(Breast cancer: triple positive)*

I actually did not experience kidney or bladder problems as a side effect to my cancer treatment. However, I have a lot of experience there because I have always been very prone to getting UTIs (urinary tract infections) ever since I was a child. After many years of speaking with the urologist, we finally came to the conclusion that I should take a low dosage of the antibiotic Nitrofurantoin as a preventive measure. Whenever I think I'm going to have a urine infection, whether it's after intercourse or after a long trip or whenever, I simply take that pill, and it has been a lifesaver.

ADVICE: If you're experiencing kidney or bladder problems, ask your doctor for a prescription of the antibiotic Nitrofurantoin. It has been a lifesaver for me.

LEG, FOOT OR TOE CRAMPS

A cramp is a sudden, involuntary muscle contraction or over-shortening; while generally temporary and non-damaging, they can cause significant pain, and a paralysis-like immobility of the affected muscle. Onset is usually sudden, and it resolves on its own over a period of several seconds, minutes or hours. Cramps may occur in a skeletal muscle or smooth muscle. Skeletal muscle cramps may be caused by muscle fatigue or a lack of electrolytes such as low sodium, low potassium or low magnesium.

* Amor T. *(Breast cancer, Ovarian cancer)*

My toe cramps were something I was kind of used to. However cramps on my feet and calves were something different. I thought it was because I did not drink enough fluids and I was dehydrated. Those charley horses on my feet are really painful! I try not to overextend my feet to where they will cramp. When they do happen, I immediately stand and slowly walk around to get my blood circulation going. Sometimes, I massage the area that's stiff with firm, but gentle rubs and that helps.

ADVICE: When you get foot, leg or toe cramps, immediately stand to get blood flowing down to that area. It also helps to massage the stiffness down with gentle rubs.

* Cindy L. *(Kidney cancer)*

I did get foot cramps, and we didn't know why because my magnesium and potassium levels were right on target. When I first started getting cramps, I would stand straight, hop out of the bed, and just cry; it hurt so bad. The bottoms of my feet just camped so badly. I wasn't dehydrated; I drank between 75 and 100 ounces of water a day to help my kidney functioning. Yes, oh yes. I was like a camel; I drank a lot of water, so the cause of my cramping was a mystery.

What I found helped take care of my foot cramps was Greek yogurt with vitamin D; a lot of it! In fact, I ate Greek yogurt three to four times a week. Greek yogurt, the real thing with vitamin D; not the sugary or sweetened yogurt. I did add Truvia or honey to sweeten my Greek yogurt and also added some vanilla and freshly sliced almonds. It was one of my favorites.

I am also on 3,000 IUs of vitamin D3 per day, per my doctor's orders, as my D3 level is low.

ADVICE: **For foot cramps, try eating Greek yogurt with vitamin D for three to four times a week. Eat the real Greek yogurt with vitamin D; not the sugary or sweetened kinds. Get the real thing. If you want it sweetened, add some Truvia or honey. You can also add some vanilla and freshly sliced almonds. It's one of my favorites. I recommend that you have your D3 level checked.**

* Yesi L. *(Breast cancer: triple positive)*

During treatment, I did not deal with cramps. However, an after-treatment side-effect I'm now dealing with are severe foot cramps. Aside from that, both my feet get very, very, very cold. When cramps happen, I soak them in warm water. Unfortunately, it usually happens in the middle of the night.

ADVICE: **Try soaking your feet in warm water when you get feet cramps. It worked for me.**

LEUKOPENIA / NEUTROPENIA (LOW WHITE BLOOD CELL COUNT)

Leukopenia is a decrease in the number of white blood cells (leukocytes) found in the blood, which places individuals at increased risk of infection. The terms leukopenia and neutropenia may occasionally be used interchangeably, as the neutrophil count is the most important indicator of infection risk

* Amor T. *(Breast cancer. ovarian cancer)*

I had to go through chemo every three weeks for six months from May through September. The day after, Bill would inject the bone marrow stimulant Neulasta subcutaneously into my abdomen, which I preferred, because that's where I felt the least amount of pain. Because chemotherapy lowers the number of infection-fighting white blood cells, which weakens my immune system and increases my risk of infection, my oncologist prescribed the Neulasta shots.

I feel so fortunate to have been able to get those shots, because Neulasta is a very expensive medication. I really did not think I could afford it at $6,000 per shot. I am so blessed to have my nurse case manager at the Cancer Center who arranged for me to get it free.

ADVICE: **Before chemotherapy, blood tests are done to make sure your body is strong enough to take the chemo drugs during infusion. Since strong chemotherapy lowers the number of infection-fighting white blood cells, which may weaken your immune system and increase your risk for infection, it is necessary to make sure you have enough white blood cells after chemo. Ask your doctor if you can get Neulasta and, if possible, make arrangements for you to get it free of charge. It doesn't hurt to ask and it will make you feel much better, if the arrangement works out.**

* Cindy R. *(Metastatic Breast cancer to Stomach)*

Even though my white blood cell count was low, it wasn't so low that I had to take medication for it. It was just kind of a monitored thing. Before getting chemo, I had to get blood tests done to determine if my body had enough white blood cells to take the chemo treatment and if so, what we needed to do. Fortunately, it didn't drop so low that I couldn't get my chemo infusion on schedule.

Of course, as I was going toward my next chemo treatment, I would start to feel better. But then when I went through my next chemo infusion, my white blood cell count dropped again. I knew that it was part of the process. The day after my chemo infusions, I had to return to see my doctor who would give me the Neulasta shots to raise my white blood cell count. Since I had a double mastectomy and lymph nodes were removed, he couldn't inject me in my arms, so he injected the Neulasta into my thighs.

ADVICE: Chemotherapy will cause your white blood cell (WBC) count to go down, which will make you feel weaker. It's expected. Your doctor will closely monitor your WBC count, especially before you're scheduled for your chemo infusion. When it drops to a certain point, your doctor may inject you with Neulasta, a bone marrow stimulant that helps the body make white blood cells.

* Rev. Linda S. (Pancreatic cancer 3x)

Whenever my labs show low blood platelets, oncology sends me home and I try again the following week and again, if necessary, before I can get my chemo. There's nothing I can do about it but let my body rest to increase my WBC count. In the meantime, I will prep dinner for tonight and tomorrow night, eat lunch while watching the last episodes of "The Chew" and take a nap. Afterwards, I will jot down notes for my lesson this Sunday. Making lemonade out of lemons ...

I get Neupogen shots to increase my white blood cell count. Unfortunately, because they dig deeply into my bone marrow to stimulate white blood cell growth, I have to suffer the side effects of bone and joint pain.

ADVICE: When you're faced with a situation you cannot control, you just have to accept it, move on and focus on doing things that make you happy; even simple things like watching TV or taking a nap. You need to do what you can from getting stressed. Same goes for those times when you're in pain. Take medication for relief or just deal with it. It will eventually go away.

* Sondra W. (Ovarian cancer 3x)

There were times when my white blood cell count (WBC) got down so low, I had to have booster shots called Neulasta. They really helped me. On the night of my first infusion, my WBC was so low that they had to give me the Neulasta for five days in a row, which was too much. After that, they learned that I only needed to have three or four shots; not five. This happened during a three-month stretch of winter and the flu season, and I had to stay in the house by myself in isolation. Oh, that was hard.

By the way, when they gave the shots, they always asked me, "Do you want it in your arm or your belly?" And, I'd say, "arm" because I didn't know what it would feel like getting a shot in my belly.

ADVICE: Strong chemo treatments lower your white blood cell count, so your doctor will be monitoring that. If your white blood cell count goes down, you may get shots like Neulasta to stimulate the growth of white blood cells. Those shots certainly help you feel better because when your white blood cell count is low, fatigue and weakness will hit you harder.

* Vida B.A. (Breast cancer)

Because chemotherapy causes the white blood cell count to go down, I was given Granocyte injections (used to boost white blood cells) after my first chemo infusion and four consecutive days thereafter. Unfortunately, despite the Granocyte, I still encountered problems with low white blood cells.

I had an incident when my white blood cell count was low. It was when I had a bad case of diarrhea and a high fever too. I was rushed to the hospital and confined for four days. When they tested me, my white blood cell count was very low, so they gave me more Granocyte injections while I was there.

ACTION: Because strong chemotherapy can lower the number of your infection-fighting white blood cells in your body leading to the weakening of your immune system, you should watch your white blood cell count. If your white cell counts are very low, you may have signs of infections, e.g. fever, chills and sweating, sore throat or swollen lymph nodes. This is dangerous, so let your doctor know immediately, so you can be treated properly to increase your white cell count.

* Yesi L. (Breast cancer: triple positive)

Having a very low white blood cell count is basically what put me in the hospital with Neutropenic Fever twice. I was placed in quarantine in the hospital until my white blood cell count came back up. I was also injected with Neulasta, a bone marrow stimulant that helped my body produce white blood cells. I actually hated the Neulasta shots because they made my bones hurt even though I knew the shots were what I needed to increase my white blood cell count.

LOSS OF APPETITE

Appetite loss is a common side effect of cancer treatment. People with poor appetite may eat less than usual, not feel hungry at all, or feel full after eating only a small amount. Ongoing appetite loss may lead to serious complications, such as fatigue, weakness from muscle loss, weight loss, not getting the nutrients that our body needs.

* Amor T. (Breast cancer. ovarian cancer)

I really just didn't feel like eating. Looking at food, it was not inviting. And, when I did eat food, it either tasted bland or it nauseated me. So, I didn't have any much appetite. Because I knew that I needed sustenance in order for my body to heal, I forced myself to eat. I had crackers, which I topped with something sweet like a little dollop of grape or strawberry jelly or my favorite, cocoa jam. The sweetness did spark interest in my taste buds.

ADVICE: Even if you don't have an appetite, just eat something, because your body needs nutrients in order to heal. If the food tastes bland, add a little sweetness, like a dollop of grape or strawberry jelly or jam to get your taste buds to wake up. Try eating 5-6 small meals a day. That way, your body stands a better chance of getting the nutrients it needs versus just eating once or when you feel like it, which is probably a rare occasion, when you lose your appetite due to cancer treatment.

* Bob G. (Soft Tissue Sarcoma, Skin cancer)

I was in the CT scan procedure for an hour and 45 minutes. The technician knew what he was looking for, but he couldn't find it. It was hidden I think. It must've been covered by a lot. When my family and I went up to Tahoe, I noticed that I couldn't eat. I tried to eat some food, but just couldn't. The next day, the problem went away. When we went to the hospital for my surgery, the doctors took their time. It looked like they weren't sure what they were going to do.

* Cindy L. (Kidney cancer)

In the first couple of weeks after surgery, I could hardly eat and quickly lost five pounds. This was due to the type of surgery I had where my surgeon, using the hand-assisted device, had to literally push all my guts out of the way to get to my left kidney. So, my guts were just bruised and tender, so that I could barely eat for a couple of weeks. After my body healed with time, my appetite returned.

ADVICE: Let your doctor and nurses know if you're unable to keep food down, so that they can guide you. It's important to understand what's happening in your body. That way, you'll know what you need to do or what to expect.

* Joan S. (Rectal cancer)

When I was going through treatment, I just had no appetite whatsoever. To make sure my body had the food that it needed to heal, I bought the super power drink from Costco, Premier Protein.

> **ADVICE:** You need food to heal. So, even if you don't have appetite, you must eat something. Try taking Premier Protein. It's a power drink, a nutrition shake, which has a lot of nutrients. You can buy it at Costco and Target.

* J.B. (Salivary gland cancer)

I definitely had a loss of appetite. This was an awful side effect. I had to go to a dietitian who recommended that I just force myself to eat even if I didn't feel like eating to keep my weight up. Because, if I didn't eat, my body would respond, and I would weaken myself. I was told to eat regular food and keep hydrated, which was very important. I was also told to eat foods that were high in protein. I was given a brand of protein milk drink, which really helped how I felt throughout the day. The brand is ORGAIN and they gave me coupons to buy it at Whole Foods. I would drink a 12 oz. bottle of ORGAIN whenever I had a hard time eating anything.

> **ADVICE:** My advice, which was given by my dietitian, is to eat even if you don't feel like eating. Eat foods that are high in protein and be sure to keep hydrated. Drinking the ORGAIN brand protein milk will also help you keep your weight up. It really helped me when I had a hard time eating anything.

* Rev. Linda S. (Pancreatic cancer 3x)

I lost my appetite during both my rounds with cancer and lost a lot of weight because of it. After surgery, I had no desire to eat for several weeks. On the days I receive chemo, I have no desire to eat. Though my appetite has been funky, I know I need to eat, as I lose a pound or two each week, which I cannot sustain. I now take Megace every six hours to stimulate my appetite and am able to eat well while maintaining my new weight of 132 lbs.

> **ADVICE:** Even you don't feel like eating, eat something. Your body needs food to heal.

* Scott M. (Metastatic Colon cancer to the Prostate & Pancreas)

One of the reasons I lost my appetite was because of the nausea I got from taking Xeloda. Another time, after going through so many procedures, I lost a lot of weight and food just turned my stomach. One day, my sister-in-law brought me a turkey sandwich for lunch. Looking at the whole plate of food was just enough to gag me. So she took the sandwich, cut a one-inch square of bread out of it, put one little, tiny, one-inch square of turkey on the bread and one drop of mayo or of mustard ... put it together ... and set it on the corner of my tray and had the rest of the food removed from the room. That tiny one-inch turkey sandwich sat on the corner of my tray, and I kept looking at it. Then I thought, "You know, I do like turkey, and that's not very much. So, I could probably try that." So, I put it in my mouth; I tasted it and I liked it! And, from that, I was able to slowly come out; reintroduce food into my system. My aversion to food might have been caused by PTSD (Post Traumatic Stress Disorder).

I had lost 70 lbs. weighing only about 130 lbs. Everybody thought I was going to die. Of course, nobody told me that then. Thank God, because that thought <u>never</u> crossed my mind! I knew that I was going to pull out of this ... it was just a matter of time.

> **ADVICE:** Sometimes, when your body is going through a lot of changes and procedures, it gets overwhelmed and decides to shut down. When that happens, it helps to reintroduce things very gradually like food. Keep in mind that your eyes play a large part in determining what food to eat. So, start with a little piece of your favorite food (for example, the one-inch piece of turkey sandwich I was given) and then work your way up in size. The biggest thing is to <u>never</u> give up. No matter how hard you're struggling, keep in mind that you're going to pull out of your struggles; it's just a matter of time.

* Susan M. *(Ovarian cancer. Metastatic Pancreatic cancer to the Lung)*

Pancreatic cancer: I didn't feel like eating at all, so I had to follow a strict diet for several months to get my stomach used to food again.

> **ADVICE:** With stomach surgery, you need to gradually introduce food in small portions. Even if you are not hungry, eat a little of something, as your body needs the nourishment to heal.

* Vida B.A. *(Breast cancer)*

Oh, I definitely experienced loss of appetite, which was caused by being nauseated from my chemo treatments. Good thing I had anti-nausea medication. I didn't eat as much as I used to. But, I tried to eat healthy food with more nutrients like rice or porridge with chicken and ginger, misua (a very, very fine rice noodle soup with meatballs), etc. Even though I didn't feel like eating, I knew I had to force myself to eat because I needed food for strength and energy to heal.

> **ADVICE:** Even if you don't have an appetite, you have to eat something. If you don't get the nutrients your body needs to get more energy and be stronger, you won't be able to heal. If nausea is what causes you to lose your appetite, ask for anti-nausea medication. Eating ginger or drinking ginger tea can also help when you get nauseated.

LUNG PROBLEMS

Chemotherapy and radiation therapy to the chest may damage the lungs. Cancer survivors who received both chemotherapy and radiation therapy may have a higher risk of lung damage.

* Amor T. *(Breast cancer. ovarian cancer)*

Pleural effusion: After my third chemo session, I informed my oncologist that when I breathed, I heard gurgling sounds; something he heard too when he examined me. So, he sent me to get a CT scan. The results showed a "large" pleural effusion (fluid buildup) in my right lung, multiple enlarged nodes in the space between both lungs (mediastinum) and around my left breast/armpit area and a 7cm soft tissues mass at the vagina cuff. My oncologist was "highly suspicious for progression of one or both" of my cancers. When I read that message, my heart sank a bit, but it didn't deter me from continuing my fight. So, I met with a pulmonologist and my OB/gynecologist for further examination of the findings. My pulmonologist then arranged for me to get a thoracentesis to remove the fluid buildup from my right lung.

Before the procedure, one of my nurses told me that the thoracentesis is quick and painless and I would need only Tylenol for any discomfort. Well, just to make doubly sure, I decided to take a vicodin. At the hospital, I had a wonderful nurse who prepped me, took my x-ray and was with me for the entire procedure. I was sitting on the exam table when the doctor came in. He described what he was going to do and told me to just still. He then inserted a hollow needle between the ribs in my back. It was a really weird feeling, especially as he slowly pushed deeper and deeper. Under my breath, I started to sing the song, "*I'm in the Mood for Love.*" Those in the room were very surprised. After all, it was a strange thing to do out of the blue. I was able to run quietly through two stanzas when my nurse gently said I should stop singing, because the doctor didn't want to make a wrong move and needed me to keep really still. I was shedding quiet tears and asked her if I could hold her hands. She said, "Of course" and that helped me through the rest of the procedure.

So what did I feel to cause me to sing or cry? Well, when I felt the needle pushing through, I immediately needed to distract myself and the first thing I could think of to achieve that was to sing. I cried, because feeling the surprising pressure of the needle going deep down into me was frightening. It was a weird feeling and even though I didn't feel sharp pains, it was a bit painful.

After the procedure, I asked to see the excess fluid that was removed and they showed me a large container filled with a yellow liquid that looked like frothy beer. The doctor had drained almost four quarts of fluid from my pleural cavity. It kind of looked like beer (yellow liquid with froth on the top). Fortunately, to date, the excess fluid hasn't returned.

Atelectasis: Since I had gone through many surgeries that required anesthesia (c-section, colposcopy, hysterectomy, mastectomy/diep flap breast reconstruction), the CT scans showed that I have atelectasis or partial collapse of my right lung. I don't really notice it, except when I try to sing in church and find that I'm easily short of breath. Hopefully, with my breathing exercises, my right lung will return to normal soon.

> **ADVICE :** Be aware of changes in your breathing and let your doctor know if you notice something is off. If you're short of breath, try breathing exercises, like this one:
> - Get into a comfortable position, e.g. lie on your back with your knees bent, sit up on a chair on bed or lie on your side.
> - Gently place your hand on your stomach and feel it rise and fall when you inhale and exhale
> - Inhale slowly through your nose and hold for three seconds
> - Exhale very slowly by blowing air out in one long, slow breath.
> - Take another deep breath and repeat five times.

LYMPHEDEMA

A condition in which extra lymph fluid builds up in tissues and causes swelling. It may occur in an arm or leg if lymph vessels are blocked, damaged, or removed by surgery.

* Aaron C. (Prostate cancer, Skin cancer)

During the surgery, my doctor removed about 20-30 inflamed lymph nodes from my groin area. He didn't want to take a chance, so he removed them. Because of that, my body had to learn to get rid of unwanted fluids that those lymph nodes were responsible for. According to my doctor, about five percent of patients will experience lymphedema due to removal of the lymph nodes. However, it'll go away after six months. So, I went through six months of swelling, especially in my ankles.

My ankles swelled, especially when I stayed on my feet for a long time, or if I ate too much salt or sodium. I had to be really careful about what I ate. Yesterday they were swollen. Today they are a little better.

> **ADVICE:** If your ankles, feet or leg swells because of the lymphedema, sit down or lay on your back and then raise your legs up a little bit. That helps alleviate the swelling. Also, watch your salt and sodium intake. Be aware of the kinds of food you eat. You'd be surprised how much sodium is in everything.

* Amor T. (Breast cancer. ovarian cancer)

Breast cancer: During my mastectomy, some lymph nodes were removed from my left armpit area. I did feel a little swelling after the surgery, but that dissipated. Where I felt the lymphedema was in my abdominal area where tissue for my diep flap breast reconstruction was taken. My abdomen was pretty swollen, so I wore a compression girdle.

Ovarian cancer. During my radical hysterectomy surgery, a periaortic lymphadenectomy, where lymph nodes in my pelvis were removed, was also done. That caused me to swell in my abdominal area. However, it didn't seem to cause me continuous problems, like lymphedema. Thank God!

> **ADVICE:** Light exercise, in which you move the affected part of your body (arm, leg, etc.) and massage encourage lymph fluid drainage. For the abdominal region, massage helps to move the lymph fluid. Compression girdles also help.

* Cindy R. (Metastatic Breast cancer to Stomach)

I did have swelling in my right arm because during my double mastectomy, they removed 12 lymph nodes from the area around my right arm. So, there were times when my arm would swell up, and I couldn't bend it, especially in the heat. The lymph nodes are the ones that take the toxins and move them throughout the body, so without them, the fluid with the toxins just sits there. It was miserable, but there were a couple of things that helped.

One was the light exercise because moving around and getting the blood flowing is important. And the other was wearing the compression sleeve on my right arm. That helped with the blood flow too. Compression sleeves are expensive. However, since they're part of my treatment, I got my insurance to pay for them. Insurance also covered the cost of my breast prosthetics too.

ADVICE: Lymphedema can be pretty miserable, especially when it's hot. However, there are ways to move the toxins and keep them from just sitting in one place (e.g. arms, legs) in your body.

1. Do some light exercise. Moving around will get your blood flowing and your circulation going.
2. If you have lymphedema in your arms, buy compression sleeves for your arms. If you have lymphedema elsewhere in your body (knees, legs, abdomen, etc.), you can get compression garments for those areas too. Check online on Amazon and similar sites. Since you got your lymphedema [from cancer], get your insurance to pay for the compression garment. Check with them before buying anything to make sure you follow their instructions for purchase or reimbursement.

Check out the American Cancer Society too. They can help you on a variety of things when it comes to your treatment. Low cost or no cost. They really help.

* Joan S. (Rectal cancer)

After surgery, I experienced swelling in my right leg. I kept my leg elevated to bring the swelling down.

ADVICE: If you experience swelling in your legs as a side effect of treatment, elevate them. That will help bring the swelling down.

* Rachel S. (Breast cancer: triple negative)

When I had a double mastectomy, they removed all the lymph nodes from my right arm and only two lymph nodes from my left arm. I got lymphedema because I no longer had lymph nodes in my right arm. My right arm doesn't have the capability anymore to push the poison fluids – for lack of a better word – from my arm, in order for me to urinate them out. So, I have to wear a compression sleeve every day for the rest of my life. There are days when I can't move my arm. It feels like there's a bar going down my arm and it's hard to straighten it. And the only thing I can do for that is to exercise and to stretch it out. It usually lasts a couple of days. And then I have to constantly massage my arm and my spine to keep the swelling down because once the arm starts to swell, it's very, very difficult to get it to go back to normal.

ADVICE: If you have lymphedema, use compression sleeves and garments to help bring down the swelling. You can also stretch it out, massage the area and also elevate it. Be proactive and do it constantly, because once you start to swell, it's very difficult to get it back to normal.

* Vida B.A. (Breast cancer)

My left arm swelled after my mastectomy, definitely one of the side effects from surgery that I had to deal with. So, my doctor suggested that I buy a lymphedema compression wrap for my arm to help with the circulation. The compression wraps are stretchable and look like a socks or leggings with openings on both ends.

Since I had lymphedema in my left arm, and I knew that the cabin pressure on the flight to New Zealand would cause my arm to swell, I bought a compression sleeve to wear on the plane. The purpose was to apply pressure on my arm to prevent lymphatic fluid from building up. Unfortunately, my arm swelled up as the plane was making its steep climb up to cruising altitude. It was so painful. So I ended up removing it, which was a relief. For the rest of the flight, I tried to relax my swollen arm and lightly massage it.

* Yesi L. (Breast cancer: triple positive)

Three of the lymph nodes around the right breast area where my cancer was found were tested and one came back with microscopic signs of cancer. So, all three were removed. Since they were considering me for a complete lymph node dissection, I begged them to bring my case up to the Tumor Board, so I could keep the rest of my lymph nodes. I had responded so well to the chemo treatment that all my cancerous tumor disappeared. I told them that I'm young, and I like to play tennis. I love to garden, and I use my right arm for everything. I completely depend on my right arm.

I understood that it's standard procedure for those who have breast cancer to remove all the lymph nodes. However, I also understood that there was no evidence to prove that doing so would increase my risk of recurrence. So I asked, "Why do I have to remove them all?" The *Tumor Board discussed my case and decided not to remove the rest of my lymph nodes. So I got very, very lucky.

[*A "Tumor Board" is a group of doctors and other specialists that meet regularly to discuss cancer cases, share knowledge and determine the best possible cancer treatment and care for certain patients.]

ADVICE: If your doctor says they need to remove all your lymph nodes even though treatment to remove your tumors was successful, ask for your case to be brought up to the Tumor Board.

MOUTH, TEETH, GUM AND/OR TONGUE CHANGES

Many cancer treatments, including chemotherapy and radiation can affect an individual's dental and oral health. Dental and oral health refers to the well-being of the entire mouth, including the teeth, gums, lining of the mouth (mucosa), and glands that produce saliva (salivary glands). Oral complications can make it difficult to eat, talk, chew or swallow. These problems can affect a patient's health and quality of life. They can even affect a patient's ability to complete treatment.

* Amor T. (Breast cancer. ovarian cancer)

During treatment, I noticed that the surface of my tongue turned pasty white. I didn't do anything about it, because it wasn't hurting and I had other, more important things to think about. I also thought it was just normal. However, when my sister, Joy, came to visit, she noticed my white, pasty tongue and said it wasn't normal. I later learned that I had oral thrush, which is an overgrowth of fungus due to the temporary impairment of the white blood cells caused by the chemotherapy. I had no idea, until my sister mentioned it. Since then, I would brush my entire tongue after I brush my teeth. Now, my tongue has a nice, healthy pink color.

ADVICE: It's easy to take the tongue for granted. After all, it just "exists" in our mouth with no apparent function, except to taste. Well, bacteria, fungi, dirt, food and dead cells can all get trapped in the tongue and cause health problems. So, brush your tongue everyday after brushing your teeth. You will be healthier because of it.

* Glenn M. (Metastatic Colon cancer to the Liver, Lungs & Adrenal Glands)

I've got dry mouth, but it's not too aggressive. It's easy to deal with. I just keep bottles of water or something to drink handy.

ADVICE: Just keep bottles of water or something to drink handy when your mouth gets dry.

* Hilda K. (Colon cancer)

My gums and my tongue turned black, one of the side effects I experienced from my chemotherapy. They were also sensitive, but not overly. They didn't bleed, or anything like that. Because my gums and tongue were sensitive to cold, I made sure I drank warm temperature water or liquids like soup. Eventually, my gums and tongue returned to their normal pink color.

ADVICE: If your gums and/or tongue turn black from the chemo, just remember that it's temporary; a side effect of your treatment. Also, they're only surface changes. Just remember to drink warm liquids to keep your gums and your tongue comfortable.

* J.B. (Salivary gland cancer)

I didn't have mouth or teeth changes, but that's because I was really conscientious about the effects of the radiation on my back teeth, which the beam kept hitting during treatment. So, I made sure to really go double time on my oral hygiene.

The medical team told me that oral hygiene was especially important because radiation therapy around the area of my mouth definitely weakens my teeth, which will then make my teeth susceptible to bacteria. Here is a mouthwash formula they gave me to use every day.

Combine one (1) tablespoon of salt with one (1) tablespoon of baking soda
Mix the salt and baking soda solution into water to make a mouthwash

To this day, I continue the practice.

ADVICE: If you'll be getting radiation treatment around your mouth area, then it's especially important to protect your teeth, so they don't weaken and attract bacteria. Use the easy mouthwash formula the medical team gave me above. It helps.

* Rev. Linda S. (Pancreatic cancer 3x)

For my second series of chemotherapy treatments, I experienced my tongue getting thick, rendering me incapable of enunciating clearly. Fortunately, it dissipated.

* Rachel S. (Breast cancer: triple negative)

When I experienced dry mouth, a friend of mine gave me this mouthwash and mouth spray, so I used that. And I just drank a ton of water, too.

ADVICE: If it's really bad, ask your doctor for a prescription mouthwash and/or mouth spray. Drinking tons of water also helps.

* Scott M. (Metastatic Colon cancer to the Prostate & Pancreas)

I did experience dry mouth, as well as mouth ulcers where my tongue and my cheeks were constantly sloughing cells. Avastin prevents new cell growth. So I got these spots on my tongue where new cells didn't form, but the old cells had already sloughed off. They looked like little pits in my tongue or on my cheeks. Since my tongue would get raw, I avoided Mexican foods, salsa, spices and jalapeno at that time. Somebody suggested that I should get the Stanford mouthwash. I researched it and found there's actually five different formulas of the Stanford mouthwash, so I have three of them. Also, there's a product that kind of keeps your mouth moist ... Biotin. I use that too; it keeps the mouth moist and it prevents dry mouth. But when my mouth gets really sore, one of the Stanford mouthwashes has lidocaine in it and some other things. It's a prescription that you have to get from a pharmacy that mixes stuff; not a regular pharmacy.

ADVICE: If your tongue is raw, avoid spicy or hot foods. Check out the Stanford mouthwash (there are five different formulas). Biotin is another product that keeps your mouth moist and prevents dry mouth. If your mouth gets really sore, one of the Stanford mouthwashes has lidocaine in it and some other things. It's a prescription that you have to get from a pharmacy that mixes stuff; not a regular pharmacy.

* Sondra W. (Ovarian cancer 3x)

I did experience dark spots on my tongue when I was going through treatment. They didn't cause any pain and didn't bother me. After chemo, they just disappeared, and my tongue returned to its normal pink color.

ADVICE: There's really nothing to do when you get dark spots on your tongue. It's just a temporary thing and will disappear after treatment.

* Vida B.A. (Breast cancer)

I had difficulty swallowing, eating, chewing and, even talking because my mouth was constantly dry. I also had canker sores in my mouth, which were painful. My doctor prescribed an ointment that I had to apply on my sores. It looked like lard, but it was really good and relieved me of the pain.

For my dry mouth, I just drank plenty of fluids and made sure I followed a strict oral hygiene to keep the bacteria away. I also kept with me a cherry-flavored lip balm that I applied to my lips every time it became dry.

ACTION: If you have any sores in your mouth, you must inform your doctor immediately. If your mouth is dry, drink plenty of fluids to keep your mouth moist and avoid dehydration. Make sure you follow strict oral hygiene, like brushing your teeth (at least) twice a day. Keep some lip balm with you, so you can apply it to your lips anytime it feels dry.

* Yesi L. (Breast cancer: triple positive)

The mouth sores for me were excruciatingly painful! I had to go into treatment for Invisalign (basically, clear braces). Because my gums were sensitive and the Invisalign tray had some hard/sharp edges, I had to remove them because they cut inside my mouth and I got really bad mouth sores. I had the Invisalign removed and resumed after completion of my cancer treatment. To treat my mouth sores, I was given a special mixture to gargle, like mouthwash. It contained liquid Benadryl, along with a prescription my doctor gave me (I don't remember the name). When I gargled it, my mouth felt like it was burning, but it definitely worked.

I also experienced dry "cotton" mouth. I just constantly rinsed out my mouth with cold spearmint tea. That really helped.

ADVICE: If you experience mouth sores, ask your oncologist or doctor for a prescription mixture for you to gargle like a mouthwash. You can get liquid Benadryl over the counter, but you'll need the prescription for the other half of the mixture. For dry "cotton" mouth, rinse your mouth regularly with cold spearmint tea.

MUSCLE PAIN / MYALGIA

Myalgias can be defined as muscle aches. They can feel like a deep, constant, dull ache, or a sharp, sporadic ache. Myalgias are often a result of some chemotherapy treatments, infections, prolonged muscle use, and other inflammatory conditions.

* Amor T. (Breast cancer. ovarian cancer)

During my treatment period, I experienced muscle pain that I would describe as "weird." They felt like quick "lightning bolts" that were hitting both my muscles and bones directly and then would twitch. I also felt prickling, tingling, coldness and numbing sensations too. There were times when, out of the blue, I would jump, because the lightning bolts would strike. Sometimes, I experienced several lightning bolts in quick succession, which were really tiring, given that my body would already be on high alert, bracing to prepare for another hit. Whew!

I experienced a lot of muscle cramps in my shins, calves, feet and toes during treatment and I still do to this day, although not as frequently. I did, however, recently suffer from charley horses (sudden, involuntary contractions of one or more muscles) in both my legs that woke me up in the middle of the night several times. Those blasted cramps are excruciatingly painful!

What I would immediately do is stand up, press down on my toes (to get them to unsnarl), walk around (to get the circulation going) and try to relax my body and muscles. Sometimes, I also rub and massage my legs and feet to soften up the muscles. Eventually, the cramps go away.

For prevention of muscle cramps, I believe that drinking plenty of water, eating bananas (high in potassium) and taking daily multivitamins, magnesium, zinc and potassium supplements.

ADVICE: For muscle cramps, drink plenty of water, eat foods high in potassium (bananas) and take multivitamins, magnesium, zinc and potassium supplements. When the cramps happen, stand up, press down on your toes and walk around to get the blood circulation going. It would also help to relax and not tense up, else it gets worse. If you're experiencing the same "lightning bolts" I experienced, you just have to tough it out. Unfortunately, it can hit you when you least expect it. Fortunately, it's fleeting and doesn't really hurt; it's just annoying and uncomfortable.

* Rev. Linda S. *(Pancreatic cancer 3x)*

Yes, I experienced muscle pain. Again, Tylenol helped.

ADVICE: Use Tylenol or whatever painkiller works for you.

* Rachel S. *(Breast cancer: triple negative)*

My muscles still get really sore. I've been trying to start strengthening my muscles a little bit more by starting to do my walks again and using the bicycle at home. Also, I started drinking 2% milk again. Cheese sticks are my go-to snacks.

* Vida B.A. *(Breast cancer)*

Yes, I experienced muscle cramps in my calves, as well as, my feet. Sometimes, I would get them when I'm in bed at 4:00am! When I got the cramps, I just tried to stretch my calves or my feet and, eventually, the cramps went away.

ACTION: If you get cramps in your calves or feet, just ty to stretch and massage the cramped muscles. The cramps will eventually go away.

NAIL CHANGES / BRITTLE NAIL SYNDROME

Brittle nail syndrome is a heterogeneous abnormality, characterized by increased fragility of the nail plate. Brittle nails affect about 20% of the population and women are affected twice as frequently as men.

Nail changes are common during chemotherapy and can include the development of lines as well as changes in the color or shape of your nails. The loss of nails may also occur, especially with chemotherapy drugs such as taxanes. If you do develop what appears to be an infection around your nails, talk to your oncologist.

* **Cindy R.** (*Metastatic Breast cancer to Stomach*)

During treatment, my nails got very brittle. They didn't turn black, but they warped and curved a little bit and then straightened out. It was a really weird sensation, but it was just cosmetic. So, I didn't do anything to them. I just noticed how strange they became.

* **Glenn M.** (*Metastatic Colon cancer to the Liver, Lungs & Adrenal Glands*)

I had quite a lot of nail changes. The worst case involved the skin bleeding on each side of my fingernails and toenails because the nails were just slicing through the thinning skin surrounding them. I got it on both my big toes really bad, and they were so painful that I was limping terribly at one point. I saw a wonderful dermatologist who, after evaluating my skin and nails, said, "I think it's the Xeloda" (one of my chemo drugs). She then put me on antibiotics and gave me a 2.5 steroid ointment to get my problem under control. It's pretty well controlled now...slowly healing. I also wear gloves to protect my hands.

ADVICE: Once you see nail changes and, especially, the skin thinning around your nails, let your doctor know, so that your doctor can prescribe an antibiotic or other medication for you. See a dermatologist if necessary. Just don't wait for the problem to get worse.

* **Hilda K.** (*Colon cancer*)

Because my body was soaked with the chemotherapy drugs, all of my fingernails and toenails turned black. They were sensitive, but not overly. I was given anti-anxiety medication to relax me when I was first given the pump. Although the medication helped me to relax in the evenings, I avoided it because I didn't want to depend on it. Eventually, I got used to the pump, and I learned to emotionally and mentally just chill and not be oversensitive about everything. I just kind of like took it easy and learned not to overthink things. I just tried to relax and kept positive because I knew my attitude would affect my recovery.

ADVICE: If your nails turn black from the chemo, just remember that it's temporary; a side effect of your treatment. Also, they're only surface changes. The main thing to do is just relax; just chill. Try to be positive about everything because your attitude will affect your recovery. So, keep it positive, as much as possible.

* **Scott M.** (*Metastatic Colon cancer to the Prostate & Pancreas*)

My fingernails and toenails chipped really easy, and they still do. They're very thin and brittle and they crack and tear really easily too. I keep them really, really short; biting them down when I don't have a nail clipper with me.

ADVICE: Just keep your nails really short, so they don't unexpectedly rip.

* **Sondra W.** (*Ovarian cancer 3x*)

Oh yeah, my nails definitely changed when I was going through treatment. They turned black! Funny thing was how my nails on one hand were darker than the ones on my other hand. So I thought to myself, "How did I do this?" After my first treatment, I noticed that my normal nail color was returning. But then, they turned black again when I had go through my second treatment. I was told that the Avastin was the one causing my hands and nails to turn dark.

ADVICE: Nail changes are just surface changes that are temporary. If it really bothers you, you can get a nice manicure to cover up your dark nails. Otherwise, don't worry about it.

* Tet M. *(Colon cancer 3x)*

My nails and fingertips darkened from chemotherapy.

ADVICE: Wear it as a badge of honor. It's a cosmetic thing and will diminish after the full treatment is completed.

* Vida B.A. *(Breast cancer)*

During treatment, my toenails and fingers turned blackish. They were also soft and brittle and very delicate. Because I wanted to protect my nails and not do anything to destroy them, I didn't apply any nail polish to them during the whole chemo process.

ADVICE: Since the chemotherapy drugs going through your entire body are toxic, they'll affect your nails. So, it's best to hold off on applying any nail polish to your fingernails and toenails to protect them. You can apply them after treatment.

* Yesi L. *(Breast cancer: triple positive)*

Yes, my nails did become brittle from the chemo drugs. One of my toe nails even fell off because it was so brittle. Before falling off, it turned kind of purplish almost like a fungal type. My fingernails were paper thin and extremely weak.

I didn't really do much for the nails. I just let it be. I knew it was a side effect of the chemo, but it wasn't really affecting me, so I just kind of dealt with it.

NAUSEA & VOMITING

Nausea is an uneasiness of the stomach that often accompanies the urge to vomit, but doesn't always lead to vomiting. Vomiting is the forcible voluntary or involuntary emptying ("throwing up") of stomach contents through the mouth.

* Amor T. *(Breast cancer. ovarian cancer)*

Breast cancer: During my weeklong stay at the hospital following my mastectomy and diep flap breast reconstruction surgery, I enjoyed wonderful, savory food from the hospital's dining room. When I landed back in the hospital because of a staph infection, I thought that I could order the same delicious, savory food I had before. When my wonderful friends and fellow lions from the Foster City Lions Club came to visit me, my delicious, savory lunch order arrived. I immediately noticed that the aroma was not making me excited, like it did before. Nevertheless, one of my friends (Chris) offered to help feed me as I was still shivering uncontrollably. After I took the first spoonful of the "delicious" shrimp stir fry I had ordered, I just gagged. Still, I swallowed the food, but then immediately, my stomach turned. I threw up everything I had eaten and then some. I was so nauseated; I did not understand why.

Following that incident, I decided to just eat simple crackers, light soup and Jell-O until I was able to take in heavier foods.

Ovarian cancer. I experienced some nausea after my hysterectomy and had to take some of the anti-nausea medication my oncologist prescribed. It wasn't too bad.

During chemotherapy, I experienced some nausea too, but not so much that I would hurl. All I had to do was eat some fresh ginger (like the one they give you when you eat out for sushi), drink fresh ginger tea, which I made myself or suck on ginger candy, which I got from the cancer center. I especially liked the ginger candy with chopped peanuts. Since I liked the ginger candy and they worked to get rid of my nausea, I bought a bunch to keep in my bags (4 per bag), my car, and of course, at home. When I was nauseated, I found that a little smidgen of jam or jelly also helped. Slowly sipping whatever I was drinking helped too.

I was given two prescription medications for chemotherapy-induced nausea medications, with the following instructions:

1. At the first sign of nausea, take Ondansetron (8mg).
2. If Ondansetron doesn't work, then take Metoclopramide (10mg).

When I took either one, I really didn't notice a difference. That is perhaps, due to the fact that my nausea wasn't so pronounced. I attribute my body's ability to cope with side effects of chemotherapy to the L-Glutamine that my oncologist instructed me to take every day.

> **ADVICE:** Before you take any medication for nausea, try eating ginger candy or anything with ginger. Keep a small supply of candy in your bags, in case you get nauseous while on the road. L-Glutamine powder is awesome in strengthening our immune system. So, please try to take it everyday to strengthen your body and heal quickly.

* Cindy L. (Kidney cancer)

My experience with queasiness was very strange. It would come about as an indescribably, odd sensation right before I got my hot flashes. Right after I got queasy, I got really hot. Then I got freezing cold for a while. Yes, it was very strange.

I never had to take anything for my queasiness because for one, it was very brief (like my stomach was just not right) and kind of just went away. Two years post surgery, I rarely get nausea except before a hot flash still, which has also decreased tremendously over time.

* Cindy R. (Metastatic Breast cancer to Stomach)

Breast cancer. The chemo drug Taxol caused my bones to ache and also made me nauseous. The one thing that really helped when I felt nauseous was eating a little something. I like grits, so I would eat a bowl of grits. When I felt nauseous in the middle of the night, I would get up and eat a little something. Then in the morning, I no longer felt nauseous. I wasn't on any kind of diet or eating schedule. I wasn't like, "Oh, I gotta cut this out and cut that out." No. Whatever I could eat to keep up my strength, I ate.

Stomach cancer. This time around, the Ibrance pill that I had to take for my stomach cancer sometimes made me nauseous. So, they gave me Zoloft, which was a "melt-away" that I placed underneath my tongue. It helped when I couldn't swallow pills because my throat hurt. They also gave me suppositories (they go up the rear end), in case I couldn't keep stuff down. Nausea is nausea. When you get it bad, it doesn't matter what orifice it [the medication] goes into.

> **ADVICE:** Since the cancer treatment drugs are strong, they can cause nausea. When you get nauseous, try eating a little something like grits. If your experience with nausea is strong, let your doctor know, so that she or he can prescribe some anti-nausea medication to help you. It may come in the form of a regular tablet, pill, capsule or melt-a-way (like Zoloft) or suppositories.

* Glenn M. (Metastatic Colon cancer to the Liver, Lungs & Adrenal Glands)

When I got nauseated and needed relief, I turned to one of my favorite meds, Marinol. I didn't really take it that much. One doctor told me, "If you're using Marinol for nausea, take two 5 mg capsules." Well, two 5mg capsules gives me a nice three-to-four hour high. Very nice. It's not like smoking marijuana or weed because it's synthetic, and they pull all the bad stuff out, so it's tuned. I think it shows promise for appetite too.

In fact, we're giving it to my 97-year old mother, and it's helping her. It helps her mood and her appetite; it's something else! We talked to her doctor and he's on board with giving her 5 mgs. Also, my brother and I figured out how to split the capsules: Freeze them solid. Then, put them in the pill-splitter, split them and take it. You might have to take them with some food. We were able to reduce her dose, so she didn't notice she was high.

* Jacki S. (Breast cancer)

I experienced nausea only with the first chemo treatment, which the nurses took care of with just one pill. After that, I was fine; no more nausea.

* Joan S. (Rectal cancer)

I got an infection, an abscess. And when I ate, I got nauseated, so I threw up all the time. They had to bring me to the hospital to check out what was going on in my body. I took anti-nausea pills when needed.

My wonderful friends and family would make my favorite dishes and, of course, I would try them. Unfortunately, the food just didn't agree with me, at that time, and I gagged and got nauseated. Everybody felt bad for me. But, that's just how it was then. Now, I can enjoy my favorite dishes again, in moderation. I am so very thankful to everyone for all they did to try to make me feel good. I am truly blessed!

* Rev. Linda S. (Pancreatic cancer 3x)

I have "tons" of anti-nausea and anti-vomiting meds to take if I need them. I have also been instructed to take them before my stomach feels sour or queasy. Instead, I've found I must take them when I have doubts about eating. During chemo, I take anti-nausea pills and the anti-nausea drug Aloxi, which is infused intravenously. They have helped to control the nausea well.

* Scott M. (Metastatic Colon cancer to the Prostate & Pancreas)

The nausea I experienced was a side effect of my taking the chemo drug Xeloda. When I was nauseous, I didn't feel like doing anything. I did have a couple of anti-nausea drugs I could take. One was Reglan and the other was Ondansetron. I gave each one an hour to work, and they didn't. So, at that point, I smoked a little pot (marijuana), and it worked almost immediately. I got it from a neighbor, so it wasn't the medical one. I personally didn't like the high it gave me, but it did work to get rid of my nausea.

* Susan M. (Ovarian cancer. Metastatic Pancreatic cancer to the Lung)

I was extremely nauseated and vomited a lot during my treatment for Ovarian cancer. After the nausea continued for about a week, fortunately, I had no vomiting. I ate a lot of saltine crackers to calm my nausea. Surprisingly, I found from Monday "doughnut days" at work that the doughnuts helped to settle my stomach. So when I got nauseated, I would buy a dozen doughnuts and eat half the box, leaving the rest for my co-workers.

> **ADVICE:** Eating saltine crackers help when you're nauseated. Also, find a food that settles your stomach, like the doughnuts that settled my stomach. If nausea medication is prescribed, take it.

* Tet M. *(colon cancer 3x)*

Anticipating a chemo session made me feel nauseated. My nausea seemed to grow as I continued receiving my chemo treatments. I can't quite explain it. I just know that at one time when the nurse was about to insert the needle into my arm, the lunch I ate before the treatment came back out.

> **ADVICE:** Try to distract yourself with hobbies. Chew gum, watch funny or uplifting movies. If you feel like it, hang out with someone who makes you laugh till it hurts (in a good way). Remember that this is only temporary.

NEUROPATHY / NUMBNESS

Neuropathy is nerve problem that causes pain, numbness, tingling, swelling, or muscle weakness in different parts of the body. It usually begins in the hands or feet and gets worse over time. It may be caused by cancer or cancer treatment such as chemotherapy. It may also be caused by physical injury, infection, toxic substances, or conditions such as diabetes, kidney failure, or malnutrition. Also called peripheral neuropathy.

Numbness describes a loss of sensation or feeling in a part of your body. It's often accompanied by or combined with other changes in sensation, such as a pins-and-needles feeling, burning or tingling. Numbness can occur along a single nerve, on one side of the body.,

* Amor T. *(Breast cancer. ovarian cancer)*

The first time I experienced neuropathy, they felt like jolts in my bones that would just come out of nowhere. I likened them to lightning bolts directly hitting my bones. All of a sudden, no matter what I was doing, I would get the jolts. Sometimes they would happen in quick succession and I would feel drained in the end. They weren't seriously painful; just really unnerving and even annoying. Imagine being quickly pricked everywhere. Yes, really annoying.

Three things I remember from having neuropathy: my feet felt like they were walking on glass shards and/or they got numb and/ or they felt extremely dry and dirty. The times my feet felt extremely dry and dirty, I placed them in a basin full of warm water and scrubbed them hard to remove the "grime". One day, I felt I had to do that three consecutive times, because there was still "grime" on my feet. But, no matter how much I soaked and scrubbed, the "grime" was still there. That was really weird.

I experienced numbness in my feet also, which was unnerving, because at times, I couldn't feel my feet that were planted on the floor. Because of it, I didn't feel stable enough to walk. I had to grab hold of the wall beside me or whatever furniture or counter was nearby. I didn't do anything in particular, except to hold my numb feet. Fortunately, the numbness didn't last. Still, since I didn't know when the numbness would strike again, I wasn't too keen about taking a walk around the neighborhood, which we did for exercise. Fortunately, Bill was encouraging and accompanied me during my walks. We walked really, really slowly at first. Then, picked up the pace gradually as I got better.

> **ADVICE:** B vitamins are useful in treating neuropathy since they support healthy nervous system function. I recommend you take vitamins B6 and B12 separately versus one B complex vitamin. If the neuropathy is causing you to feel unstable and you need to walk, have someone walk with you and walk slowly and cautiously. Use a walking stick would help for support.

* Cindy R. *(Metastatic Breast cancer to Stomach)*

Neuropathy affected my fingers only, and I was told not to touch ice or anything cold. To keep myself from just grabbing ice for my water or whatever, I actually got a magnet to attach a pair of gloves to my refrigerator. When I needed to get ice or anything from the freezer, I just threw those gloves on real quick, and it sure helped.

> ADVICE: If you have neuropathy in your fingers, protect them from anything cold. Don't touch or handle anything cold without protection. Gloves are perfect protection for your hands. Use a magnet with a hook to attach a pair of gloves to your refrigerator. That way they're always handy when you need to get something cold out of the refrigerator or freezer.

* Glenn M. *(Metastatic Colon cancer to the Liver, Lungs & Adrenal Glands)*

When I had the neuropathy, it was back when I was being treated with Oxaliplatin. At the same time, the skin on my feet were cracked, so my feet were really giving me trouble; I was limping because of it. So, I went to the foot spa several times and the people there do a pretty good job. By the time I'd gone three times, one of the nurses suggested I take a B complex vitamin for my neuropathy. I followed her suggestion and took the B complex vitamin and, at the same time, I went again to the foot spa. So, I don't know which one takes credit or if they both do. The main thing is that I got rid of the neuropathy, which made me happy.

> ADVICE: Find a good foot spa to get your feet massaged. It may take several visits, but the foot massages help take care of the neuropathy. Taking a B complex vitamin also helps. I can't remember if it's B6 or B12 or some other B vitamin. In any case, check with your doctor or nurses.

* Hilda K. *(Colon cancer)*

During treatment, I remember my feet and hands tingling and being very sensitive to cold, so I always wore socks and gloves to keep them warm as much as I could. Together with my neuropathy, I also had hypothermia because of my chemotherapy, so my whole body (not just my hands and feet) were cold.

I did feel some numbness too, but it didn't really bother me. So I just let it pass.

> ADVICE: If your feet and hands get very sensitive to cold, make sure to wear socks and gloves to protect yourself.

* Rev. Linda S. *(Pancreatic cancer 3x)*

I've experienced fleeting neuropathy in both hands with the left hand being worse than the right. One night, for the first time, cold sorbet and cold water bothered me, which is also supposed to be temporary. I felt as if I had a mouth full of burning ice crystals. The first few days after this latest chemo, my salivary glands burned briefly after taking my first two or three bites of food. These are all symptoms that should pass one day.

* Rachel S. *(Breast cancer: triple negative)*

I experienced a bit of neuropathy. I felt it more so in my fingers. Sometimes I felt it just in my thumbs. But it was on and off; it wasn't constant. All I really do is stretch out my fingers and/or thumbs. Other than that, I don't do anything for it.

> ADVICE: If you feel the neuropathy in your fingers, just stretch them out.

* Scott M. *(Metastatic Colon cancer to the Prostate & Pancreas)*

I had severe neuropathy. Hands and feet. Early on, the neuropathy was so severe on my hands that I had to wear gloves to reach into the refrigerator to get anything cold out. I could not drink anything that was colder than room temperature. No ice water; nothing cold. If I drank something that was too cold, my whole throat would feel like it was burning. So, I always had a glass of room-temperature water sitting on the counter, which I would drink and that would calm it.

Now, years later, I have neuropathy on the bottom of my feet. It feels like I'm standing on marbles. And it's constant. My foot's in the air and it feels like I'm standing on marbles. The recommended maximum dosage for the nerve medication Lyrica is 300 mg. I'm on 450 mg because I'm under doctor's supervision. Unfortunately, my feet still hurt. So, my next course of medicine would be to go on Methadone, an opioid medication used to treat moderate to severe pain. But since that's such a gnarly drug to be on, I decided that I've gotten to the point where I can tune my neuropathy out of my brain. So, I don't feel it until I talk about it or until I'm walking and my feet really start to hurt.

I'm looking into infrared technology for my neuropathy. I have a spa at home that does the whole infrared spectrum. It heats up the core to get the toxins out of the body, which helps with inflammation. You also get more of the heavy metals out of your body. Aside from that, a neighbor of mine has a medical-level infrared therapy machine for her horses when their legs and tendons are bad. We're going to test it on my feet to see if it helps. Hopefully it does.

ADVICE: Wear gloves when you need to reach into the refrigerator to get anything cold out. Keep a glass of room-temperature water out on the counter to drink when you need it. Even though there are medications to help you deal with your neuropathy, take them under your doctor's supervision only. Some of those medications are really serious and may cause adverse reactions you definitely don't want to get. For activities that require small motor skills, ask someone to help. My best recommendation here: Try and tune out the neuropathy as much as you can.

My fingertips are numb because of the neuropathy. I can't button my top button, because I can't feel it unless I'm looking at a mirror and then, I can do it. The small buttons on the sides of the sleeves, I can't button. So I would ask someone, "Hey, could you help me with the button on my sleeves?" I have issues with small motor skills and manual dexterity, because of the numbness of my fingertips.

ADVICE: When your numb fingers affect your motor skills and manual dexterity, try to adjust. Work a different way, or you can ask someone to assist.

* Sondra W. (Ovarian cancer 3x)

Oh, my experience with neuropathy was something else! I had the "electric shocks", the "walking on rocks", and the "walking on sponges". I had the "burning sensation" and the feeling of wire bands wrapped around my feet, enclosing them tightly too. I remember standing in the shower and my feet just slid out from under me. They just slid right out from under me!

There was about a month period of time when I got so weak and the neuropathy was so bad that I had to have a home health aide come in and help me take my shower since Kenneth was still working at the time. We knew I could not be in the shower alone, with no one around, just in case. So, that arrangement lasted about four weeks, and then I got better.

Now, I can shower and wash my hair and on my own. Some people don't know how BIG that is. It's like, "Oh, I'm just THRILLED to death!" I go to the bathroom and there's no bleeding. I'm just THRILLED ... My goodness, this is so much FUN!

I used Epsom salt to relieve my feet when I felt the burning sensation. I also heated up a towel and wrapped it around my feet. That worked really good at night because I would just go to sleep. During the day – Oh, here's what I learned helped – I learned that the "electrical shocks", which were prevalent then and made me feel like my feet were being electrocuted ... Well, the cause was positional, i.e. coming from my lower back.

If I were sitting down and leaning over, the feeling on my feet would be fiery. So what I did was adjust myself to sit straight on. I found that that was a very effective way to avoid triggering the neuropathy. There were also times when I was uncomfortable sitting at somebody's place, and didn't want to trigger the neuropathy. So, I would just stand up.

When I had really bad neuropathy on my feet, I got some really good shoes and an insert. Unfortunately, those shoes stopped working because somehow, my feet changed, so I bought another pair of shoes and used a cane.

The neuropathy also affected my driving because there were times it got so bad. It was like – you know when you hit your knee and your leg pops up. Well, sometimes the "electric shock" feeling got so bad that it would lift my foot off the gas or the brake. So, I had to learn to drive some distance away from the car in front of me in case the neuropathy affected my foot. That would give me time to adjust myself and "get my foot back." It was bad.

For a while there, I couldn't cook or bake because I also had neuropathy in my hands. My sense of hot and cold were so off that I had to be careful that I didn't burn myself. Fortunately, my husband Kenneth got me special gloves to use to protect my hands.

There was another instance when my neuropathy caused pain. One day when I used a knife to crack the shell of an egg, the sharp edges of the broken shell touched my hand and that was so painful...Oh my! It really was so bad! I couldn't maneuver the eggs with my special gloves, so I had to think of ways to work around them. I figured that I could just crack and open a little part of the egg, enough to get just the egg itself out or do whatever I needed to do because, mostly, I could eat only the egg whites. Even though eggs were one of the few things I could eat, I didn't want to eat too many. So, Kenneth would eat the egg yolks, and I would eat the egg whites.

ADVICE: When you get a burning sensation on your feet, get an Epsom salt foot bath. Also, if you feel the neuropathy before going to sleep, wrap a heated towel around your feet. When you feel the neuropathy during the day, notice your sitting position. How you sit may trigger your neuropathy, especially if you're leaning over when you sit. Try to sit straight up. If nothing helps when you're sitting, just stand up. Getting shoes with an insert could also provide relief.

If you have to drive, and you get a neuropathy "attack", i.e. your foot all of a sudden pops up, then drive some distance away from the car in front of you. Doing that gives you enough time to safely adjust yourself and get your foot back on the pedal.

Now, when it comes to the neuropathy causing tingling or burning sensation in your hands, there are actually special "neuropathy" gloves you can buy on the market.

* *Vida B.A.* (Breast cancer)

Unfortunately, I do sometimes get those stabbing, sharp nerve pains that feel like someone is cutting me with a knife. I experience it more when it's raining and the weather is cold. I know that it's a side effect from my chemo treatments; something to be "expected." So, I just deal with it. Fortunately, those episodes don't really last long.

ADVICE: Neuropathy is a common chemotherapy side effect. If you feel tingling, weakness, numbness or pain in your body, especially feet or hands, the experience usually won't last long. If it does, let your doctor know, so it can be looked into further. Otherwise, just deal with it. There's nothing really you can do about it. Good thing that it usually just comes and goes; it doesn't last long.

* *Yesi L.* (Breast cancer: triple positive)

I dealt with neuropathy for about two years. It felt like very sharp pins and needles. The tips of my fingers were extremely sensitive to grains and to touching sand. I couldn't stand it. Even grabbing a potato chip, because of the salt, I couldn't stand it. So, basically, I tried to stay away from those things. If I wanted to grab a chip or something with grainy texture, I used gloves or a tissue.

Also, my shoes didn't come off for years. I wore sandals with a lot of cushion like the Reef Sandals. Now, the neuropathy is gone, thank God!

ADVICE: When your feet are extremely sensitive because of neuropathy, comfort is definitely number. Get the most comfortable shoes out there with a lot of cushion. The Reef Sandals I wore were great.

PAIN

Most cancer pain is caused by the tumour pressing on bones, nerves or other organs in the body. Sometimes pain is due to your cancer treatment.

* Aaron C. (Prostate cancer, Skin cancer)

Oh, yeah, I had lot of pain after surgery. For ten days, I had to use a catheter, which was miserable, especially when I had to move. I couldn't apply pressure down in my groin area for, at least, the first three months. So, I stopped riding my motorcycle and playing my drums, because the seats were hard to sit on.

Because I couldn't sit down for a long period of time, I didn't go out much. It was just too uncomfortable. I didn't do much socializing for the first month or so, because I just couldn't sit down. It hurt to sit on hard or firm surfaces. I couldn't drive either. Just sitting in the car was miserable.

The hardest time I had with pain was the day I was released from the hospital. For whatever reason, they were so over-booked that it was really tough finding someone to help me put my pants and my shoes back on. I finally got help, but I couldn't even bend over to get my shoes on; the pain was so great. Yeah, I definitely was miserable.

I'm not a "pain med" guy. So, I toughed it out most of the time, taking the pain med only when I really needed it.

I was really sore, especially during the first three days after surgery. I haven't had pain in a while; no soreness at all. I'm even doing sit-ups!

> **ADVICE:** Don't take pain meds unless you really have to. Wear loose clothing and ask for help when you need it. You may get miserable, because you'll be limited in the things you can do. Still, you've got to tough it out. Remember that pain is part of the process, but it's temporary.

* Amor T. (Breast cancer, Ovarian cancer)

I experienced a lot of pain from both my breast cancer and ovarian cancer treatments. Yes, pain was constant, but I didn't feel like I was suffering constantly. Fortunately, with the pain meds (oxycodone and hydrocodone), I found some relief. Below are the highlights of my overall experience.

The PCA (patient-controlled analgesia). I had a left breast mastectomy and dipped flat breast reconstruction surgery that lasted eight hours. After surgery I was placed in ICU overnight. When I woke up, I was in a drugged (I call it "happy dopey") state. My nurse gave me instructions on how to use the intravenous Patient-Controlled Analgesia (PCA) attached to me, which allowed me to administer my own painkiller with just a push of a button.

She said that I should press the button I feel pain or when I feel it's about to come. The PCA pump is programmed to give a certain amount of medication when I press the button. It will only allow me to have so much medication (i.e. one release every six minutes), no matter how often I press the button. So, I won't need to worry about giving myself too much. Well, I am the type of person who does not want to depend depend on painkillers; I think I have a high threshold for pain. So, I tried to hold off on pushing the PCA button.

Unfortunately, the following day, two aides came by and told me that they were going to move me to a regular room. When they first came in, I didn't feel any pain. But then, when they tried to move me from my bed to the gurney, that's when the intense pain struck and I screamed in panic. I asked them to hold off while I pressed my PCA button and wait until the pain med took effect. Well, they didn't wait long enough (I guess they were on a schedule), because next thing I knew, they lifted me from my bed and onto the gurney, despite my screams of pain. It was really rough; they were not gentle at all and it was really scary. I sure learned a hard lesson then, i.e. when it comes to pain, follow instructions. It is CRITICAL to be proactive and be ahead of the pain; not be reactive and wait for pain to come before taking the painkiller.

Pain level of "12"! During my stay, my worst pain happened when my friend Macy came to visit. While we were talking, all of a sudden, I felt extreme and escalating pain and heaviness in my abdomen, I couldn't breathe. I was in a panic and thought of Catherine, my siblings and not being able to say goodbye to my loved ones; I felt like I was going to die right there and then; it was so frightening. The experience was so excruciating painful and my heart was racing so fast. The nurse came in and quickly asked me what my pain level was (between 0-10 with 10 being the worst). I yelled out, "12!" She worked on my PCA and I felt my pain and heaviness lessen; I was able to breathe again. Wow, what a trip!

Pain while coughing, sneezing, laughing, etc. Because of the many deep incisions in my body, I had a lot of sources for pain. Most of my pain, however, came from my abdomen when I had to cough or sneeze or laugh. Evening getting the hiccups was painful too. I eventually learned to hold my belly every time I felt the above would occur. I found that placing a little pillow on my belly and pressing on it whenever I had to cough, sneeze, laugh, etc. helped to curb the pain.

Pain getting up from the chair, bed or toilet. Throughout my hospital stay after both my breast and ovarian cancer treatment surgeries, I felt pain, although it was "muted" thanks to the painkillers. From my mastectomy/breast reconstruction/staph infection, I had a 22" horizontal incision that was made from one end of my hip to the other end of my hip. I also had a large gash on the left side of my breast and numerous stitches on my reconstructed left breast. From my radical hysterectomy, I had an 8" vertical incision that ran from the bottom of my chest plate, around my belly button and then down to the top of my pubic bone. It looks like an upside-down question mark. :-)

If I didn't move, I was fine. Pain occurred when I had to move, like shift my position in bed, hoist or pull myself up, lay myself down, sit on the side of my bed, stand up to go to the bathroom, sit on the toilet seat, then get up or try to walk around with my IV, etc. I felt sore and raw and weak.

Mind over matter. To combat my pain, I prayed constantly and kept focus on how my experience was all part of my "life adventures" AND my discomfort was temporary. I kept thinking that cancer and my physical challenges would one day be behind me. So, I should just be thankful, keep positive and take it one day, one step at a time. It also helped me when I thought good thoughts and smiled or joked around with whoever was with me. It felt good that, no matter what physical pain I felt, I still had the ability to create positive energy. Basically, "Mind over matter."

Agonizing "pinched nerves" pain everywhere. I did feel pain whenever the "lightning "I would strike my bones i.e. neuropathy. But those experiences were fleeting and not super intense. What was intense was the time when I felt I had a something that felt like a pinched nerve all over my body. That day I thought that I could just take oxycodone or hydrocodone and the pain would go away. Unfortunately as it turned out it did not. The pain persisted. My friend Sean was with me and saw my distress. He asked what he could do and I thought of ice packs for me to Leon. I sat on the recliner and lay on the ice packs, but they did nothing to relieve my pain. I was in tears by this time.

When Sean asked what else I could he could do, I prayed for guidance. I then asked him to turn on the TV and just go through the channels to see what calls out to us. We stopped on America's Funniest Videos. I found myself laughing and enjoying the show despite the intense pain I was feeling then. Looking back, I know that the distraction of something enjoyable helped me to cope with my pain versus focusing on my pain. After the show, I went to the medicine cabinet to look again for something to help. Somehow, the box of GasEx stood out from among the rest, as if to say, "Pick me! I'm the one you need!" I cannot explain why I picked the GasEx; there was no logic nor reason. However, to my surprise, after I took the GasEx, my intense pain went away. Hallelujah!

Pain from extreme constipation. I experienced a lot of pain with the constipation that came after my radical hysterectomy and it seemed to last forever. The surgical oncologist who performed my hysterectomy, suggested that I take fiber supplements like Metamucil and a stool softener. Well, I followed his suggestion, but it just made my constipation worse. It was an awful experience! I was so backed up, bloated and super frustrated. I also did not want to eat for fear of just having whatever I consumed stay in my stomach and add to my pain.

When I finally met my medical oncologist who was going to oversee the administration of my chemotherapy. I told him about my constipation serious problem he then told me to use MiraLAX instead of Metamucil or other fiber supplements. He explained...

Pain from my mediport implant. I was excited to finally get my mediport implant, because it meant no more poking my arms a "gazillion" times to find a viable vein for blood draws, infusions, etc. Unfortunately, when I got home after the implant surgery, the mediport area (located below my right clavicle and above my right breast) was really sore and painful. I did have pain meds, but every time I opened my mouth, the mediport area would move and I would feel tightness and pain. It was strange. It took longer than I thought it would for the swelling to go down. Eventually, it did. In the meantime, I just had to grin and bear it.

The importance of pain medication. After my stays in the hospital, I would always come home with prescription painkillers; serious narcotics, like oxycodone and hydrocodone/paracetamol aka vicodin. My instructions were to take them every six hours. Since I knew they were addictive, I decided to just take them as needed (i.e. when I felt pain.) Well, that kept me from moving about, because doing so would cause pain. So, no movement = no pain. When I met with my doctor for my follow-up, I informed him of my pain experiences. He then asked me if I had been taking my pain meds as directed. I expressed concern about addiction to the painkillers. He told me that wasn't going to happen, because addiction happens only after taking the medication every day for months which is what I won't have to do. He did gently scold me about not following his instructions and firmly told me that movement was necessary for my body to recover and grow stronger. So, I must take my pain meds, following the schedule he directed, not "as needed." I learned to be proactive and be ahead of the pain; not just react to it.

ADVICE: Firstoff, if you're having pain, tell someone! Don't worry about being a "bother". Doctors and nurses "measure" your pain on a scale of 0-10, with "0" being no pain and "10" being the worst pain. This helps them determine what course of action to take to relieve your pain and it also helps them know how well your treatment is working. Then, when you're prescribed narcotics for pain, take them as instructed. They're meant to aid in your recovery. If you have any concerns, you should discuss it first with your doctor; don't stop taking it, unless your doctor is aware and has another plan of action.

Pain control can help speed recovery. If your pain in well controlled, you'll be better able to complete important tasks, e.g. walking and deep breathing exercises. Keeping your pain at a tolerable level (no pain may be an unreasonable goal) will help you keep moving and speed the healing process. Just make sure to drink ample fluids along with pain medications, as they can lead to dehydration and constipation.

It is often easier to control pain if you take the medication regularly, as prescribed. Waiting until the pain is severe and then taking pain medication results in a long wait for the drug to take effect. It is better to keep the pain under control and at a tolerable level, rather than waiting until it is severe and waiting for relief. Good pain control can make it far easier to sleep, which also promotes healing

* Bob G. (Soft Tissue Sarcoma, Skin cancer)

The nurses brought me painkillers. Whenever I saw the bottle, I asked them, "What's in that little bottle?" They would take out two white pills and say, "They're painkillers." I told them that I didn't need them. I have no pain. But, they insisted that the doctor said I had to take them. So, I said, "Well then, give them to the doctor. I'm not going to take the painkillers." When they still argued, I said, "Don't argue. The message I'm getting is, you want to give me pain pills, so I will have pain for the doctor?" After that, they stopped bringing the painkillers to me. Interestingly, the same thing happened when I went to rehab. They wanted to give me painkillers. I have a high threshold of pain and really don't need painkillers.

The first few days at the hospital, I was fortunate. The machine with the IV going through it had a cocktail of drugs, which included morphine. So, I had no choice; I had to take it. One time, my early morning nurse didn't show at 4:00am and the IV meds went dry. That was my sustenance, my medicine....all in one. So then, I made a lot of noise. Another nurse ran in and said, "This is not my station, but I'm going to take care of you." And I said to her, "I don't want to see that nurse who was assigned to take care of me ever again! I could've died! I don't want to ever see her again!"

ADVICE: Communicate your needs to your doctor and nurses and don't let them force you to take anything you don't believe you need to take. They may insist or argue with you, but if they can't convince you to follow whatever they want you to do, then don't do it. It's their responsibility to explain the process or the need for the medications to you.

* Cindy L. (Kidney cancer)

I experienced tremendous post-surgery pain after my nephrectomy. Because it was laparoscopic surgery, I had a lot of gas pain due to the carbon dioxide that they used during the surgery to work on my abdominal cavity. It went into my tissues and then got trapped in my intestines. The first night I had the surgery, my surgeon came in at about 11:30 at night to make me get out of bed. He said, "This is the only time that you're going to get a high-five for farting." So yeah, he made me laugh and I thought I was going to die because I was trying to get up and fart, at the same time!

My surgeon also injected into all my incisions an anesthetic called Exparel, which would keep those areas numb for 96 hours. I had to wear a special wrist band, so that I wouldn't be given anything else for local pain for that time period.

So yes, my pain was hard to fight. My doctor had me on Oxycodone and strong Tylenol in the hospital to help with inflammation. He also gave me Simethicone to reduce my pain and discomfort from the excessive gas that I had. Actually, I learned, from a lot of people in the Kidney Support Group I joined, that they were not aware that they could've asked for the Simethicone after the laparoscopic surgery. And I don't know why doctors are not giving it more freely.

After two weeks post-surgery, I was off all pain medications. I basically just toughened up. Once in a while, I have to take a Tylenol, but that was it. I do still have periodic pain in the upper left quadrant where my kidney was. I know there's still internal healing going on and it will continue for a long time. I do still have incisional pain, although that comes more from moving wrong or doing something stupid, like trying to fix something I shouldn't be fixing or just plain overdoing it. Two years post surgery I don't have the pain in that area any longer except if I bend strangely. There is a clip in there where the kidney was so I don't know If that is what was causing the pain or not.

> **ADVICE:** If you have pain from excessive gas, especially after laparoscopic surgery, you just have to "let it rip!" It doesn't matter who's around. Just let it go, because the gas has to come out. Ask your doctor to give you Simethicone to help reduce your gas pain, bloating and discomfort.
>
> Your doctor may also prescribe you strong Tylenol or Oxycodone for your pain. If so, check side effects, since you may also need a stool softener. We know that pain can inhibit healing so it's a delicate balance in controlling the pain and preventing becoming addicted to strong opioids. Work with your doctor on this.

* Cindy R. (Metastatic Breast cancer to Stomach)

Breast cancer. Even though I had pain from the double mastectomy I went through, plus pain from the surgery to take care of an infection in the area where my right breast implant was placed, I didn't experience crazy pain. I just took the pain meds, as prescribed. I also did light exercises, because with the lymph nodes being gone and the swelling there, I had to kind of move my body to make sure the lymph fluids were not just sitting there. Those light exercises kept my blood flowing and also really helped with the pain.

Stomach cancer. Oh yeah, there was pain there for sure. It was like I felt seriously gassy all the time and I was bloated, which really hurt. So, my doctor prescribed Norco to help me deal with my pain.

> **ADVICE:** Even though you can expect to experience pain from surgery and treatment, you can manage it with the right painkillers. After surgery, you'll be given painkillers to help you move around, so that your body can heal. Let your doctor know the kind of pain you're experiencing and how much, so that he or she can give you the right medication.

* Glenn M. (Metastatic Colon cancer to the Liver, Lungs & Adrenal Glands)

I experienced a lot of pain, mostly from the skin around my fingers and toes being split by my nails as they grew. Oh, I have pain from surgeries, naturally. But, I really didn't have much pain from treatments, per se. Yes, they stuck the needles into my port, which stings for a bit, but that's it. I never really took painkillers; I'm afraid of them. I had a relative who got strung on painkillers and then went to heroine. That was really bad. Fortunately, he's off it now.

After my surgeries, they sent me home with the pain pills, but I never really paid attention to them. I toughed it out, most times. I have a high threshold of pain, which is good. I have turned to marijuana, which has been a godsend. Not only does it help with pain, it also helps with all kinds of things like appetite, attitude and nausea. I just order it from a friend and then it's delivered to me.

I used Aquaphor quite a bit on my hands and feet. It's a moisturizer that prevents drying, itchy or irritated skin. The thing I really like about Aquaphor is that it's fast and easy. My dermatologist also prescribed a 2.5% steroid ointment for me to use, in case the skin around my fingers and/or toes got really bad. The ointment put the fire out immediately. I also found that wearing gloves helped a lot. Not only did the gloves moisturize my hands, they protected them, as well. The gloves are just really easy.

> **ADVICE:** For pain, I'm a big believer in the many benefits of marijuana. It's definitely better than opioid painkillers that you can easily get addicted to. If you have pain because of thinning, breaking skin, use Aquaphor. It's a moisturizer that prevents drying, itchy or irritated skin. It's really great and it's also fast and easy. If the pain from the cuts of your thinning skin gets worse, ask your doctor for a prescription for 2.5% steroids. It'll put out the fire immediately. If the thinning skin on your fingers are causing them to be sensitive, then wear gloves. They'll protect you and they're really easy.

* Hilda K. (Colon cancer)

I don't remember having that much pain. I was very delicate to myself and I never pushed it. At the hospital, they made me get up and walk around the day after my surgery, which helped me heal faster.

There was a time, however, when I was alone in my hospital room and my pain medication wore off. I was connected to an IV that gave me control of the morphine for my pain, but didn't allow the morphine to continuously flow into me. So, I decided to give myself a shot of morphine each and every time I moved, including whenever I had to get up. Because I was afraid to feel pain, I actually went "crazy" giving myself shots of morphine. Basically, I wouldn't move, until I gave myself a shot. Eventually, doing that caught up with me. One night, around 11:00 pm, I had such a hard time breathing. My daughter Jessica was there and called the nurse who put an oxygen tube into my nose to force the oxygen into me. What a relief! Before the nurse left ... he was of Filipino descent, like me ...he said, "Ate, you shouldn't give yourself so many shots of morphine." I got busted! He went on to explain, "That's why you couldn't breathe. Just relax now. Stop giving yourself too many morphine shots." From what he said, I realized that I basically overdosed on the morphine; I had "trigger-finger." After that, I was better about my self-administration of morphine.

What also helped me was the little pillow they gave me there, like the pillows they give you on the airplane when you have a long flight. United Airlines donates those little pillows to hospitals and volunteer ladies sew pillow cases for them. Those little pillows are for people who come out of surgeries that involve the abdomen. They provide support for the patients by keeping the stomach muscles from straining and hurting when the patients have to get up or sneeze. All the patients have to do is put the pillow on their tummy when they have to get up or when they're about to sneeze. The pillow really helped me. I saved it for two years after, because it was real positive reminder that such a little thing helped me get out of bed.

> **ADVICE:** When you're given pain medication, take them only if you can't tolerate the pain. You shouldn't take it each and every time you feel a little pain, because then you'll overdose and you'll also depend on your pain medication, which will definitely not allow you to get stronger on your own. Also, the sooner you move around and walk after surgery, the sooner you'll recover. Yes, it's tough, because you'll be sore, but it's worth it. When you move around, the cells in your body become active and generate quicker healing of your wounds.
>
> If you have surgery on your abdomen, make sure to get a little pillow from the hospital to help support your tummy when you have to get up or sneeze. If they don't give out little pillows, then find one for yourself that you can carry with you. It should be soft, but firm enough to provide you extra support for you when you hold your tummy before getting up or sneezing. That little pillow from the hospital helped me a lot!

* Rev. Linda S. (Pancreatic cancer 3x)

While I was hospitalized, my pain was well managed with IV meds. During the day, I take two 325mg. Tylenol tablets, when needed, which isn't often. At night before bed, I take a Tylenol-opioid combo pill to keep pain from waking me up.

> **ADVICE:** Follow instructions from the medical team, including (if applicable) the physical therapist, to minimize pain from adhesions.

* Scott M. (*Metastatic Colon cancer to the Prostate & Pancreas*)

I experienced a lot of pain in different ways. The first time was when I was in the hospital after my colon resection. A male nurse came in to remove the 20 staples I had in my abdomen. He was so rough with me, the pain was so excruciating that I was screaming in agony! Now, I'm a big, buff guy who's served in the military. I've never, ever been an anxious person. Now, I am. I'm anxious to pain.

When I knew that I had to be sliced a second time, I told my surgical oncologist about the pain I suffered before when the male nurse removed my staples. Fortunately, she used a cream that she rubbed on the area around the staples. When she went to take them out, I didn't feel a thing!

At another time, I had to go home with a feeding tube inserted into my stomach through my abdomen, because I had trouble eating. I had to mix my food and pour the milkshake-like fluid through the feeding tube, which was about ¾" in diameter. The problem was the hole in my stomach was bigger than the tube and the tube would constantly rub against the hole in my stomach for a few months. Talk about pain! I developed a big anxiety to pain. An hour prior to having the feeding tube cleaned, I would break into a cold sweat thinking about it. So, I would take 4mg of Dilaudid (a strong pain med). Then, fifteen minutes prior to the cleaning, I would take some oral Morphine (another strong pain med). So, when the medical team came in to un-tape the whole thing to clean it, the pain meds helped with the pain.

> <u>ADVICE:</u> Try as much as you can to stay ahead of the pain. If you'll be having a procedure that you know will cause pain, take pain meds ahead of time. Let your doctor know, so that he or she can give you the strong painkillers necessary. Communicate your needs. Don't be shy in telling your surgeon, doctor or medical staff of any anxieties or fears you have. Know your body, know your fears and be vocal. Be proactive and make sure they hear you.
>
> **(ADDITION) Amor and I were just having an off-line discussion about pain and how, after her surgery, she tried to hold off pushing the morphine button for the self-administering pain medication automatic drip and I'm sitting here shaking my head thinking, "No, no, no, no, no... That's absolutely wrong!" You HAVE TO STAY AHEAD OF THE PAIN or you will never catch up!
>
> The moment you feel like pain is coming on or you're four hours into your four-hour pain med, go ahead and take it, because the pain is going to come right back. Do not let the pain get ahead of you, because you won't be able to catch up. Stay ahead of the pain. Don't try to be the tough guy or the tough girl or, you know, "macho" it out. It doesn't work to your benefit.

* Sondra W. (*Ovarian cancer 3x*)

Bladder and urinary tract pain: During my first round of treatment with the more aggressive chemo I had a lot of bladder pain, which caused me to lose sleep because I had to get up every night and go to the bathroom. At one point, I had to prop up my feet because I had a little bit of swelling. Well, that made me need to go even more, which then made me experience more episodes of pain in urinating. According to my oncologist, bladder pain and urinary tract pain is not an expected side effect of treatment. He said, "This wasn't part of the deal." Aside from that, I didn't really have a lot of other pain. So that was fortunate.

Foot pain: Almost overnight, after my first chemo infusion, I started having pain and redness on my right foot and had it checked to make sure it wasn't an infection. I found out I had "Hand-and-Foot Syndrome" caused by one of the chemotherapy drugs, Doxil. The skin on my foot was crusty and leather-like, and turned black, like it had been burnt in a fire. Since my heel also became leathery, I had to cut some of the tough skin off with a pair of scissors. The friction of the skin of my feet rubbing against my shoes caused it to be discolored, inflamed and blistered. It was so painful that even if something soft (like a pillow) touched my feet, I had to take Norco to relieve the pain! I've been wearing post-surgical sandals since. We had hoped that when I went off the Doxil over a year ago, the problem would go away. Unfortunately, it's still here today.

Pain from edema. I also experienced swelling in my legs where a lot of fluid was held, causing the skin of my legs to degrade. Because excess fluid that had accumulated in the tissues was looking for a way to get out, I developed blisters and then, my skin turned black and crusty. With all the fluid, my skin became so tight, the pain was excruciating. I took pain medication, especially at night when my legs and feet would throb, and that provided the relief that I needed. Fortunately,

I've lost 15 lbs. of fluid. Unfortunately, I still have swelling, so I have to keep my feet propped up. I also have to continue taking Lasix Furosemide, which is a diuretic to treat my fluid retention and swelling.

Pain from neuropathy. There was another instance when my neuropathy caused pain. One day when I used a knife to crack the shell of an egg, the sharp edges of the broken shell hit my hand and that was so painful...holy moly! It really was so bad! I couldn't maneuver the eggs with my special gloves, so I had to think of ways to work around them. I figured that I could just crack and open a little part of the egg, enough to get just the stuff out or do whatever I needed to do because, mostly, I could eat only the egg whites. Even though eggs were one of the few things I could eat, I didn't want to eat too many. So, Kenneth would eat the egg yolks and I would eat the egg whites.

ADVICE:
(Bladder and urinary tract pain.)
If you have bladder problems, you may be reacting to one of the medications or you may not. Whatever it is, you need to see a specialist (urologist) to look into the source of the problem and the right treatment for you. If the urologist you see can't help you, find another one right away. Move on. If the urologist recommends a treatment and that treatment doesn't work in about two weeks, you really should question it. If the urologist says that he is not sure what's happening or says that he hasn't "seen anything like it before", that is very unusual and the urologist is NOT helping you. Find another urologist who will.

(Foot pain or hand-and-foot syndrome.)
If you get changes in your feet from a reaction to one of the medications, inform your doctor so you can make sure it's not an infection. If you need to wear shoes, choose loose-fitting ones for comfort. For skin that is dry, leathery, irritated or inflamed, use Aquaphor moisturizer. For a really soothing effect, refrigerate it first, before applying it to your skin. You can also alternate, using Cetaphil lotion and coconut oil or a combination of the two; they work really well together.

After bathing, clean your dry, leathery skin with alcohol. That will help slough off dead skin cells. Then you can apply the Aquaphor or the other moisturizers to enable your skin to regain its moisture content. If you have blisters, ask your doctor for Erythromycin gel, which does a very good job of drying up the blisters. After you apply the gel on the blisters, place a light gauze over them to give them air and protect them from infection.

(Pain from edema.)
Propping your feet or legs up helps to relieve the swelling in your feet or legs. Also, wear compression stockings/leggings. They help reduce swelling, improve blood flow and prevent deep vein thrombosis (DVT), which is a blood clot that can create a very serious condition. It helps to have a podiatrist work on your feet too.

(Pain from neuropathy.)
If the cause of your pain is the neuropathy, then there are a number of solutions you can try, like giving your feet a bath in Epsom salt or wrapping a heated towel around your feet. You could also adjust your sitting position (try not to lean forward while sitting). How you sit may trigger your neuropathy, especially if you're leaning over when you sit. Try to sit straight up. If nothing helps when you're sitting, just stand up. Getting shoes with an insert could also provide relief. Massage can help, as well.

If you have to drive and you get a neuropathy "attack", i.e. your foot, all of a sudden, lifts up from the pedal, then drive some distance away from the car in front of you. Doing that gives you enough time to safely adjust yourself and get your foot back to the pedal.

Now, when it comes to the neuropathy causing tingling or a burning sensation in your hands, there are actually special "neuropathy" gloves you can buy on the market. You can "google" them on the Internet.

* Susan M. *(Ovarian cancer. Metastatic Pancreatic cancer to the Lung)*

Ovarian cancer: There was a lot pain after my hysterectomy. I had to be careful about anyone bumping into my stomach. I also had to be careful of the seat belt in the car. I put a pillow over my stomach, especially when my little daughter wanted to sit on my lap.

Pancreatic cancer: Considering the length of surgery, I had very little discomfort. I used very little pain medication.

<u>ADVICE:</u> If you had any surgery that entails a large incision in your abdominal area, using a pillow helps for comfort as well as for protection.

* Vida B.A. *(Breast cancer)*

During my first chemo infusion, I experienced an allergic reaction to one of the two chemo drugs I was given. I felt shooting pain in my nerves and sharp pain on the nerve on my big toes and tail bone, so they stopped the chemo infusion for 30 minutes. When we resumed, the pain wasn't there anymore. But then, I developed a really, really unexplainable kind of pain that wasn't physical, emotional or psychological. It was like I had a foreign body going through me and my body didn't know how to react to it. I was half asleep, moaning and groaning with this "pain' for hours. Really unexplainable. Nevertheless, I continued with the treatment. This all happened during my first chemo infusion. I didn't have the same experience for the infusions that followed.

Unfortunately, I do sometimes get those stabbing, sharp nerve pains from my neuropathy that feel like someone is cutting me with a knife. I experience it more when it's raining and the weather is cold. I know that it's a side effect from my chemo treatments, so I just deal with it. Fortunately, those episodes don't really last long.

Recovering from my mastectomy was painful. Fortunately, I had good pain medication to help. My breast implant procedure and recovery were also painful. But, I was able to tolerate it; again, with good pain medication.

<u>ADVICE:</u> During your chemo infusions, be aware of how your body is reacting to the chemo drugs. Remember that your body is not used to getting such strong drugs in your system. Let your nurse know immediately if you're experiencing pain, so they can address the problem, e.g. adjust the flow rate or stop the procedure.

Having good and effective pain medication is critical to your recovery, so take it as instructed by your doctor. That way, you'll be able to move around, which will definitely help your body heal. If you experience neuropathy as a side effect of your chemotherapy, most times it will just come and go, so just deal with it. Usually, those episodes don't last long. However, if it's causing you pain that's unbearable, do let your doctor know so you can have it checked and taken care of.

* Yesi L. *(Breast cancer: triple positive)*

I definitely dealt with pain throughout the entire treatment. After treatment, I not only felt physical pain, but emotional and psychological pain, as well. And, for me, that's something that probably will never go away. Of course, I eventually learned to deal with it. For physical pain, my go-to pain killer was Motrin.

After surgery, I remember taking Norco. And for the next couple of days, I continued to take Norco. Unfortunately, Norco gave me constipation, which was very hard on my body. So, as soon as I could get off it, I put myself on Motrin and it worked very well.

PANCREATITIS

Pancreatitis is a disease in which the pancreas becomes inflamed. Pancreatic damage happens when the digestive enzymes are activated before they are released into the small intestine and begin attacking the pancreas. There are two forms of pancreatitis: acute and chronic.

* Scott M. (*Metastatic Colon cancer to the Prostate & Pancreas*)

After removal of my gallbladder, I started getting sick and my pancreas started growing cysts the size of oranges. Those cysts blocked the stomach from letting food go into the duodenum, which is the beginning of the small intestine the pancreas is attached to in order to let the enzymes in, so that food can be digested. So, whenever I ate something, I just projectile vomited. I went through a lot of endoscopic procedures to lance these things and to figure out what was going on. Because I was also suffering from inflammation of my pancreas (pancreatitis), they worked to let the cysts out by slicing my "orifice of lodi", which is the end of the opening of the pancreas. They lanced the cysts, which were then drained and I got a little better. But, the cysts came back, because the holes filled up. So, I was operated on again. This time, my surgeon cut the cysts from end-to-end, so that there was no way they could grow back together. At the same time, I had surgery where they took part of my small intestine, routed it and attached it to my stomach. So now, I have two avenues for food to go from my stomach into my small intestine. I was in the hospital for five weeks and I haven't had pancreatitis since.

> **ADVICE:** When things happen to your body and you get sick, there's always, always a cause. It takes time to find out the cause and take care of it. No matter what, it is important to tough it out and look ahead. When all's said and done, you'll then be able to look back and say, "Man, that was really tough. But, I got through it!"

POOR SLEEP HABITS / INSOMNIA

Sleep disorders, such as difficulty falling asleep, problems maintaining sleep, poor sleep efficiency, early awakening, and excessive daytime sleepiness, are prevalent in patients with cancer.

* Amor T. (*Breast cancer, Ovarian cancer*)

Breast cancer. With four surgical drains hanging out from my torso and a deep and very long (22") incision that went from one end of my hip to the other, trying to be comfortable while I slept was really tough. Fortunately I had painkillers to help.

Trying to get myself up from bed was quite an ordeal. Because getting up from bed requires the abdomen to contract, and my abdomen was where the largest cut was made, I had to be super careful. When I got home from the hospital, I learned quickly that sleeping on my bed was not going to work. It was too soft and didn't have much support for me to grab hold of. So I arranged to sleep on the long leather couch in my living room. I also positioned a chair with tons of pillow nearby and the large cocktail table by the couch. The couch was firm and comfortable and I could use either the armrest or the back rest to pull myself up while avoiding any contraction of my abdominal muscles. I also learned to get myself up by rolling on one side, bending my knees and then using my free arm to push and raise my upper torso. At that point, I was able to move my legs to where I needed them so my feet could be on the floor.

With the drains, I had to sleep upright, on an incline or on my back (if I was able to lay down). After the surgical drains were removed, I was able to sleep on my side. That didn't happen immediately though, because I still had the large wounds from my mastectomy and reconstruction surgery to deal with. And, I had to sleep with a bra and a compression girdle on . Yes, pretty awkward times, but they're in the past now.

Ovarian cancer. When I got home after my hysterectomy, I thought I could just sleep in my bed. But my extreme discomfort from constipation got in the way. I got so bloated and filled with gas, it hurt. What did help was for me to sleep on my left side with my knees to my chest. Of course, it took some doing at first, because of the long vertical abdominal incision I had that still hadn't healed. Thankfully, the painkillers enabled me to do what I needed to do to move and adjust my positions. I also slept on the couch in the living room. Again, it helped to have the backrest and armrest there to grab on to when I needed to get up.

> **ADVICE:** If you have surgical drains hanging from your body, try sleeping upright or on an incline. Abdominal surgeries are serious business, so a lot of care is necessary to find the best way to sleep. First, make sure to take your painkillers as prescribed. They enable you to rest and move around when you need to, without worrying about

pain. If you have a long couch that is firm, I strongly recommend sleeping on that in the beginning. In most cases, the couch provides more support than the bed.

To physically get up from a lying position requires planning. First, bend your knees together and roll your body to the side you want to get up from. Then, using your free arm, push and raise your upper torso. At that point, You should be able to move your legs to where you need them, so your feet could be on the floor.

* Bob G. (Soft Tissue Sarcoma, Skin cancer)

Well, negative thoughts did enter my mind. In the middle of the night, for 3, 4 or 5 hours, I'd wake up and have a hard time getting back to sleep. I would be in a weakened condition, which made me susceptible to bad thoughts. The night fears tried to take over and it wasn't easy fighting them sometimes. I took 1-2 sleeping pills, but then I couldn't wake up in the morning. I did also play solitaire when I couldn't sleep.

What I did to deal with the night fears was think good thoughts. My good thoughts? Well, some of the nurses! I always say, "God's greatest gift to man is woman!" That's one of my favorite sayings!

Also, for men, I recommend finding a good woman. It just makes staying awake a little bit nicer!

ADVICE: The best medication for recovery is a good night's sleep. If you have night fears, think good thoughts only. If you have a hard time sleeping or getting back to sleep, try some activity, like playing solitaire. It does help to have someone stay awake with you.

* Cindy L. (Kidney cancer)

For some time, after my diagnosis, I felt highly anxious and had trouble sleeping. I was always able to just work through any kind of anxiety before. But, having cancer and the thought of losing a kidney was a little more than I could handle.

During my first ten days home from the hospital, I slept on a chair in the living room. I could not get up on my own. I had to be pulled up out of the chair with, literally, one person on each arm. I was so dependent on a lot of people.

When I was finally able to sleep in my bed, my family had to tuck me in a certain way where I couldn't move, I couldn't roll and I couldn't lie on my side. I'm a side-sleeper and not being able to sleep on my side was very difficult for me. I had a horrible time sleeping. In fact, for that period in time, Ed and I weren't been able to sleep in the same bed because I just couldn't fall asleep. After three weeks, it was a big thing and very exciting when I was finally able to lie on my left side. For some reason, I wasn't able to lie on my right side until after six weeks. That was odd, because it was my left kidney that was removed.

To help me sleep, I took Melatonin Sustained Release. Regular melatonin helped get me to sleep, but it didn't help me stay asleep, because of the very short pathways. So I took the Melatonin Sustained Release, but not every night. I took it only when needed. When I couldn't sleep, I would get up, go to the bathroom or refill my water glass, because I sleep with a water glass beside me. I would also use my tablet and watch something on Netflix or I would write a little bit too. Sometimes, it took me three hours or more to get back to sleep. Even if I'm not to get a full night's sleep, I'm usually up at 6:30am or so every morning.

Before my surgery, I was understandably anxious. My primary care physician prescribed Ativan so I could get to sleep a bit easier at night. And, during the day, I learned to do some deep breathing, some meditation, some yoga and some Pilates, just to help me to relax. As time passed, I learned to deal with my anxieties and I was able to sleep better.

ADVICE: Having cancer and losing an organ is a serious life-changing event that's very hard to deal with. I literally grieved the loss of my kidney as I would have the death of a loved one. And at times I still grieve this loss. So, having anxieties and difficulty sleeping is understandable. You need sleep in order for your body to heal. Discuss what you're going through with your medical team. Your doctor may prescribe a sedative to help you relax and sleep. Melatonin may help, but because of the very short pathways, it may not help you stay asleep. If that is the case for you, try Melatonin Sustained Release.

After abdominal surgery, it will take some time for your body to recover. Have your doctor give you a realistic post-surgery recovery timeline. Be patient and don't hesitate to ask your family and friends for support. Just think: If they were in your shoes, you would want to support them too. Also, you can't rush your body's healing process. So, if you find yourself getting anxious and emotional, it is critical that you discuss them with your doctor who may give you a prescription for a sedative, like Ativan. By the way, before your doctor gives you a prescription for a sedative, you must let him or her know if you are taking Melatonin or Melatonin Sustained Release, because they shouldn't be taken together.

* Cindy R. (Metastatic Breast cancer to the Stomach)

My poor sleep habits were due to my being so sick. I just felt so awful all over. It was weird, because when I wanted to get into a comfortable position, it would have to be the fetal position, i.e. lying on my side with my knees to my chest. It was just the weirdest thing. If I laid on my back, straight up and down, I would feel so sick. So, I just kind of kept moving myself around until I found that comfortable spot and then just go right to sleep right there. It was really crazy. I tried so many different positions to adjust myself; it was really crazy. I always had extra pillows too, especially one by my stomach to support it.

ADVICE: If you have a hard time sleeping because you're just not comfortable, try different positions. Don't just conform to whatever. Do what makes you feel relaxed and at ease. Then, be aware of what sleeping or lying position works best for your body and stick with it.

* Glenn M. (Metastatic Colon cancer to the Liver, Lungs & Adrenal Glands)

I didn't have much trouble sleeping until my chemo meds changed from Xeloda and Erbitux to Avastin and Irinotecan. I've taken the sleep-aid Ambien to help me sleep. However, when I really need them, it's like 2:30am; too late to take an Ambien. If I take an Ambien, then I'll miss the wake-up alarm, because when I sleep, I take my hearing aids off.

ADVICE: If you have trouble sleeping, try taking Ambien before you go to sleep. If you don't have to remove hearing aids while you sleep, like I do, then use the Ambien when you wake up in the middle of the night and need to go back to sleep again. Of course, talk with your doctor first about your trouble sleeping, before you take Ambien or any other sleep aid.

* J.B. (Salivary gland cancer)

I didn't really have insomnia per se. I had a hard time sleeping, which was really something I was doing to myself, because I'd be up researching online what I could about my cancer. Since my cancer is very rare, there really wasn't much information online. So, I would keep reading the same article or try to find different statistics online, like survival rates and stuff like that. That's probably what kept me up and made it hard for me to sleep. After a time, of course, I would eventually fall back to sleep.

So I would say, my anxiety caused my poor sleep habits and my anxiety was definitely strongest before any of my treatments.

* Rachel S. (Breast cancer: triple negative)

I had both a hard time falling asleep and also would wake up in the middle of the night. The hard time falling asleep was mainly because every time I would close my eyes, I got that phone call in my head again; the one where the doctor first told me I had cancer. It still happens. That experience was really traumatizing. I still hear it in my head. My doctor prescribed me the sleeping pills Ativan, which helped. But, I have a real fear of getting addicted to things. So, even with my difficulty sleeping, I use the Ativan very sparingly. Only when I went for three or four days without sleep did I find the need to take it.

ADVICE: Sleep is really important for the healing process. If you have a hard time falling asleep or staying asleep, ask your doctor for a prescription of sleeping pills. Take them only when really necessary, so you don't get addicted to them.

* Rick S. (CLL: Blood & Bone Marrow cancer)

I never slept much to begin with. So, I don't know whether my sleep habits were affected by the chemo treatment. Anyway, if I had a hard time sleeping, I would just get up and work out at the gym.

* Scott M. (Metastatic Colon cancer to the Prostate & Pancreas)

I have bad sleep apnea and am a chronic snorer. So, I did a sleep study. I also got a Continuous Positive Airway Pressure aka CPAP machine and my sleep has dramatically improved.

Before the CPAP machine, when I couldn't sleep, I'd watch Netflix at 3:00am. I got into those house-flipping shows, like "Love or List It." But then, I would wake up tired and then try to go through the day. Instead, my day would go downhill, because I would be so tired, ready to collapse, from not having enough sleep the night prior.

The fact that I'm getting forced air into me and I'm breathing and I'm sleeping the night through and I'm waking up rested has really made a huge difference to my health and energy levels. The CPAP machine has really helped me out.

ADVICE: If you have trouble sleeping and it's causing you to wake up tired and weak, get a CPAP machine. It will really make a big difference to your health and energy levels.

* Sondra W. (Ovarian cancer 3x)

I didn't really have poor sleeping habits or insomnia, per se. I think my lack of sleep was more due to having to get up at night because of my bladder and urinary tract problems. Anytime I had to go to the bathroom, I had a lot of pain.

At one point, I had a little bit of swelling. So, I propped my feet up, which made me have to get up more in the middle of the night, which caused more episodes of pain in urinating because of the bladder pain, I already had. But other than that, I was able to sleep when I didn't have to get up to go the bathroom.

* Yesi L. (Breast cancer: triple positive)

Similar to a lot of people out there, I used to sleep in the fetal position ~ everyone's favorite. But because I had bilateral mastectomy and also since I had a mediport implant in my chest, I had to readjust my sleeping position. After my bilateral mastectomy, I pretty much slept seated or on an incline. A lot of pillows and a lot of support getting in and out of bed. As I started to heal, I re-trained myself to sleep on my back and got used to it. Doctors say it's good for you. So, I still sleep on my back.

ADVICE: Adjust your sleeping position, if you cannot sleep your usual way. Use pillows for support and have something to hold on to when you have to get yourself out of bed.

POOR VEINS FOR BLOOD TESTS, CHEMO OR OTHER INFUSIONS

Poor veins are those that run deep, collapse at a drop of hat and don't flow blood fast enough. They're the veins that are challenging for the nurses, phlebotomists or lab technicians to access.

* Amor T. (Breast cancer, Ovarian cancer)

Breast cancer. My veins were nice and plump before my surgery; I donated blood regularly to the Peninsula Blood Bank. After my mastectomy, I lost use of my left arm for anything that required my veins, e.g. IV, blood draws, infusions, finger sticks, blood pressure cuffs, etc. That's because, aside from removing my left breast, the surgeons also removed some of my lymph nodes in the area to prevent the cancer from spreading. When lymph nodes are removed, there exists the potential of decreasing the body's ability to drain fluid from the arm, armpit and chest. When this happens, the lymphatic system can become overloaded and result in swelling (lymphedema). Therefore, extra caution was taken (and continues to be taken) to avoid trauma to the veins of my left arm.

When I was rushed to the ER for my high fever (101.5F-103.5F), they learned that I had a staph infection (cellulitis and sepsis) and so pummeled the veins of my right arm with some serious antibiotics. Aside from the antibiotics, they also had to use my veins there to intravenously keep my body stable with various IV fluids and medication. After a week's stay in the hospital, the veins in my right arm felt heavy; they were taxed to the max.

Since they couldn't use the veins in my left arm, the nurses or phlebotomists that had to draw my blood for follow-up tests after my hospital stays, had difficulty finding a viable vein in my right arm. So, they poked my arm a lot until they were able to find a vein they could use. I had the same experience with radiologic technicians that had to inject contrast dyes into my veins..

Ovarian cancer. When I had to go through chemotherapy, my veins were strong enough to withstand three rounds of chemo. During the third round, however I felt a sharp burning sensation shoot up my arms. I was told later that my veins were too weak. That's when I decided to get a mediport.

In pre-surgery, prepping for my mediport implant turned out to be quite an adventure. Since they had to connect me to an IV, they needed to get a viable vein on my right arm. The first two nurses couldn't do it. Then, the called their vein expert, also known as, the "nurse ninja" to find a viable vein for my IV. She too had a tough time finding a good vein to use. By this time, I had, at least, 15 holes in my arm. Finally, the anesthesiologist came by and found a vein they could use.

When I had to get a PET scan, I still had my mediport. Unfortunately the technologist wasn't trained to use a mediport and also could not find a viable vein on my right arm to inject the radioactive dye into. So, he convinced me that it would be a lot easier to use a vein on my right foot. I thought it would hurt, but it didn't. The tiny prick I felt on my foot were just like the pricks I would feel when they inject my right arm. It was such a breeze! I was surprised and wondered why this wasn't done more often. I have a ton of good strong veins on my feet. I learned later on that when veins on the feet are used for injections, there is big risk of DVT (deep vein thrombosis), which can be very, very dangerous..

In my subsequent visits to the lab to get my blood drawn for tests, I continued having experiences with some nurses or technicians thinking they found a viable vein when they did not, and then "fishing" (move the needle in and out and back and forth in the puncture site), which they are not supposed to do. This is happened during blood draws after my mediport was removed. I did some research and found some useful information. I did find a "vein finder" on Amazon which cost me around $25 but that was an absolute waste of money.

I learned that what really works is to drink a lot of water before hand and to run in place or do some physical like jumping jacks. I learned from my trainer Chris that it would also help for me to just brace my arms against my body as hard as I could. That gets the blood pumping all around especially in my arms. So far, I've done that several times and it has worked every single time. Another thing I learned is to, not only ask to have a butterfly needle used, but to inform them beforehand that I'm a "hard stick" and if they could also use a blood pressure cuff to aid in the process of finding a viable vein.

> **ADVICE:** Drink a lot of water beforehand. Brace your arms against your body as hard as you could and /or do tight shoulder rolls. That will get the blood pumping in your arms. Ask the nurse or technician to use a butterfly needle and tell them you're a "hard stick". You could also suggest they use a blood pressure cuff. If you notice they're starting to "fish" for a good vein, i.e. at the puncture site, they're moving the needle in and out and back and forth, tell them to stop and get someone else to assist.

* _Rachel S._ _(Breast cancer: triple negative)_

Since I can only use my left arm, because all the lymph nodes were taken from my right arm and cannot be used, I wound up having a port put in. They did everything, all the infusions through the port. My left arm still worked fine for my weekly blood draws.

* _Scott M._ _(Metastatic Colon cancer to the Prostate & Pancreas)_

My veins are actually getting to that point now. I had my port taken out a few years ago, so I've been getting my infusions and things in the hands and blood draws up in the arm. My veins are much harder to find now than they were when I started this. And, I got the rest of my life to go, because I've already been told that I'm going to be on maintenance chemo for the rest of my life.

There was a time they took me off of chemo for six months, because I had a lesion re-form in my liver, which they "cyber-knifed" out. So, I've already shown the propensity to have my cancer recur, if they take me off of chemo. So, I'm on the maintenance chemo to keep the cancer at bay and it seems to be working!

ADVICE: When your treatment is done, talk with your doctor about your propensity to have your cancer recur. If there's a likelihood it would recur, when they take you off of chemo, then I strongly recommend that you keep your port in; do not have it removed.

* *Sondra W.* (Ovarian cancer 3x)

Oh, poor veins for blood tests, in chemo and all the infusions…that's absolutely me! I had a mediport put in, and I was so thankful that my doctor suggested that because I have little, tiny, tiny veins. It has been a problem all my life. And my veins collapse, and they also move. They are so small. Often, more than not, the nurses or lab technicians can't access them. So I'm very glad that I had the mediport in.

ADVICE: You definitely should get a mediport, if you have poor, tiny or moving veins like me. It will definitely make you more comfortable during your treatment process. It will also make the lab draws or infusions go faster and be more effective. No more pain from all the poking and prodding, while they try to look for viable veins to use. Yes, I highly recommend getting a mediport if you have poor veins, tiny or moving veins like me.

* *Susan M.* (Ovarian cancer. Metastatic Pancreatic cancer to the Lung)

Ovarian cancer: My veins began to collapse during treatment. So, an anesthesiologist had to be called to put the needle in. **Pancreatic cancer:** After two months of chemo, I decided to have a mediport/port implanted.

ADVICE: Drinking a lot of water before chemo treatments and blood draws. It helps to pump up the veins. If your veins are poor, have a port put in, as soon as possible. It is a simple surgical procedure. The port area will be sore for a couple of weeks, but they can use the port for your treatment the day after it is implanted.

* *Tet M.* (colon cancer 3x)

My veins would collapse as my chemo infusions were about to begin.

ADVICE: Nothing much to offer here except hope to get or request for your favorite nurse who knows your veins well enough to administer chemo on small veins with minimal discomfort.

* *Vida B.A.* (Breast cancer)

After a long period of time when my veins were used for my chemo infusions, blood draws and other tests, they got really, really bad. During my last chemo sessions, the nurses had a really hard time finding a good vein; they had to try five or six times before they got a good one. Eventually, they would find a viable vein in my inner wrist area, instead of the top of my hand where they used to find some of my good veins.

It was interesting. When my veins collapsed, I wondered where they went and almost panicked. Before treatment, I had great veins that you could easily see, running from my wrist to the inner part of my elbow. But then, they disappeared from the collapse. Now, I don't notice it much anymore and I don't worry about it either.

ADVICE: If your same veins are being used a lot for injections, infusions, etc., they're going through trauma. This means they are being strained and/or damaged. Don't panic. Doctors and nurses are trained to find other veins they can use if need be. You'll get used to it, eventually.

* Yesi L. *(Breast cancer: triple positive)*

I have poor veins anyway for blood tests, so I was lucky that I had the Mediport implanted in me before I started chemo. After completing treatment, I had the Mediport removed. Since I no longer have the Mediport and my veins are still very challenging, the nurses use butterfly needles for my blood tests. They do it on my hand and they do a great job. It doesn't hurt. They know my go-to vein on my hands too.

ADVICE: If you have poor veins that challenge the nurse or technician who has to draw your blood, ask them to use the butterfly needles. Also, identify a "go-to" vein for future blood tests or infusions.

RESTLESS LEG SYNDROME

A condition in which a person has a strong urge to move his or her legs in order to stop uncomfortable sensations. These include burning, itching, creeping, tugging, crawling, or pain. These feelings usually happen when a person is lying or sitting down, and are worse at night. They can also occur in other parts of the body. Also called RLS.

* Glenn M. *(Metastatic Colon cancer to the Liver, Lungs & Adrenal Glands)*

At one time, when they gave me Benadryl before my chemo, my legs began to kick like crazy. One of the nurses told me that it's a real common reaction and it'll wear off in time. So, I just stayed there, until the drug wore off and my legs stopped kicking.

ADVICE: You can just wait for your legs to stop kicking. I also heard that you can take a hot bath and/or massage your legs to get them to relax.

SHINGLES

Shingles is an outbreak of rash or blisters on the skin. It is caused by the varicella-zoster virus - the same virus that causes chickenpox. After you have chickenpox, the virus stays in your body. It may not cause problems for many years. But as you get older, the virus may reappear as shingles.

People newly diagnosed with cancer, particularly blood cancers, and those treated with chemotherapy have a greater risk of developing shingles

* Vida B.A. *(Breast cancer)*

After my fifth chemo session, I developed shingles, probably due to my weakened immune system. At first, I thought the itchiness, rash and pain were just from mosquito bites or some insect bites. This happened during the Christmas season and I remember getting headaches and feeling so weak. When I saw my doctor, he noted that my rash had a pattern that pointed to shingles. So, he prescribed the nerve pain medication, Gabapentin, which I took immediately. Even though it was mild, it took care of the shingles, and without side effects that other nerve medications tend to have. I had to take extra to make sure the shingles didn't return.

ADVICE: Since shingles usually affects those with weakened immune systems and chemotherapy weakens our system, be aware of the symptoms of shingles, i.e. itching or prickling skin combined with pain and followed by a rash that looks like a group of fluid-filled blisters on a red, inflamed area of your skin. If you think you have shingles, let your doctor know immediately, so that you can get medication to take care of it.

Chemotherapy may damage fast growing skin and nail cells. This can cause problems such as skin that is dry, itchy, red, and/or that peels. Some people may develop a rash or sun sensitivity, causing you to sunburn easily.

* *Glenn M.* (*Metastatic Colon cancer to the Liver, Lungs & Adrenal Glands*)

I experienced a lot of pain, mostly from the thinning and breaking skin around my fingers and toes, which bled because the nails cut the skin. I used Aquaphor quite a bit on my hands and feet. It's a moisturizer that prevents drying, itchy or irritated skin. The thing I really like about Aquaphor is that it's fast and easy. My dermatologist also prescribed a 2.5% steroid ointment for me to use, in case the skin around my fingers and/or toes got really bad. They put the fire out immediately.

I had changes in my scalp. If the sun is coming through the window I can make "snow" from my dry scalp. When I thought I was okay to stop taking Doxycycline (an antibiotic), one of the nurses told me, "No, you should continue taking it." Then I discovered that because I stopped taking it, I got all "flaky"; so flaky that I could've made "snow" all day! I basically do nothing for my scalp; only for the drying skin on my face.

My hero dermatologist gave me a lotion and a nice cleanser out of her store. When I take a shower, I use the cleanser and a terry cloth. All that dry skin scrubs off. Then I put the lotion on my face while it is still wet, because it's water-soluble and will be absorbed nicely. I use the lotion heavily when I go to bed. Before going to work outside, I use more lotion and rub it into my skin a little deeper. That lotion stopped the flaking of my skin. The lotion's name is: La Roche Posay Toleriane Hydrating Gentle Cleanser. You're supposed to be able to get it at Target, in-store or online.

Vinyl gloves also offer a lot of protection. They keep the moisture in. Not only that. When I wear the gloves and put both hands in hot water when I wash the dishes, the water won't scald my skin and the dishes will still feel hot. When I pull something out of the toaster, my hands are protected. I didn't wash my hands often, because I couldn't get them dry enough to slide into the gloves. So, sometimes, I just put my gloves over dirty hands to fix dinner. I think it's clever and actually practical. I buy the vinyl gloves at Costco. There are 200 gloves in a box and you buy them as a two-box pack. So, you're getting 400 gloves and they only cost around $12.00. They are good and handy and a great deal.

> **ADVICE:** For thinning and breaking skin around my fingernails and toenails, use Aquaphor. It's a moisturizer that prevents drying, itchy or irritated skin. It's really great and also fast and easy. If the pain from the cuts of your thinning skin gets worse, ask your doctor for a prescription for 2.5% steroids. It'll put out the fire immediately.
>
> Wear gloves when the skin on your hands get sensitive. The gloves will protect you, keep your hands from drying and they're practical too. Vinyl gloves worked best for me. I bought mine from Costco at $12.00 for 400 gloves; a great deal!
>
> Finally, because it worked wonders for me, I highly recommend you check out La Roche Posay Toleriane Hydrating Gentle Cleanser, if the skin on your body or face is drying. After you wash with it, your skin will literally feel smooth and soft, like baby skin!

* *J.B.* (*Salivary gland cancer*)

As I had more radiation therapy, the skin on my cheeks became dry and a bit painful. It felt like a really bad sunburn. What I did to take care of my skin was use Vaseline.

* *Rachel S.* (*Breast cancer: triple negative*)

I didn't start seeing the effects of the radiation on my skin, until after I had been going for about three weeks. My skin started darkening. All the freckles that I had on my skin started really coming out....freckles I didn't even know I had. Just freckles everywhere. I did radiation for five weeks, five days a week, Monday through Friday. I finished on February 7, 2017 with no issues; I got through it perfectly. About a week after my last radiation, my skin started peeling. They kept telling me that it would be like a sunburn ... you know when you get sunburn and it peels, you have another layer of skin underneath it ... But, it wasn't like that at all. I had open wounds! They were big, gaping wounds that were seeping out fluid. You could see the flesh underneath. That's what it looked like in my chest. It was the most painful thing ever!

The doctor had given me an aluminum calcium powder called Domeboro, which I mixed with water, soaked a gauze pad in it and placed the gauze pad over my wound, like a burn victim. But, it didn't work! It was so difficult for me; it was such a horrible experience! Fortunately, a friend of mine gave me a special lotion that they use in France. When I used it, the following day, the open gaping wounds had a film over them; like protective film. I used it every day and saw that when my skin peeled off, it didn't leave an open gaping wound underneath it anymore. It worked wonders and got rid of everything within two days.

ADVICE: Look out for your skin peeling after going through a lot of radiation. If peeling causes your skin to reveal your flesh underneath, like an open wound, immediately ask your doctor for a prescription to heal your wounds, like the aluminum talcum powder called Domeboro.

* Rick S. (CLL: Blood & Bone Marrow cancer)

I had some itchiness on my skin, but not that much. While I was experiencing itchiness, I was also experiencing really dry skin. For my itchiness, my doctor prescribed a lotion for me to put on after my showers. It worked. I'm not sure if my drying skin was the side effect of the chemo. Nevertheless, once I used the lotion that my doctor prescribed to me, the dryness in my skin disappeared.

* Sondra W. (Ovarian cancer 3x)

The skin on my hands turned dark, kind of dark "red-like". And the skin on the bottom of my feet also darkened. My nurse practitioner told me that the Avastin would cause my skin to change and turn "red". My skin did change in color, and it became dark red.

ADVICE: Change in skin is only temporary when going through treatment. So, no need to worry or do anything about it. Your skin will return to its "normal" color in due time.

* Vida B.A. (Breast cancer)

Before I went through radiation, the skin covering my temporary implant was totally healed and looked flawless, even though I didn't have a nipple. After my radiation, however, the incision area darkened; it was burnt. The skin in my armpit area was burnt too. It felt like sunburn. Then I started itching in those areas. I was supposed to get my permanent implant after radiation, but I held off because I was uncomfortable at that time.

My doctor gave me an ointment to use and taught me how to clean the affected areas with hydrogen peroxide, apply the ointment and then dress it with gauze. I also bought a very expensive cream from France that contained a lot of skin-healing minerals and applied it to the affected areas. Since my skin got so soft, it peeled off whenever I took showers. After 2-3 weeks, my skin healed. The affected areas are still a bit dark, but not as dark as before.

ADVICE: The radiation therapy process itself is really quick; from several minutes to less than 30 minutes. It actually takes longer to wait to get into the treatment room. After you receive radiation, observe changes to your skin each time. Let your doctor know when you see darkening and/or burning of your skin, so that he or she can guide you on what to do. Even though you can expect your skin to burn and darken, there are good topical creams and ointments out in the market that can heal your skin.

STIFFNESS

Stiffness refers to the inability to move easily and without pain. It is caused by a variety of problems, including pain from muscle injury, inflammation, overuse, exercise soreness, arthritis, lymphedema or edema (swelling).

* Amor T. (Breast cancer, Ovarian cancer)

Breast cancer. After my mastectomy and breast reconstruction surgery, my body was really swollen and stiff, I could barely move. Same thing happened after my breast symmetry and nipple reconstruction surgery three months later. This was due to the many deep incisions made on my torso, caused by inflammation from the surgeries; all part of the process. As my incisions were healing, especially in my abdomen, I felt pretty stiff because it was tough to stretch out the abdominal muscles that had been cut.

Despite my stiffness, I did what I could to move around to improve circulation and strengthen my weakened muscles. I tried to sit straight and stand upright, as much as possible. Thank God for painkillers, because they really allowed me to get my body to stretch and move, so that I could heal correctly!

Ovarian cancer. I experienced a lot of stiffness from my radical hysterectomy, especially where they made an eight-inch long vertical incision from the bottom of my chest plate down to my lower pelvic bone. Again, painkillers helped me deal with them.

> **ADVICE:** If you undergo major surgery where incisions were made in your body, you can expect to feel stiffness/rigidity as your body works to recover. Painkillers will help, not just to give you relief from pain, but also to enable you to move around, which is necessary for your body to heal.

* Rachel S. (Breast cancer: triple negative)

When I had a double mastectomy, they removed all the lymph nodes from my right arm and only two lymph nodes from my left arm. I got Lymphedema because I no longer have lymph nodes in my right arm. My right arm doesn't have the capability anymore to push the poison fluids – for lack of a better word – from my arm, in order for me to urinate them out. So, I have to wear a compression sleeve every day for the rest of my life. There are days when I can't move my arm. It feels like there's a bar going down my arm and it's hard to straighten it. And the only thing I can do for that is to exercise and to stretch it out. It usually lasts a couple of days. And then I have to constantly massage my arm and my spine to keep the swelling down, because once the arm starts to swell, it's very, very difficult to get it to go back to normal.

> **ADVICE:** If you have lymphedema, use compression sleeves and garments to help bring down the swelling and stiffness. You can also stretch it out, massage the area and also elevate it. Be proactive and do it constantly, because once you start to swell, it's very difficult to get it back to normal.

SWELLING / EDEMA

"Edema" is the medical term for swelling. Body parts swell from injury or inflammation. It can affect a small area or the entire body. Medications, pregnancy, infections, and many other medical problems can cause edema. Edema happens when your small blood vessels leak fluid into nearby tissues

* Amor T. (Breast cancer, Ovarian cancer)

My body was pretty swollen after all of my surgeries (caesarean section, mastectomy, breast reconstruction and radical hysterectomy), which is to be expected anytime our body is cut open. Swelling is the result of the increased movement of fluid and white blood cells into the area of inflammation and inflammation is part of our body's immune response. I knew that the swelling would go down; I just needed to give it time. Sure enough, it did.

I did light exercise or walked to help to promote circulation needed to bring down the swelling. After my DIEP flap breast reconstruction surgery where tissue was removed from my lower abdomen and transferred to my chest to reconstruct my left breast, wearing a compression binder also helped to decrease swelling in my abdominal area. I tried to drink plenty of water to flush my system and increase blood circulation too, in order to heal properly

To avoid bruising, I avoided foods high in salicylates, like green pepper, olives, mushrooms, tomatoes, radishes, apricots, blackberries, blueberries, cantaloupe, dates, guava and raisins.

> **ADVICE:** When your body swells after surgery, take your pain meds as directed, so that you can move around (light exercise, walk, etc.) in order to promote circulation needed to bring down the swelling. If you had abdominal surgery, use a compression binder. That and drinking plenty of water will help bring your swelling down.

* Sondra W. (Ovarian cancer 3x)

I had a lot of swelling during my second round of treatment. The swelling, which was on my feet and legs, was caused by the Avastin. My oncologist did inform me that this would happen. Avastin also drives up blood pressure. So, I had to be on blood pressure medication for the last two weeks to counter this. Unfortunately, that high blood pressure medication also caused my feet and legs to swell.

Because excess fluid that had accumulated in the tissues was looking for a way to get out, I developed blisters and my skin, degraded, turning black and crusty, as if they had been burnt. With the fluid buildup, my skin also became so tight, and the pain was excruciating. I took pain medication, especially at night when my legs and feet would throb, and that provided the relief that I needed. Fortunately, I lost 15 lbs. of excess fluid. Unfortunately, I still have swelling in my legs and feet, so I have to keep them propped up. I also have to continue taking Lasix Furosemide, which is a diuretic to treat my fluid retention and swelling.

> **ADVICE:** Propping your feet or legs up helps to relieve the swelling in your feet or legs. Also, wear compression stockings/leggings. They help reduce swelling, improve blood flow and prevent deep vein thrombosis (DVT), which is a blood clot that can create a very serious condition.

* Susan M. (Ovarian cancer. Metastatic Pancreatic cancer to the Lung)

Pancreatic cancer: I had a pancreaticoduodenectomy (Whipple Procedure), which was a seven-hour, major surgery where several of my organs were removed. Fatigue set in during my 22-day stay in the hospital and continued for several months. During my second round of chemo to treat the metastasis of the cancer to my right lung, I felt fatigue for a day or two after treatment and swelling in my throat a couple of times, but nothing major. Other than that, I've been doing well considering.

For three days, before each of my chemotherapy sessions, I had to take steroids three times a day to counter any allergic reaction to the chemo drugs. They caused my face to swell up and look puffy. Since it didn't hurt, I just dealt with it as part of my treatment.

> **ADVICE:** Steroids cause swelling. Once you stop taking the steroids, the swelling goes away. The best way to deal with it is to simply accept it. The swelling will go away after your treatment ends.

TASTE & SMELL CHANGES

Cancer and its treatments can change your senses of taste and smell. These changes can affect your appetite and are often described as a bitter or metallic taste.

* Amor T. (Breast cancer, Ovarian cancer)

Breast cancer. During my weeklong stay at the hospital, following my mastectomy and diep flap breast reconstruction, I enjoyed wonderful, savory food from the hospital's dining room. When my staph infection landed me in the hospital again for another week, I ordered the same delicious, savory shrimp stir fry dish I had before. When my food order came in, my friends from the Foster City Lions Club were visiting me. I immediately noticed that the aroma was unpleasant for me, unlike before when I would salivate at the smell. Since I was still shivering a lot, one of my friends, Chris, offered to feed me. I took the first spoonful of the delicious shrimp stir fry and just gagged. After I swallowed, my stomach turned immediately and I had to hurl. I was so nauseated and I did not understand why. Following that incident, I just resorted to eating crackers, light soup and jello until I was able to take in heavier foods.

Ovarian cancer. My taste buds were blah during treatment. I didn't enjoy my food, including the delicious, savory dishes I used to enjoy. Since I didn't have much of an appetite and forced myself to eat, I just ate saltine crackers and added a dollop of sweet jam or jelly on top. I found that just a little bit of sweetness would get my taste buds to jump for joy. Now, if I had more than one dollop of jam or jelly on my cracker, my taste buds would be overwhelmed.

> <u>ADVICE:</u> Harsh ingredients in chemotherapy drugs and antibiotics damage taste buds and the distorted senses produce a metallic or bitter taste. That's to be expected. I found that just a tiny bit of sweetness added to a cracker or slice of bread is all my taste buds need to get over the bitterness or metallic tastes. Any more than a dollop would overwhelm my taste buds. I also discovered that I did better staying away from hot foods, since hot-plated foods typically carry a stronger aroma than cold foods.

> Here are other tips:
>
> - Stop using metal utensils. Instead, use plastic or wooden ones when eating.
> - Avoid canned, microwaved foods and artificial sweeteners.
> - Eat foods that are tart.
> - Take zinc supplements.
> - Stay away from restaurants, cafeterias or hot food sources with overwhelming odors.

* Cindy R. (Metastatic Breast cancer to Stomach)

From both my treatments (breast and stomach cancer), the changes in my taste buds completely affected my appetite. It was so crazy, because I had weird cravings like I was pregnant, but I was actually going through cancer.

I craved for soft chocolate chip cookies in the worst way! I craved crescent rolls, which I love. But, I couldn't get myself to even smell them, because the smell would make me feel so sick! Then, before treatment, I use to not care for tomatoes, tomato sauce, tomato paste, tomato soup and anything with tomatoes. But then, oh boy, I love that stuff now! The cool thing is that tomato is one of the top anti-cancer foods!

I also had to deal with smell changes. It was like "endless" perfume. When I was around anyone that had perfume on, one sniff and I would feel like I was going to pass out. So, I had to tell everyone around me, "Please, if there's any way possible, don't wear perfume or cologne or any fragrance."

> <u>ADVICE:</u> There's actually not much you can do when you have taste changes, except to be aware and work with the changes. It can be really interestingly weird; not necessarily a bad thing.
>
> As for the smell changes, just let those around you know if you're sensitive to certain scents or aromas. That way, they'll be aware and not wear fragrance or bring with them any smell that you're sensitive to.

* Glenn M. (Metastatic Colon cancer to the Liver, Lungs & Adrenal Glands)

Yes, I definitely had taste and smell changes that affected my appetite. I think that it could've been the Oxaliplatin that caused it, because I didn't have the problem as I stopped that regimen. There was nothing really I could do to get my sense of taste or smell back to normal. I just ate less. I used to eat ice cream, but I stopped. One time, my dogs looked at me as if to say, "Where's our ice cream?" Well, I decided to put ice cream in their respective bowls. When I did that, they looked at me as if to say, "You mean dinner is ice cream?" I then looked at the clock and noticed that it was 11:00pm and we hadn't had dinner. So anyway, I fed the dogs and then put them to bed.

> <u>ADVICE:</u> There's really not much you can do to get your sense of taste or smell back, if your medication is causing you to lose those senses. Just work with it and make sure you eat, to keep your energy up.

* J.B. *(Salivary gland cancer)*

I did lose my sense of taste halfway into the radiation therapy. It was more like a loss of the ability to taste and smell.

* Rachel S. *(Breast cancer: triple negative)*

Going through the chemo, there were things that I liked before the chemo and then, all of a sudden, I didn't. Like avocados. I couldn't stand the taste of avocados when I was going through chemo ... And I LOVE avocados! However, shortly after everything was done, my taste buds kind of started going back to normal.

> **ADVICE:** If you notice you don't enjoy your favorite foods, because they don't taste good anymore, don't worry. It's temporary. After your treatment, your taste buds will return to enjoying them again.

* Sondra W. *(Ovarian cancer 3x)*

I experienced taste and smell changes, the first time around. I had that metal kind of taste in my mouth and couldn't really taste things. That made my eating very boring and kind of hard, but I tried to eat anyway. Later, I learned to use fresh spice, especially basil, oregano and lemon juice to pump up my sense of taste. They were really simple to use. My big joy is that I didn't have those taste or smell problems the second time around. So, that was wonderful!

> **ADVICE:** Rinsing your mouth may help a bit with the metallic taste. You could also try using fresh spice, especially basil and oregano, as well as lemon juice, to pump up your sense of test. Other than that, keep in mind that it's temporary and just deal with it.

* Tet M. *(colon cancer 3x)*

When I drank water, it had a strange metallic smell and taste. Actually, to me it tasted and smelled more like onions soaked in water. Bottled water wasn't as popular back then. Perhaps this or filtered water would be a viable option? This change in taste and smell also affected my showering and cleansing routine. Basically, anytime I had contact with water, I tasted or smelled onions in water, which was not pleasant at all for me. The entire experience lasted throughout my chemo treatment period. However, it was the strongest the first couple of days after my chemo infusions.

> **ADVICE:** Try drinking bottled or filtered water instead. It may taste better for you. Take quicker showers if you wish and inhale through the mouth.

* Vida B.A. *(Breast cancer)*

For the first two weeks after chemo, I would lose my taste buds. I would just not able to taste anything, which made me not feel like eating. But, I still forced myself to eat, because I knew that I needed nutrients from food to boost my immune system and strengthen my body. Fortunately, on the third week, my taste buds and my energy would return. Yes, the third week was my "happy"' week. I didn't know it back then, but since I was on a three-week treatment cycle, after the third week, the cycle would start again where I would lose my taste buds and have it return on the third week. It's part of the process.

> **ADVICE:** Losing your taste buds during chemo treatments is common. The main thing is making sure you continue eating, even if you don't feel like it. The nutrients from food is critical to your immune system, energy and strength. Try adding turmeric spice to your food. Not only will it help with the taste, turmeric is also really good for you.

* **Yesi L.** *(Breast cancer: triple positive)*

I definitely experienced a difference in taste during treatment. Food tasted bland. But compared to other side effects, that was just one I didn't worry about too much. So I just let it be.

VOICE CHANGES

A little known side effect of chemotherapy is voice impairment, which can sometimes affects swallowing and nutrition.

* **Rev. Linda S.** *(Pancreatic cancer 3x)*

My voice is two pitches higher than normal; a side effect of chemo. This should pass.

WEIGHT LOSS

When people lose weight during cancer treatment, it is most often due to an inability to maintain good nutrition. Chemotherapy can sometimes cause nausea and a general loss of appetite, while vomiting and diarrhea can greatly impact your ability to retain nutrients from the foods you eat.

* **Aaron C.** *(Prostate cancer, Skin cancer)*

After surgery, I did lose some weight, because I lost muscle from not being able to work out and lift weights. I also lost a lot of strength. I regained my strength after some time of eating better and returning to working out and weight lifting. It took me six months to regain the strength and weight I lost in just three months.

ADVICE: Going through major surgery takes a toll on your body. So, losing weight and strength is expected. Give your body time to rest and make sure you eat, so your body gets the nutrients it needs to heal. You should then be able to regain your weight and your strength in time.

* **Amor T.** *(Breast cancer, Ovarian cancer)*

I lost 15-20 lbs. which I was actually happy about. The clothes that used to be snug on me either fit nicely or were loose. I lost weight because I wasn't inclined to eat due to my taste buds being so off. Anything I put into my mouth tasted blah, metallic or bitter. Of course, I understood that my body needed food to be able to sustain itself. So, I forced myself to eat. There were several things that helped: L-Glutamine supplements (10 grams 3x a day) taken with a glass full of diluted 100% fruit juice, eating little portions of plain rice, eggs, bread, etc. throughout the day and eating crackers with a little dollop of sweet "coco jam" or grape or strawberry jam/jelly.

ADVICE: Take L-Glutamine "powdered" supplements (10 grams 3x a day) with a glass full of diluted 100% fruit juice. Artificial ingredients cause the metallic or bitter taste, so you'll want to avoid food or beverages containing anything artificial. Eat little portions of plain rice, eggs, bread, etc. throughout the day. Eating crackers with a little dollop of sweet jam also helps.

* **Cindy L.** *(Kidney cancer)*

One of the things that will cause permanent damage to a kidney is high blood pressure. To combat my high blood pressure, I had to work to lower my weight. So I quit sugar, went on a lower carb diet and lost 48 lbs. at an alarming rate of speed and in a very short period of time. This was actually before kidney cancer diagnosis but we knew there was a problem at that time… my weight wasn't helping matters any.

My blood pressure still fluctuates and so, I have to continue to work on lowering my weight. Now, I'm at the point where I can work out more. So, I'm doing that and also going on a sensible lower carb diet… not no carbs. I eat plenty of vegetables, fruits a few times per week and I've cut out added sugars and foods with high sugar content. I also keep fats fairly low, keeping to good fats. I never add additional salt and stay at around 2300 mg a day of sodium. That is very low compared to the average American diet. I'm within 20 pounds of my normal weight. So, not too bad. I will keep working on it but not completely eliminating whole important food groups. Sugar is not an important food group!

ADVICE: If you have to lose weight to prevent your condition from worsening, like high blood pressure, then you should commit to regular exercise and healthy eating. Discuss with your physician about lowering your carbs, lowering your calories, decreasing sodium (no added salt at all) and quit added sugar. Discuss your plan with your doctor and make sure he or she is on board with it.

* Glenn M. (Metastatic Colon cancer to the Liver, Lungs & Adrenal Glands)

My weight loss is tied to my hyperthyroidism. Hyperthyroidism shortens life, because with it, our hearts beat faster. I try to make tastier food, so I eat. My oncologist said, "I don't care if you get a gallon of ice cream. Just get those g#%*m calories down!" You see, I'm already skinny. So, my oncologist was afraid that if I lost more weight (especially given my age) and something went wrong, I would just get so weak that I wouldn't be able to process the food I need to gain strength.

And here, I'm trying to gain weight and it's coming out of both ends: Diarrhea in one end and vomiting on the other end. At one time, my weight decreased from 180 lbs. when I was diagnosed to 135 lbs. I'm slowly inching up; I'm about 160 lbs. now. I eat a lot of ice cream, which my oncologist highly approves of. He said, "It's calories down the hatch."

To increase my weight, I also tried to drink a protein beverage that Costco sells that has 30 grams of protein. I forgot the name (chemo brain). Unfortunately, I didn't like drinking it, so it didn't work for me. It has been hard. Anyway, I have been eating more ice cream; eating the calories. Yeah, ice cream any time of the day…And, yeah, make it a full fat one too!

ADVICE: If you're losing weight, you need to do what you can to gain it back or else your body will get weaker. Try eating a lot of ice cream…the full fat one too. Like my doctor said, "It's calories down the hatch."

* Joan S. (Rectal cancer)

I seriously just lost my appetite and had a hard time taking in food. So, I lost 40 lbs. I did try to bring up my weight and digest something, so my body could heal. Chocolate-flavored Ensure (power drink) from Costco was my answer.

ADVICE: You need food to heal. So, even if you don't have appetite, you must eat something. Try taking Ensure. It's a power drink, a nutrition shake, which has a lot of nutrients. They have a variety of flavors and you can buy it at Costco.

After my first series of chemo treatments, I lost 44 lbs. But I was overweight, so this loss was good. For my second series of chemo treatments, I've lost a lot of weight (62 lbs. to date), but it seems to have stabilized at my current weight of 132 lbs. I'm 5'5". The dietician said I'm eating right, just eat more of it and she gave me tips on how to amp up the protein with my fruit and veggies when meat feels indigestible, such as slathering peanut butter on apple slices.

ADVICE: Talk with your dietician about your eating patterns and get tips of how to eat better. Amp up your protein with fruits and veggies, when meat feels indigestible, like slathering peanut butter on apple slices.

* Rachel S. (Breast cancer: triple negative)

I actually kept my weight pretty even. I didn't lose; I didn't gain. I think that I, maybe, gained five pounds, at most, which was really amazing to me, because everybody thinks that with cancer, you're going to lose all this weight. I knew that if I started losing weight, then I would start to lose strength, which would lead to my getting sick and things going downhill from there. So, I tried really, really, really hard ... even if I wasn't hungry... to force myself to eat something.

> **ADVICE:** It is really important to keep a check on your weight. When you're sick, you need to make sure you nourish your body with food, so that it has the strength to fight your sickness. Even if you are not hungry, force yourself to eat something, anything.

* *Rick S.* (CLL: Blood & Bone Marrow cancer)

I know I lost weight when I got double pneumonia, which was before I found out that I had CLL. I could've lost weight as a side effect of my cancer treatment, but 'm not sure.

* *Scott M.* (Metastatic Colon cancer to the Prostate & Pancreas)

There was a period of time when I lost a huge amount of weight after I went through lots and lots of endoscopic procedures. They didn't know what was going on. They opened me up ... did stuff ... They worked on my pancreas and I healed there. But, I was in a "failure to thrive" mode. Food just turned my stomach and would make me ill on the food tray. One day, my sister-in-law brought me a turkey sandwich for lunch. Looking at the whole plate of food was just enough to gag me. So she took the sandwich, cut a one-inch square of bread out of it, put one little, tiny, one-inch square of turkey on the bread and one drop of mayo or of mustard ... put it together ... and set it on the corner of my tray and had the rest of the food removed from the room. That tiny one-inch turkey sandwich sat on the corner of my tray and I kept looking at it. Then I thought, "You know, I do like turkey, and that's not very much. So, I could probably try that." So, I put it in my mouth; I tasted it and I liked it! And, from that, I was able to slowly come out; reintroduce food into my system. My aversion to food might have been caused by PTSD (Post Traumatic Stress Disorder) from all the procedures my body went through.

I had lost 70 lbs. weighing only about 130 lbs. Everybody thought I was going to die. Of course, nobody told me that then. Thank God, because that thought <u>never</u> crossed my mind! I knew that I was going to pull out of this ... it was just a matter of time.

> **ADVICE:** Sometimes, when your body is going through a lot of changes and procedures, it gets overwhelmed and decides to shut down. When that happens, it helps to reintroduce things very gradually, like food. Keep in mind that your eyes play a large part in determining what food to eat. So, start with a little piece of your favorite food (for example, the one-inch piece of turkey sandwich I was given) and then work your way up in size. The biggest thing is to <u>never</u> give up. No matter how hard you're struggling, keep in mind that you're going to pull out of your struggles; it's just a matter of time.

* *Sondra W.* (Ovarian cancer 3x)

It took me the full six weeks to recover from my hysterectomy. Unfortunately, after the surgery, I experienced a lot of diarrhea and lost a lot of weight; about 30 pounds. I just couldn't seem to get over that. My doctor kept testing me to make sure I didn't have some bacteria. But the results were always negative. Finally, weeks and weeks later, I took one test that had a positive result. Even though I was given antibiotics, I still had a lot of intestinal stuff going on. I experienced so much diarrhea, I had gone down in weight to 108 lbs. I worked with a nutritionist and as my treatment regimen changed, my weight changed, ranging from 125 lbs. to 108 lbs.

You know, I never thought the day would come when someone would tell me to eat as much as I could. Back then, when my doctor told me that, I couldn't believe it. I was like, "He told me to eat as much as I can, but I have all these intestinal problems." Then I told myself, "Gaining weight is a priority." That was an interesting experience.

> **ADVICE:** If you have a good appetite, but have trouble keeping your weight up, you need to get yourself checked for bacteria or possible intestinal problem. It is critical that you be able to eat the foods high in nutrients, which will help keep your body strong enough to cope with the challenges of treatment. Work with a nutritionist and add nutritional drinks, if you can, e.g. Boost, Ensure.

* **Susan M.** (*Ovarian cancer. Metastatic Pancreatic cancer to the Lungs*)

When I had pancreatic cancer, I lost seventeen pounds between the time I was diagnosed to the time I left the hospital, after my surgery.

> **ADVICE:** Be patient. It took a year, but I gained my weight back.

* **Vida B.A.** (*Breast cancer*)

Because I wasn't eating much, I did lose weight. However, it wasn't obvious because of the steroids I was taking that made my face look swollen and puffy. I had to take the steroids three times a day for three days before chemo.

> **ADVICE:** Weight loss is expected when you lose your appetite or taste buds, which is a side effect of chemo treatment. No matter what, you need to eat and keep yourself from losing weight, because you need the nutrients from food to boost your immune system and strengthen your body. The best way to check your weight is by weighing yourself on the scale; not by looks, because that can be deceiving.

* **Yesi L.** (*Breast cancer: triple positive*)

I am normally very thin. I've been like that all my life. I do eat well, so it's definitely not for lack of eating. I lost a lot of weight, because the treatments were so hard on my body and affected my appetite. I think I went from 115 lbs. down to 100 lbs. I weighed 100 pounds and had no hair. So, I called myself "Little Casper."

YEAST INFECTION

Yeast infection is a condition in which too much yeast grows in certain areas of the body and causes symptoms and disease. Small amounts of yeast normally live on the skin and in other parts of the body, such as the mouth, throat, and vagina. Sometimes, too much yeast can grow in these areas and cause infection. Yeast infections may also occur in the blood and spread throughout the body, but this is rare. Certain conditions, such as a weakened immune system, diabetes, pregnancy, hormone changes, and stress, and use of certain medicines may increase the risk of yeast infection.

* **Amor T.** (*Breast cancer, Ovarian cancer*)

I had developed a staph infection (cellulitis and sepsis) after my mastectomy and diep flap breast reconstruction surgeries. My fever climbed to past 103.5 F degrees and my doctors continuously "pummeled" my body with really heavy antibiotics for a week to combat the infection. Thankfully, my fever cleared. Unfortunately, when I returned home, I noticed itchiness in my privates. I ate a lot of plain yogurt and drank a lot of water to flush it out, but it persisted. When I met with my doctor, she informed me that the strong antibiotics I had been given caused my yeast infection and gave me a prescription for the antibiotic fluconazole, which took care of the problem.

> **ADVICE:** Try eating plain yogurt and drinking plenty of fluids. If that doesn't work, ask your doctor for something stronger, like an antibiotic.

~ 0 ~

Chapter 5

DEALING WITH MEDICAL TREATMENTS AND PROCEDURES

In order to rid our bodies of cancer, we may have to go through more than one procedure. Thanks to advancements in medical technology, we have many options to choose from. The wide variety of available medical treatments and procedures can be overwhelming and the unknowns of each can create a lot of anxiety.

In this chapter, we share our experiences of the many procedures we went through, so that you'll get an idea of what they entail. Just remember that, no matter how tough the experience, we overcame the hurdles and came out alive and kicking. You can too!

BREAST RECONSTRUCTION / BREAST SYMMETRY

Breast reconstruction is the rebuilding of a breast, usually in women. It involves using autologous tissue or prosthetic material to construct a natural-looking breast. Often this includes the reformation of a natural-looking areola and nipple. This procedure involves the use of implants or tissue taken from other parts of the woman's body. More often, women only need to have a single mastectomy. In such cases, having a second surgery to match the reconstructed breast and achieve symmetry is needed.

* *Amor T.* (Breast cancer, Ovarian cancer)

When I first learned that I had breast cancer, I knew I was going to have a mastectomy and breast reconstruction after, but needed to get more information. So, I did some research and learned that, aside from getting silicone or saline breast implants, I also had the option to get a DIEP flap breast reconstruction where my own tissue would be used to create a new breast. I exclaimed, "Wow!" and immediately decided that that was the procedure I wanted to have done.

My DIEP Flap Choice. Since I decided to have the DIEP flap breast reconstruction surgery I asked my plastic surgeon to explain the entire procedure to me. He did and then said that there were two advantages:

1. Since I would be using my own tissue, my body would have no problem adjusting to my new breast, and
2. I would also be getting a "tummy tuck", since my new breast tissue would be taken from the fatty tissue in my abdomen that I didn't need. (My reaction: YAY!!)

Surgery. On June 24, 2013, I had the mastectomy of my left breast with the DIEP flap breast reconstruction following immediately after. As my plastic surgeon had described prior, he made a long horizontal incision in my abdomen from one end of the hip to the other. He then took the tissue or "flap", i.e. fat, skin and blood vessels from the wall of my lower belly and moved it up to my chest to rebuild my left breast. Then, using microsurgery, he reattached the blood vessels of the flap to the blood vessels in my chest. When he closed my abdomen, he also reshaped a new navel for me. My surgery took a total of eight hours. When I awoke, I was in the ICU (intensive care unit) and quite dopey, no doubt from the painkillers I was given.

My reconstructed breast healed fine. My long, horizontal abdominal wound, on the other hand, took a bit longer. Although my abdominal muscles were not cut, the entire area was still swollen and painful from all the activity. My doctor gave me hydrocodone/paracetamol (vicodin) to take for pain every six hours, whether or not I had pain. I was also directed to walk around and be active, as much as possible. Taking the vicodin helped me to cope with my pain as I tried to walk around and be active, even if very slowly.

One of the things I had to get used to was consistently placing a small pillow firmly on my abdomen before I did any of the following: coughing, sneezing or just moving, in general. I also placed that small pillow on my abdomen to protect it when I started driving again, which was after six weeks, post-surgery.

Breast Symmetry. I met with my plastic surgeon again to discuss follow-up surgery to correct the asymmetry between my left and right breasts, as well as to reconstruct my left nipple. He gave me a choice to make my natural right breast as big as my newly reconstructed left one, but also informed me that having additional tissue in my right breast may prevent future mammograms from detecting any cancer. Upon hearing that, I chose to have a reduction of my newly reconstructed left breast instead.

On September 3rd, I had my breast symmetry surgery, along with my left nipple reconstruction. It was done on an outpatient basis and I left the hospital with an abdominal binder and one surgical drain bulb to remove excess fluid from my body after the surgery. After three months, I was able to see a micropigmentation (tattoo) artist to create my new 3D nipple. Two one-hour sessions later, I had a new, realistic-looking reconstructed nipple and my newly reconstructed left breast. Thank God for advancements in medical technology!

Insurance coverage of breast reconstruction and related procedures: By the way, I was very happy and relieved to learn that, under the Women's Health and Cancer Rights Act of 1988 (WHCRA), both my breast reconstruction surgery and the second to produce symmetrical appearance of my breasts along with the nipple reconstruction procedure was covered by my insurance. Under other circumstances, such procedures would be considered "cosmetic" and, therefore, not covered.

ADVICE: Breast reconstruction is a major decision, so it's critical that you research everything you can about your options. Review the background of your plastic surgeon and have him/her describe the procedure and related recovery timelines, so you understand what you'll be going through. Ask all the questions you need to feel comfortable with your surgeon and the entire process.

The DIEP flap breast reconstruction surgery is a complex operation that requires a highly skilled surgeon. Because tissue will be removed from your abdomen, you will have a long incision there. The incision will definitely be a source of pain. However, when you take the painkillers as prescribed, you'll be able to avoid pain, for the most part. You will need to initially take extra care when you move around too. Get a small pillow and place it firmly on your abdomen before you do any of the following: cough, sneeze, laugh or just move, in general. Use the pillow also when you drive, to protect your abdomen.

The abdominal incisions will, of course, cause scars too. Fortunately, there is ScarAway, a gel that has been proven to effectively erase scar tissue. You can buy it in drug stores and Amazon.com.

Last, but certainly not least, make sure your medical insurance carrier doesn't charge you for your breast reconstruction and its related procedures. Here's an excerpt of the law that covers you in this regard:

"The Women's Health and Cancer Rights Act of 1998 (WHCRA) is a federal law that provides protections to patients who choose to have breast reconstruction in connection with a mastectomy. If WHCRA applies to you and you are receiving benefits in connection with a mastectomy and you elect breast reconstruction, coverage must be provided for:

- All stages of reconstruction of the breast on which the mastectomy has been performed;
- Surgery and reconstruction of the other breast to produce a symmetrical appearance; and
- Prostheses and treatment of physical complications of all stages of the mastectomy, including lymphedema."

* Cindy R. (*Metastatic Breast cancer to the Stomach*)

After my double mastectomy, I decided to have breast reconstruction done. In the process, they inserted tissue expanders beneath my skin and chest muscles to stretch the area and make room for a future, more permanent implant. Then, I had to go back every week so that they could inject saline solution to gradually fill the expanders. This process allows the skin to stretch and adjust. At the time, I couldn't quite decide what size I wanted to be. Unfortunately, the right side kept getting infected.

So I ended up going through a couple more surgeries where they removed the expander on my right side, cleaned it out, cleaned the area that it was in and then putting it back to where it originally was. So, now I'm lopsided. I'm at the point where I'm like, "That's it. I don't even care. I can't take it anymore." It was crazy!

> **ADVICE:** Really think about it. Getting silicone breast implants requires more surgeries. Consider your age and future procedures necessary to replace your implants . If you decide to get silicone breast implants after your mastectomy, learn all you can about the process, especially the pros and cons. Have a good dialogue with your doctors, so you're all on the same page. My plastic surgeon knew exactly what to do when I got the infection. Sure, it was a painful and trying time. But you should do whatever you feel is right for you and your body. Whether you have breast reconstruction or not, it's your choice. If you choose to not have breast reconstruction, it's not the end of the world to have no breasts. If you do have reconstruction and come out lopsided, well, there are ways to solve that too.

* Rachel S. (*Breast cancer: triple negative*)

After my double mastectomy, I already decided to have breast reconstruction at a later date. I went with the DIEP flap breast reconstruction, because I didn't want anything foreign in my body, i.e. implants (saline or silicone gel). It also didn't make sense for me to get expanders and return for replacement implants every ten years, which is what I would have to do if I decided on implants.

Since I already had three c-sections and two laparoscopic surgeries to remove complex abdominal adhesions that had formed in my abdomen, the surgeons didn't know if the DIEP flap would be a good idea for me to go through. That's because, with DIEP flap breast reconstruction, they would use tissue transplanted from my abdomen to create my new breasts. So, they had to do a CT scan to see if I had enough blood flow there. I also had to have enough muscle to do it. Well, they found that I had both! We did have a plan B just in case they did the surgery and my tissue started to die, which was a possibility. Plan B was the implants. Fortunately, there was no need to go to Plan B.

I had my surgery on January 15th and it was supposed to last two hours with two surgeons. Instead, it lasted for eleven hours! After surgery, I was kept in ICU for four days. There, they kept me wrapped in a Bair Hugger blanket that forced warm air from a warming unit through a hose into the blanket that inflated with the warm air. They kept the room temperature 100F degrees for four days, which made me really, really hot. In addition to all that, I was not allowed to have water! When my mouth was dry, they moistened it with a wet cotton swab. The nurses came in every hour of the day and night and woke me up. They wanted to make sure my surgical wounds were healing and my tissue wasn't dying. I was miserable because I could barely sleep in between their visits.

When I checked out the results of my surgery, I saw the expected abdominal incision that literally went horizontally from one side of my hip to the other and I also saw the two mounds on my chest ... my newly reconstructed breasts. They didn't look like I thought they would, but then they were pretty swollen and were still going to be worked on. My entire midsection was sore and I felt like a punching bag. Major surgery does that.

Unfortunately, a month later, the skin around all my incisions, i.e. both my breasts and my abdomen, started to separate. The top layer of the stitches were healing, but the stitches inside were dissolving, creating scar tissue that was forcing the skin apart. There were gaps ... quarter inch gaps ... in the incisions, that were deep enough for me to put my finger into.

Treatment included antibiotics and the "wet-to-dry" dressing where I had to take a moist gauze that I sprayed with Vashe wound cleanser and pack it into the gaping wound and then cover it. Then, later in the day, I had to pull out from the open wound the gauze, now dried and filled with infected dead tissue, and repeat the "wet-to-dry" dressing again. I did this for several weeks. Fortunately, the wounds are closing and I've got the "inward scars" to deal with. I know that, in time, they will level out. For now, I'm counting on my ScarAway gel to make the scars, especially around my breast area, disappear.

* *Vida B.A.* (*Breast cancer*)

A year after my mastectomy, I decided to get an implant on my left breast. Unfortunately, it didn't have the same shape as my healthy right breast and, together, they didn't look "balanced" (they still don't), which was very disappointing. I don't want to complain about it anymore. I'm still thankful that I had it done.

The implant procedure and recovery was painful. But I was able to tolerate it. One big problem was the itchiness on the skin surrounding my implant, which I believe, was an allergic reaction. My doctor said that it was psychological, because the nerves were removed from that area. He told me to not scratch it and just put the topical steroid hydrocortisone on the area. That helped.

* *Yesi L.* (*Breast cancer: triple positive*)

Since I had a bilateral mastectomy, I had to go through numerous surgeries for breast reconstruction. My oncological surgeon and my plastic surgeon together did everything in their power to save the nipple on my right breast where the cancer was. I went into reconstructive surgery expecting to come out with no nipples, because they told me that they didn't know if they could save them. When I came out of surgery after eight plus hours, I found that I still had my nipples. It basically looked like I had a boob job done!

Part of my breast reconstruction problem was having to deal with the expanders that they put in, which were extremely uncomfortable. It felt like I was wearing an iron bra. There were times when the expanders were so painful, but I just took Motrin to relieve the pain. Unfortunately, after four surgeries on my breast, I tried to heal, but there was one little area (like a pore) that kept opening up; it was definitely infected. The doctors then had me go through Hyperbaric Oxygen Therapy (HOT). Yes, I was placed inside a hyperbaric chamber, like the one Michael Jackson had. In that chamber, I was able to breathe pure oxygen in a way that allowed my body to fight the infection I had and allow my wound to heal.

CHEMOEMBOLIZATION

Chemoembolization is a procedure in which the blood supply to a tumor is blocked after anticancer drugs are given in blood vessels near the tumor. Sometimes, the anticancer drugs are attached to small beads that are injected into an artery that feeds the tumor. The beads block blood flow to the tumor as they release the drug. This allows a higher amount of drug to reach the tumor for a longer period of time, which may kill more cancer cells. It also causes fewer side effects because very little of the drug reaches other parts of the body.

* *Scott M.* (*Metastatic Colon cancer to the Prostate & Pancreas*)

After my colon resection and six months of chemotherapy with the Oxaliplatin, Avastin and Xeloda, I was clear. The six big lesions in my liver were gone – Hooray! But, my doctors and I had already agreed that I should still go through a two-part chemoembolization of my liver to remove any remaining cancer cells in my body. In the procedure, they flooded half of my liver with chemo-filled pellets to kill the cancer two ways: (1) block blood flow from that part of the liver to kill the cancer cells, and (2) get the cancer cells to eat up the chemo fluid that they were trapped with there and die that way.

Well, I went in for the first procedure and it just knocked me on my butt. I was in the hospital for a week, with a lot of pain and my doctor said that I was such a "weenie", because he had a couple of 80-year old guys come in and just go home the next day, without any problems. But for some reason, that procedure just really knocked me out. And, for two months, I was just sicker than a dog.

After I recovered, I went back to see my oncologist and interventional radiologist and they both told me, "We don't think we should do the second half." And I said, "Hey guys, what was the plan?" And they said, "To do both halves". And I said, "Well, I'm going to survive the second one. It may be tough, but we're doing it." So, we did it and sure enough, I was in the hospital for a week, sicker than a dog, and it knocked me on my butt for two months … but, I DID IT!

ADVICE: In my opinion, you don't want to take any chances with cancer. You want to fight it with everything you've got! You want to nuke it, if you can! Sure, it may be tough and you may not have the physical strength, but you have it in you to see it through. Be determined and fight with everything you've got!

CHEMOTHERAPY

Chemotherapy is a treatment that uses drugs to stop the growth of cancer cells, either by killing the cells or by stopping them from dividing. Chemotherapy may be given by mouth (orally), injection, infusion, or on the skin, depending on the type and stage of the cancer being treated. It may be given alone or with other treatments, such as surgery, radiation therapy, or biologic therapy.

* *Amor T.* (*Breast cancer, Ovarian cancer*)

Chemotherapy schedule. Before starting my chemotherapy regimen, Bill and I attended a mandatory chemotherapy preparation meeting where the wonderful nurse practitioner gave me my treatment schedule, answers to FAQs (frequently asked questions) about the process, including when I can expect my hair to fall off due to treatment. She gave me a schedule to follow, which was really informative and made me feel comfortable, especially in seeing a timeline working towards completion of my chemo treatment. Here's a sample of my chemo schedule:

	MONDAY	TUESDAY	WEDNESDAY	THURSDAY	FRIDAY	SATURDAY	SUNDAY
Week #1	<u>Toughest Week</u>: fatigue hits hard, no energy, feeling really awful with pain and other side effects						
	Dexamethasone 8mg (2 tabs) in morning & 2 tabs in evening	**CHEMO #1** Carboplatin Taxol	Neulasta injection Stool softener Claritin 10mg x 7 days L-Glutamine (10g 3x/day)	Claritin & L-Glutamine	Claritin & L-Glutamine	Claritin & L-Glutamine	Claritin & L-Glutamine
Week #2	<u>Tough Week</u>: still fatigued and weak with pain dissipating and energy returning						
	Claritin & L-Glutamine regimen	Meet w/ MD or NP Claritin & L-Glutamine	L-Glutamine	L-Glutamine	LABS L-Glutamine	L-Glutamine	L-Glutamine

Week #3	"<u>Happy Week</u>": return of strength and energy!					
	Meet w/ MD or NP Dexamethasone 8mg (2 tabs) in morning & 2 tabs in evening	L-Glutamine	L-Glutamine	L-Glutamine	L-Glutamine	HAIR LOSS begins L-Glutamine	L-Glutamine
Week #4	Toughest Week: fatigue hits hard, no energy, feeling really awful with pain and other side effects					
	Dexamethasone 8mg (2 tabs) in morning & 2 tabs in evening	**CHEMO #2** Carboplatin Taxol	Neulasta injection Stool softener Claritin 10mg x 7 days L-Glutamine (10g 3x/day)	Claritin & L-Glutamine	Claritin & L-Glutamine	Claritin & L-Glutamine	Claritin & L-Glutamine
...and the cycles continued until the end of treatment...						

Initially, I was only supposed to go through three chemo cycles or nine weeks of treatment. Unfortunately, at the end of my third cycle, my cancer marker was still up at 361.5 (normal is 0-35), so I went through more tests, including a PET scan. Although the PET scan did not detect any cancer, my oncologist was very concerned. So, I resumed and went through three more chemo cycles or nine more weeks of treatment.

Chemo infusion activities and support. Bill was with me through all of my chemo treatments. Even though the cancer center had all the comforts I needed, I brought my own blanket, small pillow, socks, reading material, rosary and Jesus Calling book, my laptop and my iPhone. The oncology nurses there were total angels!

<u>My CA 125 History</u>

3/15/2016	430.0	pre-hysterectomy
4/21/2016	789.1	post-hysterectomy
5/13/2016	609.3	Part1: post-chemo#1
6/03/2016	396.5	Part1: post-chemo#2
6/27/2016	361.5	Part1: post-chemo#3
7/27/2016	115.1	Lab Check
8/02/2016	69.0	Part2: pre-chemo#1
8/22/2016	23.9	Part2: pre-chemo#2
9/12/2016	16.9	Part2: pre-chemo#3
10/06/2016	14.7	Part2: post-chemo (FINAL!)

Before the actual chemo, my nurse took my blood pressure, pulse, temperature and respiration rate. Then she asked my name and birth date to make sure I was the right person the chemo meds were meant for. For my first three infusions, the chemo drugs were given via IV attached to veins in either my hand or my wrist. For the last thee chemo sessions, they used my implanted mediport.

I remember that the first part of the infusion entailed flushing my veins and then giving me benadryl (for allergies). I learned really quick that if I needed to do something, I should make sure I do it before the benadryl goes into my veins, because when it does, I'm out like a light! On my first day, I thought I'd pray the rosary during my chemo session. Well, I think I was able to say "Hail Mary, full of grace..." and then passed out for 2-3 hours...waking up in time for Bill to bring me lunch. When my friends or family wanted to visit, I told them to do so in the afternoon, because I wouldn't be able to converse with them in the morning, as I would be asleep.

The only time I felt pain during my chemo infusion was after my nurse put the IV into my vein for my third chemo. I felt my vein burning up my arm and rang the bell. My nurse slowed down the drip, which didn't work. So, she did something (diluted it?), which worked. Because the drip was slower, it took longer for me to finish the chemo infusion process. After that experience, I realized that it was time for me to get my mediport implanted. The veins in my right arm were just too tired and, of course, I could not use the veins in my left arm due to my mastectomy and lymphadenectomy. The entire chemo procedure took six hours from the time they prepped the chemo drugs, hooked me up to when they removed the IV.

Cancer Center experience. The cancer center was wonderful, comfortable, full of amenities and, most of all, staffed with an amazing team of oncologists, oncology nurses, assistants and receptionists. Everyone was just helpful and friendly, which made me feel at home. They offered a bounty of snacks, like bananas, apples, oranges, crackers, raisins, health nutrition bars, cookies, etc. There were also juices, milk, and water, as well as, hot chocolate, coffee, and tea. On my first day of chemo, it was such a delight to be welcomed by a volunteer rolling a cart around filled with colorful blanket and pillow sets for me to choose from. They were created by the cancer center's volunteers for cancer patients there.

ADVICE: Make sure to get your chemo treatment schedule and follow instructions you're given. If you have any questions or concerns, you should feel free to inform your medical team. Also, let them know what you're experiencing, so they either provide you guidance or adjust your medication. Six hours may seem a long time, but if you keep yourself engaged, i.e. talking with someone, watching a video, reading a book, playing games, listening to music, etc. the time will pass by faster. Bring everything you need in a big bag.

Expect to get cold while going through chemo. Don't hesitate to ask the oncology nurses there for however many blankets and pillows you need. Wear a hat, jacket, socks, etc... anything to keep yourself warm.

For those who want to visit you, let them know that afternoon is best as you will probably be groggy or sleepy during the first part of your chemo session.

Follow your own progress. Doing so will make you feel empowered and in control. Most of all, no matter how uncomfortable you may be, think positively of how the chemo is actively fighting to rid your body of cancer. Believe in your body's ability to heal and in your medical team's ability to guide you through treatment. Still your worries and anxieties through prayer or meditation. Positivity and faith are key!

* Cindy R. (Metastatic Breast cancer to the Stomach)

Breast cancer. My chemotherapy was scheduled once every three weeks for four months. And, I had a total of eight infusions two separate times. The first round of four was for Adriamycin and Cytoxan and the second round of four was for Taxol. I always had, at least, two people with me for the six-hour session. My mom and/or my sisters gave me company.

When I received the first two rounds, which was for Adriamycin and Cytoxan, they put me in a private room. Then, when I received the Taxol, they placed me in an open room with everybody else. The Taxol pretty much put me to sleep right away. So, I was like, "Good night."

Stomach cancer. The chemo process I went through to treat my stomach cancer was very different from the chemo I went through to treat my breast cancer. My chemo infusion schedule was once a week, the drugs were different, the drip was slower and I had to bring a chemo pump home. I did that for two years (2014 & 2015), before they realized that I was misdiagnosed and that the stomach cancer was actually a metastasis of my breast cancer ten years ago; not a new cancer. So, they changed my treatment plan.

They changed my infusion schedule to once every three weeks (versus once a week) and started me on Ibrance (targeted therapy pills) and a fairly new drug, Faslodex (injections) that is working really good.

My mom and/or my sisters accompanied me to my chemo sessions again, just as they did during the chemo sessions for my breast cancer treatment. Since the sessions are about six-hours long, I always took with me extra clothes, my little bag with socks, blanket and snacks and a very special book. That book is really neat. One of my friends at work got everyone together and made a book for me of memories and things we had done. It is really sweet; a very special book that I took with me everywhere.

ADVICE: Even though with chemotherapy, your body goes through "hell", you don't have to. It's a choice. You can make the experience easier for yourself by trying to have a positive outlook and have fun and being yourself. Some patients I knew went to the chemo sessions wearing crazy hats. Then on another day, they decided to wear silly socks. Think of doing things to distract you from the infusion process. Listen to soothing music, read a fun book, have a nice conversation with other patients, etc.

The cancer center will have comfortable chairs. However, bring anything from home that will make you feel more comfortable. And, make sure you have your blanket, because it's usually cold there.

* Glenn M. (Metastatic Colon cancer to the Liver, Lungs & Adrenal Glands)

My tumor was missed in the prior colonoscopy, because it was located on the outside of the colon. Unfortunately, by the time they found it, it had metastasized to the liver: three golf-ball-sized and one baseball-sized tumors were found on my liver. The baseball-sized tumor was mostly unaffected by the six months of chemotherapy that followed, although it shrank the golf balls some.

I'm in chemotherapy now once every other week for eight weeks, for five to six hours. They changed my chemo drugs from Xeloda and Erbitux to Avastin and Irinotecan. They wanted to add magnesium to my infusion because I was low, but I didn't want to spend the extra hour it would take in the session. So, they had me try and take in orally 800 mgs of magnesium three days before my labs. Unfortunately, my body wouldn't take it. In the end, I wound up taking 400 mgs of magnesium through my port.

ADVICE: Learn about your cancer and about the chemo drugs they give you. Research and ask questions. It's your body. You're the one who will be experiencing the effects of the drugs they give you. So, learn what you can about the drugs that are going into your body.

* Hilda K. (Colon cancer)

My chemotherapy infusion schedule at the Cancer Center was every two weeks. The nurses did everything for me there. Before every infusion, they tested my blood to make sure my levels were good. When they weren't good, they sent me home and had me return the following week to repeat the blood test until the levels were good. Once the results were fine, they then took me "to the back" to prepare me for the chemo infusion.

The infusion room was an open room where they had me sit on one of the comfortable recliners they had there. The first thing they did was flush my veins using a saline solution. After that went through, they told me, "Okay, we are now going to start the drip. Just relax." Since the whole process takes about five to six hours, I mostly read magazines. You know how doctors' offices have awesome magazines? Well, I caught up on my reading of "People" ... the "crazy" reading. I enjoyed it, because it was quick and simple. Aside from reading, I also just relaxed and looked out the window at things like the trees outside. The nurses there really made sure I was comfortable.

At the infusion room, I could tell the patients who were having a tough time; I saw it in their faces. Everyone has a different dose and everyone experiences the treatment differently. Some people had a full head of hair and some came with caps on because they were bald. With all the patients, the nurses were nice and very gentle. They were always there, checking on us.

I remember the time when I unexpectedly got dizzy and felt panicky. They gave me medication to calm me down. Although I was comfortable during treatment, there were times I got a little panicky. I was told that that's to be expected. After the chemo infusions, I was sent home with a chemo pump attached to my port, which continued to dispense the chemotherapy medication over the next two to three days. They also gave me extra medication to take home, just in case I got a little panicky when I had to deal with my chemo pump. I took a little bit, but never really needed it.

ADVICE: Keep in mind that chemotherapy kills your cancer cells and will help you get better. Try to relax during treatment. Bring your favorite reading materials or read the magazines they have at the Cancer Center. You could also listen to music or work on a project or bring someone you can talk to or just sleep. Basically, you have the choice on how you spend your time. If you get panicky or uncomfortable, for whatever reason, let the nurses there know. They'll take care of you.

* Jacki S. (Breast cancer)

When I was going in for chemo, I made sure I had a short sleeved shirt on, so my left arm was available for the needle. My right arm wasn't available, because I had the lumpectomy on my right side. It was only for my first chemo appointment that I had someone accompany me, either my husband or my friend. Sorry, don't remember exactly (chemo brain!) Aside from having a little problem with nausea for my first chemo infusion, everything else was fine and ran smoothly. There were no other problems after that first chemo. So, I just handled driving myself to the hospital and back.

Something I'd like to share with everyone: Going into all my chemo treatments, I had a friend who is also one of the ice skaters I coach. She had other friends who also went through cancer and so she knew that to help out was a very positive thing for a cancer patient. So, she did something special for me. Before I went to each of my nine chemo sessions, she would hang a little gift bag containing five to seven fun pink things on my front door. There was every little pink thing you could think of, e.g.: A pink ribbon for my hair. A pink pen. A pink notebook. A pink pair of socks. A pink nail file, etc. So, before each chemo, I would open up my front door and there would be my pink goody bag! That wonderful and kind gesture definitely helped me feel better as a cancer patient and helped me cope with my chemo sessions.

ADVICE: Find a friend to go with you for support.

* Joan S. (Rectal cancer)

I started chemotherapy infusions as soon as I felt stronger after my surgery. Unfortunately, chemo and I did not agree. I could not keep anything down and I got very, very weak because I didn't eat. I also didn't move too much, which wasn't a good thing. I was scheduled for six rounds of chemo every other week and also had to take chemo pills twice a day, but stopped the treatment, because I kept getting sick.

Both my oncologist and the nutritionist at the hospital could not figure out the cause of my problems. The chemo was just making me so very sick. At one time, my visiting nurse Melissa said, "You're really pale. I want you to go to emergency." I said, "Well, let me get a good night's sleep." Well, she phoned my daughter Lori, who came and said, "Come on, Mom. You're going to go." When we got to the hospital, they found that I had an abscess in my GI (gastrointestinal) tract. I was treated and, eventually, got over that and resumed my chemo treatment.

I was in the hospital a total of seven times for different reasons. Every time I went to the hospital, they stopped the chemo, because the chemo itself weakened me. I had four of the six rounds of chemo that I was initially supposed to get.

Finally, my oncologist said to me, "As much as we want you to continue your last two rounds of chemo, your body can't handle it anymore." So, I chose not to take the last two rounds and immediately after I quit taking chemo, I started feeling better and started eating and eating. And that was a good thing. It was my choice.

ADVICE: Chemo is not for everybody. If you get a bad reaction or if you feel you're getting sick from the infusions, let your doctor know, so they can either reassure you or have you go through some other treatment.

* Rev. Linda S. (Pancreatic cancer 3x)

My first round with chemo was mild compared to others, as I was taking it only as a precautionary measure, in case undetected cancer cells were floating around my body. The 34 lymph nodes surrounding my pancreas were all cancer-free. Surgical removal of the pancreatic tail, the tumor, and the spleen (RAMPS procedure) appeared to have removed the cancer.

My second round with chemo was intense. Although, from past experience, I generally knew what to expect of the chemo infusion process, this time I also had to bring a chemo pump home with me. The chemo pump infused more drugs slowly into me as I went through the day and slept through the night for several days. Thanks to strategic placement of bed pillows, my dog Murphy was unable to harm me or the infusion pump as we slept.

My third round with chemo was tough. This chemo treatment exhausted me, caused aches and pains in places I didn't know I had, and often fogged my brain. I had to accept the fact that five days a week for three consecutive weeks, I am at the clinic for lab work, chemo and neupogen shots. Then, I'm off from all of it for one week, but only if my labs allow for the chemo. If not, the cycle stops for a week and we begin again.

As I go through chemo, I think of how the chemo drugs are kicking cancer's behind. I also realize that I tend to focus more on death during chemo week and on life during the following week of recovery. And then we start the cycle again. The infusion center is never a joyful place. So, I'm especially grateful for my Bluetooth headphones, which allow me to block everything out by listening to smooth jazz and napping periodically.

Since Murphy can't be with me here in the infusion center, I have his doppelgänger with me ~ a stuffed toy of a salt and pepper miniature schnauzer. I named her Hazel. She's my toy, a concept my dog Mr. Murphy doesn't quite grasp.

* Rachel S. (Breast cancer: triple negative)

For the first two months, I had my chemo every other week. And then, for the last three months of treatment, it was every week: Friday.

90% of the time, my husband was with me. He would take the day off from work to be with me. Twice, I had two different friends go with me; one time each. My sister also went with me one time. And for my next-to-last chemo, which happened to be at Thanksgiving, my daughter drove up from LA to be with me.

For my first two months of chemo, they gave me pre-meds to take at home before getting infused at the hospital. So, I would be awake during treatment. For the last chemo, I was passed out, because they did something different, which was for the trial study I joined. They didn't give me the pre-meds to take at home before getting chemo. Instead, they gave me the pre-meds through an IV line while I was there: a dose of Benadryl so high, it quickly knocked me out.

* Rick S. (CLL: Blood & Bone Marrow cancer)

My chemotherapy sessions were not held at a hospital, but at a hospital's "oncology lab". When I went in, the nurses had me sit on a nice beautiful, comfortable reclining chair. They raised the leg portion of the chair and had me lay there like I was in a recliner. They gave me a nice hot warm blanket and wrapped it around me. The nurses were always there, watching me and the other cancer patients. No one was going let me be alone. So, I felt that I was well taken care of.

I didn't need a bell, because I had my nurse right there, in front of me. If that nurse was out, I had another nurse behind me to call on. So, I had comfort and I had people there. And, in the oncology lab, everyone working there is like your servant. They take care of you. They smother you with love and attention.

I started chemotherapy in December 2009 and was scheduled for treatment three times a month for four months. At first, I was in a high state of anxiety. While I sat in the infusion chair, people from church came, brought me food and stayed with me. Since the hospital allowed only one visitor at a time, one visitor would come in for 30 minutes while the other goes out for 30 minutes. They were church people. So they talked with me in terms of the Bible. When we first discussed things, it would be biblically oriented, like "God loves you" and "God's here with you". After all that, we'd do general chit chat. And that's how it went for the first day of infusion. That very first day seemed really long, because my body rejected the chemo. I went in at 8:30am and was supposed to be out by 1:00pm. Instead, I was out at 5:30pm, because of the complication.

My chemo sessions were scheduled for the first, second and third days of the month for a total of four months. So, people from church lined up to take me to my chemo sessions and back. They were scheduled for one or two days, for the first day of the month, second day of the month or third day of the month.

The first day chemo session of the month was always the roughest and longest for me, because they infused into me two bags of chemo drugs at an hour and a half each and one bag that took four hours to finish. That was the most intensive; the four-hour one. And, that was the one that "killed" everything (the cancer cells). But on the second and third days, I just had the two bags to finish; I didn't have the four-hour bag. Only on the first days was I given the four-hour bag.

At one time, a lady from church brought me to my second day of the month chemo session. Her husband had died of cancer. So, she knew how to make a cancer patient like me comfortable. She walked behind me automatically, massaged my neck and shoulders and made me feel a lot better. After that, we talked. We talked about her problems and issues and I found myself giving her support. I then lost track of time and what was being done with my chemo infusion. Also, they closed the curtain on us, because she started crying. So, I tried to help her and give her some energy.

The person who brought me on my third day of the month chemo session just left me there and went to work. Since I couldn't sleep, I just sat there. I tried to close my eyes and imagine myself weightlifting or doing something I enjoy. And I love to eat. So, even though no one from my church stayed with me during chemo, the nurses were there, running back and forth bringing me all kinds of goodies from the cabinet, e.g. coffee, peanut rolls and so forth. That was nice.

* Scott M. (Metastatic Colon cancer to the Prostate & Pancreas)

Following my colon resection, I had six months of chemotherapy with the Oxaliplatin, Avastin and Xeloda to treat my stage IV colon cancer. I was also given the chemo drug Irinotecan that came in the form of pellets when I had CyberKnife surgery to lance the cysts that had grown in my pancreas.

I definitely experienced side effects, which I was already aware I would experience. I knew that I had to be strong and I knew I just had to deal with it. It's part of life and I'm grateful that it wasn't worse. I was within a quarter of an inch of having to have a colostomy. Well, I didn't have to have that, so I'm very grateful.

Now, I'm going through maintenance chemo. I'm given an infusion of Avastin on day one of week one. And, at home, I take Xeloda in pill form every morning and every night for seven weeks. Then I get two weeks off. Every twenty one days, I get an infusion and start again my seven days of Xeloda, followed by fourteen days off. The reason it works this way is to keep whatever cancer cells that are hiding in me from gaining a foothold and growing. The job of the maintenance chemo is to kill off the rest of the cancer cells, as soon as they appear. It may be slow, but it seems to be working. However, we still have to keep in mind that the scans, as wonderful as they are, can only see a billion cancer cells. That's billion with a "b". You might have a cluster of 300 million cancer cells that the scans won't see. PET scans won't see them. The CT scans with contrast won't see them. Until the scanning techniques get better and can get down to the cellular level, where they can actually see individual cells, there's always a chance there's still cancer in my body.

ADVICE: When you go through chemotherapy, you just need to be aware and accept that you will end up with some side effects; some temporary, some permanent. Even though things are tough, it's still part of life and things really could be worse. Have someone with you during your chemo sessions. You have to be strong and you have to deal with it. When it was really rough for me and (for example) my feet really hurt, I just told myself, "So what if my feet hurt? I can get some pain medication to lessen the pain." You have to find the good in life and move on.

* Sondra W. (Ovarian cancer 3x)

Before my first experience with chemotherapy, somebody gave me a little teddy bear to take with me. I also brought my headset, because I needed to listen to music while I was going through the chemo infusion. Kenneth and I always start the day praying together and sharing our thoughts. Sometimes, we also read the daily devotional from the *Jesus Calling* book. More often than not, it's our only time to talk, because during the day, we don't have that much time to talk. Yes, we talk and interact with the nurses when we're in the infusion center and we love them because they're nice to both of us. And, yes, we have a little snack and stuff there. But, once they give me the Benadryl, I'm gone...asleep. Some of my friends and family members have asked, "Why can't we sit with you?" And I answered, "No, because I'll be asleep."

So, anything I need to do, I have to do before they give me the pre-meds, because after that, that's it – I'm "down for the count" – until it's time for me to go home. I didn't know that, at first. I remember a time when I tried to send text messages after they gave me the pre-meds. The messages made no sense whatsoever; what I wrote weren't even real words! I was doped, for sure, and that was funny!

My first round of chemo treatment lasted for four months and I had it every week. They did tell me that it was an aggressive treatment, because we were going for "The Cure." Now, I learned something interesting in my experience with chemotherapy; something I didn't figure out until I was through with the treatments.

I learned that when I took steroids and Benadryl in my pre-treatment, the steroids gave me energy and the Benadryl knocked me out. Well, after my chemo treatments, I noticed that I had some energy. So, I would go around and do too much and zap myself of energy. I realized that just because I had that kind of energy, it didn't mean that my body was ready for me to use it all up. Now, this might be different for someone else. For me, however, it didn't mean that my body was able to do all the work I was trying to get it to do. And, so I believe that when the steroid wore off and my energy came down, it came down even lower than I thought it would. I had kind of exhausted my body thinking I actually had energy, which was not true. After every chemo infusion, the nurses would always say, "Go home and rest" and I didn't do that. So, I definitely took a hit for not resting after treatment.

ADVICE: Even if you feel you have energy after chemo, you can go and do stuff, but you must also be aware of how much energy you're expending and pace yourself. You must give your body time to rest, because the chemo in you is strong and will zap you of your energy. So, rest and give your body time to get strong. After treatment and recovery, you'll have the right amount of energy to do the things you want to do.

To treat the recurrence of my ovarian cancer, I received my chemo infusion every other week and alternated between the chemo drugs Taxol and Avastin. Initially, test results revealed that I had two tumors. Then, they found I had four. Still further tests showed that even more tumors were found in different areas of my abdomen. Results of the last PET scan were mixed. Some tumors got larger; a few got smaller. Some got lighter and a few got dimmer. My CA 125 dropped down, but only by 18 points. Still, it was a drop. My oncologist had hoped that my condition would stabilize. He explained that since there were no new tumors, it looked like the treatment was working and, if that's the case, then they'll just have me on "maintenance chemo." If we can really get things to go down a bit more, then, he would lower the dosage. At that time, it didn't quite go the way we hoped it would and we were both nervous that my CA 125 was going to go up again. Fortunately, it didn't. So, we were like, "Whew!"

ADVICE: Have your doctor or nurse guide you on the effects of the different medications they're giving you; take notes to help you remember. Then, plan your activities around them. Don't plan to have visitors when the medication you're taking will make you drowsy or fall asleep. The same goes for doing anything that requires thinking, like writing messages.

* Susan M. (Ovarian cancer, Metastatic Pancreatic cancer to the Lungs)

Ovarian Cancer: One of the chemo drugs I was given was Cisplatin. I don't remember the other two medications. I had six treatments over a period of six months. For the first three treatments, I had to stay in the hospital overnight, which I wasn't happy about. They administered one medication the night before, and for the remaining medications, I had to report to the emergency room for eight hours.

Pancreatic Cancer: In February 2016, I had surgery to treat my pancreatic cancer, after which I went through a total of eighteen chemo sessions. They were scheduled three Wednesdays in a row and then one week off for a period of six months. I drove myself to every treatment.

The chemo drugs also made me hungry. So, during treatment, I would eat a banana and crackers and drink a lot of water. Drinking a lot of water was very important. I would drink three to four bottles of water a day. My friends teased me about how much water I drank. Drinking a lot of water, especially before blood draws, was needed as my veins were extremely hard to find. I finally had a port put in.

In July 2018, my CT scan showed two small nodules: 6 mm in my left lung and 1 cm in my right lung, the latter of which was biopsied and found to have cancer cells. So, I went through another round of chemotherapy, this time two weeks on and one week off, which lasted four months. I had to take five pills before each session and then more pills two to three days after. For this latest round, I was given the very aggressive chemo drug Gemzar (same one I had during my last chemo sessions) and Cisplatin (one of the chemo drugs I was given when I was treated to ovarian cancer over 30 years ago).

ADVICE: Ask or read about the side effects of the chemo drugs you'll be given. Remember that you will NOT get all of them; maybe a couple. If nausea is persistent, take the anti-nausea medication prescribed to you. If you can bring a friend or family member with you, do so. Bring your computer, a good book, knitting or whatever interests you to bide your time while going through chemo.

* Tet M. *(Colon cancer 3x)*

For 52 weeks on Friday afternoons, while everyone was preparing for a fun or relaxing weekend, I was at Princess Margaret Cancer Centre, one of the world's leading hospitals for cancer care (formerly called Princess Margaret Hospital). This was my "Happy Hour" and Fluorouracil was my cocktail. As each session passed, there were times when it became increasingly difficult to cope.

ADVICE: I believe that the mind is a very powerful tool in coping. Believe that cancer will be beaten, but you have to fight to make it happen. It's not easy though. Focus on the light at the end of the tunnel. Surround yourself with people who will fight the battle with you.

* Vida B.A. *(Breast cancer)*

My chemotherapy treatment was a total of six infusions over a period of eighteen (18) weeks. It took time to get used to my chemotherapy infusions. The week of my infusion and the following week were tough, because, overall, I didn't feel good at all. The third week was "happy week", because I felt my strength return and I got my taste buds and senses back. Eventually, I learned to adjust to the weekly cycles my body had to go through.

I did have an allergic reaction during my first chemo infusion where they gave me two kinds of drugs. I felt shooting and sharp pains on the nerves of my big toes and my tailbone. The nurses stopped the treatment for 30 minutes and made some adjustments. I don't know exactly what they did, but when we resumed, the pains weren't there anymore.

I remember falling asleep through half of the session. My best friend was with me throughout my experience, which was so comforting. She told me that while I was sleeping, I was also moaning and groaning. Well, I also had a really unexplainable pain that was "emotional"; like my body didn't know how to react to how I was feeling during the chemo infusion. Since I was half asleep, I can't explain it. Nevertheless, I was able to take it. The rest of the chemo sessions, for me, were uncomfortable. It felt like my body didn't know how to react to the drugs and I kept feeling pain. It could've been an allergic reaction or psychological; I don't know for sure. I'm just glad it's done and over with.

ADVICE: Receiving chemotherapy is something your body is forced to adjust to. Observe how you're feeling during the infusion process. If you feel any discomfort, especially shooting or stabbing pains, let your doctor and nurses know immediately. You may be allergic to the chemo drugs. Your dosage may be adjusted or the chemo drugs removed altogether. It would be wonderful to have a friend or loved one with you for support. If you do, let them know that you may fall asleep during the process, because of the drugs. That way, they'll know what to expect and may bring something (book, computer, etc.) to bide the time while waiting for your session to be done.

* Yesi L. *(Breast cancer: triple positive)*

The cancer was so aggressive that the cells were reproducing at 99%! Since about a month and a half had passed from the time of discovery to the time of diagnosis, my tumor had tripled in size! Lumpectomy was not an option. I initially went into treatment feeling scared, because with no knowledge of all the drugs and infusions, all I could think of was the poisoning that was going through me. On the other hand, I also thought of the magical fluid that was going into my body and killing the cancer.

My chemotherapy consisted of Cytoxan, Adriamycin, Taxol, Herceptin and Perjeta. Those drugs saved my life! Adriamycin and Cytoxan were definitely the toughest. How I prepared was to tell myself that even though the drugs entering my veins were poison, I also thought of them as magical potions going through my body and saving my life! I got Adriamycin and Cytoxan every other week for eight weeks.

When I was given Cytoxan especially, the experience was very scary, because the nurse had to administer the drug very slowly, like over the course of 30 minutes, with a red syringe that looked like a blade. The nurse also had to wear HAZMAT protection, because the liquid injected into my body was poison.

What helped me a lot was having my dear best friend who was with me at every single chemo treatment. She is like an angel and one of the most positive persons I know. She brings me a lot of peace. So just having her there made me forget about everything.

What also helped me cope was to tell myself that it was my spa day and I was hanging out with my best friend and we talked about the European trip we did. We talked about Europe and forgot what was really going on.

After Cytoxan and Adriamycin, I was given Taxol and Perjeta weekly for ten to twelve weeks. Taxol was very hard for me and what definitely gave me Neuropathy.

ADVICE: I really think that having your best friend or family there to support you through the chemo treatments helps a lot. Also, think of your chemo infusion as having a magical potion going through your body and saving your life. That's the best way I can explain it. That's what worked for me.

CHOLECYSTECTOMY

A cholecystectomy is a surgical procedure to remove our gallbladder — a pear-shaped organ that sits just below our liver on the upper right side of our abdomen. Our gallbladder collects and stores bile, which is a digestive fluid produced in our liver.

* Scott M. (Metastatic Colon cancer to the Prostate & Pancreas)

At one point, I was having these real nasty, nasty, abdominal pains. So, my surgical oncologist went in and did some exploratory surgery. It turns out my gallbladder was dead and even turning gangrene-ish. So, then they performed laparoscopic surgery to remove my gallbladder (cholecystectomy).

COLECTOMY AKA COLON RESECTION

A colectomy or colon resection is an operation to remove all or part of the colon. When only part of the colon is removed, it is called a partial colectomy. In an open colectomy, one long incision is made in the wall of the abdomen and doctors can see the colon directly. In a laparoscopic-assisted colectomy, several small incisions are made and a thin, lighted tube attached to a video camera is inserted through one opening to guide the surgery. Surgical instruments are inserted through the other openings to perform the surgery.

* Bob G. (Soft Tissue Sarcoma, Skin cancer)

Initially, the doctors performed exploratory surgery on my left side and then on my right side. Fortunately, they found nothing. Then when I went for my first real surgery, a splenectomy where they removed my spleen and the surrounding tissue. The doctors told me what they were going to do. That surgery went very well, because back then, I was swimming three to four times per week.

The second surgery was radical surgery; an "either-you-make-it-or-you-don't" kind. In this surgery, they performed a combination radical nephrectomy-colectomy-rib resection where they removed my left kidney, 50% of my colon, one to two back ribs, plus some muscle and more tissue. I didn't know, until much later, that they did all that to remove my cancer and keep it from spreading.

ADVICE: Make sure your doctors explain what they'll be doing when they operate on you. It really helps to know what's going on.

* Glenn M. (Metastatic Colon cancer to the Liver, Lungs & Adrenal Glands)

In October of 2014, I had my first surgery, a Colectomy, to remove the cancerous tumor and about ten inches of my colon. During that surgery, they also implanted my medical port device (mediport).

* *Hilda K.* (*Colon cancer*)

It was a pretty long surgery, which took a minimum of six hours. They didn't cut open my abdomen. Instead, they cut five little incisions in my abdomen, inserted a tiny video camera into one and special surgical tools into the others. With the video camera and tools, they were able to see exactly where to go and what to get at and remove. It was very interesting!

The surgery lasted a long time, because they basically had to cut and tuck and do a lot of other things. They had to check everything around my colon area to see if anything else was affected by my cancer. If they thought something was affected, then they also had to take out all the little samples. Finally, they had to fully examine my entire system to make sure they took out all the cancer.

When I woke up from surgery, I was in my room and feeling really groggy. My whole family was there. But, I was in total pain and really out of it. So, I asked them to leave; I just couldn't give them any attention. They were sorry to leave me, but understood. My eldest daughter Jessica slept with me that night. I was hospitalized for less than a week and had a great team of nurses. Considering all that I went through with the surgery and recovery, I must say that I couldn't have asked for a better experience.

* *Tet M.* (*Colon cancer 3x*)

When my cancer was first discovered right before Christmas in 1991, the surgeons here in Toronto recommended I have a total Colectomy where they would remove the entire colon. That would have nipped it in the bud, but would have meant frequent trips to the toilet for the rest of my life. Not too thrilled about the tradeoff, my family insisted I fly home to Manila, Philippines and have the surgery performed by a great doctor who's like a father to me. He gave it his 110% and gave me a normal lifestyle by performing a Colectomy where he removed just enough of my colon to restore good health for yours truly. After the surgery, I didn't feel any symptoms of losing half of my large intestine. My bowel movement habits hadn't changed at all and I resumed life as if nothing happened, with the exception of regular checkups in the form of Colonoscopies. As a precaution, my surgeon recommended Adjuvant Chemotherapy, to ensure the cancer cells were gone. My Chemo sessions started when I flew back to Toronto.

I was diligent in having regular colonoscopies. Unfortunately, biopsies of the polyps taken out in 2005 showed they were nearing malignancy. With reluctance, I finally agreed to have a second Colectomy, so I wouldn't have to deal with another round of Chemo.

Recovering from my second Colectomy was not the breeze I experienced in my first Colectomy. Consuming certain food types would cause me to run to the bathroom sometimes sooner than later, and/or making more frequent trips, but I had learned which food to avoid. Colonoscopies had to be performed more frequently since the growth of polyps came more rapidly.

With the incredible support I received from my family and friends, I was able to cope and heal well from my surgeries.

A colonoscopy is an examination used to detect changes or abnormalities in the large intestine (colon) and rectum. During a colonoscopy, a thin, flexible, tube-like instrument with a tiny video camera at the tip of the tube (colonoscope) is inserted into the rectum and allows the doctor to view the inside of the entire colon. If a specimen is needed, the colonoscope may also have a tool to remove tissue to be checked under a microscope for signs of disease.

* *Amor T.* (*Breast cancer, Ovarian cancer*)

I had a colonoscopy ten days before my June 24th mastectomy.. The procedure was simple, because all they did at the medical center was put an IV into me, which made me quite drowsy, rolled me into an "operating" room and then I was out like a light. I didn't feel a thing until I woke up in the recovery room, where I had to wait until the doctor was able to check the results and discuss them with me. I left with a full report, complete with colored pictures of the two small polyps found and removed from my colon. The nurse wheeled me out on a wheelchair and waited until my friend picked me up by the building. The colonoscopy procedure was really quick and easy.

Preparing for the colonoscopy aka the bowel prep, on the other hand, was a bit of a challenge to go through. Basically, I had to drink a "prep" liquid in order to empty my bowels so the doctor could clearly see the inside of my colon. The day before the colonoscopy, I had to take a special laxative and drink a large volume (up to 4 liters) of special prep liquid to help me empty my bowels. Of course, that meant staying very close to the bathroom. Nothing to be ashamed of. It is what it is.

An important fact to remember is regularly performed colonoscopies will detect colon cancer in their early stages, thereby, giving you a higher chance for survival. So, please make sure to get your colonoscopy done regularly.

ADVICE: **My best advice: Just do it! The bowel prep portion, over the years, has improved a lot, so it really isn't so bad. Just think of what you're doing to keep from getting colorectal cancer. As Benjamin Franklin said, "An ounce of prevention is worth a pound of cure", meaning it's easier to stop something from happening in the first place than to repair the damage after it has happened. So, get your colonoscopy. It will save your life!**

* *Hilda K.* (*Colon cancer*)

I'm really glad that I got my colonoscopy, because that's how they found the cancer. Before the procedure, I had to drink a "colonoscopy prep" liquid several times to empty my colon and clear my bowels. I was also restricted in what I could eat and drink.

My doctor and his nurse fully prepared me for what was going to happen during the colonoscopy. They told me that I was going to have to count backwards and when I woke up, it would all be done. So, that's exactly what happened. I counted backwards in the operating room and woke up in the recovery room. I was completely unconscious during the entire procedure; didn't feel a thing! Before they could release me, they waited for me to have a good sense of where I was.

ADVICE: **Just follow the instructions, when it comes to drinking your colonoscopy prep liquid. You should stay home, as much as possible, because you'll be going to the bathroom a lot. My main advice here is to make sure you get your colonoscopy on schedule because it could be a matter of life or death.**

* *Tet M.* (*Colon cancer 3x*)

Preparing and cleansing for a colonoscopy has always been tougher for me than the actual procedure itself. I understand that this major inconvenience is common as, according to one study, getting ready for the procedure takes an average of sixteen hours, which is much longer than the three or so hours spent at a medical center during the day of the colonoscopy.

I know it's worth the hassle. Drinking the liquid that will trigger bowel-clearing diarrhea is no fun, however, I try not to let it affect me. I do stay away from any semblance of food and my family knows not to bring into the house food that will likely emit a flavorful aroma. I've been known to cuss harshly and make rude gestures at the TV when a commercial about food comes up. After the "scope" (the term I use for my colonoscopies or upper endoscopies), I would then go to the restaurant that aired the commercial and eat the food I saw on TV. It's my way of showing the restaurant that I don't hold grudges and that I'm sorry I cussed at them. Let this be our little secret.

The discomfort during a colonoscopy procedure itself is the gas pain that I feel as they pump air through my bowel for the doctor to have a better view of my insides. Expect bloating after the procedure and passing of gas at the recovery room. After the tests are completed, I'm given about an hour to sleep off the sedative.

ADVICE: Before you prep yourself for the colonoscopy, eat your favorite food, but keep in mind that you'll be dieting soon on clear liquids. Clear your room and surroundings of food and snacks during the prep period. Ask family and friends who are with you to help keep food, including the topic and the smell of food, away from you during this time.

Drinking the bowel prep liquid is not pleasant. When you're actually going through the colonoscopy prep and cleansing routine, here are some tips:

- Drink by sipping it through a straw placed far back on your tongue. This way, the liquid bypasses most of the taste buds in your tongue.
- While drinking the prep, hold your nose and drink it as quickly as possible.
- If the prep doesn't come in a pleasant flavor, you can add some Crystal Light or Kool-Aid powder (not red, blue or purple because this might be mistaken for blood or may obstruct the doctor's view during the procedure). Try this in a small batch first, like in a taste test.
- Hold a lime under your nose while you drink the liquid prep, and
- Quickly suck on a lemon slice or suck on hard candy (again, avoiding red, blue or purple colors), after you finish each glass of prep.
- Stay away from food and anything that reminds you of it, like grocery stores and food magazines. Of course, if you can walk away from the TV to avoid those mouth-watering commercials, it'll help you cope.
- Wear loose clothing and stay near a bathroom.
- Expect high-volume, high-velocity diarrhea, which will indicate that the bowel prep is working. This is just reality, folks. It's advisable to notify family members or roommates to keep the bathroom available for you as much as possible.

During the procedure, distract yourself by thinking of the delicious meal you'll have after as a reward, but don't focus on it. It's a tough balancing act. The procedure is temporary. So, keep in mind, that this too shall pass. Note that you might be asked to ease into a full meal gradually. After a few scopes, you'll get to know your body well enough to determine how soon you can treat yourself to that scrumptious meal you envisioned. Remember, each person reacts differently to sedative, if applied.

CYBERKNIFE RADIOSURGERY

The CyberKnife System is a radiation therapy device used for treating benign tumors, malignant tumors and other medical conditions. This device combines a lightweight linear accelerator mounted on a robotic manipulator and an integrated image guidance system. The image guidance system continually acquires stereoscopic kV images during treatment, tracks tumor motion, and guides the robotic manipulator to precisely and accurately align the treatment beam to the moving tumor. The system is designed for stereotactic radiosurgery (SRS) and stereotactic body radiation therapy (SBRT). The system is also used for select 3D conformal radiotherapy (3D-CRT) and intensity modulated radiation therapy (IMRT). The CyberKnife System is designed to deliver radiotherapy more accurately than standard radiotherapy devices.

* *Glenn M.* (*Metastatic Colon cancer to the Liver, Lungs & Adrenal Glands*)

I had ten sessions of the CyberKnife treatment that killed all the tumors the doctors knew about. The treatments lasted two-and-a-half hours each. That makes a total of 25 hours of CyberKnife treatments.

The way it worked was they had me fitted with a vest that had reflector tape on it. The vest helped them "target" me. Then, they surgically inserted something up my groin to reach the liver and put a "gold dot" in it, so that the CyberKnife machine could locate the target area. And then, they shot up the golf-ball sized tumors and killed them. From what I understand, they got maybe all but one of the "golf-balls," which was out-of-reach. It needs a piece of the CyberKnife again. We'll just have to wait and see.

I tend to fall asleep on the table of CyberKnife too, which isn't really a bad thing, since they want you to hold still anyway...unless you have restless legs and they start going!

ADVICE: It's a pretty effective surgery, I think. It does the job.

* Scott M. (Metastatic Colon cancer to the Prostate & Pancreas)

When I had a lesion re-form in my liver, they cyber-knifed that out. When they found that cysts had grown in my pancreas, I went through CyberKnife surgery to lance them out.

ENDOSCOPY

An endoscopy is a procedure that uses an endoscope to examine the inside of the body. An endoscope is a thin, tube-like instrument with a light and a lens for viewing. It may also have a tool to remove tissue to be checked under a microscope for signs of disease.

* Rev. Linda S. (Pancreatic cancer 3x)

I've had no problems going through endoscopies where they examine my digestive tract.

* Scott M. (Metastatic Colon cancer to the Prostate & Pancreas)

In a small window of time one summer, I had lost a huge amount of weight. So, I went through a lot of endoscopic procedures to find out what was going on. They opened me up ... did stuff ... and found out that my pancreas was inflamed. I was suffering from pancreatitis.

* Susan M. (Ovarian cancer. Metastatic Pancreatic cancer to the Lungs)

During my hospital stay after I was diagnosed with pancreatic cancer, the doctors performed an endoscopy to examine my digestive tract.

* Tet M. (Colon cancer 3x)

Just to make things more interesting, a previous upper endoscopy revealed that the roof of my stomach was lined with hundreds of fundic polyps. These go hand-in-hand with having polyps in my colon and are known to remain benign, but are closely monitored along with routine Colonoscopies just the same. Thank you, *Familial Adenomatous Polyposis, for the added attraction.

[*Familial adenomatous polyposis (FAP) is a rare inherited cancer predisposition syndrome characterized by hundreds to thousands of precancerous colorectal polyps (adenomatous polyps). If left untreated, affected individuals inevitably develop cancer of the colon and/or rectum at a relatively young age.*]

Preparing for an upper endoscopy has never been a problem. It's simply having nothing by mouth by midnight prior to the EGD. The procedure is an examination of the upper digestive tract using an endoscope. The only difficulty during the procedure is waking up unexpectedly in the middle of it and gag uncontrollably on the tube that's been inserted down my throat. [**Note**: *I always have both colonoscopy and upper endoscopy procedures performed during the same appointment.*]

In December 2009, I had a colonoscopy and upper endoscopy. It was snowing that day and I had to shovel wet snow upon reaching the house. A few hours later, I started feeling queasy. When I went to the toilet, there was blood in my stool yet again. I took a shower and packed a bag in case I had to be admitted to the hospital. Off we went for a trip to Emergency at 2:00 am. Blah, blah, blah, and with paperwork out of the way, I was sent into the inner waiting room with my mom, my aunt and my other best friend, Missy. After waiting patiently for three hours, I asked the nurse for a basin and threw up. Missy was holding it in place for me, and while I was busy gagging with my eyes closed, I heard my aunt shouting to whoever could hear her, "She's throwing up blood! Can we NOW see a doctor?" While this was happening, I could hear Missy reciting the Lord's Prayer softly as she supported my head. I opened my eyes and saw all the blood in the basin. I don't recall feeling that deathly ill, ever. I laid back on the bed and the nurses were there by then. Within a minute or two, they wheeled me into Critical Care. As they were transporting me to another section of the hospital, I was watching the fluorescent lights overhead pass by one after another and remember thinking "Hey, this is just like in the movies!"

They performed an emergency upper endoscopy, and it showed that there was an open wound on the stomach lining which was bleeding slowly yet continuously. It was the result of removing polyps for biopsy earlier that day. They put a clip on it to arrest the bleeding. I was confined in that hospital for four days to make sure I was alright. After begging endlessly, I was discharged to celebrate the last two hours of my birthday at home. Score!

ADVICE: Focus on treating yourself to a nice meal after the procedure. You deserve it. Think good thoughts throughout the scope. Try to relax and avoid moving or talking. If you think too much about what's going on, it won't help; it just makes things worse. Think about all the wonderful food you'll get to eat soon after.

HORMONE THERAPY

Hormone therapy is a cancer treatment that slows or stops the growth of cancer that uses hormones to grow. Hormone therapy is also called hormonal therapy, hormone treatment, or endocrine therapy. It is not hormone replacement therapy (HRT), which contains estrogen. Hormone therapy is the exact opposite - it blocks or lowers estrogen levels in the body.

* *Amor T.* (*Breast cancer, Ovarian cancer*)

After my mastectomy, my doctor informed me that since my breast cancer was found early enough (stage I), I didn't need chemotherapy or radiation. YAY! In September 2013, I met with my medical oncologist who put me on a hormone therapy drug called Tamoxifen. After surgery, Tamoxifen is given to those patients who received a hormone-receptor positive, early-stage breast cancer diagnosis, to reduce the risk of the cancer recurring.

I was 53 years old at the time and going through perimenopause, so I was to take the Tamoxifen daily for five years, after which my menopausal status would determine the next course of action, e.g. five more years of Tamoxifen or another hormone therapy. Side effects I experienced were bone pain, increased hot flashes and dry skin, all of which were manageable.

When I was diagnosed with ovarian cancer in 2016 (three years later), my new oncologist reviewed the pathology to ascertain if my use of Tamoxifen contributed to the cancer in my ovaries. Even though results were negative, he stated that I'm at the menopause stage and should start taking Anastrozole (brand name Arimidex) for ten years. Anastrozole is a hormone-based chemotherapy used to treat post-menopausal women. It is an "aromatase inhibitor", meaning it will limit the amount of estrogen my postmenopausal body will produce.

In 2018, I moved to my current city and met with my new oncologist who had me take a breast cancer index test to determine if continuing to take the Anastrozole would benefit me down the line, i.e. decrease my chances of recurrence. Well, results showed that my breast cancer recurrence rate was very low at 2% and that continuing to take the Anastrozole would not decrease or increase that number. Therefore, it was not necessary for me to continue taking it. I stopped taking Anastrozole on July 18, 2018, about two years after I started. It was such a relief, because I had long been suffering joint pain and problems with my fingers while gripping things, two of Anastrozole's side effects. I no longer experience them.

ADVICE: Learn about medications you're given, i.e. their purpose and ingredients, as well as, their side effects. If you've been taking Anastrozole (Arimidex), ask your oncologist if you can take the breast cancer index test. The results may enable you to be free of Anastrozole and its side effects.

* Cindy R. *(Metastatic Breast cancer to the Stomach)*

After my doctors realized that my stomach cancer was actually a metastasis of the breast cancer I had ten years prior, they placed me on Faslodex – a hormonal therapy medicine. It is given through injections and is working wonders! Every month, I get two shots: one shot in each of my butt cheeks. After I get the shots, I have to make sure I walk around for about half an hour, so that the medicine could run through me and I don't get a knot from the shots. Since the liquids injected into me are really thick, they have to be injected into me really slowly. If I don't move around after I get the shots - like if I just sat down and didn't move much, the liquid would just bunch up right where I was injected and I would feel really blah. Since I don't want to feel blah, I made it a point to move around and do something useful, like go shopping, for half an hour. Faslodex has really, really, really helped me beat the stomach cancer. It's so great!

> **ADVICE:** When it comes to medication, make sure to follow instructions and learn about how they work, including their side effects. For the Faslodex injections, if I didn't pay attention to the nurse's instructions to move around for half an hour, I would've felt really blah and really uncomfortable from the liquid being stuck in the area I received the shots in (my glutes).

* Susan M. *(Ovarian cancer. Metastatic Pancreatic cancer to the Lungs)*

To treat my ovarian cancer, I was given the hormone drug, Progesterone, to take for two years.

HYPERBARIC OXYGEN THERAPY (HBOT)

Hyperbaric oxygen therapy involves breathing pure oxygen in a pressurized room or tube. Hyperbaric oxygen therapy treats conditions such as serious infections, bubbles of air in our blood vessels, and wounds that won't heal as a result of diabetes or radiation injury. In a hyperbaric oxygen therapy chamber, the air pressure is increased to three times higher than normal air pressure. Under these conditions, our lungs can gather more oxygen than would be possible breathing pure oxygen at normal air pressure. Our blood carries this oxygen throughout your body. This helps fight bacteria and stimulate the release of substances called growth factors and stem cells, which promote healing.

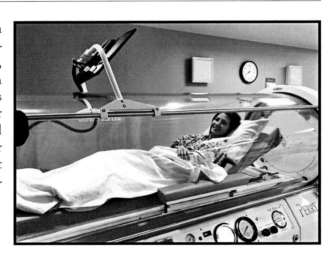

* Yesi L. *(Breast cancer: triple positive)*

After four surgeries on my breast, I was trying to heal. But there was one little area (like a pore) that kept opening up; it was definitely infected. The doctors then had me go through Hyperbaric Oxygen Therapy (HOT). Yes, I was placed inside a hyperbaric chamber, like the one Michael Jackson had. In that chamber, I was able to breathe pure oxygen in a way that allowed my body to fight the infection I had and allow my wound to heal.

> **ADVICE:** If, for some reason, you have a wound that just will not heal and looks like it is getting infection, ask you doctor about Hyperbaric Oxygen Therapy (HOT) where your body will be exposed to 100% oxygen at a pressure that is greater than normal. In that environment, the pure oxygen will speed the healing process of your wound like it did mine.

HYSTERECTOMY

Hysterectomy is the surgical removal of a woman's uterus with or without other organs or tissues. typically to treat cancer, chronic pain or heavy bleeding that has not been controlled by less invasive methods. In a total hysterectomy, the uterus and cervix are removed. In a total hysterectomy with salpingo-oophorectomy, (a) the uterus plus one (unilateral) ovary and fallopian tube are removed; or (b) the uterus plus both (bilateral) ovaries and fallopian tubes are removed. In a radical hysterectomy, the uterus, cervix, both ovaries, both fallopian tubes, and nearby tissue are removed. These procedures are done using a low transverse incision or a vertical incision.

* Amor T. (Breast cancer, Ovarian cancer)

On March 17, 2016, I had a radical hysterectomy, where my whole uterus, tissue on the sides of the uterus and the cervix were removed. At the same time, my surgeons also performed the following procedures:

- a bilateral salpingo-oophorectomy (BSO) where both my ovaries and fallopian tubes were removed;
- a bilateral ureterolysis where my ureter was isolated to prevent injury during the hysterectomy;
- a bilateral pelvic and periaortic (or paraaortic) lymphadenectomy where lymph nodes in my pelvis were removed for examination;
- an omentectomy where my omentum (thin, fatty fold of abdominal tissue that encased my stomach, large intestine and other abdominal organ and which also contained lymph nodes, lymph vessels, nerves and blood vessels) was removed;
- multiple peritoneal biopsies to determine the extent of cancer cells in the peritoneal cavity where my kidneys, adrenal glands, ureters, urinary bladder, part of the esophagus, rectum, ovaries, uterus, aorta and caudal are encased;
- an enterolysis aka lysis of adhesions where the surgeons had to break up (aka "lyse") and remove the complex web of scar tissue that had accumulated and interconnected the organs and tissues in my abdominal area from past surgeries. Here, my left ureter and some internal organs were encased in the adhesions and had to be mobilized out completely, and
- repair of injury to my small intestine, which they found during the procedure.

After the surgery, I was quite sore, as expected. In thinking about the extent of my procedure, given all that the surgeon removed from my body, I thought that perhaps I had lost, at least, five pounds. Alas, that was not realistic. You see, the ovaries and uterus together weighed .3 ozs and measured an estimated five inches...I had no idea those organs were tiny! If anything, I gained weight from the swelling. Oh well...

Recovering from my hysterectomy was really tough. Not only was my body trying to heal from the eight-inch long vertical incision from my chest plate down to my lower pelvic area, the intense constipation that followed, unfortunately, was terrible and super intense! Nevertheless, I did finally find relief with MiraLAX and have not experienced constipation since.

> ADVICE: An abdominal hysterectomy is major surgery and complete recovery can take two months, if not a bit longer. You'll stay 2-3 days in the hospital after surgery. When you're discharged, you'll be given instructions on how to take care of your wound, what you can/cannot eat and a list of activities you're restricted from engaging in, like housework, lifting, driving, and even having sex. Strictly follow those instructions and let your doctor know of any problems, like a fever, bleeding, severe pain, problems urinating, unusual vaginal discharge, etc.
>
> If you suffer from constipation, try a stool softener and a laxative. It's really best to ask your medical oncologist what's best to use, as OTC (over-the-counter) drugs may do more harm than good. MiraLAX has been touted as the "wonder drug" by so many who experienced constipation. Definitely try it.
>
> Drink lots of water and walk when you can. They both are always wise and proven ways to help your body heal smoothly, especially after major surgery.

* Cindy R. (Metastatic Breast cancer to the Stomach)

I had my hysterectomy two years after I finished chemo treatment for breast cancer and was taking the hormone pill Tamoxifen to prevent the return of breast cancer. After a couple years, results from tests they ran indicated that I was having some issues with my female parts, which concerned them. So my doctor strongly encouraged me to get a hysterectomy. He said, "Let's go in, do the hysterectomy and take you off that medicine (Tamoxifen). During the hysterectomy, they removed my ovaries, uterus ... what else is in there? Well, pretty much everything. I had the "full on". Clear it out!

The incision they gave me on my abdomen looked like a smiley face; like I got a big smile. They didn't remove my lymph nodes though.

Healing from the hysterectomy was nothing major. Thankfully, it was pretty straightforward. After surgery, I went on to take Arimidex (Anastrozole), the other breast cancer prevention pill.

> **ADVICE:** If your doctor suggests you get a hysterectomy, make sure you understand the reason. It's also really important to understand the procedure, so you know what they're removing from your body and what you get to keep. Because a hysterectomy is major surgery, communicate any concerns or side effects with your doctor, so that it can be taken care of.

* Rachel S. *(Breast cancer: triple negative "TNBC")*

Before the hysterectomy, I had to see an oncology therapist because I had sunk into a depression from thinking about how cancer was affecting my life.. I sunk even deeper when I saw the hysterectomy as a procedure that would cause me to lose myself as a woman. I thought that I had already lost my breasts and now I was going to lose all identity of being a woman. At the same time, I wasn't coping well with chemo brain; losing thoughts and memory. I was really in a dark place. Fortunately, my therapist worked through each of my issues with me; she helped me gain new perspectives. She had me comb through everything from top to bottom and made me realize that with the hysterectomy, I was actually regaining myself as a woman; not losing myself. And with regards to my chemo brain, I hadn't lost anything. I had actually gained my life!

Since the triple negative breast cancer I had is an aggressive form of breast cancer that's expected to return, my doctors have kept a very close eye on my developments. At one point, they noticed that I was bleeding lightly and immediately checked it out. Fortunately, it was nothing. Still, they strongly urged me to get a hysterectomy, as soon as possible, before the cancer returns. Doing so would, at least, remove the possibility of it returning in my reproductive organs.

So I went through a radical hysterectomy with a bilateral salpingo-oophorectomy, where they removed my ovaries, uterus, fallopian tubes and cervix via both my vaginal canal and belly button. It was laparoscopic surgery, meaning only small incisions were made in my abdomen and a special mini camera, called a laparoscope, was used to guide the surgeon. Because it was a minimally-invasive surgery, the whole procedure was quick and I only stayed one night in the hospital.

The day after I returned home from the hospital, I had to be rushed to the emergency room because of the intense pain I felt from constipation. Gas had gone up to my rib cage and I couldn't breathe without pain. They gave me morphine there and released the gas. Before I was discharged, they told me that I was going to get gas again and gave me the laxative, Dulcolax. I did experience more constipation here and there, but not as intense. After a few days, I was good.

I must say that the hysterectomy was one of the best things I could've done. It relieved me of having to worry about the cancer returning through my reproductive organs.

> **ADVICE:** If you have a choice, ask your doctor for a laparoscopic hysterectomy. It's minimally invasive and takes a shorter amount of time to heal than a regular hysterectomy that is actually major surgery.
>
> Also, Any precautionary measure done to save your life is a gain! Having hysterectomy to lessen the risk of cancer returning is definitely a gain. Just think: With hysterectomy, you're not losing your womanhood; you're gaining your life!

* Sondra W. *(Ovarian cancer 3x)*

I've had surgeries in the past. I had knee replacement on both knees and I had my appendix removed. And, with those surgeries, I always knew how they were going to turn out. My hysterectomy, on the other hand, was the first surgery that I went into not knowing what the outcome was going to be.

My doctor told me that he didn't really know how many organs were going to be affected. He also didn't know if I would have a colostomy bag temporarily or forever or not at all. And so, it was very, very different for me going into the hysterectomy not knowing anything about what was going to happen.

Everything happened so fast. However, there was a nice thing that happened on the day of surgery. A group of believers came and prayed for me. That was nice. But, what was really nice was when my doctor prayed with us too. Now, that was really great; really special!

My hysterectomy, everything went well. It was extensive, extensive, extensive! They removed my ovaries, uterus, fallopian tube, some lymph nodes and debrided my diaphragm. There were also tumors in my rectum and my bladder. It was just a lot. A lot! I remember that it was a 6-hour surgery and that I was in Intensive Care for a couple of days.

I also kind of remember my husband whispering in my ear, "You don't have a bag." Now, that was the most important thing. That was great! I did hear that. But, I didn't remember anything else, until I got out of Intensive Care.

ADVICE: Having a hysterectomy is pretty major surgery. But, it is a life-saver! Get as much information as you can to understand the procedure and what you can expect (as much as your doctor or nurse can tell you, anyway). Sure, not knowing what the outcome is going to be can be nerve-wracking. But, focus on the positive, like how the cancerous tumors, that are causing you pain, will be removed from your body. Prayer or meditation can also help to calm you before and after the procedure.

* *Susan M. (Ovarian cancer. Metastatic Pancreatic cancer to the Lungs)*

As part of my treatment for ovarian cancer, I had total hysterectomy where my uterus and cervix were removed, in addition to a bilateral salpingo-oophorectomy where my fallopian tubes and ovaries were removed.

* *Tet M. (Colon cancer 3x)*

In 2005, I had to undergo another Colectomy as a pre-emptive strike against Colon Cancer, because I was growing polyps at an alarming rate. Aside from that, they found three fibroids in my uterus ranging from approximately 3 to 9 cm. I knew I had no plans of having babies, so along with the Colectomy, I asked to have a Hysterectomy, in hopes of preventing cancer from touching those parts. I have no regrets, whatsoever, in making that decision and I'm glad I took the plunge. One ovary was left behind, so I wouldn't go into menopause. I did not experience hot flashes or anything related to menopause then. The added bonus was that menstruation ceased right after the procedure.

I'd like to point out though, that a Hysterectomy may not always be the ideal solution for certain cases, especially if the person would like to have babies. I was just lucky that it was a no-brainer for me.

ADVICE: If you do not plan on having children, think of the peace of mind of being cancer-free in that area after having a Hysterectomy.

IMMUNOTHERAPY

A type of therapy that uses substances to stimulate or suppress the immune system to help the body fight cancer, infection, and other diseases. Some types of immunotherapy only target certain cells of the immune system. Others affect the immune system in a general way.

* *Sondra W. (Ovarian cancer 3x)*

For my third round with ovarian cancer, my oncologist initially placed me on the chemotherapy drug Carboplatin and took me off of the maintenance drug Alimta, because it wasn't working. Then we kind of experimented with the drug combinations and the two weeks on and one week off schedule. Now, I'm on Keytruda and Carboplatin, which is exciting for me. Keytruda is an immunotherapy and works with my immune system to fight my cancer.

LAR (LOW ANTERIOR RESECTION) SURGERY

A lower anterior resection (LAR) surgery is a common surgery for rectal cancer and occasionally is performed to remove a diseased or ruptured portion of the intestine in cases of diverticulitis. LARs are for cancer in the proximal (upper) two-thirds of the rectum which lends itself well to resection while leaving the rectal sphincter intact.

* **Joan S.** (*Rectal cancer*)

I had the LAR surgery to remove my rectal cancer after I went through 25 rounds of radiation. During the surgery, they removed the entire rectal cancer and surrounding tissue and lymph nodes.

LYMPHADENECTOMY

Lymphadenectomy or lymph node dissection is the surgical removal of one or more groups of lymph nodes. It is almost always performed as part of the surgical management of cancer.

* **Amor T.** (*Breast cancer, Ovarian cancer*)

Along with my radical hysterectomy and several other procedures, I had a bilateral pelvic and periaortic (or paraaortic) lymphadenectomy where the lymph nodes in my pelvis were removed for examination. Although I felt swelling, numbness and pain in the surgical area after the procedure, they were manageable. Fortunately, I did not experience lymphedema.

> <u>ADVICE:</u> Anytime lymph nodes are removed, there's a risk of swelling. That's because the removal can sometimes block the flow of lymph (fluid from waste and foreign material collected from the area.) When lymph is blocked, it collects in tissue and causes swelling, the condition of which is called lymphedema. If you notice swelling, pain or numbness in your surgical area, let your doctor know, so you can get relief.

MASTECTOMY OR LUMPECTOMY

Mastectomy is the medical term for the surgical removal of one or both breasts, partially or completely. A mastectomy is usually carried out to treat breast cancer. In some cases, people believed to be at high risk of breast cancer have the operation prophylactically, that is, as a preventive measure.

Lumpectomy is surgery to remove cancer or other abnormal tissue from your breast. Lumpectomy is also called breast-conserving surgery or wide local excision because — unlike a mastectomy — only a portion of the breast is removed. Doctors may also refer to lumpectomy as an excisional biopsy.

* **Amor T.** (*Breast cancer, Ovarian cancer*)

I had my mastectomy with sentinel lymph node procedure, together with my DIEP flap breast reconstruction on June 24, 2013. This involved removing my entire left breast, without removing the axillary lymph nodes located in the armpits. Then a biopsy was performed on the lymph nodes to be sure that the cancer had not spread. Fortunately, they didn't. Also, the surgical pathology performed on the tumor revealed that I had a multifocal disease with two separate foci of invasion: grade one infiltrating lobular carcinoma and grade one infiltrating ductal carcinoma with associated a high-grade DCIS (ductal carcinoma in situ)..

When I woke up in the ICU (intensive care unit), I remember looking down at where my cancerous left breast used to be. In its place was a big glob of flesh that looked really rough and bruised and with a circular patch of skin stitched on the center. It was not a pretty sight at all. However, I was excited, because I knew that it was my "new" cancer-free boob!

Then, I looked further down and saw a very long (22") horizontal scar that ran from one end of my hip to the other end. I also had surgical drains coming out from both sides of my hip and both sides of my upper chest areas near my armpits. Because I was all drugged from the serious pain meds, I just thought, "Wow!" and drifted off to sleep. When I awoke again (still dopey), I remember seeing my beautiful daughter Catherine and feeling so very happy. Even though I couldn't move my body, I was just giddy with joy in seeing her as she had surprised me, travelling from Southern California and taking time off from her classes to be with me.

The nurse then came in to instruct me how to use my IV (intravenous) PCA (patient-controlled analgesia). She said that whenever I start to feel pain, I can easily push the button and small amounts of pain medication will be delivered through my IV line. Having that would give me control over my pain management. The only thing to remember was that the PCA would only deliver pain medication every six minutes, no more. So, I should try to not be trigger-happy.

My stay in the hospital spanned one week. During that time, my medical care team (doctors, nurses and health aides) were really awesome. I felt that they really cared for me, especially paying attention to my emotional disposition, which I think is critical to every patient's overall recovery.

The nurses regularly came in to check my vitals, wound healing and the surgical drains that were in place to remove fluids that had built up in my body after surgery. They were very reassuring on how my body and the wounds were healing, especially my reconstructed breast that, honestly, just looked awful. As a matter of fact, one of the nurses who had had a double mastectomy and was also a past patient of my plastic surgeon volunteered to show me the end result of his work. She gently lifted up her blouse and showed me her perfectly reconstructed breasts. She stated that our plastic surgeon is a "rock star" and a perfectionist. Therefore, I am in the best of hands and will be very happy with the end result. Very comforting to know.

> **ADVICE:** Having cancer is like having garbage in your body. Therefore, best way to see a life-saving mastectomy is "garbage in-garbage out." Of course, it's not easy to take on that attitude when losing a part of you that you've associated your femininity and womanhood to. However, when the circumstances are what they are, you'll benefit from seeing things in a more positive light. A new chapter where, sure you no longer have a breast or breasts you were born with, but they're not doing you any good. And, there are far, far better things you have to look forward to. Your health and your life!

* Cindy R. (*Metastatic Breast cancer to the Stomach*)

When they told me that I had stage III breast cancer in my right breast, they asked me what I wanted to do with regards to mastectomy. Since it was stage III, meaning the cancer had spread beyond the tumor and had gone to the lymph nodes, I told them, "Well, while you're in there, you might as well take it all out." That meant removing both my breasts; a double mastectomy vs. removal of just my right breast. It was a tough decision, but I know that it was the right decision, considering the cancer had already gone into my lymph nodes.

> **ADVICE:** Deciding to have a mastectomy, whether single or double, is tough. However, with the information your doctors give you, you have to look at the big picture and look at your future. Weigh the pros and cons for yourself. Sure, having breasts is important. But, much, much more important is being able to continue living for yourself and for those who love you. Besides, you can still have breasts (with breast reconstruction to replace your diseased breasts) and continue living, at the same time.

* Jacki S. (*Breast cancer*)

My doctors at the hospital were excellent, except for the first one I met with about my cancer. I did not feel comfortable with him, because he just didn't seem personable. He was very serious about everything and suggested that I have a double mastectomy, even though I didn't really need it.

I ended up having a lumpectomy only on my right breast after I got a second opinion, at the advice of my friends. When I got the second opinion, the doctor I saw was actually the head of the department. He was wonderful! I found out that he's a fisherman, like my husband. He had children. He was very personable, asking me about my life and my family. I just felt really comfortable with this doctor. He took a look at the lump and said that he felt I could just go with the lumpectomy. He respectfully asked if that would be my choice and if I would be okay with that. And, I said, "Yes!"

I did get a second surgery, after the lumpectomy, to have a little more tissue taken out. But, that was my choice. Fortunately, that second set of tissue was clear. Though I had a lumpectomy, I still have most of my right breast. Thank goodness for Victoria's Secret and Frederick's of Hollywood, no one would even know I'm missing part of my right breast. And I had that choice through my second doctor, who was respectful of my wishes, as opposed to the first doctor who wanted me to get a double mastectomy without giving me a choice.

* Rachel S. *(Breast cancer: triple negative)*

When I went in for my double mastectomy, the doctors came and tried to tell me all the side effects that were going to happen. And I told them, "You need to stop right there. Am I going to be alive?" And they said, "Yes, you are." And I said, "Well then, that's all that matters to me. Any side effects that come from this, I'll deal with at the time, because I will be alive to deal with them. I don't want to hear any more about side effects; just get it done."

The biggest fear I had was about what people were going to think. My husband looked up some stuff, but for the most part, I just knew what I needed to do. Before the mastectomy, I was between a size C and D. When I met with the plastic surgeon, he said that reconstruction for double mastectomy would result in size A breasts. I said, "I don't care. I'll be alive to be an A. How's that?" Then I asked my husband, "Do you care if I'm going to be an A?" He said, "Nope. You'll be here with me. That's all I care about!" I realized that I just had to be comfortable with myself and I had to trust that I'm making the right decision.

Everybody I talked to who had a double mastectomy were thankful that they did. For me, I'm thankful I had a double mastectomy done, because it was then that they found the other abnormal cells in my left side, which they didn't initially catch. So, I trusted myself on it and didn't go with what they said, no matter how hard they kept pushing for a single mastectomy only. Once I put my foot down, their attitude changed around it.

* Vida B.A. *(Breast cancer)*

I had a mastectomy only on my left breast. Because they removed my lymph nodes, my arms swelled. My doctor instructed me to get these special wraps for the arms – they're stretchable and look like socks or legging – that helped with the circulation. It helped to have them on when I traveled by air.

After the mastectomy, I was sent home with drain bulbs. Even though I had a single breast removed, I had two drains just dangling from the side of my breast. They didn't really bother me and I got used to them. I was even able to shower with them on.

MEDICAL PORT "PORT" IMPLANT AND REMOVAL

A medical port "port" or "port-a-cath" is a device that is placed beneath the skin and then into a vein, which will allow an easy and reliable way for your healthcare team to:

- give you intravenous (IV, through a vein) medication, such chemotherapy drugs,
- give you IV fluids,
- take blood samples from the veins, and
- give you medications continuously for several days.

Sometimes medications must be given in a vein larger than the ones in your arms. The port lets the medication go into your bloodstream through a large vein near your heart.

* Amor T. *(Breast cancer, Ovarian cancer)*

Mediport implant surgery: I had my medical port implant surgery on July 28, 2016. To prepare for it, I first had to make sure that the veins on my right (and only viable) arm were pumped enough, since they would need a good vein to use for my IV. When I got to Pre-Op at the hospital, the nurses had the darndest time trying to find a good vein. I was stuck and prodded, at least, ten times, and it felt as though my arm was full of holes! Finally, the anesthesiologist came and immediately found a viable vein. After they connected me to the IV, I was rolled into the OR ("operating room") where I greeted the doctors and nurses there. As I've done in my past surgeries, I told them that I could count from 100 down from 0 without any problem. So, they told me to start counting, and I said 100, 99... Then, I woke up in the recovery room.

My mediport was surgically implanted above my right breast and below my right clavicle. Understandably, the area was a bit sore. It also itched a little bit, but I was too doped up to pay any attention to it. I did notice that opening my mouth and turning my neck, even slightly, tugged at my Mediport and it was painful. It took awhile for the swelling to subside, but it eventually did and I no longer felt discomfort or pain. Having the Mediport was a total lifesaver, because I no longer had to suffer the pains of being pricked with a needle seemingly 10,000 times before they could find a viable vain. During chemo infusions, lab draws and port flushes, the whole process was smooth.

Port flushes: After completion of my chemotherapy treatments, I did have to to get my port flushed every month. Before each visit, I applied lidocaine pain and numbing cream onto the site and covered it with a square piece of Saran wrap. I looked forward to my monthly port flushes, because it was also a chance for me to visit with the wonderful oncology nurses who took care of me at the cancer center.

Mediport removal. Preparation for removal of my Mediport was basically the same as preparation for implant of my mediport. At (Pre-Op), they had to find a viable vein to connect me to the IV, which would carry the anesthesia that would put me under during the procedure. I remember pumping my hand as much as I could to get the blood flowing and even carried a five-pound dumbbell with me to flex my arms. I also did some jumping jacks, just to make sure. All my efforts paid off, because they found a viable vein after "only" three tries. Again in the OR, I told my doctor and the nurses there that I could easily count from 100 to 0 with no problem; I would be awake the whole time. So, I started with 100 ... Next thing I knew, I was in the recovery room! It never fails to amuse me.

> **ADVICE:** If your veins are not easy to find or if they burn during chemotherapy infusions, getting a medical port (mediport or port-a-cath) would save you a lot of pain and anxiety. When you do go for the mediport implant, ask to be put under; you do not want to be awake for the procedure. Same goes for when removal of your mediport. Ask to be put under. You do not want to be awake for the procedure.
>
> When it comes to the location of the mediport in your body, you should be given a choice. Ask your doctor what they are and then decide on what makes you the most comfortable.
>
> Before getting your mediport flushed, apply a big dollop of Lidocaine onto your port site one hour before your appointment and place a square piece of saran wrap over it and tape it to the area. That way, the numbing cream will be given time to work and will not rub off in transit.

* Glenn M. *(Metastatic Colon cancer to the Liver, Lungs & Adrenal Glands)*

I was under general anesthesia from my Colectomy when they implanted the medical port (mediport) device into me. So I didn't feel a thing and had no problem with it. I just had the discomfort of all the tubing and huge bandage afterwards.

> **ADVICE:** Having a port makes blood draws, infusions, etc. a whole lot easier. I highly recommend getting it. Just be prepared for discomfort from swelling in the beginning. Oh yeah, I'm not going to get rid of my port either.
>
> Also, if you're having surgery where you will be given anesthesia and there's a high chance you'll be going through treatment that requires infusions and lab draws, might as well also have the mediport implanted in you while you're under. You won't feel a thing and the mediport sure helps to make treatments go a whole lot easier!

* Hilda K. *(Colon cancer)*

My medical port device (mediport) was surgically implanted during my laparoscopic colectomy and was placed over my left breast, right above my heart. So, I didn't feel anything when it was put in.

After a year of my chemotherapy, I finally decided to have it removed. It was one of the most invasive experiences I've felt, aside from the surgery. At the doctor's office, they gave local anesthesia and then cut me open where my mediport was implanted. Since muscle and tissue had already grown around the mediport, the doctor had some difficulty pulling it out of me. I learned that when a foreign object is embedded into our bodies, our body's natural reaction is to deal with it and overtake it.

Because I didn't see the mediport go into me, I didn't know what it looked like. All I knew was that they had placed a mediport into me for use during treatment. Once the doctor was able to pull it out and show it to me, it looked like an insect. It was a disc with a tail; a very long tail. And that little tube was basically connected to my artery. So, anytime the chemotherapy drug went through me, it went straight to my heart and it dispensed. I mean, I couldn't believe that thing was in me. It looked like an alien!

ADVICE: Having the mediport will make receiving infusions and getting your labs done a lot easier. It is an incredible device!

* Joan S. *(Rectal cancer)*

I did get a medical port surgically implanted in me to ease my chemo infusions. It was a bit of an adjustment having it, but I had no problems with my port. Eventually, I got my port removed. I didn't expect it to be difficult or to be done in the doctor's office, because the implant was done in the hospital and I was under anesthesia. Anyway, it was done in the doctor's office and I was kind of awake. Removing the port was like a pull-type sensation. It did hurt a little, but not a lot. Also, the area was tender for a while. It does leave a scar too.

ADVICE: Just be prepared. If you haven't had your port removed, ask your doctor questions about the procedure and what to expect. That way, there are no surprises.

* Rev. Linda S. *(Pancreatic cancer 3x)*

For my initial round of chemotherapy, I had a power port implanted early in the morning and then started my first chemo treatment about an hour later. I was sedated for the implantation and had no pain from it. Halfway through my treatment series, the blood draws would not work through the port, but the chemo infusions Aloxi and Gemzar infusions still worked. From that point, the lab did all my blood draws from my arm and continued chemo infusions through my port. Shortly after completion of chemo treatment, I had my port removed.

For my second round of chemotherapy, the sedative cocktail of Versed (sedative), Fentanyl (narcotic) and Benadryl (antihistamine) was perfect. The new port implant was successful and I was ready for my chemo, which was scheduled for two days later.

ADVICE: It really helps to have a good sedative cocktail when you're getting your port implanted. Also, realistically, there are times when the port will not work perfectly. There are ways around that.

* Rachel S. *(Breast cancer: triple negative)*

Unfortunately, the placement of my port was an absolutely horrible experience, because, number one: I was awake the whole time. The doctor did give me some kind of calming stuff, but it didn't work; I felt everything. There was a technician there who told me that I should be asleep. Still, the doctor continued and injected the numbing solution into my neck, which hurt like hell! All of a sudden, I couldn't move. Then, he cut up above the neck for two entry points and then attached the tube to the vein. The whole time, I could feel them cutting! The numbing medicine had worn off completely! Seeing that I was in a lot of pain, the technician quickly talked to the doctor and I was given another shot of numbing solution to finish the job. It was really horrible. I am scared to death of getting the port taken out, because I'm afraid of going through that awful experience again.

ADVICE: If you're going get a port implanted into your body, INSIST on general anesthesia. You absolutely do not want to be awake during the procedure.

* Scott M. (Metastatic Colon cancer to the Prostate & Pancreas)

I had surgery to implant my first medical port (port) on the left side of my neck and I was placed under general anesthesia, which was no problem at all. Unfortunately, the port was placed in such a way that it kind of twisted; the nurses weren't able to get the needles in exactly straight. They had to really struggle to access my port. So, eventually, I just bit the bullet, had that port removed and had a new one implanted on the right side of my neck. That was a better port; easier to access.

ADVICE: Have the surgeon explain to you where your port will be implanted and why. If you have any concerns, let them know. Also, since it's major surgery, make sure you are under general anesthesia, so you don't feel any pain. If there are any problems accessing your port, speak up and change the location, if necessary.

* Sondra W. (Ovarian cancer 3x)

Oh, poor veins for blood tests, in chemo and all the infusions...that's absolutely me! I had a mediport put in and I was so thankful that my doctor suggested that, because I have little, tiny, tiny veins. It has been a problem all my life. And my veins collapse and they also move. They are so small. Often, more than not, the nurses or lab technicians can't access them. So I'm very glad that I have the mediport in.

The mediport procedure was really easy. I went in, got all prepared and then, went to "sleep". When I woke up, it was done; my mediport was in and everything was great. Except, a couple of weeks later, I felt this pain on my neck and thought it was from the way I had slept or something. Then, it got worse. The pain went to my chin and my ears and I thought, "Wait a minute. Am I having a heart attack? What's going on here?"

So, I went to Urgent Care where they did an ultrasound on me. They told me, "Oh, you have a big blood clot in your neck, possibly from your mediport. We can't let you get in the car and be driven to the ER, because if it starts to move and you're in traffic, there's nothing you or anyone can do." So, I ended up having to be transported by ambulance to the ER.

When I got to the ER, they confirmed that I had a blood clot from my mediport and asked me, "Do you want to go home and watch to see if anything will happen?" I answered, "No, I don't. If I could do that, I wouldn't even be here." The ER doctor said, "Oh, I can see by the look on your face that you want to be admitted." I said, "Yes."

So, I got admitted and they called in a radiologist who specializes in vascular conditions that involve the arteries and veins. He gave me an ultrasound and said, "I think that we can give you some extra shots in your stomach. Although what you're getting now should have taken care of the problem, obviously it didn't. So, we're going to up the dosage and keep you here for a few days. I'll come and make sure it works. Well, the clot got smaller, but it didn't dissolve. So I had to go on the blood thinner, Xarelto. As long as I have the mediport in, I have to take a Xarelto tablet every day. I was on this regimen for two years then stopped, because I got the bleeding ulcers from it.

ADVICE: You definitely should get a mediport, if you have poor, tiny or moving veins like me. It will definitely make you more comfortable during your treatment process. It will also make the lab draws or infusions go faster and be more effective. No more pain from all the poking and prodding, while they try to look for viable veins to use. Yes, I highly recommend getting a mediport, if you have poor veins, tiny or moving veins like me.

Side effects from mediport placements, like mine, are not the norm. Usually these procedures go off without a hitch. So, don't let my off experience keep you from getting a mediport. I'm so thankful I got one. Because of my poor veins, my treatment experience would've been much harder without the mediport.

If you have to take a blood thinner, like Xarelto, be aware of its side effects and let your doctor know if you feel any discomfort from taking it.

* **Susan M.** (*Ovarian cancer. Metastatic Pancreatic cancer to the Lungs*)

After two months of chemotherapy to treat pancreatic cancer, I decided to have a port put in, because my veins had collapsed. It was a simple surgical procedure. The port area was sore for a couple of weeks, but they were able to use the port for chemo and blood draws soon after.

> **ADVICE:** If the medical staff have a hard time finding a good vein for lab draws or infusions, you should get a medical port device implanted. It's a simple procedure and makes your treatments go by faster.

* **Yesi L.** (*Breast cancer: triple positive*)

When I had the MediPort implanted, I felt like I got hit with a bat! During the surgery, I was under anesthesia because, aside from implanting the MediPort, they performed a Sentinel Node Biopsy to evaluate the extent of my breast cancer. Basically, lymph nodes were removed from my right side and the MediPort was implanted on my left side. I definitely felt like I got hit with a bat on both sides! So, in the beginning, I needed assistance getting out of bed.

MOHS MICROGRAPHIC SURGERY (MMS)

Mohs surgery is a precise surgical technique used to treat skin cancer. During Mohs surgery, thin layers of cancer-containing skin are progressively removed and examined until only cancer-free tissue remains. Mohs surgery is also known as Mohs micrographic surgery.

* **Aaron C.** (*Prostate cancer, Skin cancer*)

To treat the skin cancer on my lower left eyelid, my doctor gradually removed all the tissue there that was cancerous. What he did was slice off the skin a little bit at a time and then checked it under the microscope to see if he got all the cancer out. He did those steps a few times, going back and forth, until he couldn't find any more cancer. I lost some eyelashes and stuff, but was glad they were able to retain the eyelid margin itself. My doctor initially thought he would have to remove a big piece of the skin and rebuild my eyelid. Fortunately, they didn't have to do that!

> **ADVICE:** Fortunately, this isn't like major surgery at all. It's done on an outpatient basis and takes only a few hours. The part that took the longest for me was waiting for the lab results of the tissue that was removed.

NEPHRECTOMY

Nephrectomy is surgery to remove a kidney or part of a kidney. In a partial nephrectomy, part of one kidney or a tumor is removed, but not an entire kidney. In a simple nephrectomy, one kidney is removed. In a radical nephrectomy, an entire kidney, nearby adrenal gland and lymph nodes, and other surrounding tissue are removed. In a bilateral nephrectomy, both kidneys are removed.

* **Bob G.** (*Soft Tissue Sarcoma, Skin cancer*)

Initially, the doctors performed exploratory surgery on my left side and then on my right side. Fortunately, they found nothing. Then when I went for my first real surgery, a splenectomy where they removed my spleen and the surrounding tissue. The doctors told me what they were going to do. That surgery went very well, because back then, I was swimming three to four times per week.

   The second surgery was radical surgery; an "either-you-make-it-or-you-don't" kind. In this surgery, they performed a combination radical nephrectomy-colectomy-rib resection where they removed my left kidney, 50% of my colon, one to two back ribs, plus some muscle and more tissue. I didn't know, until much later, that they did all that to remove my cancer and keep it from spreading.

* Cindy L. *(Kidney cancer)*

My surgeon went through everything that was going to happen during my surgery. He really made me feel that I was part of the decision as to how this surgery was going to be accomplished, whether it was going to be a full nephrectomy or a partial nephrectomy. Because the size of the cancerous tumor in my left kidney (5cms), we decided that I would need a full (radical) nephrectomy.

There are three ways a nephrectomy can be performed, i.e. open surgery, hand-assisted laparoscopic surgery (HALS) or Da Vinci robotic surgery. We chose hand-assisted laparoscopic surgery (HALS). It's a modified laparoscopic surgery where one of the incisions made in the abdomen is made big enough for the surgeon's hand to be inserted through with instruments, so that the surgeon can do whatever he needs to do in there.

During the surgery, my surgeon's hand went into the back of my abdomen to get a hold of my left kidney. He then wrapped it in a plastic bag, cut off all the blood supply and removed it through an incision they made that ran from a point below my belly button to my pubic mound. That diseased kidney was wrapped in a plastic bag to keep the cancer cells from escaping or spreading.

He also removed all the surrounding tissue. Because the cancer had not metastasized, he left my adrenal gland in there, which surprised me, because I didn't see the necessity of keeping it in there, especially when I didn't think it was functioning well, if at all.

NIPPLE RECONSTRUCTION / AREOLA MICROPIGMENTATION (TATTOOING)

Nipple reconstruction is done after the reconstructed breast has had time to heal — at least 3 or 4 months after reconstruction surgery. The nipple may be reconstructed from the surrounding skin at the site desired for nipple placement. The surgeon makes small incisions and then elevates the tissue into position, forming and shaping it into a living tissue projection that mimics the natural nipple. Some women choose to have a nipple and areola tattooed on the reconstructed breast. Other women decide to have a star, a heart, or another meaningful image tattooed on the reconstructed breast instead of a nipple. The most realistic results are often achieved with 3D nipple tattoos, which are basically real tattoos that use oscillating needles coated with pigment.

* Amor T. *(Breast cancer, Ovarian cancer)*

My nipple reconstruction took place three months after my breast reconstruction where a temporary round piece of skin taken from my abdomen was attached to the center my new left breast. Interestingly, that piece of skin was of a different color from my new left breast, so that got me curious about how my new nipple would be created out of a round piece of skin. Obviously, I didn't think far ahead enough to research this procedure before my initial breast reconstruction. Also, returning from the hospital after a two week stay, I was just not of the mindset to even turn on the computer to check.

The nipple reconstruction surgery was held at the same time as my breast symmetry procedure. For the nipple reconstruction, a small incision was made at the site of the new nipple's location. The skin there was pulled up and out to form into a nipple shape and small sutures (stitches) were used to secure the form. After the surgery, I looked down at my nipple and saw a really stiff piece of skin looking back at me. Hmm ... interesting. My surgeon explained that everything will soften and settle into place when the sutures melt and the inflammation eventually disappears with time. Of course, he was right and the end result was wonderful.

After three months, the nipple of my new left breast had healed and it was time to the 3D tattoo. Before I met with her, my surgeon had me remind her to make sure the borders of the areolas should not be perfectly round, but irregular. The micropigmentation (tattoo) artist was quite skilled, experienced and pleasant. I got to pick from a large selection of dyes; two hues, since we were going for the 3D effect. Also, she made sure that the tattooed areolas for both breasts matched. Her artistry was excellent!

> **ADVICE:** After nipple reconstruction surgery, expect to see stiff looking nipples. That's temporary. With time, the inflammation and sutures will disappear and your breast and nipple tissues will soften. For your areolas, make sure your micropigmentation (tattoo) artist creates a normal-looking areola with soft, irregular borders and without perfect lines. You will definitely want both breasts to match.

PANCREATECTOMY / DISTAL PANCREATECTOMY / WHIPPLE PROCEDURE / RAMPS

(Radical Antegrade Modular Pancreatosplenectomy Surgery)

In the treatment of cancer, pancreatectomy is the surgical removal of all or part of the pancreas. Several types of pancreatectomy exist, such as:

- Distal pancreatectomy - usually performed if we have tumors that are confined to the tail (left portion) of the pancreas. The surgeon removes the tail and sometimes part of the body of the pancreas and the spleen.
- RAMPS (Radical Antegrade Modular Pancreatosplenectomy Surgery) - a safe and oncologically superior procedure for the treatment of left-sided pancreatic cancer;
- The "Whipple" procedure also known as Pancreaticoduodenectomy - the most common type of surgery for pancreatic cancer. It is used to remove tumors that are confined to the head, or right portion, of the pancreas.

* *Rev. Linda S. (Pancreatic cancer 3x)*

Treatment for my first bout with cancer included laparoscopic surgery, specifically the RAMPS procedure. Here, they removed the pancreatic tail, the tumor, and the spleen, which then appeared to have removed the cancer. I was comforted knowing that I had the best surgeon in the region for a RAMPS procedure, although the hospital was a six hour round-trip drive from home.

* *Susan M. (Ovarian cancer. Metastatic Pancreatic cancer to the Lungs)*

When they performed the Whipple Procedure on me, it was a seven-hour procedure where several of my organs were removed. After the surgery, fatigue set in during my 22-day stay in the hospital and continued for several months.

PAROTIDECTOMY

Parotidectomy is the name of the surgery used to remove a benign or cancerous tumor in the parotid gland (a large salivary gland located in front of and just below the ear). This operation requires particular care and expertise on the part of the surgical team, because the facial nerve and other structures are nearby.

* J.B. (Salivary gland cancer)

The surgery I had was called parotidectomy. It was an in-patient surgery and usually takes two hours, depending on the grade of the cancerous tumor. The grade of my tumor was a bit higher, so my surgery took four hours.

During the surgery, the doctor cut near my right ear and down along the jawline. That then opened up a space for them to take out the right parotid gland, which is one of the two biggest salivary glands. And at the same time, they tried to also remove the cancer that was kind of sticking along the cervical gland (located in the neck region) and the salivary gland areas. After they removed the cancer, they just kind of stitched me back up. This was all done while I was under general anesthesia. I was given prescription painkillers, but I didn't need to take them, because I have a high threshold of pain.

PROSTATECTOMY / ROBOTIC SURGERY DA VINCI SYSTEM)

Prostatectomy refers to the surgical removal of all or part of the prostate gland. This operation is done for benign conditions that cause urinary retention, as well as for prostate cancer and for other cancers of the pelvis. There are two main types of prostatectomies. A simple prostatectomy (also known as a subtotal prostatectomy) involves the removal of only part of the prostate. Surgeons typically carry out simple prostatectomies only for benign conditions. A radical prostatectomy, the removal of the entire prostate gland, the seminal vesicles and the vas deferens, is performed for malignant cancer.

* Aaron C. (Prostate cancer, Skin cancer)

After I was given my prostate cancer diagnosis, I researched my options for treatment. I looked at radiation, but learned that if they found more cancer after my first radiation treatment, I would have to go through the radiation again, because they won't be able to perform surgery on me once I go through radiation. However, if I have surgery first, then I would have the option of radiation treatment if the surgery doesn't completely rid my body of the cancer.

Before the two and a half hour surgery, they anesthetized me. So, I was out. Then, they cut small incisions – most of them, about an inch and a half in length - in several places in my abdomen: one above my belly button, two on my right side and two on my left side. The robotic arms went in through those incisions. They also inserted a tube and inflated my abdomen, using nitrous oxide. The purpose is to bloat the cavity area and get a view of everything in there. When the surgeon uses the equipment, he looks through a machine that has a little camera already inside the abdominal cavity area. The robotic arms also have fingertips that are controlled separately. In the end, the robotic arm went through the biggest incision, which was right above my belly button, and "pulled" my prostate out. It's amazing technology and a million dollar piece of equipment.

During the surgery, my doctor also removed about 20-30 inflamed lymph nodes from my groin area. He didn't want to take a chance of any of them carrying cancer, so he removed them. When I woke up after, the catheter was already in place. My surgery was scheduled for 7:00 am and I was out by 11:00 am. I stayed overnight in the hospital and left for home the following afternoon. I was sore from the surgery and had to keep the catheter on for ten days. It was miserable.

ADVICE: If you have the option, I highly recommend getting robotic surgery. The incisions are smaller, which result in a reduced risk of infection. Scarring is minimal. Pain and discomfort is reduced. Hospital stay is shorter and there is less bleeding. You'll still be sore after the surgery, but that happens after all surgeries. The biggest advantage is that you'll recover faster.

RADIATION THERAPY

Radiation therapy uses precisely focused, high-energy beams to kill cancer cells. It is usually given from a machine outside the body (called external-beam radiation therapy), most often in the form of x-rays but sometimes as protons or other types of energy. Radiation therapy can also be delivered internally by placing radioactive material in the body near tumors (called brachytherapy).

* Bob G. (Soft Tissue Sarcoma, Skin cancer)

After my second operation, I asked the surgeon if I would lose my hair. He said, "Oh, we're not going there." And then, using purple ink, he mapped out a diagram on my abdomen for the radiation to follow. I don't remember drinking any dye; I think they injected it. In any case, my radiation was for two weeks. Sometimes my wife drove me there and sometimes I drove myself. The radiation was quite an experience and I'm fortunate that staff at the hospital was very good.

For my second round with radiation, I had to go through 30 treatments, which was radiation five days a week for six weeks. The only interruption I had was during the holidays. The treatment itself was very short; like one minute. The wait, actually, takes longer. I don't remember the details of the procedure itself, because it was so very long ago!

For my 30 radiation treatments, I drove to the hospital for the first two weeks. For the next two weeks, my wife drove me there. After, I drove myself the rest of the time.. Recovery after the radiation treatments seemed much slower. I couldn't deal with much activity. I walked more slowly and I remember we did go to a movie. But, other than that, we just stayed home.

For the treatments, I clearly remember that I kept thinking, "Let's get it done!" The doctors seemed to be taking their time and I was getting frustrated, because I wanted the cancer out! I also kept thinking that my kids weren't prepared for me to leave this earth.....and I STILL feel that way!

ADVICE: This might be contrary to some, but I believe that if there's cancer in your body, then just get it out! For skin cancer, it may take from 20 to 29 surgeries.

* Cindy R. (Metastatic Breast cancer to the Stomach)

I had radiation treatment every week day for eight weeks. It was an interesting experience; not bad at all. When I saw that I had twelve tiny dots tattooed on my chest, I thought, "Oh, that's the earth floating in space." During radiation, the radiation technologist uses those dots as markers to map where they're going to shoot the laser. The radiation tattoo markers were, actually, my very first tattoos.

As I received more radiation, I felt like I was getting a real bad sunburn. I didn't put lotion or anything on it. I just kind of dealt with it. The one thing I remember that was really neat was when, after eight weeks, on my last day, one of the nurses at the office gave me flowers. It was like a graduation; such a neat thing. I was like, "Wow, thank you!"

ADVICE: Radiation therapy is pretty straightforward. They put marks (tattooed dots) in the area that needs to be treated, they radiate you in those areas and then you're done. The preparation takes much longer than the actual radiation process. You won't really feel anything during the radiation. After several treatments, however, those radiated areas will feel like sunburn. Let the technologist or your doctor know if you're feeling uncomfortable or if you feel any pain. That way, they can give you something for relief.

* Jacki S. (Breast cancer)

I had radiation treatments once a week for 36 weeks and drove myself to the hospital and back home (except for the first radiation treatment). Each session lasted about two hours, including prep time. To prep, I had to get into a dressing or hospital gown and I had little markers placed on my chest. Basically, they made little tattoos where the radiation was going to be heading into my body and, each and every time, the radiation went into the exact same place it went into the last time. I laid down for, I think it was, a half an hour, for each one of those sessions. Once the session was done, I just went on with my day. I picked up my daughter from school or the bus stop. If it was a day I was scheduled to work at the ice rink, then I went to teach at the ice rink after my radiation treatment.

Throughout treatment, I still took care of getting my 12 year old daughter up and ready for school. I also made her breakfast and drove her to the bus stop to go to her middle school. Then, I continued my routine, which was based on a schedule I coordinated between my job as an ice-skating instructor and my radiation and chemotherapy appointments. There were times when I had to give lessons on the days I had my radiation treatment. I didn't have any side effects or anything. So, I went on with my regular day.

Something fun that I experienced when I had no hair was getting the free hats when I went in for radiation. Because there are so many patients that go in for radiation and don't have their hair yet, there's a special group of women (I don't know who they are; they're just angels) who make hats for patients who need them. What they do is they put these hats in a basket right inside the office. Before you go in for your radiation and, if you feel like you need a new hat or you would like to have a hat for another occasion, the hats are in the basket for you to take, free of charge! So, that was very nice. I did have a bunch of them. But then, I brought some back to the radiation department and some I took to the Salvation Army, because there's always someone who could use them.

ADVICE: Find a friend to go with you for support. Enjoy the little gifts given to you by cancer supporters.

* Joan S. (Rectal cancer)

After being diagnosed with cancer, I went through 25 rounds of radiation. My schedule was five days a week for five weeks. I got fatigued from the radiation therapy I received. But, that didn't stop me from my regular activities, except for short time I was fatigued, which lasted about one and half hours.

* J.B. (Salivary gland cancer)

I had my radiation treatment every weekday (five days a week) for seven weeks. For me, the doctor created a plan or a map for the machine to target a very specific area located along the side of my head by my cheek. Then, I had a plastic mold created of my face. They had to align my face correctly. That mold was then placed over my face and strapped onto the table I was on. It kind of looked like a mask from Phantom of the Opera. It was hard plastic but it looked like mesh. The mask was very tight on my head, so that I couldn't move my head at all. Then the machine went around me, beaming the radiation on my cancerous parotid gland.

Preparation for the radiation therapy took a whole lot longer than the actual radiation treatment, which lasted about 10 minutes. The worst part was when I had to breathe through my nose, because the mask was on so tight that I couldn't open my mouth. There was one day when I had a bunch of allergies and it was hard to breathe through my nose. That was the worst feeling. But, I dealt with it accordingly. I made sure that I took allergy medication with me.

During the later parts of the radiation treatment and even after, I felt that my skin was drying up. Yes, there was pain, but it was mild, more like a bad sunburn. I used Vaseline on my skin and that took care of the problem.

ADVICE: The whole process really isn't too bad. The good thing is that it's fairly quick, compared to other treatments. If you have any problems, the medical team is there to help you. If you feel you have allergies coming on, you should bring allergy medicine, so that you can breathe through your nose. Use Vaseline on your skin if you feel like it's drying up.

* Rev. Linda S. (Pancreatic cancer 3x)

I had to go through radiation to treat the recurrence of my cancer. I consulted with the radiologist and the dietician and felt good about the customized radiation process. They tattooed the skin of my abdomen two weeks before my radiation treatment, for which I was to go through five days of radiation for 90 minutes each.

The first radiation treatment failed before it began. We experienced a glitch. The Ativan (a sedative) worked beautifully to eliminate my anxiety from claustrophobia. The pain pill, however, was not strong enough to do its job without putting me to sleep. If I slept, I couldn't respond to the commands from the radiologist and technician. So I was awake and in excruciating pain that radiated from my left to right side on the abdomen and on both sides of my lower back. After about 20 minutes, I squeezed the bulb for help and asked them to raise my knees higher, thinking that would decrease the strain on my abdominal muscles. They placed towels between my knees and the riser they rested on, to no avail. Another 20 minutes went by before I squeezed the bulb again. We had to stop. There was no way I would last another 50 minutes in that degree of suffering. All the meditative and visualization techniques I knew were useless. I leaned into the pain so deeply, you would think that I would have moved through it but it only intensified.

I asked the radiologist, "Will this set me back?" He replied, "We'll stay ahead of it." I learned later that they scheduled me for chemo the next day.

* Rachel S. *(Breast cancer: triple negative)*

I had to go to radiation therapy for five weeks. The first time I went in, they did x-rays and made a mold of my head. Then, they made a mold of my head and arms. The purpose for the mold was for them to have me in exactly the same position, every single time I went in, so that they can make sure the radiation went into the right places of my body. So, every time I went in, I lay on the table and positioned my arms above my head, inside the mold they made, and I had to lay there exactly the same way. When necessary, they adjusted my body to make sure that all the points hit.

I have three tattoos, one on either side of my body and one in the center of my chest, which they used to align the radiation heat. I didn't feel it at all; I just laid there perfectly still. The whole procedure took about 10 minutes.

* Scott M. *(Metastatic Colon cancer to the Prostate & Pancreas)*

Of all the treatments I've had, radiation therapy was probably the most difficult. It snuck up on me. I only had the radiation therapy for the prostate cancer. I went through radiation for 43 days in a row and for only for fifteen minutes at a time. My radiation treatment was 360 degrees, meaning they had to roll my body twice, 360 degrees one way and then 360 degrees going back the other way, to hit the prostate. But, two weeks after treatment was completed, it was like I drove a car 60 mph into a brick wall. I just had no energy. I was completely, completely drained, and it lasted for several weeks. I think that's normal.

> **ADVICE:** Even though the radiation procedure may take a small amount of time, recovering from it may take a bit longer. Radiation is draining, so just be prepared to be really tired and feel completely drained. It's to be expected.

* Vida B.A. *(Breast cancer)*

I received radiation therapy on my left breast after the reconstruction. My schedule was every weekday for one month. Before radiation, the skin on my left breast was totally healed and looked flawless. Even though I didn't have a nipple on the reconstructed breast then, that was fine with me.

The radiation itself took only a few minutes; not even 30 minutes. The waiting took longer than the radiation. During the radiation, they first focused on the surface of my left breast area. Then, they moved to the area behind my left armpit. Since results of my PET scan showed something underneath my chest bone, they had to radiate the middle of my chest too.

In the beginning, I was going through the radiation like a breeze. As I completed more treatments, however, I found that the skin on my breast and armpit areas darkened from the burn of the radiation. Although I didn't really feel pain, I did itch a lot in those areas. It felt like sunburn.

My doctor gave me an ointment to use and taught me how to clean the affected areas with hydrogen peroxide, apply the ointment and then dress it with gauze. I also bought a very expensive cream from France that contained a lot of skin-healing minerals and applied it to the affected areas. Since my skin got so soft, it peeled off whenever I took showers. After 2-3 weeks, my skin healed. The affected areas are still a bit dark, but not as dark as before.

> **ADVICE:** The radiation therapy process itself is really quick; from several minutes to less than 30 minutes. It actually takes longer to wait to get into the treatment room. After you receive radiation, observe changes to your skin each time. Let your doctor know when you see darkening and/or burning of your skin, so that he or she can guide you on what to do. Even though you can expect your skin to burn and darken, there are good topical creams and ointments out in the market that can heal your skin.

* Yesi L. *(Breast cancer: triple positive)*

Aside from chemotherapy and targeted therapy, I also had to have radiation. I went through 24 rounds of radiation every weekday, Monday through Friday. It was very quick and took only about 20 minutes.

To prepare me, they actually tattooed my skin with tiny dots, which they called "markers". I got four tiny dots on my skin to guide the radiation beams to go to the exact same area each time. It made like a whole quadrant. The markers were just on my right breast.

I definitely experienced skin irritation from the radiation; it felt like sunburn, at first. Then, as it progressed, it felt like a really, really bad sunburn. The oncology team had a care package for me that included Eucerin. They applied a thick lather of the Eucerin on the treated area after the Radiation and told me to not touch it and don't put anything else on it. Sometimes the irritation got so bad that I ended up with a little blister. So they gave me some topical antibiotic.

RADIOEMBOLIZATION / Y-90

A type of radiation therapy used to treat liver cancer or cancer that has spread to the liver. A thin, flexible tube is used to inject tiny beads that hold the radioactive substance yttrium Y 90 into the main blood vessel that carries blood to the liver. The beads collect in the tumor and in blood vessels near the tumor, and the yttrium Y 90 gives off radiation. This destroys the blood vessels that the tumor needs to grow and kills the cancer cells. Radioembolization is a type of internal radiation therapy. Also called intra-arterial brachytherapy.

* *Glenn M.* (*Metastatic Colon cancer to the Liver, Lungs & Adrenal Glands*)

The baseball-sized tumor was too big for the CyberKnife treatment. So, I went through two radioembolizations also known as Y-90 treatments. A radioembolization (Y90) is a minimally invasive procedure that combines embolization and radiation therapy to treat liver cancer.

Y-90 is the particular radiation they put into glass microspheres one-third the diameter of a human hair; a half tea-spoon is about a million of them. They went in through my groin to find the artery feeding the tumor itself. Then, they dumped the entire load of Y-90 glass microspheres inside the tumor, which started plugging up the capillaries. The Y-90 only penetrates about three-eighths of an inch, but it can't miss because it's inside the target. It's kind of like shooting fish in a barrel. That pretty much killed my "baseball."

SPLENECTOMY

Splenectomy is a surgical procedure to remove your spleen. The spleen is an organ that sits under your rib cage on the upper left side of your abdomen. It helps fight infection and filters unneeded material, such as old or damaged blood cells, from your blood.

Removing your spleen is a major surgery and leaves you with a compromised immune system. For these reasons, it's only performed when truly necessary. The benefits of a splenectomy are that it can resolve several health issues such as blood diseases, cancer, and infection that could not be treated any other way.

* *Bob G.* (*Soft Tissue Sarcoma, Skin cancer*)

Initially, the doctors performed exploratory surgery on my left side and then on my right side. Fortunately, they found nothing. Then when I went for my first real surgery, a splenectomy where they removed my spleen and the surrounding tissue. The doctors told me what they were going to do. That surgery went very well, because back then, I was swimming three to four times per week.

The second surgery was radical surgery; an "either-you-make-it-or-you-don't" kind. In this surgery, they performed a combination radical nephrectomy-colectomy-rib resection where they removed my left kidney, 50% of my colon, one to two back ribs, plus some muscle and more tissue. I didn't know, until much later, that they did all that to remove my cancer and keep it from spreading.

> **ADVICE:** Make sure your doctors explain what they'll be doing when they operate on you. It really helps to know what's going on.

Targeted therapy is a type of treatment that uses drugs or other substances to identify and attack specific types of cancer cells with less harm to normal cells. Some targeted therapies block the action of certain enzymes, proteins, or other molecules involved in the growth and spread of cancer cells. Other types of targeted therapies help the immune system kill cancer cells or deliver toxic substances directly to cancer cells and kill them. Targeted therapy may have fewer side effects than other types of cancer treatment. Most targeted therapies are either small molecule drugs or monoclonal antibodies.

* Cindy R. *(Metastatic Breast cancer to the Stomach)*

Faslodex: I was diagnosed with stomach cancer in 2014 and was treated with chemotherapy for two years. When they realized that my stomach cancer was actually a metastasis of my breast cancer from ten years prior (2004), they put me on the Faslodex (hormone injections) and Ibrance, which is targeted therapy; not traditional chemotherapy.

My doctor gave me a special pill organizer for the Ibrance, because I had to follow a specific schedule, i.e. three weeks on and one week off. Although the pills were color coded, the pill organizer was really invaluable. Otherwise, it would just be confusing. Aside from the Ibrance, I had to take a daily pill. So I programmed an alert on my cell phone to remind me to take it. The pill organizer and alarm really made a difference for me. They're so great, because once I get started on my day, I'll tend to forget, if I didn't have those tools.

> **ADVICE:** First, you have to be really strict about following the schedule for taking your medication. Since taking the targeted therapy pill Ibrance is so specific and can be confusing, you have to use a pill organizer. Use your calendar too, if necessary. You risk forgetting if you think you can just remember on your own. Aside from talking with your doctor about how to take your medication, ask him or her about side effects and what you can expect Also, if you forget to take your pill, let your doctor know immediately. That way, he or she is aware and can guide you on what to do.

* Scott M. *(Metastatic Colon cancer to the Prostate & Pancreas)*

Chemoembolization: After my colon resection and six months of chemotherapy with the Oxaliplatin, Avastin and Xeloda, I was clear. The six big lesions in my liver were gone – Hooray! But, my doctors and I had already agreed that I should still go through a two-part chemoembolization of my liver to remove any remaining cancer cells in my body. In the procedure, they took and flooded half of my liver with chemo-filled pellets to kill the cancer two ways: (1) block blood flow from that part of the liver to kill the cancer cells and (2) get the cancer cells to eat up the chemo fluid they're trapped in and then die that way.

Well, I went in for the first procedure and it just knocked me on my butt. I was in the hospital for a week, with a lot of pain and my doctor said that I was such a "weenie", because he had 80-year old guys come in and just go home the next day, without any problems. But, for some reason, that procedure just really knocked me out. And, for two months, I was just sicker than a dog.

After I recovered, I went back to see my oncologist and interventional radiologist and they both told me, "We don't think we should do the second half." And I said, "Hey guys, what was the plan?" And they said, "To do both halves". And I said, "Well, I'm going to survive the second one. It may be tough, but we're doing it." So, we did it and sure enough, I was in the hospital for a week, sicker than a dog, and it knocked me on my butt for two months ... but, I DID IT!

* Sondra W. *(Ovarian cancer 3x)*

Avastin. Avastin was my targeted therapy medication. Its job was to block a protein called VEGF (vascular endothelial growth factor), which helped to prevent the growth of blood vessels that feed tumors. It was administered intravenously, in combination with my chemo drugs.

> **ADVICE:** Targeted therapy is not for all cancer patients. Check with your doctor if you meet the specific criteria for targeted therapy.

* Yesi L. *(Breast cancer: triple positive)*

Herceptin. Along with the chemo drugs Taxol and Perjeta, I was also given Herceptin, which is a targeted therapy drug. I had thought that I was going through more chemo, but they corrected me and said it was actually Targeted Therapy I was being given. They explained that it was because I was HER2 positive, which means the cancer cells I had were producing too much of the protein known as HER2, making the cancer aggressive. Herceptin has been proven to be an effective drug for treating my cancer. It was also administered just like chemo. Fortunately, the side effects were not as harsh.

THORACENTESIS / PLEURAL TAP

Thoracentesis, also known as thoracocentesis or pleural tap, is an invasive procedure to remove fluid or air from the pleural space for diagnostic or therapeutic purposes. A cannula, or hollow needle, is carefully introduced into the thorax, generally after administration of local anesthesia.

* Amor T. *(Breast cancer, Ovarian cancer)*

After my third chemo session, I informed my oncologist that when I breathed, I heard gurgling sounds; something he heard too when he examined me. So, he sent me to get a CT scan. The results showed a "large" pleural effusion (fluid buildup) in my right lung, multiple enlarged nodes in the space between both lungs (mediastinum) and around my left breast/armpit area and a 7cm soft tissues mass at the vagina cuff. My oncologist was "highly suspicious for progression of one or both" of my cancers. When I read that message, my heart sank a bit, but it didn't deter me from continuing my fight. For my lung issue, I met with a pulmonologist who performed a thoracentesis to remove the fluid buildup.

One of my nurses told me that the thoracentesis is a quick and painless procedure; I would need only to take a Tylenol, if that. Well, just to make doubly sure, I decided to take a vicodin. I had a wonderful nurse who prepped me, took my x-ray and was with me for the entire procedure. I was sitting on the exam table when the doctor came in. He described what he was going to do and told me to just be still. He then inserted a hollow needle between the ribs in my back. It was a really weird feeling, especially as he slowly pushed deeper. Under my breath, I started singing the song, "I'm in the Mood for Love." Those in the room were very surprised. After all, it was a strange thing to do out of the blue. I was able to run through two stanzas of the song, when my nurse gently told me to stop singing, because the doctor didn't want to make a wrong move and needed me to keep really still. I was in tears and asked her if I could hold her hands. She said, "Of course" and that helped me through the rest of the procedure.

So what did I feel to cause me to sing or cry? Well, when I felt the needle pushing through, I immediately needed to distract myself and the first thing I could think of to achieve that was to sing. I cried, because feeling the surprising pressure of the needle going deep down into me was surprisingly frightening. Even though it wasn't a sharp pain, for me, it was painful.

After the procedure, I asked to see the excess fluid that was removed and they showed me a large container filled with a yellow liquid that looked like frothy beer. They told me that the doctor had drained almost four quarts of fluid from my pleural cavity. I was so amazed! Fortunately, to date, the excess fluid hasn't returned to my lungs.

> **ADVICE:** Before and after the thoracentesis, x-rays will be taken of your lungs. During the procedure, you'll be asked to sit up, while the doctor inserts a hollow needle between the ribs in your back. I strongly suggest that you ask for a painkiller stronger than tylenol or aspirin, because the process is definitely not painless; you will feel a strange, uncomfortable sensation as the needle goes deeper into our body.

TURP (TRANSURETHRAL RESECTION OF THE PROSTATE) SURGERY

Transurethral resection of the prostate (TURP) is a surgery used to treat urinary problems due to an enlarged prostate. A combined visual and surgical instrument (resectoscope) is inserted through the tip of your penis and into the tube that carries urine from your bladder (urethra).

* *Glenn M.* (Metastatic Colon cancer to the Liver, Lungs & Adrenal Glands)

To take care of my prostate issues, I had TURP surgery and stayed overnight at the hospital. I had a Foley catheter with three tubes, so that they could flush my bladder and prostate. By the time they let me go home, they got 22 liters of saline flushed. My ability to void was blocked up the following night and my wife had to take me to the hospital at 2:00am to get my bladder drained, because even the catheter wouldn't open up. The doctors were able to unclog the catheter and push it out with a syringe to get me going. I could have kissed them!

* *Rick S.* (CLL: Blood & Bone Marrow cancer)

While I was still undergoing chemotherapy treatment, I became ill with benign prostatic hyperplasia (BPH) aka enlarged prostate. So, my primary doctor scheduled me for a TURP (transurethral resection of the prostate) surgery to take care of the problem. Three days before my scheduled operation, my oncologist found out about it and said to my primary doctor, "Wait a minute. I have to take him off of chemo first for two weeks. You can't perform the operation for, at least, another two weeks." So my surgery was rescheduled for three weeks from that time.

During TURP surgery, they cut away the prostate tissue that's laying up against your urethra. The enlarged prostate is what causes the urethra to be restricted. That's why males have to go to the bathroom a lot at night. Once the tissue is trimmed away from the urethra, the surgery is done. Fortunately, the procedure does not result in a lot of bleeding.

ADVICE: If you're going through chemotherapy and you need to have surgery for a separate condition, you must make sure both doctors treating you communicate with each other. It's mind-blowing to think that if my oncologist hadn't found out about my TURP surgery and I continued with my chemotherapy at the same time, I would've been in serious trouble.

~ o ~

Chapter 6

GETTING A HANDLE ON SCANS, BIOPSIES AND OTHER PROCESSES

Doctors depend on scans and tests to find out what's going on in your body and there are processes that will help you, the patient, with your bodily functions. Sometimes you'll have to juggle as you go from tests to scans to biopsies. Whatever you need to do, just think of these processes are stepping stones towards better health.

BIOPSIES

The removal of cells or tissues for examination by a pathologist. The pathologist may study the tissue under a microscope or perform other tests on the cells or tissue. There are many different types of biopsy procedures. The most common types include: (1) incisional biopsy, in which only a sample of tissue is removed; (2) excisional biopsy, in which an entire lump or suspicious area is removed; and (3) needle biopsy, in which a sample of tissue or fluid is removed with a needle. When a wide needle is used, the procedure is called a core biopsy. When a thin needle is used, the procedure is called a fine-needle aspiration biopsy.

* *Aaron C.* (*Prostate cancer, Skin cancer*)

Before I had prostate biopsy, I asked to be put out for the procedure, because just the thought of what they were going to do made me cringe. You see, for the biopsy, they insert a device with needles up the rectum. Those needles then go through the rectum wall into the prostate and take about twenty samples. The samples are then placed under a microscope where they do a pathology to see how much of the samples have cancer. The findings are about 98% accurate and there is a 1% chance of getting an infection for which antibiotics are given, because the biopsy itself is actually a surgical procedure. So, I told my doctor, "I want to be unconscious for this." He said, "Okay, sure."

After the biopsy, I found blood in my urine, because they put "holes" in me. Also, when I ejaculated, I was shocked that blood also came out. It was the weirdest and just gross! But then, that all cleared out and, eventually, went away. Aside from elevated PSA levels, there was no indication that I had cancer; I had no lumps or anything on my prostate. However, results from my biopsy confirmed that I did have cancer.

ADVICE: **Insist on being put out; you don't want to be awake for prostate biopsy. Expect some blood in your urine and semen. They'll clear out and, eventually, go away.**

* Amor T. (Breast cancer, Ovarian cancer)

Breast cancer. After my mammogram, I was asked to stay and wait for the radiologist to determine that the images are sufficient and nothing else was needed. This has happened just about every time I had a mammogram. Well, this time was different. The x-ray technician informed me that the radiologist would actually like to check further on something she saw.

I went through a bilateral ultrasound and that revealed bilateral breast cysts with the left breast having an irregular hypoechoic area, which is indicative of breast cancer. My radiologist then decided it necessary to perform an ultrasound guided core biopsy to look deeper. The results were atypical ductal hyperplasia which, although not a form of breast cancer, suggests a very high risk of developing breast cancer. So, I had to have more tests and my radiologist scheduled me for a stereotactic biopsy.

The stereotactic core biopsy was really interesting, because the examination table was different. It had a large hole. I was asked to lay on my stomach and then place my left breast through that hole. Then, I felt the examination table slowly rise up to the ceiling ... Whoa! My radiologist positioned herself below the raised table and proceeded to remove tissue from my breast to be biopsied. I don't remember feeling pain; just some tugging. It helped to be engaged with my radiologist and her assistant; both of who kept me in the loop of what was happening during the procedure. In the end, the stereotactic biopsy revealed moderately differentiated DCI (ductal carcinoma in situ), which was hormone receptor positive.

Ovarian cancer: During my hysterectomy, my surgeon also performed multiple peritoneal biopsies to determine the extent of cancer cells in the peritoneal cavity where my kidneys, adrenal glands, ureters, urinary bladder, part of the esophagus, rectum, ovaries, uterus, aorta and caudal are encased.

On July 21, 2016, I had a CT-Guided Vaginal cuff (v-cuff) biopsy to identify the 7cm vaginal cuff mass found in my CT scan. The biopsy showed fiber muscular tissue where there were blood vessels and a ganglion as well as a small piece of the nine squamous epithelium resembling that and all squamous epithelium. Since there was no inflammation or malignancy, there was no need to do anything.

> **ADVICE:** Since biopsies are invasive (some more than others), make sure the doctor explains the procedure to you, including what you can expect. A numbing cream should be applied. If not enough is applied and you feel pain, let your doctor know immediately. At the end of the procedure, it's always good to ask if anything was found and what is the next step. Asking questions lets the doctor know that you are someone who takes initiative and wants to be informed.

* Cindy R. (Metastatic Breast cancer to the Stomach)

I went through two needle biopsies on my right breast before I was diagnosed with stage III breast cancer. They were done in the doctor's office and, unfortunately, they were painful! I pretty much tried to think good thoughts throughout the procedure. But, this was the funny part...My mom was with me and she does not do pain, needles or anything like that. So, I was like grinning and bearing it and getting through the procedure when mom went (boop!) on the floor ... passed out cold. The doctor had to tend to her and I was like, "Hey, wait a second. I'm the patient here."

It was really sweet of my mom to be there with me, knowing she didn't do pain or needles or anything like that. But, when she became the patient for awhile, I laughed so hard, because it was just too funny. That was definitely a bonding moment for my mom and me.

> **ADVICE:** During any procedure, let your doctor know when you're feeling pain; don't just take it. Another thing you can do is just focus on good thoughts. Try to keep it light, because when you get tense or upset, it doesn't make things better; you just make things harder for yourself.

* J.B. (Salivary gland cancer)

The biopsy was a bit scary. The doctor, a head & neck specialist, had a giant syringe and just poked the tumor that was in my cheek and drained fluid from it. He actually had to poke the tumor three times. Since they numbed the area, it wasn't painful.

To prepare myself, I actually researched what most biopsies for this type of tumor required. I did expect some sort of syringe. I didn't feel it was necessary to have someone with me, so I just went to my appointment alone.

* Rev. Linda S. (Pancreatic cancer 3x)

I was sedated for the procedure and felt nothing.

* Rachel S. (Breast cancer: triple negative)

The first biopsy I had was done after I went through my ultrasound and mammogram. When the doctor came in, he biopsied two places. He biopsied the left side and then he biopsied the lymph nodes.

The next biopsy I went through is not usually done. It was what I call the "nipple test". Actually, it is called "sentinel lymph node biopsy", which is performed before or during breast cancer surgery to help figure out if the cancer spread to nearby lymph nodes.

My doctors knew that the lymph nodes on my right side had cancer. Since they didn't know if the lymph nodes on my left side had cancer, they wanted to have them checked. So, before I had my double mastectomy, they took me into the Radiology Department and injected me with this nuclear medication. Here is a description of what they did: They injected the fore point around my nipple with this nuclear medication, which is drawn to abnormal cells. It was THE most painful thing! The doctor was really good though; she did it really fast, like boom … boom … boom. Still, it was the most painful thing. My nipple couldn't be numbed at all because numbing it would cause the veins to collapse. So, my nipple couldn't be numbed, and I also couldn't be sedated. Nothing. I could have absolutely nothing in me.

> **ADVICE:** Biopsies can be uncomfortable and some, unfortunately, can be painful. In some biopsies, you will just feel something like a pinch. If you have a low threshold of pain, you can let your doctor know that you need more lidocaine or painkillers than most patients.
>
> If they have to do the "Nipple Test" aka Sentinel Lymph Node Biopsy on you, you unfortunately don't really have much of a choice, because you can't have any medications in you that would cause the veins to collapse, like painkillers do. Just try to take your mind off of what's happening and think of something positive and calming.

* Rick S. (CLL: Blood & Bone Marrow cancer)

During my biopsies, I just told myself to relax as they inserted the needle into my skin very gently. It didn't bother me at all. When my lymph nodes had to be biopsied, it was just a matter of them putting me to sleep. So I never felt a thing. They biopsied once in my left armpit and once in my right armpit.

I didn't ask many questions other than when and how I could prepare for the biopsies. The basic answer is you don't. You just prepare your mind to deal with it.

* Scott M. (Metastatic Colon cancer to the Prostate & Pancreas)

I'm one of those guys who need extra numbing medicine or I'm going to feel it. The prostate biopsies were extremely painful. When I told my urologist how painful they were, he said, "Well, you shouldn't really be feeling anything." He upped the dose of numbing medicine the next time I had a biopsy and I didn't feel a thing.

> **ADVICE:** Even if the doctor tells you, "you really shouldn't feel anything", if you know you need extra numbing medication, just speak up. No reason to go through pain, if you can help it.

* Susan M. (Ovarian cancer. Metastatic Pancreatic cancer to the Lungs)

Before my surgeries for Ovarian Cancer and Pancreatic Cancer, the doctors biopsied the tumors that were found in my abdominal area.

A follow-up CT scan in October showed a large nodule on my thyroid and a biopsy was done in November to test it. Fortunately, it was benign and my doctor scheduled yearly checkups for my thyroid. In the meantime, a recent follow-up CT scan showed two small nodules (6 mm in my left lung and 1 cm in my right lung). A biopsy of my nodule in my right lung, unfortunately, tested positive for cancer. So, I went through another round of chemotherapy.

* Tet M. (Colon cancer 3x)

Biopsies of the polyps taken out during my 2005 colonoscopy showed they were nearing malignancy.y. With reluctance, I finally agreed to have the second colectomy so I wouldn't have to deal with another round of chemo. This was over a decade ago and my life hasn't been the same since.

I had a core needle biopsy to remove the suspicious tissues from my breast. During the procedure, I couldn't look at my own breast. I just kept looking at the monitor of the biopsy machine where I was able to see the mass. It looked really big, because they enlarged the focus on the tumor. I was able to see when they pulled a trigger and the core needle removed the tissue samples they needed. It wasn't painful at all, because of the anesthesia.

ADVICE: A core needle biopsy is a simple procedure where they remove sample tissues from your breast to test for cancer. You'll be given anesthesia or similar. If you're uncomfortable or anxious, let the doctor or nurse know. Watching the activity in the monitor during the biopsy will help in taking your mind away from whatever discomfort you're feeling.

* Yesi L. (Breast cancer: triple positive)

During the initial biopsy I had, they didn't give me general anesthesia; just local anesthesia. I was able to see on the machine's screen this thick needle going inside of me. For me, it was on the right breast and I felt a lot of pressure. It was painful during and after the procedure. But, basically, I toughed it out. I took a deep breath and focused on the screen. I know for other people, it helps to just focus on something else, like a focal point somewhere on the wall.

BLOOD TESTS

A procedure in which a needle is used to take blood from a vein, usually for laboratory testing. A blood draw may also be done to remove extra red blood cells from the blood, to treat certain blood disorders. Also called phlebotomy and venipuncture.

* Amor T. (Breast cancer, Ovarian cancer)

Before cancer, I donated blood on a regular basis. My veins were healthy and so was my blood. Unfortunately, that's changed. When I lost use of the veins in my left arm due the removal of lymph nodes during my mastectomy, plus the veins in my right arm collapsed from overuse, before I got my mediport, I would get really anxious about getting my blood drawn. That's because I had too many experiences where a nurse or phlebotomist had to stick the needle in my arm multiple times and even "fish" (something they're not supposed to do) to find a viable vein. I was traumatized by all that. Fortunately, getting my mediport made the blood draws a whole lot easier. Just "plug and play!"

After my mediport was removed, I initially got anxious about getting blood draws. But then, I found some surefire ways to get my veins pumped up for smooth access. Basically, what I did was tense my arms against my body until I felt the rush of blood in my arms. I also did jumping jacks, ran in place, did tight arm curls, and then did long and quick swim strokes, stretching my arms out alternately in front of me and then in back of me, as if I was in a race. Right before the nurse or phlebotomist would try to find my vein, I held the tensing of my arms against my body, until they told me it was time. These ideas have worked for me ever since.

ADVICE: If you have poor veins and they'll be needed for regular draws or infusions (like chemo), I strongly suggest getting a mediport. If you just need to get through blood draws, then try these easy ways to pump up your veins: (1) Tense up your arms against your body really hard, as if bracing yourself. You should feel the rush of blood in your arms, (2) do jumping jacks or run in place to get your heart rate up, (3) do tight arm curls, with or without a dumbbell, and (4) while standing, do long and quick swim strokes, stretching your arms out alternately in front and then in back of you, as if swimming in a race.

* Cindy L. *(Kidney cancer)*

When I experienced very strange itching in July of 2015, the doctor I was seeing then had me take some blood tests. When we met to discuss the results, she said that my bilirubin was high so I was jaundiced, my triglycerides tripled, but my cholesterol levels were fine. Then she said we should just wait until next year to see if my itching will stop. I said, "No, I don't think so" and left. Then, I changed doctors.

I went through so many blood draws to check my kidney function, my levels of magnesium, potassium...those sort of things. As a rule, I'll have blood draws once every six months for my follow-ups for the first three years post-surgery. And then, a follow-up once a year after ten years post-surgery. After that, I can decide, along with the doctor I'm with at that time, whether I should continue to be tested or if we just call it a day. At that point, we'll just have to wait and see.

ADVICE: In a nutshell, blood tests help doctors evaluate how well your body is functioning. They also help them diagnose your condition and determine your health risk factors. Blood tests, therefore, are necessary. When your doctor gives you the results of your blood tests, ask questions, so you can understand what's going on with your body. If the answer is unclear or doesn't sit well with you, ask for a clearer explanation.

* Hilda K. *(Colon cancer)*

Blood tests were continuous for me, because they had to make sure my blood count was good before I could continue treatment. I didn't experience any problems when they drew blood from me.

* Rev. Linda S. *(Pancreatic cancer 3x)*

I had them just before chemo every two weeks and several times while hospitalized. My veins are great so I had no problems.

* Rick S. *(CLL: Blood & Bone Marrow cancer)*

Because I had good veins from weight lifting, the blood draws didn't affect me at all.

* Scott M. *(Metastatic Colon cancer to the Prostate & Pancreas)*

Blood draws are easy. It's all on the phlebotomist. You know, the little tiny needles that they use now? Well, half the time, I don't even feel the needle going in.

ADVICE: If you're afraid of the pain you'll feel when you get your blood drawn, let the phlebotomist know. They have those little tiny needles they can use.

* Sondra W. *(Ovarian cancer 3x)*

My veins are not good for blood draws. That's why I'm glad I had the mediport, because when I got blood draws before, I was always all bruised up. They would go from one arm to the other and then from one hand to the other, just to find a viable vein they could use to draw my blood. It got so very tedious and painful, until I finally got the mediport. The mediport just made my experience so much easier and quicker.

ADVICE: I don't have any advice, except to get a mediport if the nurse or lab technician has problems finding your veins to draw blood for tests.

* Susan M. *(Ovarian cancer. Metastatic Pancreatic cancer to the Lungs)*

Ovarian cancer. During my treatment, I had blood draws several days before my scheduled chemo infusions.

Pancreatic cancer. During my treatment, I had blood draws every day while in the hospital and several days prior to my chemo infusions.

* *Tet M.* (Colon cancer 3x)

Growing up, I wasn't afraid of needles and I wasn't about to start now. Watching the needle penetrate my skin was my way of telling cancer and Chemo, "I'm not afraid of you. I'm going to beat you."

> **ADVICE:** Look at the needle as one of your weapons against cancer. It's being used to draw blood that will be tested in your fight against cancer. If needles really bother you, strike up a conversation with the lab technician/nurse so your attention isn't on the blood draw.

CATHETERIZATIONS

Urinary catheters are used to drain the bladder. Your health care provider may recommend that you use a catheter if you have: urinary incontinence (leaking urine or being unable to control when you urinate) or urinary retention (being unable to empty your bladder when you need to).

* *Aaron C.* (Prostate cancer, Skin cancer)

Before surgery, the hospital had me go through a two-hour class to learn everything I needed to know about what to do prior to surgery and after surgery, how to take care of my catheter, what to be aware of when it comes to erections, bladder control, etc. They were really up on all that stuff. That was good, because then I understood the importance of my catheter.

During the prostatectomy, my doctor, essentially cut my urethra tube when he removed my prostate and then sewed it back together. He informed me that it usually only takes three or four days to heal, but he didn't want to take a chance. So, I had to keep the catheter on for ten days before he removed it. Yeah, I went home from the hospital with the catheter and had to keep it on for ten days, which was miserable for me. I was sore and couldn't move too much, because every time I did, the catheter tube moved too. It would yank on me. Also, they had a bottle attached to my leg. At the end of the bottle was a drainage bag. I had a small bag for use during the day and a larger bag for use at night.

For the first few days, I had to sleep on my back. I was really limited to what I could move while sleeping. I had to be positioned a certain way, because of the urinary drain bag I had to wear. I had to lay on the left side of my bed, so that the drain bag attached to my catheter, which was strapped to my left thigh, could hang over that side of the bed. That positioning allowed the fluids (residual from surgery) to flow down naturally. I was barely walking around during those ten days, because I was just so uncomfortable with all the stuff. Aside from the urinary drain bags, they gave me a bag to drain my urine into. I had to measure that. I also had a drainage tube with a pump or a bulb. When I squeezed it, the pressure drew any internal fluid (like blood, water, etc.) that stemmed from my surgery into the bulb. Then, I had to drain the bulb once or twice a day, depending on how fast it filled up. All this was necessary to keep out excess fluids and make sure my catheter didn't cause an infection.

By the way, I bought a tube of liquid KY Jelly because the head of my penis was getting irritated by the catheter. So I put some KY Jelly around the head of my penis and that kept it from getting irritated.

When they, eventually, took out my catheter, it was weird. They pulled the drainage tube and the catheter out of my spot at the same time, which was horrible! It was a really weird feeling. And, they didn't numb the area, either. They just said, "Take a deep breath" and then they pulled that sucker out. I was like, "Ah, Sh*t!" When I had the catheter, I slept okay. But once that was out, I slept much better.

After removal of my catheter, I had to retrain my bladder muscle, because at that point, it was hypersensitive; all the nerves are frazzled. I needed my bladder muscle to hold the water, which takes a while. For the first six months, I didn't have any expectations of having any normal bladder control. Then, nine months later, I started to see a big difference in my bladder function, like being normal again. I was able to control my flow. Still (and this is funny...), if I fart too hard or if I strain, I'll leak, sometimes. If I'm running and bouncing, I'll leak, because my bladder is still not 100% healed. So,

I still have to wear a urinary control pad. I used to go through two or three pads a day. Now, I don't even fill a single pad up in one day. I've got a lot more control. I'm definitely getting stronger. Like I said, it's a month by month movement.

ADVICE:

- First, make sure you attend an educational class that will provide you all you need to know about your surgery, treatment plan and any medical equipment you'll be needing, like a catheter;
- Allow yourself time to adjust to your catheter. It's probably not going to be easy, but you just need to accept its importance and tough it out. It'll eventually become a thing of the past, like it is for me now.
- If your penis gets irritated by your catheter, just get some liquid KY Jelly to rub on to the head of your penis. That will take care of the irritation.
- Before they remove your catheter, ask them to numb the area. If they don't do that, then ask them to be gentle, so it doesn't become a negative experience for you.
- Don't expect normal bladder control to return anytime soon. Expect occasional leaking, especially when you strain, fart too hard, run, bounce or have sex.
- Keep a good supply of urinary control pads.
- Measure your progress by months, not weeks or days.

* Amor T. (Breast cancer, Ovarian cancer)

Breast cancer: The first time I was told that they had to put a urinary catheter into me, I was afraid that it would be really painful. My nurse reassured me and said that she would be gentle and put it in slowly. She did and it really wasn't as bad as I thought it would be. Her reassurance really helped to make this first experience of mine with a catheter easier than I imagined it could be. Urinating through a catheter meant I didn't have to get myself up from the bed to go the bathroom; it made the whole experience efficient and easier for my body. When my condition stabilized and my body grew stronger, the time came for them to remove my catheter. I pleaded with them to let me keep it on. Amused, they gently told me that keeping it on wouldn't help me. To heal and grow stronger, I need to become independent. The catheter would get in the way of my independence. Even though I felt bummed, I knew they were right and so, I worked on becoming independent of all the medical devices I had grown attached to.

Just one day after I was discharged from the hospital after my mastectomy and breast reconstruction surgery, I had to be rushed to the hospital's emergency room. I had developed a high fever, which quickly went from 101.5F to past 103.5F and I was shivering like crazy. When the emergency room nurse asked me if I needed anything, I told her (with teeth visibly chattering) that I needed a catheter. She said that she could help me to the bathroom nearby. I told her that I could barely move because of my abdominal surgery and urgently needed a catheter…"Please!" She then immediately gave me a catheter. Aaaah….relief!

Ovarian cancer: After my hysterectomy, I noticed that I had a foley catheter attached to me and smiled, because it has helped me so much in the past. Again, when the time came for the nurse to remove it, I was saddened, but then I would have to work to go to the bathroom. Yes, the catheter "spoiled" me!

ADVICE: Catheters are great, because you can easily get relief without having to go through the hassle of getting disconnected from the machines, pushing aside the "gazillion" blankets and pillows around you, scooting yourself up the bed to sit on the side, gingerly placing your feet on the floor while trying to get stable enough to stand, shuffling your feet towards the bathroom while connected to your IV drip, etc. etc. etc. Yes, I'm exaggerating a bit. But for the most part, it's true. Anyway, if they say you need a catheter and you've never had one before, don't worry. It's there to really help you. When the time comes for your catheter to be removed, that means it's no longer helping you. Once it's removed, you'll become independent again, and that's a good thing.

CT (COMPUTERIZED TOMOGRAPHY) SCANS

A procedure that uses a computer linked to an x-ray machine to make a series of detailed pictures of areas inside the body. The pictures are taken from different angles and are used to create 3-dimensional (3-D) views of tissues and organs. A dye may be injected into a vein or swallowed to help the tissues and organs show up more clearly. A computerized tomography may be used to help diagnose disease, plan treatment, or find out how well treatment is working. Also called CAT scan, computed tomography scan, computerized axial tomography scan, and CT scan.

* *Amor T.* (*Breast cancer, Ovarian cancer*)

I've gone through so many CT scans, both with and without contrast. The procedure itself is painless and doesn't take very long. What does take long is the preparation, especially if the contrast dye is used, because finding a viable vein in my arm to inject the contrast dye into takes times. To make the process smoother, I first schedule my CT scans for as early in the morning as I can. Usually, they have me fast. So, the quicker I get the procedure done, the sooner I can eat again. Then, before I leave the house, I make sure to remove my jewelry and wear clothes that have no metal objects (buttons, belt buckles, decor). Instead, I wear sweatpants and long-sleeved t-shirts. Sometimes, even though I already made sure I removed metal objects, the technician asked me to wear a hospital gown. That's fine.

Most times, I had a contrast dye ordered for my abdominal CT scan . The contrast dye was necessary to highlight soft tissues, such as organs, blood vessels and other structures for my doctor. To prepare, I couldn't eat or drink anything within four hours of my exam, except for smell sips of water with my medications. Then, at the radiology center, I would either be given a large glass of very cold oral contrast to drink or have the contrast dye injected directly into my vein to help my soft tissues and blood vessels stand out in the image. A couple of times, they gave me a straw to help manage the taste. However, I've found that just downing the liquid as quickly as possible was easier. With the cold drink and the cold temperature at the imaging center, I found it necessary to ask for a warm blanket, which they happily provided me.

The only pain per se I experienced was during the injecting of the contrast dye into my arm. They could only use my right arm to locate a viable vein, because lymph nodes were removed from my left arm during my mastectomy rendering my veins there unusable. One time, the radiology technologist pierced my skin so many times (as many as ten times) with the needle before finally finding a serviceable vein. Ugh! In the meantime, what I did was just look away at a nice picture on the wall and prayed or daydreamed good thoughts.

After the contrast dye was set, the exam table I was on moved slowly into the doughnut-shaped CT machine. There was a lot of whirring, buzzing and clicking sounds. The machine's voice guided me through the process, telling me when to breathe or hold my breath. During my abdominal CT scans, I remember feeling a warm rush go down to my pelvic area, making me feel like I need to pee. That's the contrast dye at work to illuminate the organs in that area. The process takes anywhere between 15 - 30 minutes, depending on prep time. After the scan, I'm always told to drink plenty of fluids to help my kidneys remove the contrast material from my body.

ADVICE: If you'll be instructed to fast, have your CT scan scheduled for early morning, so you can get it done and eat sooner than later. Make sure you wear clothes without metal, e.g. buttons, zippers, decor, etc. and skip the jewelry. Even if you wear clothes with metal, you'll be asked to wear a hospital gown.

Before the CT scan, you may have to drink a very cold contrast drink. The quicker you can down it, the better. You can ask for a straw too, if you prefer to drink it that way. Because the drink is very cold, you'll feel really cold after. Since it will take 30 minutes for the dye to course through your body, you'll have to wait. Ask for a warm blanket to use while you wait.

During the CT scan, you may or you may not be given another dye (this time, injected). Procedures here vary. When you the machine's exam table, you should get as comfortable as you can and then lay very still. When your exam table moves into the machine's doughnut hole, you'll hear whirring, buzzing and clicking sounds. You'll also hear a voice guiding you when to breathe and when to hold your breath.

After the procedure, drink plenty of fluids to help your kidneys remove the contrast material from your body.

* Bob G. (*Soft Tissue Sarcoma, Skin cancer*)

I was in the CT scan procedure for an hour and 45 minutes. The technician knew what he was looking for, but he couldn't find it. It was hidden, I think. It must've been covered by a lot. When my family and I went up to Tahoe, I noticed that I couldn't eat. I tried to eat some food, but just couldn't. The next day, the problem went away. When we went to the hospital for my surgery, the doctors took their time. It looked like they weren't sure what they were going to do.

At another time, while sitting on the examination table during one of my appointments, I asked my doctor when I'll get another CT scan. He said that it takes several weeks to get a CT scan, unless it's an emergency. I told him that I wanted one as soon as possible. He said that I'm not due another CT scan for six months. He assured me that I would get a CT scan, but not just yet. I looked at him hard and said that I wanted my CT scan NOW! We discussed it and I told him that when I came in to see him, I was very sick. Now, I feel great; I'm in good shape, back to swimming and just don't want to wait until I get sick again. I told him that I wanted the scan on a regular basis. He saw how determined I was and it worked! I got my CT scans scheduled sooner and on a regular basis.

ADVICE: It is really important to be ahead of the game; to get examined on a regular basis. You don't want to wait to get sick to see your doctor. Be proactive!

* Cindy L. (*Kidney cancer*)

When I had to go in the emergency room, they did a CT scan without contrast. That's because I have a heart issue that could cause me problems with a particular contract that is used with CT scans.

ADVICE: When you get CT scans, you'll be asked if you're allergic to a special dye, also known as contrast, which they use to highlight the areas of your body being examined. CT scans can be done without them too. It's just that having the contrast will allow for a clearer scan. To be safe, let them know if you have had negative reactions to dyes or contrasts in the past.

* Cindy R. (*Metastatic Breast cancer to the Stomach*)

Before the CT scan, they had me drink a certain liquid and, through my mediport, they injected into me a dye for the procedure. That dye traveled through my veins and warmed me up "down there". It made me feel like I was peeing. I was like, "O...kay....(?)" I felt like asking them to unstrap me so I could go pee.

ADVICE: If you've never gone through a CT scan before, ask your doctor what you can expect and also how you should prepare for it. During the procedure itself, you can expect some warming up of the area being scanned. If it's in the abdomen, then you can expect to feel a warming sensation in your pelvic region; like you need to go pee. Don't worry; it's normal.

* Glenn M. (*Metastatic Colon cancer to the Liver, Lungs & Adrenal Glands*)

I had a lot of CT scans and PET scans. So, I pretty much know what to do. Basic rules are:

- Don't eat anything after midnight
- Wear loose, comfortable clothing, like sweats, that don't have metal in them

I also bring my eye mask with contours on the sides, so I can open my eyes and it's still dark. They're better than placing a regular face towel on my eyes. Either way, I tend to fall asleep.

ADVICE: Follow whatever directions they give you, especially what you can or can't eat or drink and when you should stop eating or drinking. Scans are different for everyone. Definitely wear loose and comfortable clothes;

* Hilda K. *(Colon cancer)*

For me, going through the CT scan procedure itself was simple and easy. However, there is one thing that's "scary." It is not knowing what the result is going to be, because you want it to be clear.

After treatment, I had to continue getting CT scans every month. Now that I have passed my five-year milestone, I need to get a CT scan only once a year. It's been quite a haul and my birthday is my remembrance!

ADVICE: The CT scan procedure itself is simple and easy. Just make sure to follow instructions, especially if you have to fast before-hand. Try not to think too much about the results too much. You'll just create unnecessary anxiety for yourself. Keeping a positive attitude always helps, no matter what.

* Joan S. *(Rectal cancer)*

I remember having to fast two days before the CT scan and then drinking a quart of dye before the procedure. I have to have CT scans every three years now.

* J.B. *(Salivary gland cancer)*

The CT scan wasn't too bad. Actually, it was interesting. They had to attach something like an IV into me, in order to inject a dye for contrast. After that, while I was laying down, I was moved into this machine that was kind of like a cave; it also looked like a doughnut. When I went inside, there was this voice that told me not to swallow and then I heard the sound of the machine spinning around.

* Rev. Linda S. *(Pancreatic cancer 3x)*

I went through CT scans to determine if the mass I had in my pancreas was scar tissue or a tumor. For the CT scan procedure itself, I experienced no problems.

* Scott M. *(Metastatic Colon cancer to the Prostate & Pancreas)*

Going through the CT scans and the big "doughnuts" were never a problem for me. I'm not claustrophobic. It's just part of my life.

* Susan M. *(Ovarian cancer. Metastatic Pancreatic cancer to the Lungs)*

In January of 2016, I was rushed to the emergency room, because I was quite jaundiced and felt pain in my abdomen. Tests showed that my liver blood count was very high, so they ran a CT scan. From the results, I was given a diagnosis of stage II pancreatic cancer. After completion of my chemo treatments, I was scheduled for CT scans every six months.

In July 2018, my CT scan showed two small nodules (6 mm in the left lung and 1 cm in the right lung). So, I went through and completed four months of chemotherapy. Another CT scan was done and showed that the nodules remained the same and that the nodules were actually not lung cancer, but a metastasis of my original pancreatic cancer. At this time, I am off chemo for another two months before I get another CT scan done. From there, my doctors will determine the best course of action.

* Tet M. *(Colon cancer 3x)*

Going through the CT scans wasn't an unpleasant experience for me, as the procedure itself wasn't invasive. However, drinking the dye/contrast that I had to drink prior to the scan was a bit of a challenge for me, but definitely manageable.

CYSTOSCOPY

Cystoscopy is the examination of the bladder and urethra using a cystoscope, inserted into the urethra. A cystoscope is a thin, tube-like instrument with a light and a lens for viewing. It may also have a tool to remove tissue to be checked under a microscope for signs of disease.

* *Sondra W. (Ovarian cancer 3x)*

I had the problems, for sure, during my first treatment, i.e. bladder bleeding and pain. No kidney problems; just bladder problems. I finally saw a urologist. He first examined me in a procedure called cystoscopy where he inserted a hollow tube (cystoscope), equipped with a lens, into my urethra and slowly advanced it into my bladder. After that, he conducted an intravesical bladder instillation, where he injected medication directly into my bladder via a urethral catheter. It was a very painful procedure. But since I was already in so much pain from my bladder problems, the pain from the instillation was okay. And, boy, I tell you, I was thankful for my urologist!

DEXA SCAN

A DEXA scan is a non-invasive test that measures bone mineral density to assess if a person is at risk of osteoporosis or fracture. DEXA stands for dual energy x-ray absorptiometry—a mouthful of a term that actually tells a lot about this procedure, in which two X-ray beams are aimed at the bones.

* *Amor T. (Breast cancer, Ovarian cancer)*

I went through my first DEXA scan after completion of my chemo treatments. It was a quick and painless procedure. All I had to do was lie on my back on an x-ray table. The technician made sure that I did not have any metal on my clothing and then made sure my arms and my legs were positioned properly, including using cushion blocks to keep my feet straight. There was an x-ray arm above that moved alongside the x-ray table as it scanned by body.

ENEMA (FLEET)

An enema introduces liquid, often mineral oil, salt water, or laxative, through the user's anus to the large intestine. In addition to treating constipation, an enema may be used to administer medicines or barium. An enema may also be used to empty the user's bowel before a procedure such as a colonoscopy.

* *Amor T. (Breast cancer, Ovarian cancer)*

After my hysterectomy, I experienced a lot of gas and then constipation. I initially thought nothing of it, because I experienced constipation before. However, my constipation grew worse with each passing day and I grew more and more bloated; it became really painful. I took fiber supplements, but they didn't work at all. As a matter of fact, they seemed to make matters worse. When I informed my first doctor (a gynecologic oncologist), he said I should just take the fiber supplements (Benefiber or Metamucil) together with a stool softener. I did that and, unfortunately, things just got worse! I didn't want to eat anymore, because I was so painfully bloated! Someone suggested I use fleet enema, which Bill helped me with. The combination action of the liquid softening my impacted stool and the enema nozzle loosening my rectum stimulated the bowel movement that I so desperately needed.

After getting relief from the enema, my constipation, unfortunately, returned and I was in such a quandary. When I met with my new doctor (a medical oncologist) and informed him about my constipation woes, he immediately suggested I use MiraLAX. He explained that I didn't need extra fiber to create bulky stool, which is what Benefiber and Metamucil do. What I really needed was something to help "grease" my colon to enable my impacted stool to smoothly flow out of me and that's what MiraLAX does. After one use, relief was immediate and also permanent.

ADVICE: When you're constipated, enemas do help to soften your impacted stool and stimulating them to create a bowel movement. The directions are easy to follow. You can do it yourself or get someone to help you.

INTRAVESICAL BLADDER INSTILLATION

The procedure is also referred to as bladder instillation, intravesical treatment, intravesical therapy. These guidelines use the term intravesical instillation. Immunotherapy aims to eradicate disease by provoking or enhancing the host immune response.

* *Sondra W. (Ovarian cancer 3x)*

I had the problems, for sure, during my first treatment, i.e. bladder bleeding and pain. No kidney problems; just bladder problems. I finally saw a urologist. He first examined me in a procedure called cystoscopy where he inserted a hollow tube (cystoscope), equipped with a lens, into my urethra and slowly advanced it into my bladder. After that, he conducted an intravesical bladder instillation, where he injected medication directly into my bladder via a urethral catheter. It was a very painful procedure. But since I was already in so much pain from my bladder problems, the pain from the instillation was okay. And, boy, I tell you, I was thankful for my urologist!

Initially, the medication for my bladder lasted only three days. So, I went through another dose of treatment and that lasted five days. After that, I returned for yet another round of medication, which then lasted a week. Finally, my bladder wall softened up and got better. Unfortunately and despite the several bladder instillations, we couldn't get rid of the bleeding. We got rid of the pain and the urinary tract infections, but we could never get rid of the bleeding.

MAMMOGRAM / MAMMOGRAPHY

An X-ray of the breast that is taken with a device that compresses and flattens the breast. A mammogram can help a health professional decide whether a lump in the breast is a gland, a harmless cyst, or a tumor. A mammogram can cause pressure, discomfort, and some soreness that lasts for a little while after the procedure. If the mammogram result raises suspicions about cancer, a biopsy is usually the next step.

* *Amor T. (Breast cancer, Ovarian cancer)*

My breast cancer was found early because I, consistently, got screening mammograms every year since I turned 40 years of age. I prepare by choosing to wear coordinates, i.e. a skirt and top or a pair of pants and a top. That's because it'll be easier to just remove my top for the procedure versus having to change out of a whole dress into a hospital gown.

During the procedure, the technologist positions my arm and shoulder to rest on the machine, while she positions my breast on the machine's plate and then turns a knob, which moves another plate towards my breast to flatten it ... yeah, ouch! Then she quickly goes behind the protective screen, tells me to hold my breath and takes the x-ray picture of the breast. She does this several times until the images are satisfactory.

ADVICE: Wear coordinates (separate top and bottom) to you appointment, so you'll need to only remove your top and be able to keep your bottom on and not have to change into a hospital gown. Prepare to be guided by the

technologist. They're always friendly and gentle. The discomfort of having the breast "flattened" is no fun, but it's tolerable. Just think that it can save your life, like it did mine.

MRI (MAGNETIC RESONANCE IMAGING) SCANS

A procedure in which radio waves and a powerful magnet linked to a computer are used to create detailed pictures of areas inside the body. These pictures can show the difference between normal and diseased tissue. Magnetic resonance imaging makes better images of organs and soft tissue than other scanning techniques, such as computed tomography (CT) or x-ray. Magnetic resonance imaging is especially useful for imaging the brain, the spine, the soft tissue of joints, and the inside of bones. Also called MRI, NMRI, and nuclear magnetic resonance imaging.

* *Amor T.* (Breast cancer, Ovarian cancer)

MRI of the breasts: To better characterize the extent of cancer in my left breast, I went through an MRI. Unlike a mammogram which uses x-rays to create images of the breast, a breast MRI uses magnets and radio waves to produce detailed 3-dimensional images of the breast tissue. Before the test, they had me change into a hospital gown and remove all my jewelry. Then, I was asked to lie face down on the MRI table where there were two holes for me to place each breast through, allowing them to hang uncompressed. It was a bit awkward, so the technician guided me and added some pillows for support. What followed was the injection of a contrast solution (dye) into my arm through an IV line to enhance the appearance of tissues or blood vessels on the MRI pictures. The MRI table then started to slowly move into the narrow tube in the middle of the machine until I was completely inside. The technician gave me instructions over the system, including how long each imaging session would take and when I should stay absolutely still.

The thing I remember most was the noise, more like a loud clanking (pipe hitting pipe) noise, along with whirling, clicking and bumping sounds that resemble a loud washing machine. Initially, it was quite unnerving and I really annoying, because the machine was so loud. But then, I knew I had to just tough it out and figure a way to go to my happy place to drown out the noise. I first tried to relax my breathing, which was tough, because I was laying on my stomach and it was rising as I breathed. But I continued trying and learned to breathe in relaxed way while in that odd position. Then, I started thinking happy thoughts and singing happy songs in my head. It wasn't easy to do, at first, but I persisted and it worked. Next thing I knew, 45 minutes had passed. I was so relieved!

MRI of the knees: Since I had been experiencing bone pain and deterioration from my chemotherapy, I went through an MRI to determine the reason why I was having pain in my knees. The experience was far different from my last experience for my breast. This time, I wasn't injected with a contrast dye and I was given a nice set of headphones with music of my choice, plus a built-in system for the technician to give me instructions. When I laid on the exam table, they positioned my knees with a lot of support pillows to keep my entire legs still. Then the exam table moved towards the machine, but only to where my knees were inside the "doughnut" hole. My upper torso was still outside, which meant the loud clanking, whirling, clicking and bumping sounds weren't loud at all.

> **ADVICE:** MRI experiences will vary depending on the part of the body to be examined. If you need an MRI for your breasts, practice beforehand how you'll breathe lightly while on your stomach. It's tricky, because your weight in on your diaphragm. Be prepared to be injected with a contrast dye. If you'll head will be going into the MRI machine, you'll hear very loud noises continuously (like a very loud washing machine), which could be rather annoying. Bring your ear plugs or ask the technician for some overhead music. If neither are available, try to go to your "happy place" in your mind. Sing songs in your head or daydream happy thoughts. Let your mind drift and take you away from the crazy loud environment that is the MRI machine.

* *Cindy L.* (Kidney cancer)

Since I have a heart issue that could cause me to have problems with the particular dye/contrast that they use with CT scans, my doctor and I felt that Gadolinium, the dye/contrast used with MRIs, would be better handled by my heart.

Within a couple of hours of the MRI, I got word from him that they were referring me out to a urologist, because there was about a 95% possibility that I had cancer in my kidney.

I'm claustrophobic, so I requested a wide or open bore MRI machine, which has a much larger opening than a regular MRI machine. Those machines, as with regular MRI machines, are noisy and I don't think there's really any getting away from it. What I do is ask them to choose a chill radio station and crank the music up.

So I agreed to an MRI once a year for my follow-ups. I wouldn't agree to any more than that, because they are finding evidence that Gadolinium lies around in the brain. So as you can see, "damned if you do; damned if you don't." Since I'm stage 1, grade 1, I'm willing to take the chance. It is my body and I'm willing to take the chance that the risks of having these contrasts far outweigh the benefits for me.

> **ADVICE:** MRI machines are noisy. I don't think there's really any getting away from it. What I recommend is that you go in knowing your favorite radio station or XM Sirius station that you like to listen to and ask them to crank it up. Whether it is soft music or rock and roll or heavy metal that relaxes you, ask them to crank it up, because you'll need it to drown out the noise from the machine.
>
> If you're claustrophobic, let your doctor or medical team know and ask for a wide bore or open bore machine. Tell them to find one for you. If they say, "Well, we don't have it here." You can say, "Then please find me a hospital or facility that has one and get me a referral for it." Also, before they put you into the MRI machine, most technicians will ask, "Are you claustrophobic?" If you say, "Yes", they'll give you a washcloth to cover your eyes. If they don't ask you, then you ask for a washcloth. Put it over your eyes and don't take it off until you are out of that machine.
>
> Gadolinium is the dye/contrast that normally used with MRIs. If you're allergic, you need to let your doctor and technician know.

* Cindy R. *(Metastatic Breast cancer to the Stomach)*

When I had the MRI for my breast, I just lay on my back while they scanned my breasts. The process was pretty simple, mainly … just relax, don't move … just relax … Then, loud bang … click, click, click, click … dang, dang, dang, dang, dang … It really annoyed me. So, I decided to go to my "happy place." To go to my "happy place" I just close my eyes and tell myself to relax, as soon as I lay down. And then, I would go to Disneyland or I would be home with my dogs playing … or just go somewhere in my memory of times that made me happy.

> **ADVICE:** Before your scheduled MRI, think of happy places or activities you'll go to in your memory during the procedure. When you lay down on the patient table of the machine, just close your eyes, breathe calmly, tell yourself to relax, ignore the sounds and go to your "happy place."

* Rev. Linda S. *(Pancreatic cancer 3x)*

Because I am claustrophobic, I took a small dose of Xanax before having the MRI. But, the dose should have been stronger, because ten minutes before the imaging was complete, I was anxious and close to screaming, "Get me out of here!" I think I did ask, "How much longer?"

> **ADVICE:** If you're claustrophobic, it helps to ask for a stronger dose of Xanax or anti-anxiety meds.

* Rachel S. *(Breast cancer: triple negative)*

I did go through a full-body MRI to make sure my cancer didn't metastasize.

* Rick S. *(CLL: Blood & Bone Marrow cancer)*

After going through MRIs that made me quite uncomfortable and anxious, I finally had to tell them to do my MRI using the "doughnut" (open MRI machine) and not the "tube" (traditional MRI machine), because I was claustrophobic.

* Scott M. (*Metastatic Colon cancer to the Prostate & Pancreas*)

The MRIs I went through were really loud. I was given ear plugs, but they were still loud.

* Yesi L. (*Breast cancer: triple positive*)

Going through an MRI was a little claustrophobic for me. The noise was like loud chiseling. To deal with the noise, I got earphones. What also helped was trying to think of it as therapy; some type of spa session. I knew I had to be very, very, very calm.

PET (POSITRON EMISSION TOMOGRAPHY) SCANS

A positron emission tomography (PET) scan is an imaging procedure that allows your doctor to check for cancer in your body. The scan uses a small amount of a special dye containing radioactive glucose (sugar) tracers. These tracers are either swallowed, inhaled, or injected into a vein in your arm depending on what part of the body is being examined. A scanner is then used to make detailed, computerized pictures of the areas inside the body where the glucose is taken up. Because cancer cells often take up more glucose than normal cells, the pictures can be used to find cancer cells in the body.

* Amor T. (*Breast cancer, Ovarian cancer*)

I had to fast before my appointment and was told to come in 30 minutes earlier than my scheduled time, because I had to drink a very cold contrast dye and it needed time to course through my body before the procedure. I then changed into a hospital gown. When it came time to inject me with the radioactive drug (tracer), the technician had difficulty finding a viable vein. After several tries, he asked if he could use the veins in my feet (since those in my left arm were rendered useless after my lymph nodes were removed there.). I cringed and hesitated, staying that it would hurt. The technician said that it would actually feel the same as if he were injecting my arm. Since I was curious, I told him to go ahead. He immediately went for a fat, healthy vein in my right foot. When he injected my foot, he was right ... it felt the same as if he had injected my arm!

After the injection, I asked to use the bathroom before the scan. The technician pointed me towards the "radioactive" bathroom and warned me not to use the regular bathrooms at this time. He explained that the radioactive tracer in me would leak out into the toilet and may affect someone who's pregnant or shouldn't be around any radioactivity. After I used the bathroom, I imagined the toilet bowl glowing!

The PET scan process was pretty much like the CT scan process. I laid on a padded exam table that moved into the machine's "doughnut" hole and laid very very still as I heard whirring and clicking sounds. I just closed my eyes and went to my "happy place" with happy thoughts, dreams and music. After the scan, I used the "radioactive" bathroom and drank a lot of fluids as instructed, to wash away the tracer from my body.

detailed, the contrast dye used in different too. For the PET scan, you'll be injected with a radioactive dye, which you need to be aware of when you use the restroom.

* Glenn M. (Metastatic Colon cancer to the Liver, Lungs & Adrenal Glands)

I was off the chemotherapy for almost six months and six new tumors appeared in the scans. They were so small; about .22 inches or less than a quarter inch in size. They barely showed up on the PET scan. My oncologist wasn't even sure they were cancer. So, now I'm back on chemotherapy, which includes infusion with Erbitux every other week and oral Xeloda one week on and one week off. My tumors are now stable and my oncologist still doesn't think they're cancer.

I had a lot of CT scans and PET scans. So, I pretty much know what to do. basic rules are:

- Don't eat anything after midnight
- Wear loose, comfortable clothing, like sweats, that don't have metal in them

I also bring my eye mask with contours on the sides, so I can open your eyes and it's still dark. They're better than placing a regular face towel on my eyes. Either way, I tend to fall asleep.

ADVICE: Follow whatever directions they give you, especially what you can or can't eat or drink and when you should stop eating or drinking. Scans are different for everyone. Definitely wear loose and comfortable clothes; you want to be as comfortable as possible. Also, don't wear clothes with any metal in them, like metal buttons or zippers or decorations. Otherwise, you'll have to remove them and wear the loose gown; the one with the open back.

* Hilda K. (Colon cancer)

It was a really interesting experience, because it wasn't just a CT scan; it was a stronger scan. To prepare me for the PET scan, they gave this drink that tasted terrible. Then, the technician brought out this cylinder with a radioactive symbol on it and injected into my vein a radioactive liquid. I also remember that the technician had a shield in front of her to protect herself, because she was dealing with radioactivity. After a few minutes, they ran me through the PET scan, which is a crazy, but amazing technology.

ADVICE: Even though the PET scan procedure involves radioactive material, it's very similar to the CT scan. Drinking the terrible-tasting prep liquid is just one of those thing you have to drink. Just do it and get it over with. If you think too much about it, you'll just make it harder for yourself.

* Rachel S. (Breast cancer: triple negative)

Because I wasn't too sure about the procedure, I felt a lot of anxiety before going through my first PET scan. I wondered if it was going to hurt. So the first time I did it, I was scared. But the second time I went through the PET scan, it was easy. Both times I went, I just went on my own; I didn't have anybody with me. I just thought that for procedures like this, it doesn't really matter whether you bring someone with you or not, because they can't go in the room with you when you're going through the procedure.

ADVICE: Before you go through a PET scan or any procedure, it's best to ask your doctor or the medical staff at the imaging center, what the procedure will involve and you can expect. You can also research information on the procedure, so you'll be prepared and know, more or less, what's going to happen.

* Scott M. (Metastatic Colon cancer to the Prostate & Pancreas)

Going through the PET scans and the big "doughnuts" were never a problem for me. I'm not claustrophobic. It's just part of my life. The one interesting thing that I learned was: I thought the PET scans would see everything. But, they don't.

The PET scan will only see a cluster of one billion or more cancer cells....that's billion with a "b". So, if you have a cluster of 300 million cells, it's not going to be seen on the PET scan.

* Sondra W. (Ovarian cancer 3x)

At one point in time, we thought my CA 125 level went down to 10. So it seemed like everything was really good, right? When I had a PET scan, everything was clear there too. And so, I went off and started the Living Strong, Living Well program, trying to get back to "normal." As a matter of fact, Kenneth & I were looking for a new place to live. We went to Denver, San Diego and Albuquerque and looked. What a blessing! That was a special period of time for me to do that. Because, two days after we returned from our travels and decided to move to Denver in August, I went to my scheduled PET scan appointment. And then...BOOM! Results showed that the cancer was back. I was like, "What??" And then, I thought, "God said, 'Not yet', sister." I realized that the timing was a blessing in disguise and said, "Thank you, Lord!" I wouldn't have wanted to go to a new place or see a new doctor who didn't know me or who didn't know the sensitivity of my system. I also wouldn't know how they would treat me. So I was like, "Wow! Thank you!"

All the "hot" spots on the PET scan showed that I'm still in remission, which is a good thing. But then, three new spots were found in my liver. My oncologist changed my "maintenance chemo" regimen. She removed the chemo drug Alimta and keeping me on Carboplatin and Keytruda. For now, we're experimenting every week to see what will work.

The plan is for me to continue the PET scans every two months until my liver spots are gone. They do shoot the radio-active stuff into my veins, but they use my mediport. Fortunately, I haven't had to drink any glucose solution beforehand.

> **ADVICE:** Follow the specific directions that the doctor gives to help you prepare for your PET scan; mostly fasting instructions. The PET scan itself is simple and doesn't really take long.

* Susan M. (Ovarian cancer, Metastatic Pancreatic cancer to the Lungs)

During my treatment for pancreatic cancer, I had a PET scan before my surgery to evaluate how my tissues and organs were functioning.

* Vida B.A. (Breast cancer)

Going through the PET scan was like going through the CT scan. It was an easy process. Before the scan, I was given a really sweet liquid to drink that kind of tasted last Mountain Dew and I was also given a radioactive medication with glucose through an IV (intravenous) line in my arm.

> **ADVICE:** Your doctor's office will give you instructions of how to prepare for the PET scan, including what you can or cannot eat and drink, what to wear, etc. It's an easy and painless process.

* Yesi L. (Breast cancer: triple positive)

For my PET scan, they injected a dye directly into my right breast. That was painful. So, I just took a deep breath and looked as they injected me with the dye. I have a high tolerance for pain, so I was able to look. I knew it was just temporary and I knew it was important for my overall treatment.

> **ADVICE:** When they inject the dye into you, take a deep breath and think positive, like how the PET scan is important and also focus on things that make you happy.

When a medical port *aka* mediport, port-a-cath or port is implanted under the skin to inject drugs or draw blood samples, flushing the system is essential to prevent clot formation and catheter occlusion. Normal saline is used to flush fluids through, a heparinized saline solution is used to maintain patency while maintaining access or to discontinue access.

* Amor T. *(Breast cancer, Ovarian cancer)*

After completion of my chemotherapy treatments, I did have to to get my port flushed every month. Before each visit, I applied a small dollop lidocaine pain and numbing cream onto the site one hour before my appointment and covered it with a square piece of Saran wrap. I looked forward to my monthly port flushes, because it was also a chance for me to visit with the wonderful oncology nurses who took care of me at the cancer center.

> **ADVICE:** Before your scheduled port flush, apply a small dollop of lidocaine pain and numbing cream to your port site, cover it with a square piece of Saran wrap and tape it down. When you do this, you'll barely feel anything when the nurses flushes your port.
> Port draws are easy for blood tests, because it's basically a "plug-and-play." The nurse attaches (plugs) the catheter to your port and the blood starts flowing.

* Cindy R. *(Metastatic Breast cancer to the Stomach)*

My port flushes and draws were mainly smooth. There was only one time when they weren't able to draw blood out through it and I got a small clot. So, they had to put de-clotting medicine right in there and we had to wait a half hour before trying to draw the blood out again. It worked. The clot happened only once. Everything else was fine; a piece of cake.

> **ADVICE:** Port flushes and draws are really a piece of cake. If something gets stuck, the nurse or technician handling your port are trained on how to take care of it. So, it's a simple process.

* Rev. Linda S. *(Pancreatic cancer 3x)*

I did not have any problems with my port during my first round of treatment. During my second round, however, they had a hard time drawing blood through my port. They were still able to use my port for the chemo infusions, however. They just had to use my arms to draw blood. I have good veins in my arms, so that worked.

* Rachel S. *(Breast cancer: triple negative)*

Before I go for my Port Flush, I numb my port area with a huge dollop of lidocaine and cover it with saran wrap, the "Press-n-Peel" kind of saran wrap. It's the absolute perfect thing, because I don't need to tape over it. The "Press-n-Peel" kind of saran wrap doesn't budge, while the regular saran wrap does.

Also, I get two packages of graham crackers to eat while the nurse comes over to flush my port after chemo. The graham crackers take away the nasty aluminum taste from my mouth, which a lot of patients taste when they're getting their ports flushed.

> **ADVICE:** When you're done with your chemo session and the nurse comes over to flush your port, eat graham crackers. It will take away the nasty aluminum taste in your mouth; a taste that a lot of patients get when their ports are being flushed. Some hospitals actually put graham crackers or saltine crackers on the counter for patients to eat. See if your hospital does the same thing. If not, get some and bring it with you to your chemo treatment.

* Scott M. (Metastatic Colon cancer to the Prostate & Pancreas)

Ultrasounds are simple procedures. The technician applies gel on you and then uses a device connected to the computer to scan the area of your body that needs to be scanned. Of course, since the gel can be cold, it's always good when they warm up or rub the gel before the procedure.

> ADVICE: Ask the technician to warm up the gel, before applying it on you.

* Sondra W. (Ovarian cancer 3x)

During the brief time that I was off of chemo, I went once a month to the Cancer Center to get my mediport flushed. This happened twice and I never experienced any issues. Recently, there was a time when my oncology nurse had to apply ice to numb my mediport area and keep it from bruising. So I jokingly told her that I see she's having fun and "practicing" on me.

> ADVICE: Port flushes on the mediport are quick and don't hurt. The oncology nurses are trained and they help you get comfortable. To lessen any feeling in the area and prevent bruising, you can ice the area to numb it.

* Susan M. (Ovarian cancer, Metastatic Pancreatic cancer to the Lungs)

After completion of my chemo treatment for pancreatic cancer, they scheduled my port flushes for every six weeks.

* Yesi L. (Breast cancer: triple positive)

When they use the mediport for chemo infusions and port flushes, it feels like having a push pin pushed into you. So, basically, it is painful. I just take a deep breath and think positive thoughts. For everything hard, that's what I do. Deep breaths and positive thoughts.

> ADVICE: It really helps to take deep breaths and think positive thoughts. I know that some patients put numbing cream or ice on the mediport area one hour prior to the infusion or port flush to numb it. I didn't need it, but I heard it does help.

ULTRASOUND / SONOGRAPHY

A procedure that uses high-energy sound waves to look at tissues and organs inside the body. The sound waves make echoes that form pictures of the tissues and organs on a computer screen (sonogram). Ultrasound may be used to help diagnose diseases, such as cancer. It may also be used during pregnancy to check the fetus (unborn baby) and during medical procedures, such as biopsies. Also called ultrasonography.

* Aaron C. (Prostate cancer, Skin cancer)

I had to get an ultrasound on my bladder to make sure it was normal and I could hold and release water. It was an easy procedure and my bladder functions were normal.

* Amor T. (Breast cancer, Ovarian cancer)

I've experienced an ultrasound on my breast when cancer was suspected and an ultrasound of my abdomen when ovarian cancer was suspected. Everytime I had an ultrasound, they put gel or "goop" (as I call it) in the area. The technician or radiologist rolled the transducer over the goop to create the images on the ultrasound screen. Sometimes they swirled the transducer around my breast or abdomen, stopping every once in awhile to mark certain areas. Sometimes, they would ask me to turn slightly to the side, so they can get a better scan of my liver and other organs that also wrap towards the back. The process if fairly simple and I can see what's on the screen. The only thing is, I never really understood exactly what I was looking at; it looked like a hazy image to me.

ADVICE: The gel or "goop" can be cold when first applied to your skin. Ask the technician if they can warm the gel beforehand.

* Cindy L. *(Kidney cancer)*

My doctor ordered an abdominal ultrasound and checked my liver. Everything was fine. Then he said, "Oh, by the way, there's a cyst on your left kidney. Don't worry about it. These things are usually benign."

Well, something in the back of my mind said, "No, we ARE going to worry about this." So, I said, "I'm going to wait six months and then we're going to look at it again." This was in December of 2015. So in July of 2016, I went back to my doctor and requested the ultrasound. Within two hours of that ultrasound, he was on the phone and said, "We need to see what this is." After meeting with him again, we decided that I would get an MRI of my kidney versus a CT scan. That's because I have a heart issue that could cause me to have problems with the particular contrast that they use with the CT scan; we felt the contrast with the MRI would be better handled by my heart. Within a couple of hours of the MRI, I got word from him that they were referring me out to a urologist, because there was about a 95% possibility that I had cancer in my kidney.

ADVICE: Ultrasounds help doctors diagnose certain conditions. They're faster procedures, because they're done in real-time with you, the patient, there and conscious. When you believe that something is not right with you and your doctor cannot explain it, then request for an ultrasound. Fortunately, it doesn't require the use of dyes/contrast.

When you are informed that you have a cyst in your kidney and that cysts are "usually benign", do not rest on that. You have to be vigilant and let your doctor know that, until tests prove your cyst is benign, you are taking the cyst seriously. Then, schedule to meet and be re-tested after a reasonable period of time, e.g. six months.

* Cindy R. *(Metastatic Breast cancer to the Stomach)*

When I noticed a lump on my right breast, the doctor didn't want me to go through a mammogram, because the tumor in my breast was very large. So, they did the same thing they do for pregnant women; they had me go through an ultrasound where they spread gel on my breast and ran the transducer over the area to examine the massive lump. It was the size of a golf ball. The procedure wasn't painful at all.

ADVICE: Since they don't stick anything into you (like a needle), ultrasounds are simple and painless. Just expect them to place gel on your skin, which may be cold. Other than that, the process is really simple.

* Rev. Linda S. *(Pancreatic cancer 3x)*

I didn't experience any problems while I went through ultrasounds. The only thing I noticed, however, was how the technician's facial expression telegraphed when the ultrasound found something unusual.

ADVICE: Don't look at the technician's face during the ultrasound.

* Sondra W. *(Ovarian cancer 3x)*

A couple of weeks after my mediport was implanted, I felt this pain on my neck and thought it was from the way I had slept or something. Then, it got worse. The pain went to my chin and my ears and I thought, "Wait a minute. Am I having a heart attack? What's going on here?" So, I went to Urgent Care where they did an ultrasound on me. They told me,

"Oh, you have a big blood clot on your neck, possibly from your mediport. We can't let you get in car and be driven to the ER, because if it starts to move and you're in traffic, there's nothing you or anyone can do." So, I ended up having to be transported by ambulance to the ER.

Because I was having many issues with my legs, I have since had to have ultrasounds done on them also to ensure there are no blood clots. While I'm laying down during the position, they adjust my position several times several times to make sure they see every part of my legs.

ADVICE: The ultrasound procedure is quick and painless. The technician will instruct you on how you should be positioned and sometimes will reposition you, as needed. Then, some gel will be applied onto your skin, so the handheld probe or paddle that the technician will use can glide on the area being examined.

* *Susan M.* (*Ovarian cancer. Metastatic Pancreatic cancer to the Lungs*)

Ovarian Cancer: Before my hysterectomy, I had an ultrasound that revealed the tumor that was in my ovaries.

Pancreatic Cancer: When the first CT scan, after completion of my chemo treatments, showed that I had nodules in my thyroid, my doctor ordered an ultrasound for my thyroid. When I saw my endocrinologist, she also used results of the ultrasound to do a biopsy. Fortunately, the nodules were benign. My endocrinologist checks my thyroid every year.

~ o ~

Chapter 7

ADAPTING TO PERSONAL CANCER TREATMENT DEVICES & ACCESSORIES

During treatment, there are many gadgets and accessories available to assist us through the process. They may be used as extensions of our treatment outside the hospital or to aid us in our daily functions or to help us cope with side effects or to provide support as we work out way towards healing. For some, they may be a challenge to deal with. Whatever the case may be, we hope that in sharing how we adapted to our personal cancer treatment devices and accessories, you will find good ideas on how to work with yours in positive ways.

CATHETERS (URINARY)

A urinary catheter is a hollow, partially flexible tube that collects urine from the bladder and leads to a drainage bag. Urinary catheters come in many sizes and types. They can be made of rubber, plastic (PVC) or silicone. Catheters are generally necessary when we can't empty our bladder. If the bladder isn't emptied, urine can build up and lead to pressure in our kidneys, which can results in kidney damage. Most catheters are necessary until we regain the ability to urinate on our own, which is usually a short period of time. Elderly people and those with a permanent injury or severe illness may need to use urinary catheters for a much longer time or permanently.

* *Aaron C. (Prostate cancer, Skin cancer)*

Before surgery, the hospital had me go through a two-hour class to learn everything I needed to know about what to do prior to surgery and after surgery, how to take care of my catheter, what to be aware of when it comes to erections, bladder control, etc. They were really up on all that stuff. That was good, because then I understood the importance of my catheter.

During the prostatectomy, my doctor, essentially cut my urethra tube when he removed my prostate and then sewed it back together. He informed me that it usually only takes three or four days to heal, but he didn't want to take a chance. So, I had to keep the catheter on for ten days before he removed it. Yeah, I went home from the hospital with the catheter and had to keep it on for ten days, which was miserable for me. I was sore and couldn't move too much, because every time I did, the catheter tube moved too. It would yank on me. Also, they had a bottle attached to my leg. At the end of the bottle was a drainage bag. I had a small bag for use during the day and a larger bag for use at night.

For the first few days, I had to sleep on my back. I was really limited to what I could move while sleeping. I had to be positioned a certain way, because of the urinary drain bag I had to wear. I had to lay on the left side of my bed, so that the drain bag attached to my catheter, which was strapped to my left thigh, could hang over that side of the bed. That positioning allowed the fluids (residual from surgery) to flow down naturally. I was barely walking around during those ten days, because I was just so uncomfortable with all the stuff. Aside from the urinary drain bags, they gave me a bag to drain my urine into. I had to measure that. I also had a drainage tube with a pump or a bulb. When I squeezed it, the pressure drew any internal fluid (like blood, water, etc.) that stemmed from my surgery into the bulb. Then, I had to drain the bulb once or twice a day, depending on how fast it filled up. All this was necessary to keep out excess fluids and make sure my catheter didn't cause an infection.

By the way, I bought a tube of liquid KY Jelly because the head of my penis was getting irritated by the catheter. So I put some KY Jelly around the head of my penis and that kept it from getting irritated.

When they, eventually, took out my catheter, it was weird. They pulled the drainage tube and the catheter out of my spot at the same time, which was horrible! It was a really weird feeling. And, they didn't numb the area, either. They just said, "Take a deep breath" and then they pulled that sucker out. I was like, "Ah, Sh*t!" When I had the catheter, I slept okay. But once that was out, I slept much better.

ADVICE:

- First, make sure you attend an educational class that will provide you all you need to know about your surgery, treatment plan and any medical equipment you'll be needing, like a catheter;
- Allow yourself time to adjust to your catheter. It's probably not going to be easy, but you just need to accept its importance and tough it out. It'll eventually become a thing of the past, like it is for me now.
- If your penis gets irritated by your catheter, just get some liquid KY Jelly to rub on to the head of your penis. That will take care of the irritation.
- Before they remove your catheter, ask them to numb the area. If they don't do that, then ask them to be gentle, so it doesn't become a negative experience for you.

* Amor T. (Breast cancer, Ovarian cancer)

Breast cancer: The first time I was told that they had to put a urinary catheter into me, I was afraid that it would be really painful. My nurse reassured me and said that she would be gentle and put it in slowly. She did and it really wasn't as bad as I thought it would be. Her reassurance really helped to make this first experience of mine with a catheter easier than I imagined it could be. Urinating through a catheter meant I didn't have to get myself up from the bed to go the bathroom; it made the whole experience efficient and easier for my body. When my condition stabilized and my body grew stronger, the time came for them to remove my catheter. I pleaded with them to let me keep it on. Amused, they gently told me that keeping it on wouldn't help me. To heal and grow stronger, I need to become independent. The catheter would get in the way of my independence. Even though I felt bummed, I knew they were right and so, I worked on becoming independent of all the medical devices I had grown attached to.

Just one day after I was discharged from the hospital after my mastectomy and breast reconstruction surgery, I had to be rushed to the hospital's emergency room. I had developed a high fever, which quickly went from 101.5F to past 103.5F and I was shivering like crazy. When the emergency room nurse asked me if I needed anything, I told her (with teeth visibly chattering) that I needed a catheter. She said that she could help me to the bathroom nearby. I told her that I could barely move because of my abdominal surgery and urgently needed a catheter..."Please!" She then immediately gave me a catheter. Aaaah....relief!

Ovarian cancer: After my hysterectomy, I noticed that I had a foley catheter attached to me and smiled, because it has helped me so much in the past. Again, when the time came for the nurse to remove it, I was saddened, but then I would have to work to go to the bathroom. Yes, the catheter "spoiled" me!

ADVICE: Catheters are great, because you can easily get relief without having to go through the hassle of getting disconnected from the machines, pushing aside the "gazillion" blankets and pillows around you, scooting yourself up the bed to sit on the side, gingerly placing your feet on the floor while trying to get stable enough to stand, shuffling your feet towards the bathroom while connected to your IV drip, etc. etc. etc. Yes, I'm exaggerating a bit, but for the most part, it's true. Anyway, if they say you need a catheter and you've never had one before, don't worry. It's there to really help you. When the time comes for your catheter to be removed, that means it's no longer helping you. Once it's removed, you'll become independent again, and that's a good thing.

Chemotherapy "Chemo" pumps are one of the ways we can have our chemotherapy. They allow us to have chemo in a controlled way. They are attached to either ports or catheters, and can be either outside or inside our body. We can discreetly carry an external pump around with us during the weeks we're having treatment. Chemo pumps are also called infusion pumps. When we have chemo through a central line or a PICC line, a nurse can attach a pump.

* Cindy R. (Metastatic Breast cancer to the Stomach)

The treatment I went through for my stomach cancer was different from the chemo treatment I went through for my breast cancer. I started with weekly chemo infusions and then I also had to bring a chemo pump home with me. I did that for two years (2014 & 2015), before they realized that I was misdiagnosed and that the stomach cancer was actually a metastasis of my breast cancer ten years before; not a new cancer like they first thought. It was a really bad experience. So, they changed my treatment plan.

At first, I had to keep the chemo pump with me 24/7 for three days. The second time around, they increased it to five days. Yeah, it looked like I was wearing a fanny pack. The fanny pack held the little canister with the chemo drug, which was attached to my port. I remember the name of the medicine clearly. We laughed about it, because it was called 5-FU. And so we were like, "Alright cancer. FU!"

Whenever I brought the pump home from my recent chemo, I couldn't get it wet. To be able to shower with it, they instructed me to place the chemo pump outside the shower, cover my port with saran wrap (the press-n-seal type) and then put a little tape around it. That will keep it dry and it did.

I slept with my chemo pump and everything. Even though the port didn't really bother me, the chemo pump it was hooked up to did, because it was on my side. So, when I wanted to turn, I had to adjust and do it very carefully. I placed a small pillow by my pump, so that I wouldn't roll over on top of my pump.

Thankfully, my chemo pump didn't hum or make noise or even vibrate. However, I could definitely tell it was there, because of all the tubing. Even though it didn't make any sound, I could tell when it was working, because of the liquid that I could see running through the tube. It just did its thing quietly. I still had to wear the fanny pack with the pump when I slept.

> **ADVICE:** Having a chemo pump will be awkward, at first. But you'll learn to adjust and get used to it. You can actually do a lot of things while you have your chemo pump on without anyone really noticing you've got it on. That's because the chemo pump is small and looks like a fanny pack and you can wear it under a top shirt or jacket.
>
> To sleep with your chemo pump, place a small pillow by the pump. That will keep you from rolling over it.
>
> To shower with your chemo pump, hang it somewhere outside your shower (in the fanny pack), cover your port with saran wrap (the press-n-seal type) and then put a little tape around it. That should keep it dry.

* Hilda K. (Colon cancer)

Before every chemo infusion, I prepared myself by taking a shower. That was because I knew that when I came home, I would have the chemo pump with me for the next two to three days and didn't want to worry about taking a shower. I psyched myself to <u>not</u> look at the chemo pump as a "burden". I slept with it and my family was comfortable with it. It became like an accessory to me; like a bag. No one, outside my family, knew that I was walking around with my chemo pump; they couldn't tell.

When it came to sleeping, I slept with my pump next to me. I made sure I didn't turn while sleeping by placing pillows next to me. So, basically, I slept on my back and was able to be comfortable and sleep regularly.

So, I find the chemo pump amazing; one of the things they thought of, so patients like me could lead a "normal" life. It was connected to my port underneath my blouse and was strapped around me. It was black in color and the size of a handbag – 8"x 11." It actually looks more like a "man-purse." Every time I had it, I could hear it quietly turn on and turn off. I wore a jacket over my blouse and looked "normal." The chemo pump allowed me look normal, while it continued to dispense the medication.

I could've taken a shower with the pump, by holding the pump out like an IV drip, while showering. But, I chose not to. When I worked out at the gym, I cleaned myself by washing myself, holding the pump away from me. It was easy! I'm telling you...this experience with the pump was really easy!

The fact that I didn't have to go to work helped tremendously. I mean, I lived in sweatpants, t-shirt, jackets and tennis shoes. I was really comfortable and I know that contributed to my recovery.

ADVICE: The more you know about your chemo pump, the more you'll learn how to be comfortable with it. No one has to know you have a chemo pump, because you can hide it under your clothes. If you have to shower or wash yourself with it, just hold the pump out with one arm, like an IV drip. When you sleep, sleep on your back with the chemo pump beside you. Keep several pillows around you, so you don't turn.

Some people get anxious about dealing with their chemo pump; that's okay. If it helps to take anti-anxiety medication, as your doctor for it and take it, as needed.

The main thing is to not see your chemo pump as a "burden". That attitude just doesn't help you. See it in a positive light, as an "accessory" for you and work with it. You'll get used to it and find it's actually easy.

* *Rev. Linda S.* (*Pancreatic cancer 3x*)

My second round with chemo was intense. Although, from past experience, I generally knew what to expect of the chemo infusion process, this time I also had to bring a chemo pump home with me. The chemo pump infused more drugs slowly into me as I went through the day and slept through the night for several days. Thanks to strategic placement of bed pillows, my dog Murphy was unable to harm me or the infusion pump as we slept.

ADVICE: If you sleep with your pet or someone at home and you have a chemo infusion pump, try strategically placing bed pillows around you, so that you nor your pump will be harmed while sleeping.

COLOSTOMY BAGS

A colostomy bag, also called a stoma bag or ostomy bag, is a small, waterproof pouch used to permit sanitary collection and disposal of bodily wastes. During a surgical procedure known as a colostomy, an opening, called a stoma or ostomy, is formed between the large intestine (colon) and the abdominal wall.

* *Joan S.* (*Rectal cancer*)

After surgery, I had to get a colostomy bag. They showed me how to empty and change it. The first time I saw it, I completely threw up. The entire process and having it in me was such a shock! Even though it was a shock, I eventually got used to it. Honestly, I hate it. But, I do tolerate it, because it's something I have to live with. It's a part of my life now.

There are monthly support group meetings for those who have to live with colostomy bags. Some people need the support groups to cope and some don't.

ADVICE: Even though you may not like having to live with a colostomy bag, it's a fact of life. So, just do what you have to do with it. Try not to think too much about it, because it's not going to change anything or make things better.

FEEDING TUBES

A gastric feeding tube (G-tube or "button") is a tube inserted through a small incision in the abdomen into the stomach and is used to supply nutrition when you have trouble eating. Feeding tube insertion is also called percutaneous endoscopic gastrostomy (PEG), esophagogastroduodenoscopy (EGD), and G-tube insertion.

* Cindy R. (*Metastatic Breast cancer to the Stomach*)

When I had my medical port implanted into me, I decided to have the feeding tube put in at the same time. My doctor recommend I get it as a precautionary measure, just in case I couldn't eat on my own. Fortunately, I was under anesthesia for the entire procedure.

The feeding tube was placed right next to my belly button. They actually cut an incision above my belly button and inserted the tube through the incision. I'm not sure exactly what the tube was attached to. There was kind of more to it than just putting in a feeding tube. So, I was in the hospital for a couple of days afterwards.

Just having the feeding tube in made me really sick. I couldn't eat and just felt really bad for a few days, going in and out of the hospital. I hope no one ever has to go through it. I had it in for about a year and didn't have to clean it. If I needed to, I could use it at home or at the doctor's office or wherever. Thankfully, I didn't have to use it at all; I was able to eat on my own the whole time. That's probably why I didn't have to clean it.

To remove it, I didn't need to have surgery. One day, when I went in to see my doctor, he said that I was doing so well and asked me if they could remove the feeding tube. When I said yes ... Boom! They just pulled it right out! It was crazy! They didn't give me any numbing cream or anything for pain. They just had me lay down and then they pulled it right out. They didn't even sew me up. It was the craziest thing! I was expecting this whole big procedure and everything, but nope. Just "Here you go..."

ADVICE: If you can't eat or drink through your mouth, then you will need a feeding tube. Yes, it's really uncomfortable, but it's necessary for you to take in food, which you definitely need to recover and gain strength.

When they ask you if they could remove your feeding tube, have them explain to you first how they're going to do it, so that you'll be prepared and there won't be any surprises.

* Scott M. (*Metastatic Colon cancer to the Prostate & Pancreas*)

At one time, I had to go home with a feeding tube inserted into my stomach through my abdomen, because I had trouble eating. I had to mix my food and pour the milkshake-like fluid through the feeding tube, which was about three quarters of an inch in diameter.

The problem was the hole in my stomach was bigger than the tube and the tube would constantly rub against the hole in my stomach for a few months. Talk about pain! I developed a big anxiety to pain. An hour prior to having the feeding tube cleaned, I would break into a cold sweat thinking about it. So, I would take 4mg of Dilaudid (a strong pain med). Then, fifteen minutes prior to the cleaning, I would take some oral Morphine (another strong pain med). So, when the medical team came in to un-tape the whole thing to clean it, the pain meds helped with the pain.

ADVICE: A feeding tube is necessary when you have trouble taking in food. It can be uncomfortable and painful. Before you get a feeding tube, learn everything you can about how to use it, clean it and any problems to look out for. If you feel pain, be sure to stay AHEAD of the pain, e.g. take the pain medication before any activity you know that will trigger pain.

LYMPHEDEMA COMPRESSION SLEEVES & ABDOMINAL BINDERS

A lymphedema compression sleeve is an elasticized garment that is worn to reduce the swelling and pain caused by lymphedema. They resemble "knee socks" for your arms and come in a variety of colors and designs.

An abdominal binder is a compression garment that fits tightly around your abdomen to decrease swelling, improve blood circulation and oxygen levels at the operative site, provide support throughout the recovery process, shape the body and accelerate the healing process.

* Amor T. (*Breast cancer, Ovarian cancer*)

After my DIEP flap breast reconstruction surgery, my body was quite swollen. The only thing I could do was be patient and allow my body time to process through the torment that it had just gone through. Three months later, I had a second surgery; this time to restore symmetry of my breasts. Again, my body took a beating.

Even though my body was sore and literally black and blue, I felt positive knowing that the inflammation was part of the body's immune response without which my wounds and damaged tissues from surgery would not be able to heal.

After my open wounds healed, I wore an abdominal compression binder. Purpose of the binder was to provide compression and support to my abdomen, improve blood circulation, decrease postoperative pain, promote deep breathing, help reduce swelling and promote the healing process.

In the beginning, breathing was difficult, because of how my diaphragm would move download towards my injured abdominal muscles as my lungs filled with air during inhalation. The compression binder helped to support the process, thereby allowing me to breathe without much pain.

I wore it as much as I could, even while sleeping. I had two compression binders, so that I could use them alternately. They were very comforting and became a part of me while I was healing. As swelling in my body decreased, I was able to compress my abdomen more and more. The end result was a nice, slimmer looking abdomen.

> **ADVICE:** Compression binders are great, because they'll actually "hold everything together" so that you can move around better without feeling that your sutures are going to come apart. I suggest using it as much as you can while you're healing. It, not only provides compression and support, but also improves blood circulation, decreases postoperative pain, promotes deep breathing and helps reduce swelling. The compression binder will also provide stability to your abdominal region and help your wounds heal faster leading to a quicker recovery. Highly recommended.

* Cindy R. *(Metastatic Breast cancer to the Stomach)*

I did have swelling in my right arm because, during my double mastectomy, they removed 12 lymph nodes from the area around my right arm. So, there were times when my arm would swell up and I couldn't bend it, especially in the heat. The lymph nodes are the ones that take the toxins and move them throughout the body. Without them, the fluid with the toxins would just sit there. I was miserable with the swelling, but there were some things that helped.

One was the light exercise I did, because moving around and getting the blood flowing is important. The other was wearing the compression sleeve on my swollen arm, which helped with the blood flow too. Compression sleeves are expensive. However, since they're part of my treatment, I got my insurance to pay for them. Insurance also covered cost of my breast prosthetics too.

> **ADVICE:** Lymphedema can be pretty miserable, especially when it's hot. However, there are ways to move the toxins and keep them from just sitting in one place (e.g. arms, legs) in your body.
>
> 1. Do some light exercise. Moving around will get your blood flowing and your circulation going.
> 2. If you have lymphedema in your arms, buy compression sleeves for your arms. If you have lymphedema elsewhere in your body (knees, legs, abdomen, etc.), you can get compression garments for those areas too. Check online on Amazon and similar sites. Since you got your lymphedema, get your insurance to pay for the compression garment. Check with them before buying anything to make sure you follow their instructions for purchase or reimbursement.
>
> Check out American Cancer Society too. They can help you a variety of things when it comes to your treatment. Low cost or no cost, they really help.

* Rachel S. *(Breast cancer: triple negative)*

When I had a double mastectomy, they removed all the lymph nodes from my right arm and only 2 lymph nodes from my left arm. I got lymphedema because I no longer have lymph nodes in my right arm. My right arm doesn't have the capability anymore to push the poison fluids from my arm, in order for me to ~ for lack of a better word ~ "urinate" them out. So, I have to wear a compression sleeve every day for the rest of my life. There are days when I can't move my arm. It feels like there's a bar going down my arm and it's hard to straighten it. The only thing I can do for that is to exercise and to stretch it out. It usually lasts a couple of days and then I have to constantly massage my arm and my spine to keep the swelling down, because once the arm starts to swell, it's very, very difficult to get it to go back to normal.

* Vida B.A. *(Breast cancer)*

My left arm swelled after my mastectomy, definitely one of the side effects from surgery that I had to deal with. So, my doctor suggested that I buy a lymphedema compression wrap for my arm to help with the circulation. The compression wraps are stretchable and look like a socks or leggings with openings on both ends.

Since I had lymphedema in my left arm and I knew that the cabin pressure on the flight to New Zealand would cause my arm to swell, I bought a compression sleeve to wear on the plane. The purpose was to apply pressure on my arm to prevent lymphatic fluid from building up. Unfortunately, my arm swelled up as the plane was making its steep climb up to cruising altitude. It was so painful, so I ended up removing it, which was a relief. For the rest of the flight, I tried to relax my swollen arm and lightly massage it.

MEDICAL PORTS (MEDIPORTS) / PORT-A-CATH

In medicine, a port is a small medical appliance that is installed beneath the skin. Under the skin, the port has a septum (a partition separating two chambers), through which drugs can be injected and blood samples can be drawn many times, with very minor discomfort, if any. Ports are used mostly to treat hematology and oncology (cancer) patients.

* Amor T. *(Breast cancer, Ovarian cancer)*

I thought that I would be able to go through all my chemo treatments without having to get a mediport. On my third round of chemo, however, my veins started to burn and that was my wake-up call. My doctor told me that since the veins in my right arm had been heavily used in the past (they were pummeled with heavy antibiotics to fight off my staph infection), they were too weak to continue being used.

My doctor gave me a choice on where I'd like to have my mediport located and explained it should be in an area that would be easily accessible for infusions. I chose to have it above my right breast and below my right clavicle. Sure, it would be visible to others, but that didn't matter to me. During the mediport implant surgery, I was anesthetized. Having the mediport made my treatment experience easier, because I no longer had to suffer the pains of being pricked with a needle seemingly 10,000 times before they could find a viable vain. During chemo infusions, lab draws and port flushes, the whole process was smooth. I didn't have to do anything special with my mediport. It looked like a small bump below my right clavicle. I did have to careful about applying pressure on it, like the car's seat belt, as it would irritate the skin. I also had to protect it from any blunt force.

After completion of my chemotherapy treatments, I did have to to get my port flushed every month. An hour before each visit, I applied lidocaine numbing cream onto the site and covered it with a square piece of Saran wrap (the press-n-seal type). I looked forward to my monthly port flushes, because it was also a chance for me to visit with the wonderful oncology nurses who took care of me at the cancer center. Two years after my last chemo infusion, I had my mediport was surgically removed and,, again, was anesthetized for the procedure.

also be able to choose the location of your mediport, which of course, should be accessible to the professionals. However, it's important that you be comfortable with its location too.

Before your mediport is to be used (for infusions, draws or flushings), apply a small dollop of lidocaine numbing cream on the area one hour ahead of time That way, you won't feel a thing when they access it. When it comes time to remove your mediport, have them anesthetize you too. It's so much easier that way.

* Cindy R. (*Metastatic Breast cancer to the Stomach*)

For both my breast cancer and stomach cancer treatments, I got a port. Actually when they did the mastectomy, they placed the mediport above my left breast, on the upper left hand side, right underneath my collarbone. It was like, "Do whatever you need to do. I'm under. So, go ahead."

When they removed my first port, I felt it all. I knew what was going on. It was just like, "You've got to be kidding me! Yes, I could feel everything!" Only then did they put more numbing cream there. Yeah, I knew exactly what was going on and it was not fun.

The second time around, for treatment of my stomach cancer, I had the port implanted at the same time they had the feeding tube put in. I still have the mediport in me. Since it looks like things are going along so good, I might get it removed soon. We'll see. Yeah, this time, when they remove my port, I will tell them that I want to be under, because it's like, "Hey, I just don't want to know what it feels like."

By the way, just something that I decided to do for myself … When I turned 50, my mom and I went went on a Disney cruise to Mexico and the Panama Canal and we also got to swim with the dolphins. So, I got a tattoo over the original spot where the port was. It's a tattoo of a dolphin, the breast cancer ribbon that says "Survivor" and lots of waves over where the port was. I just wanted my tattoo to be something really, really special at my 10-year mark that says: Yeah, I'm a survivor!

ADVICE: Having a medical port aka "medi-port" will really makes chemo infusions and lab draws easier for you when you're going through treatment. You should be under general anesthesia when they implant it. Before the procedure, ask your doctor to explain the procedure and ask questions like, what to expect, how to clean it, where the medi-port will be placed and why. When it comes time to remove your mediport, insist they put you under general anesthesia too, because you don't want to experience the pain of removal at all.

When they remove the mediport, you'll have a little scar. You can have something nice tattooed on it, if you like. You can use it to remind yourself that you are a survivor and you are proud of it!

* Hilda K. (*Colon cancer*)

My medical port device (mediport) was surgically implanted during my laparoscopic colectomy and was placed over my left breast, right above my heart. So, I didn't feel anything when it was put in. After a year of my chemotherapy, I finally decided to have it removed. It was one of the most invasive experiences I've felt, aside from the surgery. At the doctor's office, they gave local anesthesia and then cut me open where my mediport implanted. Since muscle and tissue had already grown around the mediport, the doctor had some difficulty pulling it out of me. I learned that when a foreign object is embedded into our bodies, our body's natural reaction is to deal with it and overtake it.

Because I didn't see the mediport go into me, I didn't know what looked like. All I knew was that they had placed a mediport into me for use during treatment. Once the doctor was able to pull it out and show it to me, it looked like an insect. It was a disc with a tail; a very long tail. And that little tube was basically connected to my artery. So, anytime the chemotherapy drug went through me, it went straight to my heart and it dispensed. I mean, I couldn't believe that thing was in me. It looked like an alien!

ADVICE: Having the mediport will make receiving infusions and getting your labs done a lot easier. It is an incredible device!

* Scott M. (*Metastatic Colon cancer to the Prostate & Pancreas*)

I had surgery to implant my first medical port (port) on the left side of my neck and I was placed under general anesthesia, which was no problem at all. Unfortunately, the port was placed in such a way that it kind of twisted; the nurses weren't able to get the needles in exactly straight. They had to really struggle to access my port. So, eventually, I just bit the bullet, had that port removed and had a new one implanted on the right side of my neck. That was a better port; easier to access.

PROSTHESIS (BREAST)

A breast prosthesis is an artificial breast form worn to simulate a woman's natural breast after mastectomy. You can simply slip one prosthesis or two prostheses into your bra to fill the space where your breast or breasts were. Many women choose breast prostheses over reconstruction. And then there are also women who choose to not have either. Choose whatever option is the most comfortable for you.

* Cindy R. (Metastatic Breast cancer to the Stomach)

Before I got my permanent implants, I used breast prosthesis aka "falsies" and had some funny experiences because of them. One time, I was at my sister's wedding with all my family around me when, all of a sudden, bloop! ... one of my falsey things slipped out of my dress! Well, in front of everyone, I simply picked it up and put it back in. It was so funny; we all laughed so hard!

By the way, because having breast prosthesis was part of my treatment, I got my insurance to pay for them.

SURGICAL DRAINS / JP DRAIN TUBES & BULBS

A Jackson-Pratt or JP drain is a surgical drain. A surgical drain is a closed-suction medical device that is commonly used as a post-operative drain for collecting bodily fluids from surgical sites. The device consists of an internal drain connected to a grenade-shaped bulb via plastic tubing.

* Amor T. (Breast cancer, Ovarian cancer)

After a week in the hospital, I was sent home with four JP (Jackson-Pratt) surgical drain bulbs hanging from my body: one by each breast and one by each side of my hip. The drains removed the fluid that had built up in my body after surgery. A nurse instructed me how to clean the wounds in those areas and also measure and record the fluid collected in the bulbs every day. I remember watching as she showed me how to properly collect the liquid by first pinching the part of the tube closest to my body and sliding it down towards the bulb. This was to squeeze as much liquid as she could out of the tube and into the bulb. After recording the liquid, she completely emptied the bulb until it was "flat" and reattached the bulb to the drain tube.

Choosing clothes to wear when I had the four surgical drains hanging from my sides after surgery was tough. I really had to be creative. So, I searched my entire wardrobe for loose clothes with garters or ties. I wore wraps or sarongs and even large scarves that I could use as a wrap. This is because I needed to be able to have each of the surgical drains hang out from my body while being able to access them also. I couldn't wear pants at all, in the beginning, because of the drains hanging from both sides of my hips. With the loose wraps or gowns and using safety pins, I hung the drain bulbs with the tubes and attached them to the sides of the wrap's or gown's material. When I had to leave my home to visit the doctor, I wore very loose cardigans or long sleeve tops which I used to attach the drain bulbs to.

Since showering with the four drain bulbs hanging from me was a bit awkward, I chose to just give myself daily sponge baths. I also used baby wipe to clean myself. Three weeks after my mastectomy and DIEP flap breast reconstruction surgery, my first set of drain bulbs were removed. After my follow-up breast symmetrical and nipple reconstruction surgery, I had two drain bulbs, one beside each breast. Those were removed after two weeks.

> **ADVICE:** Definitely pay attention and take notes, if you can, when you're given instructions on how to care for your surgical drains and bulbs. It would help for the nurse to train you and then watch you clean your wound and measure liquid in the drain bulb before you leaving the hospital.
>
> Because the bulbs and tubes stick out of your body, you have to be creative in choosing clothes to wear. Loose wraps and gowns work best, since you won't have to put them over your head. If you absolutely have to wear pants, wear super loose ones with drawstrings. By the way, when you're out in public and you're conscious about having drain bulbs hanging out of your body, put those thoughts aside. You just went through major, life-saving surgery. What other people think should be of no consequence to you, meaning not important.

* Cindy R. *(Metastatic Breast cancer to the Stomach)*

My surgical drains were located on both sides of the area where they removed my breasts, next to the armpits. I remember that I had to measure the liquid that came out through the drains and into the bulbs. When I had the drain tubes, I wore loose clothes and anything that buttoned up in front, like guy's shirts.

It was around Christmas time and my sister made me a really loose, button-up top with prints of dogs dressed in Christmas attire all over it. It was fun to wear. I know I hooked up the drain tubes and bulbs somehow to my blouse, but I don't remember exactly where or how right now.

> **ADVICE:** Your doctor or nurse will give you specific instructions on what to do with your drain bulbs and how to measure the liquid that drains out into the bulbs. Since they protrude out from your body, you'll have to wear a loose top to cover them up. They're temporary and will be removed after no more liquid comes out of the area you were operated on.

* Vida B.A. *(Breast cancer)*

Recovering from my mastectomy was painful. Fortunately, I had good pain medication to help. After surgery, I was sent home with two drain tubes and bulbs dangling from the side of my left breast area. They were placed there to collect excess fluid from my surgery. They didn't really bother me. I was even able to take showers with them.

> **ADVICE:** When you're sent home from the hospital with drain tubes and bulbs, make sure to listen to the instructions they give you and then strictly follow them. They'll be removed from you after there is no excess fluid to collect from your surgery area. You should still be able to take a shower with them on. Check with your doctor first, before you do.

WIGS AND OTHER HEAD COVERS

Chemotherapy has been known to cause alopecia, which is baldness or the partial or complete loss of hair. You have a array of head covers to choose from, be they wigs, hats, caps, beanies, scarves or turbans, to conceal your lack of hair. Those of us who've gone through alopecia were able to find creative and fun ways to cover our bald heads. Doing so definitely helped to make what could easily be considered a grim experience, interesting and even, fun.

* Amor T. (Breast cancer, Ovarian cancer)

My wonderful sister Joy generously bought me a beautiful, quality wig that looked like my original long hair. Along with it came the necessary accessories, like a mesh wig cap liner, a wig band, wig shampoo, wig conditioner, wig comb, wig stand, etc. The ladies at the wig salon referred me to a stylist who was skilled at cutting and styling wigs. When I met with her, I described exactly how I wanted my wig to look like my original hair and she did a great job!

When I was bald, I used the mesh wig cap liner that covered my entire head, to secure the wig onto my head. When my hair started growing, the wig cap liner couldn't grip my head, because my growing hair was creating a "slippery" surface. That's when the wig band came into the picture. It had a very wide band with velcro fasteners at each end and it did the trick of securing my wig to my head.

Initially, I thought that I would use my wig all the time, but discovered that I actually didn't need to. I wore my wig when I had to go to social functions, e.g. church, movies, meetings or dining out. Other occasions, like visiting family and friends, grocery shopping, going to the hospital, etc. I didn't feel were necessary for me to wear my wig. Collecting a bunch of head covers was fun. I got a lot of chemo caps made of different materials. Some were plain colored and some had designs. I had the basic neutral colors of black, white and tan. Sometimes I wore them as is and sometimes I used them as a base, placing on top of them a designed cap that was complimentary. For me, it added to my look, especially when I coordinated my clothes with my head covers. I also collected a lot of scarves - I mean, a LOT of scarves! There were so many ways to twist and tie them; I really enjoyed finding creative ways to cover my head.

Being bald caused me to get cold easily, especially at night when I slept. So, I wore a nightcap; something I never thought I had to wear. And no, I'm not referring to the alcoholic drink some people have before going to bed (smile!).

ADVICE: After you lose your hair, you definitely have options. Research different kinds of wigs and headcovers (beanies, scarves, caps, etc). Get creative and coordinate not only your clothes to your headcover, but try coordinating one headcover with other headcovers. For example, placing a beanie with a paisley design over a black beanie or wearing an orange beanie over a red beanie, letting a little bit of the orange serve as the lining for the red beanie. This will give an extra layer for comfort/warmth plus add a sleek lining for your "double-beanie" fashion statement.

Since body heat escapes mostly through the head, when it's exposed (without hair), it's important to wear a headcover when it's cold outside. You'll notice getting colder going through treatment. So, wear a cap at night when you're sleeping. During the day, you can keep your head warm with caps, hats, scarves, etc. and your wig, if you did decide to purchase one.

Regarding wigs, I suggest just getting one first to see if you like how it feels on you. If you purchase one, you can have it styled to your liking with a stylist who has experience with wigs. Learn everything you can about wig care and get the accessories you need to take care of it. You'll need to purchase wig grooming items, like wig shampoo, wig conditioner, wig comb, wig stand, wig bands and wig caps. As for storing or transporting wigs, here's what I learned.

1. Turn your wig inside out and gently place long locks inside the wig top.
2. Put a hair net around your wig to keep everything in place.
3. Wrap your wig in a silk scarf - a cotton or synthetic scarf will make your wig and wig cap frizzy.
4. Place it in a zippable plastic bag or a wig packing bag and seal it to avoid moisture.
5. At this point, you can put your wig in your suitcase or your carry-on.

---

* Cindy R. (Metastatic Breast cancer to the Stomach)

Breast Cancer: I lost my hair completely when I was going through chemotherapy to treat my breast cancer. Every follicle of hair on my body, I lost. I had super long hair before chemo. Since I knew my hair would fall off eventually, I got it cut really short, at first, because I didn't know if I just wanted to shave it all off yet. Then when it started falling out, I thought, "Well, I should just shave it now."

I did use a wig, but I did not like it, at all. It just was the most uncomfortable thing, so I just wore a scarf. I also wore chemo caps at night or whenever it got cold. And I was always so cold. I wore a lot of caps and scarves to cover my head, because I didn't like to wear the wig I had. I only wore my wig on occasion, like the time my sister got married and we went to Hawaii. I was part of the wedding party and I wanted to, at least, look halfway normal. It was so uncomfortable for me. So, I took it off whenever I could and put it back on only when I really needed to. I was more comfortable wearing bandanas, caps and those kinds of things.

My sister and I actually had some fun making our own little hats too. They were almost like babushka hats that you can tie around. We sewed them from different materials to be creative. I just wanted to have fun with it.

Stomach Cancer: This time with chemotherapy, I lost some hair, but not all of it, like I did the last time when I was being treated for breast cancer.

By the way, the American Cancer Society has a program that's called "The Look Good, Feel Better" program that helps women with cancer, manage the appearance-related side effects of treatment. There, trained volunteer beauty professionals teach cancer patients simple techniques on skin care, makeup and nail care and give practical tips on hair loss wigs and head coverings (scarves, caps, turbans, etc.). Workshop participants receive a free cosmetic kit and style tips. The workshops are free to women undergoing chemotherapy, radiation or other forms of treatment. I also got a free wig from them.

The program is a great resource, especially for those patients who learn that treatment will cause them to lose their hair and won't know what to do and where to go when that happens. It's really helpful.

> <u>ADVICE:</u> If your treatment calls for chemotherapy, you will most likely lose your hair; maybe some, maybe all. Whatever the case may be, just look at it as a temporary change. Getting angry or sad about losing your hair to chemo won't help you. What will help is seeing it as an opportunity to have fun wearing different hats, scarves, caps, turbans, wigs, etc.
>
> Ask your doctor about the American Cancer Society's "The Look Good, Feel Better" program that helps women with cancer, manage the appearance-related side effects of treatment. There, trained volunteer beauty professionals teach cancer patients simple techniques on skin care, makeup and nail care and give practical tips on hair loss wigs and head coverings (scarves, caps, turbans, etc.). Workshop participants receive a free cosmetic kit and style tips. The workshops are free to women undergoing chemotherapy, radiation or other forms of treatment. The program is really a great resource, especially if you do lose your hair and need to know what you can do or where to go when it happens It really is helpful.

* *Hilda K.* (Colon cancer)

At the Cancer Center where I was treated, they had a program to help patients deal with physical changes, like a dermatologist, a cosmetologist to teach you how to put on makeup or someone to teach you how to tie scarves. I was prepared to have a "shave day" and a "scarf day" with some of my family members, but I ended up not having alopecia per se or losing all of my hair. That's because the way they administered my chemotherapy wasn't hard-hitting or aggressive; the dosage was dispensed gradually. I learned that each cancer has different levels of treatment. So, with my colon cancer, I did lose hair, but as soon as I lost some hair, new hair was also growing back. So, I never went completely bald.

Although I still had hair, it was thin. That, along with my chemotherapy treatment, made me feel cold a lot. So, I did wear hats or caps. At my oncologist's office, there was a basket of gloves, hats and scarves that were knitted and donated by someone. If I forgot my hat, I didn't have to worry, because I could get a knitted hat there. And, every time I went there, I got a different color.

> <u>ADVICE:</u> Whether you are completely bald or have thinning hair, you're bound to get cold, because that's a side effect of Chemotherapy medication. To keep yourself warm, cover your head with a hat, cap or scarf.

* *Jacki S.* (Breast cancer)

I did opt for a wig versus wearing head scarves. For me, head scarves are very noticeable on cancer patients and they would draw more attention to me than if I wore a wig. So then, after that one shower, when I realized I lost a lot of hair, I let my daughter cut the rest of my hair off. She loved that, because she got to style-cut my hair in whatever way she wanted. That was a fun little episode we had out in the garage. I put a hefty garbage bag over my head (I cut a little hole in it, of course) and sat on the chair. My arms weren't available. So, I just let my daughter have the scissors and she cut as much as she wanted. She styled it first and then cut the rest off. She really enjoyed that and it put a smile on my face, because it made her happy. And in a way, your daughter (or son or other family member) is having to deal with this, just like you are.

And sometimes, it's harder on the kids than it is on the adult going through it. I knew my daughter was also a very strong individual, trying to help me out. So, our beauty session in the garage was a fun, humorous time for us. After that, I went to Supercuts and let them do the buzz cut all the way ... cut all the rest of it ... Gone!

Something fun that I experienced when I had no hair was getting the free hats when I went in for radiation. Because there are so many patients that go in for radiation and don't have their hair yet, there's a special group of women (I don't know who they are; they're just angels) who make hats for patients who need them. What they do is they put these hats in a basket right inside the office. Before you go in for your radiation and, if you feel like you need a new hat or you would like to have a hat for another occasion, the hats are in the basket for you to take, free of charge! So, that was very nice. I did have a bunch of them. But then, I brought some back to the radiation department and some I took to the Salvation Army, because there is always someone who could use them.

Everybody has to make their own decision about what to do when they lose their hair. I bought wigs and my husband was so supportive. In fact, he liked the way I looked when I lost my hair from the chemo. I did buy a wig that was pretty expensive and then I had some fun cheap ones as well. But my husband liked me without the wig and he liked me to make kind of wild makeup, because he said I looked like Cleopatra. I had a good looking head without hair on it, which I guess doesn't happen for everybody. So, my family was very supportive and he gave me compliments on how I looked.

ADVICE: Do whatever makes you comfortable. It's your decision whether to wear wigs or scarves or caps or hats. It's your decision to make, no matter what anybody says. You have options and whatever you decide to do, just do it for you and do it your way.

* Rev. Linda S. (Pancreatic cancer 3x)

I went through chemotherapy three different times. The first time, chemo straightened my hair. In subsequent times, it thinned my hair. Since one of my chemo treatments began in September and ended in March, I wore scarves and hats to keep my head warm. For spring and warmer weather, I wore a wig for social occasions or church services. I chose not to shave my head because of the cold weather. For my second round with chemo, I decided to shave my head after I noticed small strands of my hair on my iPad screen. The weather is warmer too. No matter what the weather, I know that I have choices with scarves and hats and wigs for social occasions or church services.

ADVICE: Again, I advise patients to do what feels right for them.

* Rachel S. (Breast cancer: triple negative)

I originally was going to have a wig made, but I did some research and I found out how they feel so heavy and can also feel itchy. Also, I learned that they're hard to take care of. So, I just came to the realization that, you know what, I don't care what people say right now. I'm going to do this; I'm going to be comfortable. So, I didn't wear a wig; I went around bald. I really didn't care. I did wear scarves and chemo caps, but not all the time.

ADVICE: If you were told you'll lose your hair, the best way to deal with it is to accept it. First of all, it's temporary and will grow back after treatment. And, second, you really don't need hair. So, don't care what others think. They're not going through what you're going through; they're not you. No matter what you have covering your head, your smile can be the main feature. Your positive attitude also can be your main feature. Besides, you can be creative and try on different scarves or caps. Or, you can get fashionable wigs, if you want.

* Sondra W. (Ovarian cancer 3x)

My hair loss happened within a couple of weeks after my first chemo infusion. At first, some hair came out in small clumps. But then, I believe, on the third week, I put my comb in there and then big, just BIG chunks just came out. I was like, "Well, she had that right." Then I thought, "Okay. Well, I'll just have some fun with this. I'll get different scarves and hats and wigs and just have a little fun with it." Since I couldn't get wigs made of real hair, I got the synthetic ones. Unfortunately, they made me perspire so much that I would just get drenched. Even when I wear it for only five minutes,

I would just be wet. I had two wigs that I was not able to wear. It was winter and it was cold. So, I thought the wigs would help me stay warm. Well, they didn't work that way, because they made me perspire and I just got wet. So, I gave up on the wigs and, instead, used carves and different caps.

Now, the chemo caps were something I could be fashionable with too. I wore them all the time, even in the house, because I was so cold. My head was so cold. I know some people thought, "Oh, it's okay for you to be without your hair. You can leave your cap off." And I would explain, "No, no. It's not that. My head is freezing and I'm really cold." I think it was hard for people to understand. Well, heat does leave through the head and the extremities, our fingers and toes too.

ADVICE: When you lose hair, just think of it as temporary. It will grow back. In the meantime, have some fun with it. Get some wigs, hats, scarves and caps. You can be fashionable and change colors every now and then. The main thing is to keep yourself warm by keeping your head covered.

* Vida B.A. *(Breast cancer)*

Since it's usually hot and humid here in the Philippines, I didn't wear anything to cover my bald head, if I wasn't going anywhere. At home, my head was bare. However, when I had to go out, like when I had to attend a wedding and other social functions, I had a variety of head wraps and wigs to choose from to cover my head.

I decided to enjoy wearing head wraps and wigs and collected different ones in a wide variety of colors. It was my way of coping, because sometimes my self-esteem was low and I felt ugly. With my collection of headwraps and wigs, I could put makeup on, try to look nice and not look sick. Being able to do that made me happy. I chose to make the best of what was happening to me.

ADVICE: To cover your head, there are so many different kinds of head wraps and wigs ... so many designs, colors, lengths you can choose to wear when you go out. Taking some control over how you look with head wraps and/or wigs and makeup will help you cope better with your situation and make you feel good. Focusing on what you can do is much better than focusing on your sickness and your hair loss.

* Yesi L. *(Breast cancer: triple positive)*

Losing my hair was definitely the first major side effect I had to deal with. From my research, I read that it would happen 14 days after treatment and I was absolutely right. Before all that happened, however, I already told myself that I was not going to let cancer take my hair. I was going to proactively take my own hair away. Before treatment, my hair was down to my waist: long, beautiful, healthy hair. I definitely did not want it to be a sad thing. I wanted it to be something that wasn't frightening for me or for my daughter, Zoe. I wanted her to be part of my choice. So, we had a "Hair Party." It was very intimate. Just my husband, my daughter, my best friend and my hairstylist, who is a good friend.

ADVICE: If you know you'll be going through hair loss, try to rock it. Whatever comes your way, just rock it. So, for me, it was a time to wear colorful scarves. I didn't bother with buying expensive, fancy wigs. I found them extremely uncomfortable. If you are considering a wig for yourself, there are a lot of places that donate them like Cancer CAREpoint and Bay Area Cancer Connections.

There may be those times when you have to go to a special event and you do not want to wear a scarf. I had those times and so I did wear, what I called, my "party wig". The wig was itchy, but it was just for partying. Other than that, around the house, I would have absolutely nothing on my head. For cold weather, I would have just a beanie or a scarf.

~ 0 ~

Chapter 8

WRESTLING WITH NATURAL NEGATIVE EMOTIONS

Cancer is a word that brings about negative emotions that are natural for any human to feel. Processing through them can be very challenging, because there is so much of the unknown for you to grasp. You know that, with cancer, you will have to face difficulties. How you adjust to this new reality is personal to you. You will work through your feelings in your own way and in your own time. No matter what, please remember to always validate your emotions and be kind to yourself.

In this chapter, we provide you with how we were able to successfully rise above our negative emotions. For sure, tough emotional battles were fought. However, we came out triumphing in the end.

ANGER, BITTERNESS, DISGUST, RESENTMENT

* *Cindy L.* (Kidney cancer)

When I learned that I had kidney cancer, I got angry. Yes, I was crying, but I was mad. My daughter was having problems in UCF Orlando. She was having serious medical issues; kept fainting and we didn't know why. She was taken to the emergency room three times in an ambulance and she would faint. We didn't know if was her heart, her brain, or what. And, I was headed down the very next day to see her. So, yes. When I found out I had cancer, in the middle of everything that was going on, I got pretty upset.

Four days later, they thought I was experiencing a pulmonary embolism (PE). I was taken back to the hospital. I remember being angry because they put ultrasound gel all over my body and I just had my first shower since surgery on that day. And I remember being upset because I wasn't able to get a shower the next day. But at least, I didn't have a PE, so that was the good news.

During treatment, I kept getting angry that I got cancer. I had the pity party of "why me?" Sometimes, I wondered if it was because of the adrenal gland or if my menopause caused it. I felt that I just got angry over nothing. Since I had a hard time asking my family for support, I would just snap at them, expecting they could read my mind and know what I needed. I was so angry and frustrated, because I couldn't even get up out of my chair to go to the bathroom by myself, without help.

So, I found a psychologist who taught me how to deal with my anger and frustrations. I learned, first of all, to validate my humanity and allow myself to vent. However, I shouldn't unpack and live in my anger. I should deal with it, get over it and move on. I learned to practice to pause, which was to shut my mouth, shut my mind, take some deep breaths and don't say anything until I've calmed down. It hasn't been easy, but I keep practicing. And, to this day, it's helped me become a stronger person.

ADVICE: First, it's never easy to learn you have cancer, especially when you have other matters to deal with. It's natural to get angry and cry. So allow yourself to vent. Validate your humanity. Don't let anyone invalidate you or minimize how you feel; whether right, wrong or indifferent. You're entitled to it. Just don't unpack and live in your anger. Deal with it. Get over it. Then, move to someplace else.

To handle your anger or any upset feelings, the biggest advice I can give you is: <u>Practice to pause</u>. Shut your mouth. Shut your mind. Take some deep breaths and don't say anything, until you calm down and are able to get a handle on your anger. Not easy to do, but practice makes perfect. Take one step at a time. You'll find that you may have to keep on practicing it. Practice to pause. When you get that down, you'll be glad you did.

* *Cindy R.* (Metastatic Breast cancer to the Stomach)

When I felt a little anger, I tried to turn it around and say, "This isn't going to be a bad thing. It's going to be a good thing." Every once in a while, I experienced the "Why me?" emotion. But for the most part, I was like, "You know what? I'm going to be a chronic cancer survivor. And, everything's going to be okay."

<u>ADVICE:</u> Being angry is part of being human. But, staying angry won't do you any good. It certainly doesn't feel good and it definitely won't make you get better either. Push yourself to think positive. You're more likely to get better faster with that attitude than being angry and negative.

* *Rev. Linda S.* (Pancreatic cancer 3x)

When I was diagnosed with stage II Pancreatic Cancer in July 2016, I was upset, quite upset. I had just bought a house, retired and moved to Illinois from California two months prior. I was looking forward to enjoying retired life with my family and friends, especially my mother, Ma Mere, who has Alzheimer's. Having cancer and going through treatment was the exact opposite of what I had envisioned. So, I was really shocked and angry when I received the diagnosis. I had suspected cancer, but <u>not</u> Pancreatic Cancer. Thankfully, I had good friends there with me when I was given the diagnosis; they saved me from hysteria. When I finally calmed down, I mobilized myself to do what I needed to do to address it – physically, emotionally, mentally, and spiritually.

Then, when I was told that my cancer had returned, the same surgeon who said last year that I was more likely to die from old age than Pancreatic Cancer, now says it's common for tumors to return in a year or less. Pissed me off.

<u>ADVICE:</u> As much as possible, have someone with you when you're given the diagnosis. If you receive upsetting news, allow yourself time to process it. After, mobilize yourself to do what you need to do to address it – physically, emotionally, mentally and spiritually.

* *Rachel S*. (Breast cancer: triple negative)

For a long time, I was very angry with God. Why would He allow this to happen? I had a lot of people who came and prayed with me and stuff like that. But, whenever I felt bad, I just turned to my family and friends. My anger with God didn't really last that long.

There's a lot to be said about attitude. My whole life is my kids. Going through everything....whenever I was upset or sad or whatever, I would go find myself with my kids. I'd turn on music....we'd sit there and do silly things and stupid dances ... We would turn on the "wiggle" and start dancing to the "wiggle"... One day, I was dancing in the car and my son said, "Mom, stop." So I said, "You know, one day, you're going to look on this moment and you're going to think about me. And, this is what you're going to remember." I continued, "This is how I want you to think of me." And he said, "You just engulf yourself with what you love". And, that's <u>exactly</u> what I do!

<u>ADVICE:</u> Getting angry is natural. But, don't let it consume you; it only drags you down and does not help you at all. There is a lot to be said about attitude; a positive attitude, a fighting attitude. You want those you love and those who love you, to feel your love, not your anger.

* Rick S. (CLL: Blood & Bone Marrow cancer)

I wasn't angry or bitter. I was just disgusted at the whole thing because I had always taken care of myself. I ate well. I exercised for six hours a day, and I watched what I ate too. I couldn't figure out for the life of me how I ended up with Leukemia. I also had disgust for myself, because I would just sit on my chair for three hours, which didn't do my physical fitness any good. I did that for months, which drained my energy.

ADVICE: You can be angry or bitter or disgusted, but don't spend all your time thinking about it. If you just sit on your chair or stay in your room for hours doing nothing, but think about how bad you're feeling, then you're not doing yourself any good. Go out and do something you enjoy.

* Scott M. (Metastatic Colon cancer to the Prostate & Pancreas)

I was really angry when I found out that I was misdiagnosed a year before I found out I had cancer. I wondered what that delay of one year cost me. If I had done a colonoscopy a year earlier, would I have been a stage III as opposed to a stage IV and improve my chances of survival? So I went through that anger. I even sought the advice of a medical attorney to see if I had a medical malpractice claim. But, for the state of California, it's a "he said-she said" or "he said-he said" kind of thing. At the place where I was diagnosed, they had "canned verbiage", like a boilerplate kind of verbiage that said that they had advised me to do the colonoscopy when, in fact, they hadn't advised me of anything. So, I was pretty angry. But, at the same time, I'm a fighter. I was 23 years in the military; very disciplined. Failure is not an option. So, I had the strength and fortitude mentally to say we're going to beat this.

ADVICE: It's natural to feel anger, when you think you were wronged or when you think life is unfair. So, it's okay to be angry at the situation. But, what doesn't work is when you let that anger take over you and bring you down. Move past it and focus on getting better.

* Susan M. (Ovarian cancer, Metastatic Pancreatic cancer to the Lungs)

When I learned I had pancreatic cancer, I was honestly angry, because I had just retired at the end of December 2015 and really looked forward to enjoying retirement. I felt like I was going to be cheated out of my retirement life.

ADVICE: It's natural to feel angry, especially after working for so long and looking forward to a peaceful and relaxing life of retirement. Still, you can't let your anger overwhelm you and keep you from what you need to focus on, which is healing and beating cancer!

* Tet M. (Colon cancer 3x)

Surprisingly, I did not experience anger, bitterness or resentment when I was told I had Colon Cancer. Instead, I felt relieved that it had happened to me and not to anyone else in my family. Not once did I utter the words "Why me?" I'm not the most religious person around, but this experience made me realize that I was up against a formidable opponent, and it brought me closer to God, knowing He was going to be here by my side. And He hasn't failed me since.

ADVICE: If you are the religious type, surrender yourself to your faith and let it take all the worries away. If you are not the religious type, you may want to seek counseling from therapists. Surround yourself with positive people who truly care about you. Distract yourself with hobbies or activities that make you happy.

* Aaron C. (Prostate cancer, Skin cancer)

Well, I experienced the regular anxiety of not being able to function normally. It's very frustrating, as a male, to not get normal erections like I did before. Those are the worst side effects. It gets depressing sometimes and I get moody. I get more irritable because I have to wear a diaper. Actually, I have to wear a pad all the time, pretty much. At night, I don't wear one. You know, it's the most private area of a man's body and it's the most affected by it.

> **ADVICE:** You know, you've got to look at the big picture. And, stay healthy. Keep exercising. When you exercise, you're forcing the blood to flow through your whole body. So stay active and do your Kegel exercises. Also, don't waste your time buying those diaper underwear pants; they're ridiculous! Just go right to the (incontinence) pads. Those are a lot easier to deal with and that's all you need.

* Amor T. (Breast cancer, Ovarian cancer)

Breast cancer: I had a left breast mastectomy and DIEP flap breast reconstruction surgery that lasted eight hours. After surgery I was placed in ICU overnight. When I woke up, I was in a drugged (I call it "happy dopey") state. My nurse gave me instructions on how to use the intravenous Patient-Controlled Analgesia (PCA) I was connected to, which allowed me to administer my own painkiller with just a push of a button.

She said that I should press the button when I feel pain or when I feel it's about to come. The PCA pump is programmed to give a certain amount of medication when I press the button. It will only allow me to have so much medication (i.e. one release every six minutes), no matter how often I press the button, so I won't need to worry about giving myself too much. Well, I am the type of person who does not want to depend on painkillers; I think I have a high threshold for pain. So, I tried to hold off on pushing the PCA button.

Unfortunately, the following day, two aides came by and told me that they were going to move me to a regular room. When they first came in, I didn't feel any pain. But then, when they tried to move me from my bed to the gurney, that's when the intense pain struck and I screamed in pain and panic. I asked them to hold off while I pressed my PCA button and wait until the pain med took effect. Well, they didn't wait long enough (I guess they were on a schedule), because next thing I knew, they lifted me from my bed and onto the gurney, despite my screams of pain. It was really rough; they were not gentle at all and it was really scary. From that experience, I developed anxiety. Everytime I felt, even a tiny bit of pain, I pressed the PCA button. I definitely didn't want to feel that excruciating pain again.

Ovarian cancer: There were times when I my bone pain would be constant, I would get anxious about falling or breaking my bones. I also experienced anxieties when neuropathy hit and I didn't feel stable enough to walk, or even stand. Those anxieties didn't last long, because I was always reminded that, no matter what, God is with me.

> **ADVICE:** When you're anxious, in a panic or paranoid, you're worrying excessively about losing control, especially if it's based on a past painful experience. Best thing to do to put those emotions aside is to distract yourself with pleasant and positive thoughts. Your physical circumstances are your physical circumstances. You actually have the power within you to rise above them with your spirit and focus on thoughts that benefit you...good, happy thoughts.
>
> By the way, if you were given instructions (like when to use the PCA), follow those instructions. That way, because you'll be ready, you won't develop anxieties about pain occurring when you're not ready.

* Cindy L. (Kidney cancer)

For some time, after my diagnosis, I felt highly anxious and had trouble sleeping. I was always able to just work through any kind of anxiety before. But, having cancer and the thought of losing a kidney was a little more than I could handle. When I met with my urologist, who is wonderful and a highly skilled surgeon, he saw that I was highly anxious and very emotional. So, he prescribed the sedative Ativan to help me sleep and relieve my anxiety.

I learned to do some deep breathing, some meditation, some yoga and some Pilates, just to help me to relax. I went for walks and changed whatever activity I was doing when I got anxious to something else, like getting back out to nature, going for walks on the beach or taking pictures. I physically changed the activity I was doing. That really helped me with my anxiety.

I used to get panic attacks years ago; it kind of runs in my family. For whatever reason, they stopped. I don't have panic attacks now, but I tend to have anxiety. Anxiety over things that I feel I should be handling better. Silly little things like, "Oh, my gosh. I've got to go home and take the trash out!" Now, that's silly enough. But to me, I got anxious over strange things. Maybe it's something that came with my menopause. Or maybe some of my natural, negative emotions were magnified by what I went through with kidney cancer and this was part of the physiological effects. I've been discussing this with my doctor and my psychologist.

ADVICE: Talk to your doctor about the anxiety you're feeling. It's natural to go through such emotions when you're dealing with a serious illness. Your doctor may prescribe you a sedative like Ativan to help relieve your anxiety. Deep breathing, meditation, yoga, Pilates and similar activities help too. When you feel you're getting anxious, change whatever activity you're doing to something different, like getting back to nature, taking pictures, etc.

* Cindy R. (Metastatic Breast cancer to the Stomach)

I had some anxiety or panic, especially when my doctor was telling me, "Oh, I only saw this patient twice and haven't seen him since." I was like, "Oh my God! Maybe this is it!" But then, I would tell myself, "No, no, no ... I'm going to fight it. I don't want to be one of the stats. I don't want to know that I have an expiration date. I'm just going to fight this and do everything in my power; everything in my spiritual power; everything in my nutritional power to fight it!"

ADVICE: When your mind tries to pull you into being anxious and panicky about the unknown or awful negative outcomes, break out of that thinking and fight it with everything you have. When you have the determination to beat these negative emotions, you'll come out of your challenges stronger and win against cancer.

* Glenn M. (Metastatic Colon cancer to Liver, Lungs & Adrenal Glands)

I did panic when I first learned I had stage IV colon cancer. I kept saying, "Sh*t! Sh*t! Sh*t!" because I didn't know what I was going to do. Good thing my wife, Barbara, was there to support me and calm me down.

I also had anxiety at work when I was operating without updated records. I think about all sorts of "what-ifs"; things that could go wrong while I was waiting for the updated records and what I could lose. Fortunately, my oncologist helped me out. He's my hero!

ADVICE: It's easy to panic when you get really bad news that throws you for a big loop. You get confused and your mind goes all over the place really fast. Have someone you trust be with you to help calm you when you receive the news.

On anxiety, it helps to stop over-thinking things, especially in negative ways. Those "what-ifs" don't help. Just work with what you've got. Do what you can.

* Hilda K. (Colon cancer)

Only on a couple of occasions did I experience anxiety or panic. The first time happened during my chemo infusion. For some unknown reason, I got dizzy and started panicking. The nurses told me that it happens and gave me extra medication to calm me down. In the other incident, I forgot that with my hypothermia, I had to stay away from taking in anything cold. Well, instead of drinking warm water; I drank cold water. Immediately, I felt I was suffocating, because my throat was constricting and I couldn't breathe. So, my husband called emergency. However, I was able to calm down and breathe normally. It was just one of those panic moments. Learning from that episode, I became more aware of the temperature of what I drank or ate; I avoided anything that was cold.

* J.B. (Salivary gland cancer)

Anxiety caused my poor sleep habits and they were definitely strongest before any of my treatments. I had a hard time sleeping, which was really something I was doing to myself, because I'd be up researching online what I could about my cancer. Since my cancer is very rare, there really wasn't much information online. So, I would keep reading the same article or try to find different statistics online, like survival rates and stuff like that. I probably shouldn't have read as much as I did. But, it was just a way to numb myself; a way to cope.

I tend to look for the worst that could happen. I wanted to just deal with it and say, "OK, so let it be. This is what it is. If it's going to be that way, then so be it." Like I said earlier, I basically numbed myself with the knowledge. But I think there's a fine line between the anxiety and the numbing. The initial anxiety went away after a while. I had a lot of support from my girlfriend. I'm not really the type to seek emotional help from other people.

* Rachel S. (Breast cancer: triple negative)

I dealt with anxiety, panic and paranoia pretty much the same way I dealt with depression. I shoved them aside, as much as I could.

Of course, I experienced anxiety. I had thoughts about...God forbid this treatment doesn't work, what will happen to me? What if my cancer comes back? What are my kids going to do? It was an awful feeling. So, I made a decision early on that I was <u>not</u> going to let these negative thoughts eat me alive, and I was going to make life as good for my kids as I possibly can. Because, if I don't survive this, I wanted them to have good memories; not bad memories. I was really determined about that. I just was not going to leave this world and have them think of me as always being upset. When they think of me, I want them to think: my mom was very positive and my mom was happy.

The other thing that I did was take to Facebook in a big way. I did so for three reasons:

1. My Facebook community gave me the support I felt I needed;
2. Whenever I was upset, it helped to read back on my posts and my friends' caring comments, and
3. I received positivity and encouragement through Facebook.

* Rick S. (CLL: Blood & Bone Marrow cancer)

I went through a little anxiety about what was going to happen to me. But, nothing ever happened to me. I built it up in my own mind.

When I started chemo, I was initially in a high state of anxiety. So people from church would take me to the oncology lab where my chemo sessions were at and, most times, would stay with me. Then, the nurses always took care of me, smothering me with love and attention. They had me sit on a nice beautiful, comfortable reclining chair. They raised the leg portion of the chair and had me lay there like I was in a recliner. They gave me a nice hot warm blanket and wrapped it around me. The nurses were always there, watching me and the other cancer patients. No one was going let me be alone. So, I felt that I was well taken care of and didn't feel that high state of anxiety anymore.

* Scott M. (Metastatic Colon cancer to Prostate & Pancreas)

I used to be a high-strung, Air Force pilot type person with a high threshold for pain. However, when I experienced excruciating pain from some of what was done to me while I was being treated, I developed an anxiety to pain. So, I learned to just communicate my anxiety to pain with my doctor, who gave me anti-anxiety meds, as well as painkillers. The anti-anxiety meds helped keep me chill.

* Sondra W. (Ovarian cancer 3x)

I had nocturnal anxiety, which is a panic attack that awakened Kenneth from sleep. I had anxiety because there was so much to do when I got diagnosed such as making arrangements to send my 95-year old mother, who I had been taking care of, to my brother in Ohio and placing her in a facility there. There was so much going on and so much to do to get all her stuff together. I just got overwhelmed with what I was being asked to do for her move, while at the same time, having to deal with my diagnosis. Eventually, I realized that I couldn't do it all, and I had to focus on my health. When that got cleared, I didn't have those anxieties anymore.

* Susan M. (Ovarian cancer. Metastatic Pancreatic cancer to the Lungs)

Even though I experienced anxieties during treatment for pancreatic cancer, I didn't have them very often. I tried to stay busy and relied on my faith. I also took up yoga.

* Tet M. (Colon cancer 3x)

Ever since I found blood in my stool, I would be concerned that every time, I would detect a discoloration of my stool. And yes, since I was 27, I would always look at what's in the toilet bowl after each and every bowel movement.

* Yesi L. (Breast cancer: triple positive)

I definitely had a lot of anxiety and paranoia just dealing with the possibility of recurrence or what was going to happen. I had a lot of uncertainty, thinking "how am I going to get through this?" and "how can my body continue to take the treatments?" Especially after being hospitalized, it was definitely scary. So psychologically, emotionally it was very, very draining.

I was not prepared for the struggling I had with all the emotional side effects of having cancer and the treatments. I understand that they mostly came from me. And, they got a lot worse after treatment was over.

CONFUSION

* Amor T. (Breast cancer, Ovarian cancer)

My confusion was actually from my chemo brain. Not remembering things, not being able to multitask, not being able to focus on things or conversations ... all those thinking skills I was able to easily do before, I had difficulty doing. I remember asking myself, "What? What just happened?" I was confused and at a loss. I thought something was wrong with me and didn't know why. Fortunately, I later learned that I was going through "chemo brain" and it will eventually pass.

ADVICE: If you're confused about anything, just remember that your entire body, which includes your brain, is going through cancer treatment. Be kind to yourself; don't judge yourself for your confusion. If anyone has a problem with you being confused, don't let it affect you. It's their problem, not yours.

* Glenn M. (Metastatic Colon cancer to the Liver, Lungs & Adrenal Glands)

I've gotten to the point where, at the end of the day, I evaluate the day by how much time I spent trying to find things I misplaced, like my phone. With my hearing loss, it doesn't help a lot to call my phone when I misplace it. I have to actually see it with my eyes. Misplacing my phone has caused me a lot of confusion and it's so frustrating. So, here's what I did to solve that problem.

I basically have a long, stretchy string attached to my phone that's also attached to my pen. You know what it is? It's a "Chums." Chums have these strong elastics that help you hold on to your eyeglasses that is strung around your neck, so you can dangle your eyeglasses. So, to be able to find my phone, I have one end of the Chums elastic string attached to my pen and the other end attached to my phone. When I want to use my phone, I just pick up my pen.

There was an incident during my first infusion when my chair "ate" my phone. I had to get my nurse KB to call my phone, so I could find it. That was before I thought of the Chums elastic attachment that helps avoid confusion and frustration.

When it comes to thinking about how much time was spent...oh, like three hours looking for stupid stuff and I know it's in the house somewhere. It's self-defense. I don't like losing stuff. I don't like feeling confused.

ADVICE: Well, this is what I tell myself: "Don't get confused!" Seriously. Try to calm down and relax. You think better and clearer when you're not all worked up. And, getting all worked up doesn't help. Get someone to help find things or figure things out.

* J.B. (Salivary gland cancer)

I did not have any anger, but I did have confusion. I felt a whole bunch of emotions all at once, which I think came from all the constant research and planning that I was doing. I really wanted to know of cases similar to mine and where my situation applied. I also researched the hospital's website where I was able to ask doctors and nurses online the questions I had about my cancer and my options. I did a lot of that. So, of course, with all the information I got as well as with all the unanswered questions (due to the rarity of my case), I got confused.

* Scott M. (*Metastatic Colon cancer to the Prostate & Pancreas*)

Confusion came with my chemo brain; it's extremely noticeable. When I was new to cancer and before I read any magazines about it, I told my doctor, "Hey doc, I have this like chemo brain." I thought I came up with a new term. He then pointed at a magazine that read, "Chemo Brain: How to Deal with It". And I went, "Oh, so I guess I'm not the first one to go through it." It made me feel better that I wasn't the only one experiencing chemo brain. But, it did create confusion, in the beginning.

> <u>ADVICE:</u> It's so important to reach out to others. They may not have exactly the same experiences as you, but they have already navigated those waters and may be able to help you with a technique to cope or understand.

* Sondra W. (*Ovarian cancer 3x*)

There was confusion when sometimes, I didn't realize it was me who was confused. At that time, my husband Kenneth was working long hours, different shifts, and commuting to Oakland for work. He wasn't getting much rest, because when he'd get home, he had to spend all that time with me. It was exhausting and, so he took a hit. At one point, he just couldn't do it all. And so, we both experienced confusion with what we needed to do for ourselves and for each other. I finally realized that I just had to slow down and not think too much; not try to do too much. I learned that I needed to take one step at a time; one day at a time.

> <u>ADVICE:</u> When you're confused, pull back and see things from an objective point of view. Slow down and try not to think too much or do too much. And then, just have extra conversations. Communicate.

DEPRESSION

---

* Amor T. (*Breast cancer, Ovarian cancer*)

I remember a really sad time when I was at home trying to recuperate from my mastectomy and DIEP flap breast reconstruction surgery. At the time, I was dating someone who I thought cared for me. When I asked him for some assistance, he yelled at me. That really took me aback, because I was in pain and felt so helpless. I am the type of person who really tries not to ask for assistance or help, unless I really need it. Well, after he yelled at me, I quietly cried and got really depressed. It was like I was trapped, both physically and emotionally. After that episode, I stayed quiet and pretended I was strong, when in reality, I was in pain and struggling. I did not ask for his help anymore. Even though, with him, I was not alone physically, I felt that it would've been better if I were. It was like I was trapped, both physically and emotionally.

What I did to lift my spirits up was talk with God and lean on Him for the comfort and peace of His Love. With God in me, I no longer felt alone. God also constantly reminded me to be thankful; there are so many people who love me, no matter what. There are also so many in this world who are suffering far worse circumstances than I am. I also thought of the many reasons I have to be thankful. When I was down, I remember looking around thanking God for everything I saw, e.g. the sky, the blanket, my clothes, the trees, the birds, etc. It was sometimes hard to do, because I hurt so deeply inside. Still, I continued the practice being thankful for everything I saw with my eyes and, eventually, the darkness lifted and I felt joy and peace again.

> <u>ADVICE:</u> However this example of depression was not caused by having cancer per se, it is part of the reality that sometimes comes with dealing with cancer. Defined, depression is a mood disorder that causes a persistent feeling of sadness and loss of interest and can interfere with your daily functioning.
>
> If you're going through depression, you're having thoughts that are disempowering; thoughts that are not happy thoughts that lift your spirits. Every time a disempowering thought tries to bring you down, replace it with a happy thought. Remind yourself that you want to be happy. Whatever the cause(s) of your unhappy, disempowering thoughts, e.g. dealing with cancer, people who hurt you, not being able to control your circumstances, etc... replace them with reasons to be happy and thankful. Do things to distract you from your depression, like chat

with friends, watch a fun movie, enjoy a good book, etc. Also, try practicing looking around and being thankful for everything you see. Sure, it may be silly, but it works to lift your spirits. Being "silly" is much better than being depressed.

Get professional help. They're trained, educated and have helped those in your similar situation. Please don't let your pride get in the way. Talking with professionals can be the eye-opener you need to lift you out of your depression. If you're spiritual, talk with God...and open your mind and heart to really listen to Him. With God, you can really find the Peace and Joy you're looking for. You just have to believe.

* Glenn M. (Metastatic Colon cancer to the Liver, Lungs & Adrenal Glands)

I think it might be in my blood, because my dad had depression and it wasn't covered by Medicare. For treatment, I think he had 30 electric shock treatments that cost him $30,000. I said, "Just give him $30,000 and he won't get depressed anymore!"

Anyway, I don't think of depression. I'm spiritual. I'm also religious, but not overly religious. I think it does help to be spiritual when I get depressed. I think God loves me. I think that and it makes me feel good.

ADVICE: I think that depression sets in when you can't control things and there's so much in life you can't control. So why try to control it and get all depressed when you can't? Try looking beyond. Being spiritual and thinking that God loves you, no matter what, will help you get out of your depression.

* Rachel S. (Breast cancer: triple negative)

Although I fought to shove depression and other negative emotions aside, there were times when they would hit me. When that happened, I would go to my Facebook page and read the supportive words of encouragement from my friends and family and they would pick me up.

I have people who criticize me for taking to Facebook the way did (and do). But, Facebook has helped me get through a lot. So, their criticism can't stop me from using Facebook.

ADVICE: It is understandable to feel depression or other negative emotions. But, it is important not to dwell on them, because they only bring you down and do not help you feel better at all. You can get help from your family, community or medical team. You can also use Facebook (or other positive social media sites) to distract you from the negative and pick up your spirits when you are feeling down.

* Rick S. (CLL: Blood & Bone Marrow cancer)

I did have depression and I also felt frustration, because I couldn't do what I did before. And, I guess I felt those emotions because I let my mind take me places where it shouldn't have taken me. I let my mind defeat me. I should've gotten up and mowed the lawn. I should've gotten up and gone to the gym. I should've just fought my frustration and depression and done those things.

ADVICE: When you're feeling frustrated and depressed, fight it! Don't go there. Instead, get up and do something like mow the lawn, exercise, meet with your friends, take a walk, listen to music, or some activity you enjoy. Just don't allow your mind to take you to dark places that don't help you.

* Scott M. (Metastatic Colon cancer to the Prostate & Pancreas)

I'm now on anti-depressants. I'm in a vulnerable time in my life, so I'm at a weakened state. I'm also on anti-anxiety meds; they help keep me chill. One of my mottos is: "No Stress". So, I try and avoid stress, whenever possible. With all the meds I'm taking, I feel like I'm a representative for "better living through pharmaceuticals."

* Sondra W. (Ovarian cancer 3x)

Oh, no, no. That's not me at all. It's so funny because you know when you go in for your appointment, and they ask you, "Do you have any thoughts of harming yourself?" Well, I answered, "You've got to be kidding me! You see how hard I'm working? No way!"

ADVICE: Yes, having to deal with cancer is challenging. However, you are important, and your health is worth fighting for. So, don't use up your energy getting depressed focusing on your cancer. Use your energy to fight it every way you can. You may be physically weak, but you can be strong spiritually and emotionally. So, keep the faith! In doing so, you will beat cancer!

* Vida B.A. (Breast cancer)

There were moments after chemo when I felt so down and depressed. I tried not to feel that and show it to the world. But, of course, I couldn't avoid feeling it, so I really tried hard not to make a big fuss about it. The week of chemo and the week after were the times when I was down and out. I experienced numbness and pain and was sensitive until after that time passed and I got my senses back. After those two weeks...Well, the third week was my "happy" week. I didn't fully realize it at the time, but those feelings came in cycles.

One of the things that depressed me was having to be confined to my room for those first two weeks after chemo. To cope, I tried not to think about my situation and just accept it. There were definitely times when I was down and just turned off the lights to go to sleep. However, for the most part when I felt depressed, I tried to distract myself with things to do throughout the day, like play games and read Facebook posts. After a while, I got the hang of it.

ADVICE: When you feel down and out, try to stop your mind from focusing on your illness, as much as possible. That doesn't do you any good. Instead, try to distract yourself with things to do throughout the day or night, like play games, read Facebook posts, watch a movie, talk with your family or friends, etc. You'll eventually get the hang of it. Of course, there will be times you just don't feel like doing anything and that's okay. Focus on your blessings and all the positive around you and don't let your situation control you.

* Yesi L. (Breast cancer: triple positive)

Depression hit me really hard. I sometimes lived in a void during treatment. But definitely, after treatment, I was in a void.

ADVICE: Keep in mind that your family and friends love you and focus on that, no matter what. If you find that you still don't feel any happiness, especially, if you feel very agitated or resentful on that of that, then you must seek professional help. You may have a psychological issue caused by the trauma of your treatment. Reach out to a psychological therapist.

FEAR

---

* Amor T. (Breast cancer, Ovarian cancer)

Breast cancer. The only times I felt fear were during the times I felt intense pain while being treated for breast cancer. One episode occurred in ICU when the hospital aides moved me from my ICU bed to the gurney and my painkiller had not yet taken effect. My screams of fear and panic seemed to fall on deaf ears as they transported me to my regular room. I feared the pain would never end.

The other episode happened while I was having a conversation with my friend, Macy, who was visiting me at the hospital. I felt a pain that jabbed me so hard in my abdomen, an intense heaviness set in and I couldn't breathe. I remember being very afraid that I would not be able to see my daughter Catherine again. I felt both fear and deep sadness. Those were frightening experiences for me.

Ovarian cancer. This time around with ovarian cancer, fear did not grip me like it did before with breast cancer. That's because, I had grown stronger as a woman and my faith was stronger. I also had (and still have) my amazing life partner Bill who, not only completely supported me in all my needs, he made me feel safe and protected.

During the times I felt my body just getting weaker and I didn't know if I was going to make it, I turned to God for comfort and peace. Having faith really kept my fears away. This is when I started to read the daily message from the "Jesus Calling" book that my awesome friend Val gave to me and recite the Holy Rosary every day. To this day, I continue and it always gives me comfort and peace.

> <u>ADVICE:</u> Fear is normal when you're going through a serious life changing illness. Don't ignore your fears or criticize yourself for being afraid. That will only make things worse. Talk with someone about your fears, like a loved one, friend, or professional (therapist, doctor, nurse, etc.) Being able to vent will help release the negativity that comes with fear or any negative emotion.
>
> If you're spiritual, talk with God. Vent to Him. Say whatever you need to say, without restricting yourself. Then, listen with an open heart to hear what God says to you. Feel His comfort and love. Thank Him for your blessings, no matter how afraid you're feeling. When you do, you will find peace envelop you and your fears will go away. When you practice this every time you feel afraid, your fears will eventually disappear and be replaced by peace and goodness.

* *Cindy L. (Kidney cancer)*

Yes, I experienced the fear of, "What if it comes back?" That sort of thing. But, then I think, "What if I go out on Highway 98 and get hit by a truck?" So, I've learned to put that fear into perspective. I tend to be able to tuck that fear away until Sunday night or Monday night; the night before my blood draw, my MRI or the following Sunday night before I meet with my doctor. That's when high anxiety and fear hit me. Right before those tests, I start asking, "What if? What if? What if?" And then afterwards, my emotions return to normal.

To calm my fears, I first recognize it for what it is and put it into perspective. It's not based on anything factual. Deep breathing and stretching help. I also find someone to talk to. Having someone to talk to, I think, helps the most.

> <u>ADVICE:</u> Take deep breaths and put your fear into perspective. That fear isn't based on anything factual. Stretch your body too, however way you want. It gets the blood circulation going and your helps keep your mind from thinking too much. Most of all, find someone to talk to.

* *Cindy R. (Metastatic Breast cancer to the Stomach)*

I felt fear the second time around when I was diagnosed with stomach cancer, but not the first time around when I received my breast cancer diagnosis. When I found out I had stomach cancer, I initially thought, "Is this really the end? Oh my gosh, this is not good."

The first time around (breast cancer diagnosis), it was weird, because I was like, "Okay, I have cancer. Okay let's just take care of it and get it out of my body."

To cope with my fear, I had to internalize it myself. I saw the look of fear in my mom's face that seemed to say, "Oh my God, I might lose my daughter." But I was like, "No, I'm not going to let it happen. I've got so much to do and so much to live for. I'm not going to let this get to me."

For the most part, I tried to stay positive. I even got involved in ladies groups, even though I was sick. I belonged to four or five different ladies groups. I also have my dogs that I play with all the time and I have to take care of them; I can't be sick. So, that was my mindset in dealing with my fear. My life had purpose and I was living my life with purpose.

* Hilda K. (Colon cancer)

After surgery, my whole family ... everybody came to the hospital, including my brother-in-law from Hawaii. My sister Nita, who had cancer twenty years ago, was also there. I think she was the most fearful of all, because she experienced it herself. Crazy...it was crazy! They were all there and I was shocked when I woke up. My brother-in-law came from Hawaii to support my sister and to support everyone, because they were totally scared...I mean, literally scared. I couldn't believe how fearful they were and I was trying not to be scared. But, they made ME scared, because THEY were scared. It was as if they were telling me "goodbye." So, I just said, "See you guys later. I'm going to go to sleep."

Whenever I feel fear and uncertainty, I always go back to prayer and my faith in God. When I prayed, I felt that my prayers were being heard and I believed that God would help me through this challenge. I asked Him for strength and to help me to live as long as I can.

When the doctors told me that I had Colon Cancer and the worst that could happen would be for my entire colon to be removed and to live with colostomy bag for the rest of my life, I remember praying to God, "I don't mind the worst. Just let me live as long as I can, so that I can be with my children and get old. I will live with the bag forever; just, please, give me some more time." That was my realization. That was my acceptance.

For me, my faith in God and my trust that He would guide and strengthen me, helped me conquer my fears. I knew that I also had to keep positive, no matter what. I couldn't let the negative feelings, like loneliness or self-pity, take me down. I also knew that I could only depend on myself to be strong through this challenge. That definitely helped me heal, because I was in good spiritual and mental health and I was determined too.

* Jacki S. (Breast cancer)

When I learned I had cancer, I was scared and in shock. I couldn't believe I had cancer. I followed what my doctor advised me to do and talked with other cancer survivors.

* Joan S. (Rectal cancer)

I had a fear of the unknown. I was afraid of what could happen. It wasn't easy. What helped me was prayer, keeping positive and being thankful. Prayer helped me feel calm. Keeping positive made me feel better about my situation; it gave me hope. And, being thankful, just reminded me of how blessed I am.

* Rev. Linda S. (Pancreatic cancer 3x)

When I was first diagnosed, the only things I feared were uncontrollable pain and leaving my elderly mother, for whom I am her primary caregiver. My faith, family, and friends helped me cope. Then, when I was informed that the pancreatic mass I thought was removed by surgery and eighteen chemo treatments had returned in less than a year and had actually grown during six months of chemotherapy, I was really frightened.

ADVICE: Try to keep the faith and allow family and friends to be there for you, as much as possible.

* Rick S. (CLL: Blood & Bone Marrow cancer)

I didn't have fear that something was going to happen to me, because I had a good doctor. However, I did have fear that I was going to lose my strength.

* Scott M. (Metastatic Colon cancer to the Prostate & Pancreas)

There is fear of the unknown. I talk it out with people and then come to my own conclusions. I do know that there is less fear with me talking with the nurses and the doctors here at the Cancer Center about the similar cases they have that are positive and the ones that they are winning. So, I focus on those and that tends to allay my fears.

ADVICE: It's natural to have fear, especially when you're feeling vulnerable and in a weakened state. However, you have to talk it out with people. Talk with your doctors and nurses about the positive cases that are similar to yours and the ones they're winning in. Focus on the positive and your fears will be relieved.

* Sondra W. (Ovarian cancer 3x)

I experienced fear of the unknown. Initially and for a brief period of time, I was feeling afraid, but couldn't pinpoint why. So, I stopped to really think, "Okay, what am I afraid of?" Eventually, I realized that, with all that was going one, I was afraid of the unknown. To deal with my fear, I did scripture reading and I used music to kind of slow myself down too. I also gathered information to better understand my situation.

ADVICE: Having fear when you're diagnosed with cancer is natural. You need to think of exactly what you're afraid of. That will help you come to terms with it. Then, think of ways to calm your fears like using prayer, meditation, research, or whatever activity you find helps.

* Susan M. (Ovarian cancer, Metastatic Pancreatic cancer to the Lungs)

Ovarian Cancer: It was December 1984 when I was diagnosed with stage II ovarian cancer, after my hysterectomy. Although I was somewhat surprised, I knew it was hereditary, because my mom had it. The worst part was the gripping fear I felt thinking I would never see my then eighteen-month old baby grow up. However horrible I felt, I knew that I had to really focus on recovery for my family's sake.

Pancreatic Cancer: Having cancer again was a horrible feeling and definitely scared me. I prayed a lot and tried really hard to stay positive.

ADVICE: Fear can paralyze you, if you allow it to take over your emotions. Although it's natural to be afraid, try to focus on what you <u>can</u> do to get better and heal, for your sake and for those who love you. If you need to, get professional help.

* Yesi L. (Breast cancer: triple positive)

I had a lot of fear of the cancer coming back, not fear of the treatments or pain. It's definitely gotten better, but it's not gone. I think that's just natural. I knew my fear was psychological. So, I did get a lot of help from therapy.

* *Amor T.* (*Breast cancer, Ovarian cancer*)

I experienced frustration with my health condition and with billing and insurance challenges that came my way. Instead of staying frustrated, I just looked at the facts and do what I could to resolve whatever situation was causing my frustration. If the cause was my cancer, I knew it would take time to heal, so I just needed to be patient and bear the pains. If the cause was something like complicated billing errors, I researched what I could and, using facts and reason, calmly dealt with the billing source. I never stayed frustrated, because I always reminded myself of those who are less fortunate than me, especially innocent children who are suffering.

ADVICE: When you're in pain or just not feeling well, it's easy to feel frustrated. A lot of frustration is based on expectation, especially when you've experienced things working and being better. It's important to see frustration for what it is. A natural human emotion. It's also important to not let it get out of control. If you're frustrated about your health condition and you're getting treatment, think of how your treatment will get you better with time and then, be patient. If your frustration stems from other causes, focus on what you can do to change or resolve it with facts (objectively), not hypotheses (subjectively).

* *Bob G.* (*Soft Tissue Sarcoma, Skin cancer*)

For the treatments, I clearly remember that I kept thinking, "Let's get it done!" The doctors seemed to be taking their time and I was getting frustrated, because I wanted the cancer out! I also kept thinking that my kids weren't prepared for me to leave this earth ... and I STILL feel that way!

ADVICE: Let your doctor or nurse know if you're frustrated about anything. That way, they can explain the process or their plans to you and you'll get some answers, if not all.

* *Cindy L.* (*Kidney cancer*)

I had a lot of frustration when I was going through treatment. And I still get frustrated because of my physical weight. One of the biggest frustrations was not being able to pick up my granddaughters, even the eight-month old baby who weighs 24 lbs. Yes, I did try to pick her up at one point, but I paid for it. I was really sore the next day.

I was in the hospital for only two and a half days. Yes, it was a pretty quick stay. I was in a step-down ICU the whole time I was there. I was fortunate that I had one-on-one nursing care and I actually had two medical technicians all to myself. I had a urinary catheter for a short time. Once they removed it, of course, I had to walk to the bathroom, which was very difficult.

I couldn't bend over because of the incisions in my abdomen; it was so frustrating. And they were putting so many fluids into me, especially Ringer's Solution (a special solution of salts), to force my remaining kidney to get real active. So I felt like I had to pee every 15 minutes, but I could barely get to the bathroom. It was really a struggle.

The first night after surgery, I remember experiencing a lot of discomfort. I wanted to brush my teeth. So, the tech stood behind me, because I was pretty unsteady. Obviously, a tall person made the sink, because I couldn't get high enough to reach over to spit into the sink. I'm 5'1" and a half. I'm very long-waisted and my legs and arms are shorter that a person who is the same height as me. Anyway, I remember getting so frustrated, the tech grabbed me a little basin to spit into. It was the small basin the hospital has for patients to vomit into when in bed. Good thing the tech was swift-thinking, because I was about to gag and just couldn't reach the sink. After, I said, "Boy, this sucks. I can't even reach the sink in here!" Yes, really frustrating.

ADVICE: When you have abdominal surgery, your abdominal muscles will be weak and you'll feel pain when you do anything that requires movement in your abdomen, like coughing, sneezing or getting up from your bed or chair to walk to the bathroom or wherever. Get a pillow or a rolled-up towel and use it as a split every time you're about to move. Just press it firmly but gently on your abdomen as you're about to move, and then move. Sure, feeling pain and not being able to move is frustrating, but start slow and get assistance. Be patient and allow your body to heal. Getting all worked up isn't going to make things better. Take deep breaths and try to be positive.

* Glenn M. (Metastatic Colon cancer to the Liver, Lungs & Adrenal Glands)

I've gotten to the point where, at the end of the day, I evaluate the day by how much time I spent trying to find things I misplaced, like my phone. With my hearing loss, it doesn't help a lot to call my phone when I misplace it. I have to actually see it with my eyes. Misplacing my phone has caused me a lot of confusion and it's so frustrating. So, here's what I did to solve that problem.

I basically have a long, stretchy string or cord attached to my phone that's also attached to my pen. You know what it is? It's a "Chums." Chums have these strong elastics that help you hold on to your eyeglasses that is strung around your neck, so you can dangle your eyeglasses. So, to be able to find my phone, I have one end of the Chums elastic cord attached to my pen and the other end attached to my phone. When I want to use my phone, I just have to pick up my pen.

There was an incident during my first infusion when my chair "ate" my phone. I had to get my nurse KB to call my phone, so I could find it. That was before I thought of the Chums elastic attachment that helps avoid confusion and frustration.

When it comes to thinking about how much time was spent...oh, like three hours looking for stupid stuff and I know it's in the house somewhere. It's self-defense. I don't like losing stuff. I get frustrated when I do.

ADVICE: Try to calm down and relax. You think better and clearer when you're not all worked up. And, getting all worked up doesn't help. Get someone to help you find things or figure things out with you.

Also, try this. If you keep losing things you need handy (like your cell phone), get a strong, elastic cord, like the ones they sell to attach to eyeglasses or sunglasses, so you can wear it like a necklace with your glasses dangling from it. Chums is the brand I used. Attach one end of the cord to a pen or something that you reach out for often. Then attach the other end to the object you keep losing, like a cell phone (or whatever).

* Rev. Linda S. (Pancreatic cancer 3x)

Whenever I got frustrated by the many things I could not make sense of or control, like waiting, I released and re-released my delusion that I was in control.

ADVICE: The sooner you release thinking you can control people or the process, the sooner you'll feel better.

* Rick S. (CLL: Blood & Bone Marrow cancer)

I felt frustration and got depressed, because I couldn't do what I did before. And, I guess I felt those emotions because I let my mind take me places where it shouldn't have taken me. I let my mind defeat me. I should've gotten up and mowed the lawn. I should've gotten up and gone to the gym. I should've just fought my frustration and depression and done those things.

ADVICE: When you're feeling frustrated and depressed, fight it! Don't go there. Instead, get up and do something like mow the lawn, exercise, meet with your friends, take a walk, listen to music, or some activity you enjoy. Just don't allow your mind to take you to dark places that don't help you.

* Scott M. (Metastatic Colon cancer to the Prostate & Pancreas)

I get frustrated because of my chemo brain, which makes me forgetful. It's almost a form of a dementia, in a way. One day, early on in my chemo treatment (the first six months, which was the worst, because I had the Oxaliplatin), I got up; I got dressed; I got in my car; I drove to the end of my street....At the end of my street, there's a T. You either turn left or you turn right. I didn't know which way to turn, because I had no idea where I was going. I turned around, drove home and I never did figure out what I got up to go do. I just got up, got dressed in business clothes and I was supposed to be someplace. Of course, I didn't make it and I couldn't remember it. So, I got frustrated and a little bit hopeless. I thought, "Gee, is this what lies in my future?" But then, I just kind of said, "Oh well…" and laughed it off. I told myself, "If it's that important, someone will get in touch with me. They'll get a hold of me."

ADVICE: It's natural to be frustrated when you're going through a rough time. But, it's important to not dwell on what's frustrating you and just move on, especially if it's something that can't be changed. Laugh it off too, if you can. It'll help too.

* Sondra W. (Ovarian cancer 3x)

It was more frustration during the times I thought we just made some headway in our move activities or whatever we had to do, but then something would come up. I eventually realized that something is always going to come up and the frustration happens when I don't expect anything to come up. So, I told myself, "Okay, if something doesn't come up, that's great. But, if something does come up, that's not unusual." I learned to be accepting and after that, I didn't experience frustration like I used to.

ADVICE: Learn to accept that everything's not going to turn out like you want it to. If things work out, then that's great. If they don't, then it's not unusual. If you learn to accept that, then you won't get frustrated. Be careful when setting expectations of yourself and others.

* Tet M. (Colon cancer 3x)

My main frustration was handling the anticipation of an upcoming Chemo session. I understood that feeling frustrated was unnecessary and my mind was making matters much worse than they actually were. I knew I was stronger than this, being a fighter all my life, but many times, I found it to be such a difficult challenge. Although my frustration would wear me down, the feeling was temporary and I would, again, get up and tackle it with all my might.

ADVICE: Try to be more positive about the whole experience. Mind over matter could definitely make a difference. And, of course, prayer and faith moves mountains. If you feel worn and beaten, remember that you are human. Give yourself a little time to process and then, pick yourself up and count your blessings. The magnitude of your frustration is based on the energy you give it. Again, mind over matter.

* Yesi L. (Breast cancer: triple positive)

I felt so frustrated at times, because I felt I lost complete control over my body. I felt so vulnerable. I know a lot of us feel that way when we go through illness or something like this. We're not okay with feeling vulnerable. But then I found out that feeling vulnerable is not necessarily a bad thing. I mean, we are human after all. And, it's okay for others to take care of us.

ADVICE: When you're frustrated, because you feel you lost control, just tell yourself that it's okay. Tell yourself that you are only human and it's okay for others to take care of you. Be kind to yourself and let others take care of you.

GRIEF, LOSS, HOPELESSNESS, SADNESS

* Amor T. (Breast cancer, Ovarian cancer)

During my breast cancer experience, I was with someone who made it known that he would rather be somewhere else than with me. There were times he got annoyed with my requests for assistance. One clear memory was of him yelling at me when I asked for something. That really hurt deeply and I quietly cried by myself. I didn't want to depend on him, but

I felt helpless. I could barely move, because of my wounds and I felt such a depth of sadness that pierced me. From that experience, I learned that, even if I'm sick, it's best to only be with those who want to be with me because they really care for me, not because they feel obligated to be with me. If they would rather be somewhere else or if they demonstrate that they don't want to be with me, then I really don't need to be with them either.

What I did to lift my spirits up was talk with God and lean on Him for the comfort and peace of His Love. With God in me, I no longer felt alone. God also constantly reminded me to be thankful; there are so many people who love me, no matter what. There are also so many in this world who are suffering far worse circumstances than I am.

ADVICE: Having cancer can certainly bring about sadness and hopelessness. Not being able to feel good or move about like you used to ... or having to depend on someone who clearly does not want to be with you ... is sad. First, validate your sadness. That means, recognize it for what is: a natural human emotion. Cry, if you need to. That will release pent up negative energy. After crying, you'll be able to think clearly and objectively about what you're going through. Then, focus on what you can do versus what you can't do.

If you're spiritual, lift your problems up to God and lean on Him for comfort and peace. "Let go and let God" is so applicable when you're down and feeling so broken. Think of all you've been blessed with and thank God for every one of them. When you do, you will feel strength and peace and joy in His Love.

* Cindy L. (Kidney cancer)

I'm coming to terms with the loss of my kidney, the emotion I felt was grief. It was like grieving a death really. You see, before my kidney was removed, it was still functioning totally normal. There was not one blood test that showed that anything was wrong with it. Aside from the cancer that was in there, my kidney function was perfect. So, I struggled with losing it.

It's taking me a while to work through my loss; it's taking time to process. Talking about it helps and I'm starting to understand how my body is functioning on one kidney.

ADVICE: Grieving the loss of one of your organs or body parts is normal. So, nothing to be ashamed of. You have to process through the grief though and live in it. It will take time; you just have to move forward and learn to live with what you have. Two years later I still sometimes grieve. It has gotten easier or I guess I've learned how to respond in a different manner.

* Rev. Linda S. (Pancreatic cancer 3x)

I felt them all – grief, hopelessness and profound sadness ~ without guilt or self-recrimination.

ADVICE: Allow yourself to go through the process of grief, hopelessness and/or sadness. Do not suppress them.

* Rick S. (CLL: Blood & Bone Marrow cancer)

I felt sad because I felt alone. Even though I lived in a retirement community with many people, I still felt alone. There were church people who would drop over to visit and I'd get involved in conversation with them and my friends would visit too and we'd talk awhile and my good friend Bill would drop in at just the right time and we'd enjoy our conversations together. Unfortunately, time with my visiting friends are temporary. In the end, I was back to feeling alone. I did meet with therapists about this aloneness that I had been feeling and we're still trying to work it out.

When I felt the sadness of being alone, I tried to get involved in as much as I can handle. I would go for a walk. Get out. Go to the gym or water some plants. I believe it's really important to just get active. Sometimes, with activity, I was able to get rid of my sadness. I tried to do my memorization of Bible verses and I did pretty well. Sometimes, however, they jumbled up in my mind. But, I memorized about 50 or 60 Bible verses, so that definitely helped. After all that, I found that the best thing to do was get out of my house. Just get out. See what's going on. Let the wind blow on my face; something that took away the sadness of being alone.

* Sondra W. (Ovarian cancer 3x)

The first time I felt the deepest sadness was after I heard the diagnosis that I had ovarian cancer. Then, in my mind, I thought Kenneth and I were going to grow old together and maybe we're not. That was really sad for me. Whenever I felt that deep sadness, I would tell Kenneth who would listen and comfort me and pray for me and us as a couple. And from that, my sadness was lifted.

I had to watch myself still. Sometimes, I would fall into a deep sadness, like I really needed comfort. So, I just put a time limit on it. I would tell myself, "Okay...all right...you're allowed to be this way, but only for the next three minutes or so. After that, that's it! I really don't have time for self-pity, and it sure doesn't help me!"

I did avail myself of some classes offered by Cancer CARE Point, a non-profit organization in the area that provides a variety of free services for cancer patients. The first one I took was on relaxation techniques. The second one I took was on tapping, a stress relief technique. I also took a self-hypnosis class and a class on the reiki healing technique.

Tapping for me is a really good technique to learn for this kind of thing because – and this is huge! – it gives us the affirmation we need to cope. The instructor showed us the points and explained how everything works in opening up these energy points. In the practice session, I thought, "Okay, let me go right to the heart of my thing." So, what I said as I tapped (and you only speak in terms of how you feel; not who you are) was, "*Right now, I'm feeling sad because I might not live as long as I expected. But, for today, right now, I am here and I'm fine.*" That really made a big difference for me when I kept saying it, while going through all my tapping points. It just put me in a different frame of mind by using these energy channels. And that was really good.

* Susan M. (Ovarian cancer. Metastatic Pancreatic cancer to the Lungs)

Pancreatic Cancer: There were times hopelessness and deep sadness overcame me. They came with the feelings of weakness and loss of control. Praying really helped me and gave me hope and peace. Also, I tried hard to stay positive every day. It wasn't easy, but I was determined. I knew these negative feelings weren't helping me. So, I just focused on the positive ones that did.

* Tet M. (Colon cancer 3x)

I had scheduled to have my weekly Chemo session fall on a Friday, so I could recover from any possible sickness or debilitation during the weekend. It worked out for me, except there were times I fell into the trap of feeling sorry for myself, knowing everyone else was out on picnics, barbecues, hanging out and such. This spanned 52 weeks.

ADVICE: I may sound like a recording, but try to concentrate on the positive side, which is recovering and beating cancer. Imagine the cancer cells dying because there is no place for them in your body. None.

* Yesi L. (Breast cancer: triple positive)

I definitely experienced grief. I think grieving is huge; a very important part in the recovery process. I acknowledged my grief and then was able to let it go.

Regarding sadness, I felt so much sadness with the simple thought of not being there for my daughter; possibly not seeing her grow up.

ADVICE: It's okay to grieve. It's natural. Allow yourself to grieve for your situation. But then, let it go. The same with sadness. It's natural and part of the process. But then it's really important to let it go after a time and not dwell on the grief or sadness.

GUILT, SELF-CONDEMNATION

* Cindy L. (Kidney cancer)

I didn't feel guilty, at all, about having cancer. I did kind of feel guilty about my husband not being able to get the double hip replacement he needed when the opportunity would have presented itself in his work schedule, in our family activities and everything else. He was looking at getting that done when I ended up having cancer. I also felt guilty that we had to stop our regular walks when I had to go through treatment, because walking helps him to strengthen that area.

ADVICE: Feeling guilty about having cancer is completely unnecessary. It doesn't benefit you at all. So don't give it another thought. Feeling guilty about putting your loved ones through the challenge with you is understandable. However, it also doesn't benefit you or your loved ones. So, don't give that any of your energy either. Just focus on getting better, so that you can all enjoy each other when you finally recover.

* Joan S. (Rectal cancer)

I felt guilt, because I didn't get a colonoscopy when I should've. I realize now, it's so important.

ADVICE: If you are 50 years old or older, make sure to get your colonoscopy and then follow the schedule for your next colonoscopy, which depends on what (if anything) was found in your previous colonoscopy. Having a colonoscopy could mean the difference in whether your cancer is found early or late and what treatment you'll need.

* Scott M. (Metastatic Colon cancer to the Prostate & Pancreas)

My family was directly affected by my cancer and I recognize that they had to adjust their lives because of me. Still, I didn't feel guilt. I know they have a huge role and I'm very grateful.

ADVICE: Don't be guilty about anything. Just know that your spouse (if you're married), significant other or caregiver has a huge role and their lives are going to change. Don't feel guilt. Just be grateful for their support.

* Aaron C. *(Prostate cancer, Skin cancer)*

The skin cancer I actually had was first misdiagnosed as a stye by my doctor. So, I had it for about a year until a dermatologist looked at it and told me that it wasn't a stye, but skin cancer. The dermatologist said that my doctor should've caught it. Of course, I was irritated and upset by the misdiagnosis.

> **ADVICE:** It's natural to be irritated and upset by a misdiagnosis. However, you have to keep your focus on what treatment you'll be getting and what you need to do to get rid of your cancer.

* Glenn M. *(Metastatic Colon cancer to the Liver, Lungs & Adrenal Glands)*

My employees would tell you, I get irritated. I'm aware of this. So what I do is participate in things like the Chemo Brain Talk and go out and meet people; engage with them and strike up a conversation when I can.

    During that first chemo session when I lost my cell phone and my nurse KB was taking care of me, helping me to find it, she picked up that Scott (the cancer patient in the chair next to me) and I had things in common we could talk about. So, she pulled out the divider between us, folded it and took it away. Scott and I hit it off and started talking non-stop. We didn't care about what was happening on the floor. When we had to, we just dragged the chairs around and, before we knew it, we're there half an hour after they unplugged us both from our infusions.

> **ADVICE:** When you find yourself getting irritated or impatient, find something interesting to do that will engage you and take your mind off of stuff. Participate in things like the Chemo Brain Talk or Art Therapy classes. Engage with people you have similarities with, like Scott and I did. Share jokes or poems or stories...anything to get you smiling and laughing. Activities like that will keep you from getting irritated.

* Joan S. *(Rectal cancer)*

I had to get a colostomy bag. Because it took me a long time to change it, I got impatient or irritated.

> **ADVICE:** You'll have a visiting nurse who will train you on how to empty the colostomy bag. If you're not happy, ask for help and then, <u>pay attention!</u>

* Rev. Linda S. *(Pancreatic cancer 3x)*

When I experienced impatience or irritation, it was only with occasional delays and unclear communication in the medical system and with well-meaning people who felt their words were helping and not hurting me. I wanted people to listen to me and not to give me advice, unless I asked for it. Ultimately, I had to directly let them know.

> **ADVICE:** Be clear about what you need and feel free to speak up about it.

* Rachel S. *(Breast cancer: triple negative)*

I remember feeling irritation and impatience. There was a time when I tried to tell my son something and he didn't focus or pay attention. In the back of my head, I was thinking, "I don't have a lot of time for this." But, I also knew that I was pushing him a little much and it wasn't fair to him. I tried to be aware of my behavior and how my irritation and impatience affected my family. I knew they were affected by my cancer, too.

> **ADVICE:** When you feel irritation or impatience, just be aware of your behavior. It wouldn't be fair to take it out on those around you.

* Sondra W. *(Ovarian cancer 3x)*

I never used to be irritable or impatient; I never used to be that way. But I think during treatment when I got too tired, I felt like somebody was pressing me. So, I'm sure I sounded irritable. And, I realized that I was also impatient because my priority or urgency wasn't everybody else's, so I didn't blame them.

Since my cancer diagnosis, however, there are now some things that have an urgency to me and an importance to me that weren't there before. So in that regard I think I can get impatient if something gets in my way. I realized that I just had to stop, breath, and just settle down; I had to pull back because I could work myself up, and that, certainly, didn't help.

I learned to give grace and accept that not everybody is in the same place as I was. They didn't feel the same urgency I did. And, what was important to me was not necessarily important to them. I had to respect other people and where they were and not get all worked up over their not having the same urgency as me.

ADVICE: When you get impatient or irritable, take a deep breath and just accept that not everybody is in the same place as you are. They can't quite get where you're coming from. Respect other people and where they are and don't judge them for not having the same urgency as you. Also, remember that if you were in their shoes (if the "tables were turned"), you probably wouldn't understand "you" either!

* Tet M. *(Colon cancer 3x)*

Irritation and short temper were born out of frustration. My support system took the brunt of it: My family and closest friends were my emotional punching bags, which was totally uncalled for.

ADVICE: Your support group (family, friends) understand what you're going through, even if it's not fair how they end up paying a price for it as well. If you cannot keep your temper in check, at least apologize after the episode and maybe treat them to a meal or do something nice in exchange. If you aren't feeling too well, a smile will do; it can make a difference. Above all, beating cancer will be the most rewarding payback not only to yourself, but also to your support system. THIS is what you should focus on.

* Vida B.A. *(Breast cancer)*

I got impatient and irritated, not only because of my situation, but also because some of the medication I was given made me really grouchy. There were times I yelled at someone, because I just wasn't in my right mind. Looking back, I realize that my impatience and irritability would happen during the first two weeks of chemo; the same days when I felt weak and frustrated. The third week would be my "happy" week when I was back to being my very positive, happy self. Since my treatment schedule covered six cycles, I went through the same feelings six times.

ADVICE: Take note of how your medications affect your behavior or mood. Ask your family or friends to take note too, so that everyone is aware and will be more understanding. The main thing is to know that getting impatient or irritated is a *temporary* side effect of the chemo drugs.

* Yesi L. *(Breast cancer: triple positive)*

Yes, I definitely felt impatience and I absolutely felt irritation. When I was feeling extremely fatigued and did not want to feel fatigued, I tried to push myself to do things. Well, even when I was able to do things, my feeling fatigued just irritated me, impacting those around me. And, they only have so much patience for my behavior.

ADVICE: Definitely be aware of your behavior and attitude. Seek professional help, when you realize you're impatience or irritation is affecting those around you. I cannot emphasize that enough.

* Amor T. (Breast cancer, Ovarian cancer)

There were times when I felt lonely, even though I wasn't physically alone. Aside from having to deal with trying to move with my deep wounds, I had to deal with the man I was dating at the time who made it obvious that he didn't really want to be with me. Of course, with my mastectomy, I also felt "broken" and, therefore, undesirable. With this man, I felt so alone. When I was with others, it was the complete opposite. I felt loved and valued. At the time, I decided not to say anything to this man, because I needed to reserve my strength and just focus on healing my body. When I finally healed, we respectfully parted ways.

ADVICE: If you're feeling lonely, even if you're not physically alone, first be kind to yourself. If you're with someone who doesn't want to be with you, try not to depend on that person for any support, especially emotional. Call those who clearly love you and want to support you. Allow them to lift your spirits. Don't waste your energy on someone who clearly doesn't deserve your energy, especially when you're sick.

* Cindy L. (Kidney cancer)

When I was first diagnosed, I felt the loneliness. But then, as my support team came in and as I talked to more survivors, I quickly lost that feeling of loneliness. I felt I wasn't alone in my battle.

ADVICE: It helps to talk with survivors who have been in your shoes and share the same experiences.

* Rachel S. (Breast cancer: triple negative)

I felt loneliness in the beginning. I remember that I would, all of a sudden, feel like I was completely alone. I had thoughts that my husband just didn't understand. I needed him to be with me and not at work all the time. Of course, those thoughts and feelings of loneliness didn't last, because I knew I had the support of my husband, my family and my friends.

ADVICE: Just focus on the positive and cope with those feelings, as much as you can.

* Sondra W. (Ovarian cancer 3x)

I used to experience some loneliness when my husband Kenneth had to work all those long hours. But now, he is retired from that job, and I don't feel the loneliness as much. When I do experience it, what I do to cope is to read scripture. I just refresh and remind myself that God is always with me; I'm not by myself. God is always here with me, for me, and before me; walking before me and beside me. And, He is showing up all time. I just have to pay attention and be thankful for the amazing support system God has provided me. That's what I do to cope.

ADVICE: When you're experiencing loneliness, it's important to do something that will keep you engaged and focused on something positive. Prayer and meditation help to clear your mind of worries, definitely, put you in a peaceful and comfortable place.

* Susan M. (Ovarian cancer. Metastatic Pancreatic cancer to the Lungs)

Pancreatic Cancer: Loneliness set in at times when I was emotionally spent and felt that I was going through everything on my own. Even though I knew my family and friends were there for me, they weren't experiencing what I was experiencing. So, I prayed hard to stop those feelings of loneliness that I knew were just weighing me down. I tried hard to stay positive focusing only on good things; things that made me happy. I also made sure I accomplished several things every day. That helped.

* Yesi L. *(Breast cancer: triple positive)*

At times, there was loneliness because everyone was living their normal lives. When I was in the house alone, I experienced it a lot because I was used to working and being active.

MOODINESS

* Yesi L. *(Breast cancer: triple positive)*

Breast cancer treatments can put women into menopause, because our hormones will go all over the place. That's what happened to me at the early age of 32. And the hormones were sort of like a roller coaster. I wasn't aware of my moodiness, until someone told me.

NIGHT FEARS / NIGHTMARES

* Amor T. *(Breast cancer, Ovarian cancer)*

There were many times I laid awake at night thinking of the "what ifs" and worst case scenarios. When that happened, I either prayed or thought happy thoughts, which included daydreams of fun times (past and future) with those I love. I did what I could to banish those fears that threatened to paralyze me and bring me down. I knew that they were not real and, therefore, were replaceable with happy, positive thoughts.

Of course, there were times when I had actual nightmares when I slept. I found they occurred whenever I slept on a full stomach, which didn't give time for my food to be properly digested. When I stopped doing that, the nightmares went away.

* Bob G. *(Soft Tissue Sarcoma, Skin cancer)*

Well, negative thoughts did enter my mind. In the middle of the night, for 3, 4 or 5 hours, I'd wake up and have a hard time getting back to sleep. I would be in a weakened condition, which made me susceptible to bad thoughts. The night fears tried to take over and it wasn't easy fighting them sometimes. I took one to two sleeping pills, but then I couldn't wake up in the morning. I did also play solitaire when I couldn't sleep.

What I did to deal with the night fears was think good thoughts. My good thoughts? Well, some of the nurses! I always say, "God's greatest gift to man is woman!" That's one of my favorite sayings! Also, for men, I recommend finding a good woman. It just makes staying awake a little bit nicer!

ADVICE: The best medication for recovery is a good night's sleep. If you have night fears, think good thoughts only. If you have a hard time sleeping or getting back to sleep, try some activity, like playing solitaire. It does help to have someone stay awake with you.

* Cindy L. (Kidney cancer)

I experienced a lot of nightmares. I spent a total of 40 days not knowing what we were dealing with, i.e. 30 days before my surgery and, because I had to wait for the final report to come out, 10 days after my surgery. During that period, I had the night demons, the nightmares and a lot of night fears of whether they had gotten it all, what kind of kidney cancer it was, what stage, what grade.

I still get them every once in a while at night. When I wake up, I would get that feeling of dread. So I turn on my tablet and watch something to take my mind off of it and it works!

ADVICE: The best thing you can do is just take your mind off of those negative thoughts. If you can, go somewhere; do something to occupy your mind, like I do watching movies on my tablet. Read a book, talk to someone, listen to music you enjoy, take a walk outside, etc. Go to your happy place. Doing that will take care of your nightmares.

* Rachel S. (Breast cancer: triple negative)

I had them all the time. I just tried to fall back to sleep.

* Sondra W. (Ovarian cancer 3x)

When I first went through treatment, the nights were hard for me. I think it was, generally speaking, due to the fact that I thought there was nothing I could do to distract my thoughts without going overboard. When I read, listened to music, did my coloring, etc., I got all wired up and could not settle down. So, I had to learn to fight those night fears.

Now, I settle down faster. What I learned to do was tap into my sense of humor. I would think about something funny and then latch on to it. Another thing I learned to do was be aware of what I give myself attention to. If I read, listened to music, did my coloring, etc., I learned that the type of music I listen to and the kind of material I read affects my emotions. So, I chose to listen to relaxing music for meditation and to read inspirational articles or re-read thoughtful cards sent from friends. I was also careful about the type of movie I watched at night before going to sleep. That made a big difference for me.

ADVICE: Think of something positive or funny, like jokes or a funny experience, and then hold on to it. Also, be careful of what you watch at night before going to bed. Keep it light and positive; nothing scary or negative. Listen to relaxing music for meditation, read inspirational articles, or re-read thoughtful cards your friends sent you. Choosing light, positive materials will help you sleep at night.

NUMBNESS, INDIFFERENCE, PASSIVENESS

---

* Rachel S. (Breast cancer: triple negative)

There was a point where I just got numb to what people thought of me. I didn't care if they condemned me for things I liked doing, like going on Facebook a lot. I didn't care what I looked like. If people didn't like the way I looked, then I'd tell them "Don't look at me". Before, I cared about what people thought and I didn't have this confidence. But, now I do and

I just don't care about stuff like that anymore. And now, you know.....I have no hair....sorry. I've got no chi-chis ... sorry. Stuff like that just doesn't matter. I don't feel I need anyone's approval anymore. So, there was a numbness in emotion.

ADVICE: Be yourself and be comfortable with who are you. You don't need anyone's approval.

* Vida B.A. *(Breast cancer)*

During those weeks when I felt weak and helpless, I tried not to show it, even though I was in pain. I really didn't want to make a big fuss about it. There were times when I, basically, numbed myself to my situation. It was like an escape from reality, so to speak. Fortunately, those times were temporary and didn't happen often.

To cope, I tried to distract myself with things to do throughout the day, like play games, read Facebook posts, watch a movie or talk with family or friends. It also helped to think positive thoughts and focus on my blessings.

ADVICE: It's normal to numb yourself from your situation when it brings you down, because it helps you to escape and get some relief. That relief, however, is temporary and you have to face reality in order for things to get better. To cope, try to stop your mind from focusing on the negative, as much as possible. That doesn't do you any good. Instead, try to distract yourself with things to do throughout the day or night, like play games, read Facebook posts, watch a movie, talk with your family or friends, etc. You'll eventually get the hang of it. Of course, there will be times you just don't feel like doing anything and that's okay. Focus on your blessings and all the positive around you and don't let your situation control you.

* Yesi L. *(Breast cancer: triple positive)*

Passiveness: That was huge, in my case. My then fiance, now husband, described me as passive-aggressive during treatment. I just was not happy. After treatment, I lived in a void for a little over a year, not able to process my emotions. I didn't have any guidance. I felt lost. I felt like this whole void was taking over me and I didn't know what to do with myself. I retreated because I lost control of my body. I didn't feel like I was in control.

ADVICE: Seek psychological help, keep an open mind and listen to those around you. You don't have to be in control all the time. It's okay. Let it go. Being passive-aggressive is not healthy.

RESIGNATION

---

* Amor T. *(Breast cancer, Ovarian cancer)*

Both times I received my cancer diagnosis, I was stunned. Of course, no one wants to hear they have cancer. However, since that was my reality, I calmly accepted it and thought of what actions I could take to rid myself of cancer. I did not concede defeat nor give up on myself, which is what resignation is all about.

I let go of trying to control life and researched what I could to learn everything about the disease and all treatment options. I wanted to keep my focus on getting the cancer out of my body and then living a healthy life. I believe there is peace and freedom in accepting life's trials and doing what I can to learn and grow from them.

ADVICE: Don't give yourself up to cancer! Feeling defeat and resigning yourself to cancer will just make things worse when you could actually make things better for yourself, despite having cancer. The key is acceptance, followed with action on what you can do about it.

Start with a positive mindset and determination to rid your body of the disease. Think of the many things you can do to get your health back, like following your doctor's instructions, getting plenty of rest, eating healthy foods and exercising to stimulate your immune system, avoiding negative thoughts that don't benefit you at all and focusing on all the positive you have around you, including the little things. As psychologist and author William James said, "Acceptance of what has happened is the first step to overcoming the consequences of any misfortune.

* Cindy L. *(Kidney cancer)*

I remember thinking like that even before I was formally diagnosed. I just remember sitting in the office with my husband; I had resigned myself to the fact that I had cancer. And I was just waiting to hear the words from my doctor. And as soon as he came in, I said to my husband Ed, "See? Look at his face. I can tell you now, the ax is going to fall." My doctor just kind of looked at us, pulled up his computer where he was going to bring up the slides with information and was about to talk to me when I started crying and said, "I have to go pee."

So I got up and left; I just needed a minute by myself. I went down the hall to the bathroom and left those two in there. When I came back in, I said, "Okay. Well, I'll tell you what. I'm leaving tomorrow to go out of town to take care of my daughter. "What has been going inside of me didn't just start overnight. It has been here for a long time and it's not going to go anywhere for the week that it's going to take me to see my daughter." At that point, I guess I was resigned to the fact that I cancer, even before my doctor gave me the official word that I had cancer. But then, I was also resigned to the fact that I had something more important to do, which was to go take care of my daughter who needed me.

> **ADVICE:** Resignation isn't necessarily a bad thing, as long as you don't give up on yourself. It's just accepting a hard reality and dealing with it.

* Rev. Linda S. *(Pancreatic cancer 3x)*

I accepted whatever was coming my way as dealing with reality. I do not see that as being resigned to anything.

SELF-PITY

---

* Amor T. *(Breast cancer, Ovarian cancer)*

The rare occasions I felt self-pity were brief, but they still reared their silly heads to tempt me. I prepared myself by praying and thanking God for the abundance of blessings I've been given. I also asked my family and friends to give me five minutes to ride my "pity wagon", if my emotions got the better of me and I needed to vent. However, when the five minutes is up, I asked them to gently tell me to get off of my "pity wagon" and focus on the many things that are going right in my life, including having them in it! I didn't have to vent that much, because I kept thinking of those less fortunate than me, especially the little children suffering from cancer.

> **ADVICE:** "Why me?" is an understandable question to ask when you're suffering from cancer or any life-threatening illness. It is very important to vent; to ride your "pity wagon." However, staying on it will just have you go on a downward spiral. So, ask your family and friends who support you to allow you to vent for five minutes (yes, they should time you) and when your five minutes is up, they should tell you to get off. You'll find that when you're able to vent, you'll feel better and lighter, having shared your heavy emotions.
>
> Do try to keep focus on all the wonderful things that are going right in your life, including little things like having a TV to watch or shoes on your feet or food to eat, etc. Think of those less fortunate than you, especially little children suffering from cancer. Doing so will help you realize your blessings.

* Cindy L. *(Kidney cancer)*

At first, I was really angry that this happened to me; the "why me?" pity-party. I kept asking, "Why did this happen to me?" But then, I had to keep telling myself, "Well, it did and there's nothing I can do about it. And lying down in the dump isn't going to help." So, when I started feeling sorry for myself, I would go out, take a walk, go watch a movie...do something. I liked walking through Walmart or wherever. I'd see people who were much worse off than I was. That always helped take me right out of my pity-party, because it straightened out my little attitude.

I always tell my children, "When you feel sorry for yourself; when you think you've got life bad, take a look around you. There's always somebody much worse off than you."

* J.B. *(Salivary gland cancer)*

I did feel a bit of self-pity. When I isolated myself, it was just a coping mechanism and took me time to process and digest. Fortunately, it was a temporary process. I think that a little bit of isolation is not a bad thing. However, I think it becomes a negative thing when you worry others. That was a big thing with my girlfriend. She didn't like the fact that I knew my situation affected her, yet I didn't share my feelings with her. At that point, I realized that when my isolation obviously affects someone else, then it's probably time for me to snap out of it.

ADVICE: Feeling self-pity is natural and so is isolation. However, when your keeping isolated obviously affects those who love you, then it's probably time for you to snap out of it and open up to them a bit more.

* Rev. Linda S. *(Pancreatic cancer 3x)*

Not applicable. My attitude was, "Why not me? People get cancer all the time."

* Rick S. *(CLL: Blood & Bone Marrow cancer)*

I did go through a period of self-pity, because I was a champion all my working career. I worked hard. I always jumped out of bed and ran my ten miles and I did my job and I was applauded at work and then all of a sudden, I've got nothing but four walls surrounding me. That's how I went through my period of self-pity. It's passed now and I've learned that it doesn't benefit me and that there are things I can do to focus my mind on; not self-pity.

* Scott M. *(Metastatic Colon cancer to the Prostate & Pancreas)*

ADVICE: You're going to feel self-pity and it's okay. Just feel your emotions and let your emotions play out to conclusion. Don't try to suppress anything. Just let it out, be yourself and talk with people about it. There are a lot of people out there who want to help you.

* Sondra W. *(Ovarian cancer 3x)*

I had to watch myself. Sometimes, I fell into that. If I felt like I really needed to pity myself, then I just put a time limit on it. I would tell myself, "Okay...all right...you're allowed to be this way, but only for the next three minutes or so. After that, that's it! I really don't have time for self-pity and it sure doesn't help me."

ADVICE: Having cancer is very challenging. So, feeling self-pity is natural. Allow yourself the freedom to vent and feel self-pity. But, don't go overboard, or else you'll drown. Give yourself a time limit, like three minutes, to get it all out. After that, stop and focus on something else that's positive. Self-pity will not make your health or your situation better. As a matter of fact, it will definitely make it worse.

* Yesi L. *(Breast cancer: triple positive)*

I didn't allow myself to go there, because I felt that would explore a side of me that I didn't like. It just doesn't help. So, I just did not allow myself to go there.

ADVICE: My advice is just to keep positive. No need for self-pity. It just doesn't help.

SHAME

* Amor T. (Breast cancer, Ovarian cancer)

I remember times when I looked sick as I made my way to the doctor's office. Whenever I caught people staring at me, I just smiled at them. Yes, my body was weak, but my spirit wasn't. And I have absolutely nothing to be ashamed about, no matter what anyone says. I also caught some people looking at me with judging eyes, but their opinions or judgments did not phase me at all. If my wig fell off to reveal my bald head, I would actually be laughing so hard, because to me, that would be really funny; not embarassing or shameful.

When Bill and I went to Hawaii, I looked at my selection of bathing suits and chose to wear my bikinis. Sure, the scar of the long, jagged, vertical incision from my hysterectomy would be exposed, but so what? It's absolutely nothing to be ashamed about. As a matter of fact, a couple of kids there stared at my scar. I told them that I had major surgery that saved my life and voila!, the scar is my souvenir. They said "Wow, that's awesome!" After that, we all smiled together. That was a wonderful experience.

ADVICE: There should be no shame whatsoever in having cancer, no matter what anyone says or thinks. If you didn't exactly live a healthy lifestyle and you got cancer, then … you got cancer. Period. End of story. Too often, people have stories about what caused cancer or other illness or misfortunes, etc. and then they judge. You don't need that at all. So, ignore any stigma about having cancer and don't feel any shame, whatsoever, for having it. When people say negative things that mean to shame you, ignore them. Don't waste your time or energy on them. Instead, focus your thoughts and energy on the positives, what you can do to get stronger and beating cancer. When you focus on what makes you happy, you'll have plenty of ammunition to fight cancer.

* Cindy L. (Kidney cancer)

I never felt any shame for having kidney cancer. Why should I? I didn't do anything to bring this on.

I did, however, feel a bit of shame when I had to use one of the little electric scooters at Walmart while I shopped. This happened the first couple of weeks after surgery. It seemed that people looked at me and I felt I needed to explain why I was using the scooter. I also felt that I was taking the scooter from someone who actually needed it. But then, I realized that I actually needed it because our Walmart is huge and I physically couldn't walk around without assistance from the electric scooter.

ADVICE: First off, you should never feel shame for having contracted a deadly disease. If anyone suggests that, do not listen to them. You should never feel shame for getting sick. Second, if you need to move around and your body is still recovering from surgery, don't feel ashamed about using the electric scooter in the store, if they're available. Because of your condition, you have a valid reason to use it.

* Rev. Linda S. (Pancreatic cancer 3x)

Never!

ADVICE: Never feel shame for having cancer!

* Rick S. (CLL: Blood & Bone Marrow cancer)

I never felt shame. And, no one should feel shame for having cancer.

ADVICE: There's no need to feel shame. You didn't cause your cancer. There's no reason to be ashamed, because it happened to me. I didn't cause my cancer.

* Scott M. *(Metastatic Colon cancer to the Prostate & Pancreas)*

ADVICE: No matter what, you shouldn't feel shame for having cancer.

* Sondra W. *(Ovarian cancer 3x)*

Well, that's interesting because I know some people have asked me, "Do you not want me to share that you have cancer or not say anything?" I have never felt ashamed of having cancer. Why should I be? As a matter of fact, I find that in sharing that I do have cancer, I give and I get back. So I'm like, "Oh no! No, it's okay. It's really okay."

ADVICE: Cancer is never something you should be ashamed of, no matter what anyone says. It's a disease and a fact of life. It's a battle that you're fighting to win. Never bring shame into the picture. It is absolutely not something to be ashamed of, (again) no matter what anyone says.

* Yesi L. *(Breast cancer: triple positive)*

I did not feel shame. I know I didn't have hair. I didn't have eyelashes. My eyelashes were my biggest source of pride and I lost three sets of them. Still, I never felt shame. I knew that my looks didn't define me. I knew who I was and accepted myself throughout the experience.

ADVICE: Cancer and everything that goes with it does not define you. When you accept yourself for who you are, then those around you will do the same.

SHOCK / STUN

---

* Aaron C. *(Prostate cancer, Skin cancer)*

More of what I felt was shock, when I found out I had prostate cancer. Before she passed, my mom had figured that I would, eventually, get prostate cancer, because supposedly, one in seven men will get it. However, from one book my first urologist recommended I read, the odds, for those under 55 years of age to get prostate cancer, are one in fifty. So, I was in shock.

ADVICE: No one wants to get unexpected news, especially if it's about cancer. But, you just have to put things into perspective and realize that, at least, the cancer was detected early enough to get treatment that will remove it, so you can heal and return to living a normal life again.

* Amor T. *(Breast cancer, Ovarian cancer)*

When my doctor called and told me that the test findings were positive for breast cancer, I was shocked. I couldn't speak for a couple of seconds. But then, I gathered my thoughts and calmly asked her for more information. This was an interesting experience, because with all the tests I was going through (ultrasound, CT scans, MRI, multiple biopsies), I did suspect that I had breast cancer. I guess I didn't think I would hear it confirmed. Thus, my shocked reaction. The shock didn't last long at all, because I focused my thoughts and energies on learning what I could about my cancer as well as all the treatment options out there for me.

* Cindy L. *(Kidney cancer)*

I was shocked when I learned that I had kidney cancer. I mean, here I was, doing everything I could to take care of myself, lose weight and get into shape. Things were looking good and bright for the future. I was back out looking for jobs and then WHAM! They told me I had cancer. So yeah, I was shocked. But I quickly got over that and replaced it with being mad, which I kind of got over too, as time passed.

ADVICE: It's normal to experience shock when they tell you that you have cancer. It is a deadly disease and you know that you can expect serious changes in your life; something you do not want to hear, especially when you have plans for the future. Give yourself time to process, but focus on getting over it, because staying in that space will not benefit you, at all.

* Jacki S. *(Breast cancer)*

When I learned I had cancer, I was scared and in shock. I couldn't believe I had cancer. I followed what my doctor advised me to do and talked with other cancer survivors.

ADVICE: Breathe and learn about your cancer. It also helps to talk with cancer survivors to understand the experience and what you can expect.

* J.B. *(Salivary gland cancer)*

When my doctor told me that the biopsy he took of the tissue of my salivary gland was malignant and cancerous, I was shocked and confused. It was definitely surreal and took me a while to process, before I could talk with anybody about it. Of course, my family was shocked too, especially given my age and the rarity of the cancer.

* Rev. Linda S. *(Pancreatic cancer 3x)*

I suspected I had cancer but not Pancreatic Cancer, so I was shocked but grateful that a good friend was with me when the doctor gave me the diagnosis. Having her and her husband there saved me from hysteria.

ADVICE: As much as possible, have someone with you when you're given the diagnosis. If you receive upsetting news, allow yourself time to process it.

* Rick S. *(CLL: Blood & Bone Marrow cancer)*

I was shocked at the news that I had cancer, because I had always taken care of myself. What I did after I found out was I worked out.

* Sondra W. *(Ovarian cancer 3x)*

When I was informed that I had ovarian cancer, I was stunned because I had mentioned to my doctors that I thought something was wrong. I had had a pelvic ultrasound, and they had assured me that nothing was wrong. With that, I felt relief. But then, Boom! Something was definitely wrong. I didn't feel anger for their having misdiagnosed me. I just couldn't believe I had cancer.

> **ADVICE:** Keep in mind my doctor's statement: "That was then. This is now." It helped me to face the reality of my situation and not go back to what could have or should have been. When you have cancer, you have cancer. Thinking of how or why it happened doesn't make it go away. So just think of your present situation and how you'll move forward.

* Tet M. (Colon cancer 3x)

Upon being told I had colon cancer, one of the first things I did was to go to my workplace's Human Resources department to inquire about life insurance coverage. My initial thought was, what will happen to the people I will leave behind if I pass away?

> **ADVICE:** My reaction followed by action, while normal, was in a way funny, because it showed how naïve I was of the advancement in medicine. It also showed my lack of faith in God and in myself. I eventually recovered from this. Faith in yourself, in your doctor(s) and above all, faith in a Supreme Being is what will quietly help you move forward.

* Yesi L. (Breast cancer: triple positive)

I was absolutely shocked by the news that I had cancer. I was in denial at first, but then I processed it by being with nature (hiking). Being in contact with nature is peaceful and looking or listening to water is soothing. The sound of water; the greenery, smelling the flowers..... It was and still is just the biggest picker-up.

> **ADVICE:** Try turning to nature. It brings peace and is very soothing. It helps take the shock of bad news and helps you move forward.

STRESS / OVERWHELM

---

* Amor T. (Breast cancer, Ovarian cancer)

This was an interesting experience. During both my breast and ovarian cancer battles, it was overwhelming trying to digest information about my cancer and treatments, at the same time, trying to understand why my body was doing what it was doing and how to cope with it all. Dealing with the medical bills, statements, appointments, and correspondence with my doctors, hospitals, pharmacies and insurance companies was also overwhelming. Trying to keep my worried family and friends abreast of developments was overwhelming too. I felt like I was caught up in a whirlwind and wanted to rest, but just couldn't stop. I had to go with the flow and do what I could. I definitely learned a lot about my strengths and the available resources out there for use.

I knew, going in, that dealing with cancer and the myriad treatments, would be overwhelming. So, mentally, I prepared myself. However, when I completed chemo treatments, I was really surprised by how overwhelmed I got with certain conversations, including those with my amazing, everloving family.

Until I looked into how chemotherapy affects the brain, I had no idea that I had "chemo brain." I found myself getting confused and having problems focusing, multitasking, remembering things, learning new things and finding words. My inability to follow conversations was apparent whenever my siblings and I would have video conference calls and I would just get overwhelmed, trying to follow who said what and how to respond. When my wonderful family came to visit, there were so many conversations going on at one time that I tried to keep up, but just got overwhelmed. Several times, when I felt my heart racing, I retreated to my bedroom to rest and take deep breaths.

Feelings of overwhelm can continue after treatment. To date, I've been in remission for 2½ years and realize that I can sometimes get overwhelmed by simply looking at the words on my screen as I write this book. The state of crazy overwhelm has calmed down a bit, but the reality is still there. The only thing that I know to do when I'm overwhelmed is to take a deep breath, close my eyes, clear my mind and relax. I also get up from my desk and do some stretches while looking out my window for a change of scenery. When I return to my computer, the words on my screen make sense and no longer overwhelm me.

The mental state of overwhelm can cause a lot of anxiety, because things seemingly are out of control. However, because it's a mental state, I believe that in recognizing it for what it is - a mental state - I actually can, mentally, tell myself to not worry and just chill! Then, I refocus on what really matters. It takes a lot of practice, but it does work.

> **ADVICE:** The overwhelm that you experience when dealing with cancer is to be expected and not to be trivialized. You can feel like your life just went out of control, because your normal routine is disrupted. Aside from trying to understand your treatment options, processes you'll have to go through, how you'll be able to function without the cancerous organ removed (if such is the case), coordinate who'll take care of your kids, your job, our elderly parent, the bills, etc., you also need to focus on healing and getting stronger. Sometimes, the medication you're given to help you recover causes your brain to "hiccup" every now and then...All that and then some.
>
> Firstoff, take a deep breath when you start to feel overwhelmed and take it one step at a time. Actually, take a step back and look at what you're dealing with as a whole, which is A LOT! When you're looking at it, calmly tell yourself, "Everything will work out." You're just going to do what you can do and you're also going to ask for help. And then, do it. Don't be afraid to ask questions or ask for help.
>
> Practice taking yourself out of situations that overwhelm you. For example, if you're overwhelmed by not being able to finish what you're reading or if you're overwhelmed by multiple conversations happening around you at the same time, step away. Go to another room, if necessary, and take a deep breath, close your eyes and clear your mind, i.e. think of something peaceful, like a sweet song or a beautiful prayer. After you take that much needed break (a retreat, actually), you can then return to what you were doing and feel better about it.

* *Cindy L.* (Kidney cancer)

Gadolinium is the dye/contrast that is normally used with MRIs. As part of my future ongoing check-ups, I'll have to get MRIs with gadolinium, so that they can see any microscopic cancer cells. I would agree to that once a year, not any more than that, because they are finding evidence that gadolinium lies around in the brain. So as you can see, you're damned if you do, damned if you don't. Since my cancer was found at stage 1, grade 1, I'm willing to take the chance to discontinue it. It is my body. I'm willing to take the chance that the risks of having gadolinium and other contrasts in my body far outweigh the benefits for me. This was one of the major things that stressed me out. So, I worked with a psychologist to deal with it. Once I made the decision that I was not going to continue with the gadolinium and other contrasts, I got a sense of peace.

I also experienced feeling overwhelmed at times, during treatment. Everything just seemed to be coming at me all at once; they tended to happen really fast. So I just got totally overwhelmed. What I learned to do to cope was tell myself to slow down. Then I would tell myself to start at the top and see what we're going to do to deal with the situation to avoid getting overwhelmed. Now, that's how I look at all situations, when I go from "house fire" to "house fire". I grab the bull by the horns and just deal with it. And then I march on. I know that's all I can do and it's worked for me.

> **ADVICE:** When you get stressed or overwhelmed, you need to slow yourself down. See a psychologist, if necessary. To slow yourself down, first take a deep breath. Then tell yourself to start at the top and figure out what you're going to do to deal with the situation to avoid getting overwhelmed. Grab the bull by the horns, deal with the situation and then march on.

* *Sondra W.* (Ovarian cancer 3x)

I definitely experienced feeling overwhelmed during the time I found out I had cancer and also when I had to make arrangements to send my 95-year old mother I had been caring for to my brother in Ohio and place her in a facility within two weeks. There was so much going on and so much to do in getting all her belongings and medical records together. I just got overwhelmed with what I was being asked to do for her move while at the same time having to deal with my diagnosis. There were appointments with my gastroenterologist, a gynecological surgeon, an interventional radiologist and my primary doctor. It was exhaustion that helped me realize that I couldn't do it all, and I had to focus on my health.

Because I only had so much energy and there was so much I had to do, I learned to let people help me. I didn't have the stamina to push through on my own anymore. I just got kind of overwhelmed with everything that was happening. People were really nice texting me, emailing me, calling me ... I just couldn't seem to handle it all. You know what I mean? So, I learned to rotate what I had to do, who to talk to, etc. because I couldn't do everything in one day. I also learned I needed to be specific with people about what I needed to have done.

What I found most stressful was in dealing with my and others' expectations of me. Interestingly enough, one of the most stressful situations has been people's reactions to my recently being declared in remission. Some people thought that meant chemo was over and that I was instantly "well." They were inviting me to lunch and dinner and expecting to see me back at church that very week and planning trips and other activities. They didn't realize I needed to be on a maintenance chemo and that my body needed time to recover from the very treatment that had put me in remission. They just didn't know.

I realized I needed to reset people's expectations. But first, I needed to do some adjusting myself. After 2 ½ years of praying for the miracle of "remission" it was being declared after only three treatments with a new combination of chemo and immunology medications. Both my husband and I were stunned! It took us a few days to really take it in and begin the transition of "fighting" mode to "living" mode. What will this part of the journey look like? How do I reset others' expectations without taking away their joy and excitement about this "remission" miracle and seeming ungrateful or unbelieving of this great "favor" shown to me by God? I think knowledge and information about this phase of the journey shared from a realistic but optimistic perspective is the key for me and family, friends, and others with whom I interact.

ADVICE: When you're in a situation where there's so much going on, you need to learn to let go of the thoughts of trying to get everything done. Break activities into smaller segments that match your level of energy. Ask for and accept the help you need. Use your energy to clear your mind of worries. Get a good night's sleep because you need everything you've got to beat cancer! Identify a "go to" place within yourself or literally that fosters balance, calmness and optimism whether it's meditation, music, a walk, the ocean, scripture, whatever soothes you and gives you peace. Seek the level of knowledge and information that helps you cope. This differs for each of us and whatever it is for you is okay as long as it doesn't become stressful. There are little "gems" of pleasure and beauty hidden in each day - look at them. Each day holds some type of blessing - acknowledge them, be thankful for them, enjoy them!

* Yesi L. (Breast cancer: triple positive)

Yes, the experience was definitely overwhelming! I mean, just the treatments themselves could be very overwhelming.

ADVICE: Allowing yourself to be taken care of is probably the best advice I can give.

UNCERTAINTY

* Amor T. (Breast cancer, Ovarian cancer)

When I had to manage (separately) both my cancer diagnoses and treatments, I experienced bouts of uncertainty. Most of the time, I use my logic in dealing with problems in life, because, for me, focusing on facts and being objective helps me to think clearly and reach my goals. Physical pain or extreme discomfort, however, sometimes threw my logic out the window, which enabled uncertainty to come through the door. It had me question my circumstances and tried to get my pity-party going.

Good thing my spirit was strong and did not (still doesn't) depend on logic or emotions. Because of my strength of faith, during times I felt distressed, my spirit gently reminded me of all my many blessings. It also reminded me that uncertainty is a state of mind that involves imperfect or unknown information and dwelling in the unknown or imperfect does not benefit me, especially my health. So, I learned to ignore uncertainty and focus on all my blessings.

* Cindy L. (Kidney cancer)

Gadolinium is the dye/contrast that is normally used with MRIs. As part of my future ongoing check-ups, I'll have to get MRIs with gadolinium, so that they can see any microscopic cancer cells. I would agree to that once a year, not any more than that, because they are finding evidence that gadolinium lies around in the brain. So as you can see, you're damned if you do, damned if you don't. Since my cancer was found at stage 1, grade 1, I'm willing to take the chance to discontinue it. It is my body. I'm willing to take the chance that the risks of having gadolinium and other contrasts in my body far outweigh the benefits for me.

This was one of the major things that stressed me out. So, I worked with a psychologist to deal with it. Once I made the decision that I was not going to continue with the gadolinium and other contrasts, I got a sense of peace.

Of course, I have uncertainties about my future. And, at least partially, I am scared too. No one knows what's going to happen in the future. We're just fine examples and proof that we don't. And so, we could have the best laid plans and it could all be for naught.

* Cindy R. (Metastatic Breast cancer to the Stomach)

I definitely have some uncertainty during my second round (stomach cancer diagnosis) because when you get that diagnosis, it's like, "Oh boy!" It was crazy, because they actually did give me an "expiration date, saying, "You have three months to live." But, on the other hand, it wasn't 100% guaranteed either. It was the craziest feelings.

I kept telling myself, "Okay wait, I only have today really. Whether or not I have cancer, I have today. So, what I'm going to do is make it good for me and to make it good for others too, as much as I can." I really tried not to think about, "Oh my gosh, I'm sick or I might be dying. I might be this, I might be that ..." No, that's just not a good thing to do.

* Hilda K. (Colon cancer)

Whenever I feel fear and uncertainty, I always go back to prayer and my faith in God. When I prayed, I felt that my prayers were being heard and I believed that God would help me through this challenge. I asked Him for strength and to help me to live as long as I can.

When the doctors told me that I had Colon Cancer and the worst that could happen would be for my entire colon to be removed and to live with colostomy bag for the rest of my life, I remember praying to God, "I don't mind the worst. Just let me live as long as I can, so that I can be with my children and get old. I will live with the bag forever; just, please, give me some more time." That was my realization. That was my acceptance.

For me, my faith in God and my trust that He would guide and strengthen me, helped me conquer my fears. I knew that I also had to keep positive, no matter what. I couldn't let the negative feelings, like loneliness or self-pity, take me down. I also knew that I could only depend on myself to be strong through this challenge. That definitely helped me heal, because I was in good spiritual and mental health and I was determined too.

ADVICE: Uncertainty crops up when you don't know what's going to happen and you're not sure what you're going to do, in case something happens. It affects us when we're hit with life-changing news, especially when it comes to our health. My advice is to be prepared for anything, including the worst. Come to terms with who you are, where you're at, what could happen, where you'll be and all that. When you are prepared, then you're more accepting and can deal with life's challenges better. Being determined to be strong, despite your uncertainties, will enable you to heal faster and move forward in good ways.

* J.B. *(Salivary gland cancer)*

Because there aren't many findings on my type of cancer, I experienced a lot of uncertainty. I dealt with the uncertainty by looking at information of my cancer as "sample sizes" versus percentages. Statistics information found in my research were very low, so they were "sample sizes." In thinking about the risk of recurrence, I thought about the fact that it may happen. Even if the chances weren't fifty-fifty, I just accepted the fact that recurrence may happen; no one knows for sure. Rather than look at statistics of recurrence like 30% or 15%, I just told myself that it either happens or it doesn't. And then I planned accordingly. The doctors did give me advice when it came to my uncertainty. They did a lot to reassure me that because I'm young and healthy, my chances of recurrence are pretty low. I'll give them that.

WITHDRAWAL, RETREAT, RECLUSIVENESS

* J.B. *(Salivary gland cancer)*

When I learned I had cancer, I did withdraw a bit and become reclusive. It was just a coping mechanism and took me time to process and digest. Fortunately, it was a temporary process. I think that a little bit of isolation is not a bad thing. However, I think it becomes a negative thing when you worry others. That was a big thing with my girlfriend. She didn't like the fact that I knew my situation affected her, yet didn't share my feelings with her. At that point, I realized that when my isolation obviously affects someone else, then it's probably time for me to snap out of it.

ADVICE: Withdrawing and isolating yourself is natural. However, when you stay withdrawn from those who love you, it hurts them. When you see that it affects them, then it's probably time for you to snap out of it and open up to them a bit more.

~ 0 ~

Chapter 9

CARRYING ON WITH DAILY LIFE ACTIVITIES

When you have cancer ... or when anyone has cancer, for that matter ... the world doesn't stop turning. Life continues, just in different ways. Some adjustments may be necessary, but you have options and the tasks or activities could still be doable. In this chapter, we share what we've done to demonstrate the ways we've been able to carry on with our daily life activities, whether in active treatment or post-treatment. It's amazing how much we could still do. We just have to create the opportunities for ourselves and move forward with what we've got.

APPOINTMENTS

* *Aaron C.* (*Prostate cancer, Skin cancer*)

I absolutely asked my doctors questions. I wasn't afraid to ask personal questions about erections, sex ... all that kind of stuff. I knew he'd tell me, because he's already seen it. I knew I had to find out what's normal and if my recovery is on par for what the doctor has seen. I asked questions like: "What is normal?" "What isn't normal?" And, I made sure to keep asking lots of questions. I researched and read a lot. I didn't take notes; I just remembered. Before meeting with my doctor, I wrote down questions I wanted to make sure I asked him. No one accompanied me to my doctor's appointments.

ADVICE: Don't be afraid to ask personal questions of your doctor, e.g. about sex, erections and all that kind of stuff. Your doctor has seen a lot of cases similar to yours and so would tell you. Before meeting your doctor, write down your questions so you don't forget to ask them. Ask questions like: "What is normal?" "What isn't normal?" And keep on asking questions throughout your treatment, so you know what's going on. Take notes, if it'll help you remember the doctor's answers to your questions. Research on your cancer and your options, so you're aware. Having someone accompany or not accompany you to your doctor's appointments is your choice. Do what makes you comfortable.

* *Amor T.* (*Breast cancer, Ovarian cancer*)

Breast cancer: I went alone to my appointments most of the time, because I didn't feel it necessary to "bother" anyone, if I could physically do it on my own. After my surgery, however, my wonderful friend Martha, accompanied me to my appointments. It really meant a lot to have her support.

Ovarian cancer: My awesome boyfriend Bill accompanied me to all of my doctor appointments, as well as all of my chemo sessions, lab draws, scans, etc. If he couldn't be with me in the imaging rooms (MRI, PET, CT scans), he patiently waited for me in the waiting room and brought some reading material to bide his time. His presence made a world of difference for me. Not only did he support me emotionally, he also gathered information, asked questions on my behalf, helped me remember details and kept me focused on healing.

By the way, there were many appointments where the doctor's office or imaging center needed me to complete forms and provide information about my medical history, medications and supplements, past medical procedures, etc. I compiled all that information in my iPhone's NOTES app and just brought it up to refer to when filling out the forms. Sure beat trying to remember everything.

ADVICE: Having someone to accompany you to your appointments and support you would really help to make your experience with cancer treatment more manageable. Sure, you may be a strong individual and can go it alone, but having cancer in itself is already a hard reality to face. Allow your loved ones to be with you for support. Not only will it enable them to understand what's going on, you'll both benefit in learning how to navigate through the system together. If necessary, they can speak on your behalf. They can also help you remember information that will be thrown at you from all directions. Remember the saying, "two heads are better than one." Besides, if your roles were reversed and your loved one had cancer, you would want to accompany and support them too.

Since cancer treatment usually entails seeing other specialists and going to imaging centers, keeping a list of all your medications and supplements, past procedures and your medical history to refer to will help make things easier for you. If you have a smartphone, you should be able to store it there for easy access.

* Bob G. (Soft Tissue Sarcoma, Skin cancer)

While sitting on the examination table during one of my appointments, I asked my doctor when I'll get another CT scan. He said that it takes several weeks to get a CT scan, unless it's an emergency. I told him that I wanted one as soon as possible. He said that I'm not due another CT scan for six months. He assured me that I would get a CT scan, but not just yet. I looked at him hard and said that I wanted my CT scan NOW! We discussed it and I told him that when I came in to see him, I was very sick. Now, I feel great; I'm in good shape, back to swimming and just don't want to wait until I get sick again. I told him that I wanted the scan on a regular basis. He saw how determined I was and it worked! I got my CT scans scheduled sooner and on a regular basis.

ADVICE: It is really important to be ahead of the game; to get examined on a regular basis. You don't want to wait to get sick to see your doctor. Be proactive!

* Cindy L. (Kidney cancer)

My husband Ed accompanied me to all my medical appointments, whether it was meeting with my doctors or getting my blood tests, scans, etc. Being a nurse, I would do my research and prepare my questions, if any, before my appointment. Also, as much as possible, I would try to schedule all my appointments in one day. That way, I save time and energy. If my appointments can't be scheduled on the same day, I would schedule them as close to each other as possible. For example, I would get my blood test and chest x-ray done on the same day. Then, I would schedule my MRI for the next day. For all appointments, I always have someone with me, because it helps me cope with everything that's going on. Also, it helps to have another person there to help me remember the information I was given.

During appointments, I always take notes and if my doctors tell me something I don't understand, I let them know. If a question comes up in my mind after my appointment, I know that I can always email or call my doctor with that question.

ADVICE: Get all your appointments scheduled on the same day, as much as possible. If they can't be scheduled that way, then try getting them scheduled as close to each other as possible.

Make sure you take someone with you. Don't try to do it all yourself, especially the first couple of times, because there's always going to be a follow-up. Having someone with you not only helps with remembering the information that was given to you, it also helps you cope with everything that's going on in this challenging time.

Also, take notes while you're there. Most doctors won't let you record them. So taking notes while you're there is always a good idea. And, don't let the doctors make you feel rushed. If you don't understand something, ask or say, "I didn't quite understand what you just told me and I have some questions. Is it okay to email you or call you?" As a nurse, I know that you have the right to call or email your doctor and they have to get back to you with answers to your questions. Remember that your doctors and nurses are there to take care of you and they can't read your mind. So, if you have concerns or questions (no matter what you think they might say), you need to speak up.

* Cindy R. (Metastatic Breast cancer to the Stomach)

Someone was with me for all my appointments, especially in the beginning. The first time around, I was so numb like "Okay, what do I ask? What do I do?" I just had no idea. Thankfully, my sister was super strong and she had questions, which were basically my questions. And she took notes for me and everything. She remembered every little step, because I just couldn't. I just didn't know and I couldn't remember. So, thankfully, my middle sister Karen was such a huge help. She was just great throughout. My mother also came with me to all my appointments.

ADVICE: Having someone accompany you to your appointments is really critical. Your doctor or nurse will give you a lot of information that can be overwhelming. Going through cancer treatments is already overwhelming on its own. So you need to have someone (family or friend) with you to help you take in the information, get instructions, ask questions, etc. This is not the time to rely on your memory or your smarts because, with your sickness, you are most likely to forget and even miss out on important details. So, do yourself a favor and make sure someone accompanies you to your appointments.

* Joan S. (Rectal cancer)

My daughter Lori and my friends, Barbara, Mary and Jody accompanied me to my appointments. At the appointments, I was given handouts, which I kept. Anytime I had questions about my treatment, I definitely asked questions, like, "Why am I so sick?" "Why am I not eating?" etc. I asked questions because I needed to understand what was happening.

ADVICE: It helps to have someone accompany you to your appointments. You feel their support, waiting for the doctor doesn't seem so long when you have someone to talk to and you have a second pair of ears to retain information that was given to you.

* J.B. (Salivary gland cancer)

When I communicated with my doctors, it was mostly over the computer. Then, they would respond in writing. It was really necessary to have that open communication.

When I went to appointments, I did take notes on my computer. I also asked my doctors a lot of questions about my chances of recurrence, statistics, etc. I didn't worry about the procedures I had to go through as much as I worried about my long-term chances. I usually went to my appointments by myself, because most times, my appointments would be scheduled around lunch time and it was difficult for people to take time off to accompany me.

* Rev. Linda S. (Pancreatic cancer 3x)

I'm usually behind the wheel for six hours, round trip, for a 30-45 minute appointment. Family and friends accompany me. But, I drive, unless I have to be sedated or am under heavy narcotics. I am immensely grateful for all my family and friends and so thrilled that several of my local friends have stepped up to the plate to provide practical help, like transportation to and from medical appointments, even when they have full lives of their own, retired or not.

Usually, my sister (a retired nurse) or a trusted friend accompany me and help me sort out what I heard during the medical appointment. I do not remember the questions I asked but, in general, they were about the procedures, the expected outcomes, and my prognosis. I rarely took notes. While waiting, I chatted with whoever had accompanied me that day.

* Rachel S. (Breast cancer: triple negative)

When I first started going to my appointments, I would ask a lot of questions like: "What is that?" "What are you doing?" I needed to know every step of what they were doing and they were really good about telling me. After a time, I saw the doctor once every few weeks. So, it was important for me to talk with the nurses and let them know what's going on. I didn't wait to see the doctor.

During the appointments after surgery, my husband was the one who took notes of our visit, because I physically couldn't write. Because my lymphedema was so bad, I couldn't form the letters to write. I was like a first grader learning to write for the first time, like ... up ... down ... around. I mean, I literally had to tell myself to write like that. I had to relearn writing.

* Rick S. (CLL: Blood & Bone Marrow cancer)

When I had appointments with my doctor, the biggest question I asked was, "After all my work in physical fitness, is this chemo going to cause other problems for me later on?" He just answered, "Not that we know of." When he said that, I was somewhat relieved.

I didn't really ask too many questions at my appointments. And, I didn't take notes, due to problems I have writing because of my Cerebral Palsy. I just remember.

* Scott M. (Metastatic Colon cancer to the Prostate & Pancreas)

Whenever I went to my appointment (and I must say that the medical team, here at the Cancer Center, has been exceptional), I was given information on what to expect early on, i.e. medicines I was going to be on, what their side effects would be, things to avoid while I'm taking those medications so as not to decrease their efficiency /efficacy in the body, etc. I never took notes, but I listened. I also had a lot of friends who came. One time, they got in trouble for "partying" in the wait room, because someone smuggled in a bottle of wine. Anyway, they were living.

* Sondra W. (Ovarian cancer 3x)

To prepare for my appointments, I had to write my questions down. I quickly learned that when I got to my appointments, I forgot things, even the most important things. Then I would walk out of there without the answers I needed.

So now I write down anything new that happened since my last visit. I write my questions down, and I also write down the answers because I do forget those too.

While I'm waiting in the lobby for my appointment, I actually look at the brochures displayed there to see what classes are going to go on. And, if there's anybody there that wants to talk or someone I already made a connection with, then I have conversations with them while I wait. Sometimes, I bring a book to read or read the magazines there like "Conquer" and "Cope." If my husband Kenneth is with me, then we use that time to catch up and talk. So that's what I do.

ADVICE: It really helps to jot down questions for your doctor or nurse and their answers too. That way, you'll be aware and knowledgeable about your treatment. You can also bring a friend or family member with you to be your second pair of ears and eyes. He or she can help you remember the important things.

To bide your time while you're waiting, there are many things you can do, like read or write, or talk with someone. You can keep yourself busy with things that interest you; that's if that's what you want to do.

* Susan M. (*Ovarian cancer, Metastatic Pancreatic cancer to the Lungs*)

Ovarian Cancer: I was alone when my doctor told me that the tumor I had in my ovaries was positive for cancer. My dad and husband attended the follow-up appointment at the first hospital and my dad accompanied me to my appointment at the other hospital.

Pancreatic Cancer: I took notes. Both my husband and daughter accompanied me to my first appointment. For subsequent appointments, my daughter and a friend came with me. Since chemo started, I went to the doctor appointments on my own.

ADVICE: Always bring a friend or family member to appointments. You just won't hear or comprehend everything the doctor is saying. Take notes or ask the doctor if you can tape your conversation, so you could go back and review what was discussed. My daughter taped my first visit with the oncologist after my surgery.

* Tet M. (*Colon cancer 3x*)

Initially, I wasn't sure what questions to ask the doctor. Fortunately, in time, Google became our friend.

ADVICE: Now that we have the Internet, research on the type of cancer you are diagnosed with. Remember to visit reputable, reliable sites only. Don't extract information from blogs published by self-proclaimed experts operating from his/her basement.

Ask the medical practitioner hard questions such as, survival rate, recovery period from surgery and what to expect after, the length of your hospital stay, the chances of recurrence, etc. If applicable, ask about the number of radiation and/or chemo sessions, as well as, possible side effects. And please try to have a companion or two with you to be the extra pair of ears, to scribble down notes or even to ask follow up questions.

* Vida B.A. (*Breast cancer*)

Going to my medical appointments, I was always prepared to wait, sometimes for over an hour. The waiting was the only thing I hated. But then, I didn't have a choice, so I would find things to do to keep myself busy while I wait, like browse the internet on my iPhone. My helper was always with me; she's really my angel. Since there were a lot of restaurants in the hospital's lower level, I would send her to buy something to eat and then, we would have a picnic while we wait.

During my appointments, I always took notes. Of course, I followed instructions my doctor gave me. But, I took notes, because I wanted to be able to remember what we discussed.

ADVICE: Be prepared to wait in the reception area whenever you have any appointment. Instead of just sitting there, you could keep yourself busy by reading, playing games on your smartphone, talking with your companion. If you don't have a companion, try talking with other people in the waiting room with you. Since having cancer and going through treatment is already a lot to deal with, taking notes during your appointments will help you remember what's happening in your treatment and how you're progressing. You don't have to try to remember; just refer to your notes.

* Yesi L. (Breast cancer: triple positive)

Appointments are something that can definitely be very overwhelming and experiences definitely vary from hospital to hospital. I was very fortunate to have had a Nurse Navigator at Cancer Center who actually planned all of my appointments, because of my diagnosis. Since I wasn't working at the time, my schedule was wide open. So, that made it very, very easy for them to schedule me for just mornings. I'm a morning person, so that worked perfectly for me.

I researched my cancer and treatments, so I was prepared with questions to ask. I wanted to know what was going into my body and what the treatments were going to do to my body. It helped to have the knowledge so that I could process the experience better. I tried to stay only with the internet sites that ended in ".org", like www.cancer.org for the American Cancer Society. Internet sites that do not end in ".org" just have a lot of misleading information.

Since gathering the information was overwhelming, my Nurse Navigator took notes for me. It was like I had my own personal assistant to help while I was undergoing treatment.

I definitely had my husband, my mom or my friends accompany me to the important appointments, like CAT scans, MRIs or new procedures like my first Radiation treatment. I needed them with me, because I didn't know how the treatments were going to affect me.

ADVICE: Definitely ask questions and research what you can about your cancer, so you can ask questions about your treatment. Avoid internet sites that do not have ".org" at the end. Those sites just have a lot of misleading information.

For your appointments, especially the important ones, have someone who is dear to you; someone you really trust, be there with you. They may be your spouse, your significant other, your mother, your best friend, etc.

ARTS & CRAFTS, HOBBIES, WORKSHOPS, CLUBS

* Aaron C. (Prostate cancer, Skin cancer)

One of my hobbies is playing my drums. For the first three months after my surgery, I couldn't play them, because the drum stool was a hard surface that would apply pressure down in my groin area if I sat on it and cause a lot of pain. It was so painful to sit on hard surfaces, at that time. I couldn't even ride my motorcycle, because the seat was hard to sit on.

ADVICE: You'll be really sore and experience pain after surgery. So, try to relax and give yourself time to heal. You'll be able to return to your normal activities and hobbies after your body gets stronger and your treatment is over.

* Amor T. (Breast cancer, Ovarian cancer)

Breast cancer. Right before I learned I had breast cancer, I was an active member of the Foster City Lions Club. I was very involved in our club's many fundraising and service activities, because volunteerism is a favorite activity of mine. When we were at the Lions 4C4 District Convention in Sacramento, I remember receiving my doctor's call telling me that she strongly suspected that I had breast cancer, but needed for me to get an MRI to confirm her suspicion. I kept my calm.

After the convention, I went on a personal leave of absence and put my activities with the Lions Club on hold, so I could just focus on my health. Well, even though I stopped attending the meetings, my fellow Foster City Lions became active in taking care of me and following up on my progress. I felt so very loved and valued and remember thinking how much God has blessed me with my fellow Lions. When I went into remission, I immediately returned to participate again in the Lions activities that I enjoyed so much..

Ovarian cancer. Bill and I had been shuttling between our home in Santa Clara and our newly-purchased home in Penn Valley and were working on projects in both houses. When my gynecologist called to inform me that I had ovarian cancer, we knew we had to take a good, hard look at the situation. We then discussed our plan of action and decided to hold off on the jaunts between our two homes and just focus on my treatment and getting my health back.

I also attended personal training sessions at My Core Balance twice a week, which I really enjoyed. When I started treatment, I had to stop. Fortunately, I was able to resume my training less than a month from my last chemo session. It was tough to start again with my body at such a weakened state. However, with persistence, determination and awesome trainers, I was able to regain my strength and core alignment.

ADVICE: Putting your activities on hold to focus on your health and treatment should be a priority. You can always return when you've completed treatment. Of course, if your activities can be done at home, you can adjust and just do them on the days your body has the energy for it. Main thing is to not drop it altogether, especially if it's something that brings you joy.

* Cindy R. (Metastatic Breast cancer to the Stomach)

During the time of my diagnosis, I was training my dog. She was actually going to be in a show and I had a trainer who was able to come to my house, whenever I was feeling really bad, and help me train her. When I felt better, I'd go to his place or I'd go to the park and train her there with a group. So, I adjusted the scheduling of the training, depending on how I was feeling at the time.

Unfortunately, I couldn't continue with her training, because I got so sick to the point where I just couldn't do it, no matter how hard I tried. The worst part was when I was in bed all the time, thinking that this might be the end. I watched a lot of TV, which helped me get my mind off things. I tried to watch a lot of comedies so that I could laugh. My dogs would climb in bed and snuggle up with me, while I pet them. At the time, that was all I could do with them.

I also enjoy making jewelry. Whenever I had my good days, I would pull out my jewelry sets and spread them all around me. Then, I would look online and check out what there was. I would say, "Oh, that's a neat thing" and maybe print it out to work on later when I felt like starting a new jewelry project.

Thankfully, with the help of my friends, I was able to continue with my ladies groups. For activities, I would go to the monthly luncheons and my friends would help me out with that. I was actually on the board at one time, but had to take a step back, because I got really sick. Now that I'm feeling better, I'm back on the board and doing more; getting more involved.

ADVICE: Just do what you can. Don't give up the activities you enjoy. For sure, don't give them up, because if those activities are things you enjoy, then they're what's going to help you get better. They'll help keep your mind engaged and interested. All you have to do is adjust the activities to fit your needs. People will want to help too. So, allow them to assist you. Do what you can, even if it's just looking at pictures online of things that you might want to do or make later on. It'll keep you interested and engaged and your mind active, instead of focusing on being sick, which doesn't help at all.

* J.B. (Salivary gland cancer)

For the most part, I was able to continue with my hobbies and things that I enjoyed, although there were times I had to adjust. When I felt fatigued, it limited the amount of time I could do the things I enjoyed. I did plan around the times fatigue would get to me.

ADVICE: You can still enjoy the things you like to do. Just plan around the time fatigue gets to you, which, for me were the evenings.

* Rev. Linda S. (*Pancreatic cancer 3x*)

I enjoy playing word games on my Kindle, reading, and coloring. I love cooking but had neither the energy to cook nor the desire to eat for several weeks after surgery and on the days I received chemo. However, when I did have the energy and the time, I enjoyed cooking for myself, as well as for others.

ADVICE: **Continue to do what you enjoy when you have energy.**

* Scott M. (*Metastatic Colon cancer to the Prostate & Pancreas*)

I have my horse (Tucson) and riding my horse was really good therapy for me when I was going through treatment. It was also good exercise, because you do get to a point when you feel very weak. There were times when it was almost all I could do to just "tack up" and saddle my horse. Then I had to pick his hooves, brush him out and all that kind of stuff. Other than that, I didn't really have any hobbies, while I was going through treatment.

Before cancer, I loved to read novels. I have a hard time reading now, because I forget what I've read due to my chemo brain. So, unfortunately, I don't read as much as I used to.

ADVICE: **If there's something you enjoyed before cancer, you will have to adjust in order to continue enjoying those activities. Don't focus on what you can't do. Focus on what you <u>can</u> do, instead.**

* Sondra W. (*Ovarian cancer 3x*)

I was glad to be able to do the Living Strong, Living Well strength and fitness training program for adult cancer survivors. That was really good. They had exercises and all kinds of creative movements to make you use your muscles. When I went through the program, it was at my own pace because I actually was behind everybody in the class, energy-wise. I was so worn down. The instructors didn't mind that. They always told me how I could do things to adjust. They were also aware that I had my knee issues, and I had really bad neuropathy, which threw off my balance, as well. So, they showed me how to adjust. Because of the extent of my condition, I could not use any equipment. I had a little exercise routine that I did down the hall while all the rest were doing the weight training part of the regular program. I learned a lot and built up some stamina, and that's a really good thing.

ADVICE: **Even if you feel you don't have the energy or just don't feel like getting back to your hobbies or going to workshops, fitness programs, etc. it's really important to gradually get out and get engaged on some form of activity. Those activities will help your overall sense of self and get you out of focusing on your body's weakness. Simple walking is a great first step.**

* Vida B.A. (*Breast cancer*)

While I was going through treatment, a lot of people gave me coloring books. I thought I would enjoy them, because I'm an artist. However, when I started on it, I only completed one page and didn't feel like doing it again. Fortunately, I found an app on my iPhone that was like a coloring book where I used my fingers to color the pictures on the screen. I liked it much better; it was faster and I could see the results right away.

I also enjoyed playing mahjong with my friends. It's really good therapy for me, because it keeps my mind going and thinking; using strategy to make my moves.

ADVICE: **When going through treatment, it's therapeutic to have a hobby or art activity you can work on. Playing games with friends or family is fun too. Whatever you do, choose something that will keep you active and busy. That way, you distract yourself from your sickness, which actually helps you to heal faster.**

* Yesi L. *(Breast cancer: triple positive)*

I enjoyed gardening. Plants and greenery make me happy. It's very relaxing. I was actually very fatigued most of the time. But, I did have a bit of energy to continue with my gardening.

Cancer Center had the *Art & Soul* workshop, but I did only one. I was just too fatigued to continue.

ADVICE: Do what you enjoy. But, if you are fatigued, listen to your body and rest. You can continue your hobbies, etc. when you have more energy.

CHILDREN

---

* Aaron C. *(Prostate cancer, Skin cancer)*

I have a healthy relationship with my daughters and I'm very honest with them. I didn't get into too many details, because they're young. I, basically, said that I had prostate cancer and I'm going to be okay. When they heard that, they got worried and thought I was going to die. I told them, "No, I'm not going to die. I'm going to have surgery." Then I said, "I'm going to be a little bit out-of-commission for a while, but your dad's going to be fine."

When my kids came over to be with me, we just hung out and watched movies and stuff. There were a few things I couldn't do, like run and chase them for a few months, like I used to. One day, they saw the bag attached to my leg. So, I had to explain to them that I had to urinate into the bag. Then I told them, "I need you to help me do this and this..." At first, they got grossed out by it. But then after, they were totally cool with it, because they wanted to help me. You know, help their daddy.

The first ten days after surgery, when I couldn't do anything because of my catheter. I had my ex-wife take our kids to school or wherever they needed to go. I didn't tell her about my cancer; I didn't want her to know. I try to keep my privacy private. I just told my ex, "Hey, I can't" or whatever excuse I used. The good thing is that most of this happened around July when they were out of school for the summer, so the timing was right. Now, I'm able to have fun with my daughters and chase after them, like I used to do before I had cancer.

ADVICE: If you have a slow-growing cancer, meaning you don't need immediate treatment, time the surgery, so that it's held during the time you don't have a lot of things going on. You can expect to sit at home and do absolutely nothing, but watch TV and, maybe, walk around a little bit in your house for the first ten days.

Be as honest as you can with your children and, definitely, consider their age. If they're not adults, they don't need to hear details. What they need is reassurance that your illness and treatment period are temporary and that you're going to be okay.

* Amor T. *(Breast cancer, Ovarian cancer)*

Breast cancer: In 2013, when I was diagnosed with breast cancer, my daughter Catherine was away at college. She was 22 years old at the time and was really calm when I told her that I had breast cancer. I remember calling her and just focusing on the facts of the matter, saying, "I have breast cancer on my left breast. I'll first have a mastectomy to remove my left breast and then a breast reconstruction to create me a new left breast, using my own body's tissue. It will take me some time to recover from the surgery, but I'll be fine. Nothing to worry about. All I ask for is your prayers." I didn't put much emotion into my conversation with Catherine. I knew that how I explained my situation to her would influence how she took the news and digested it. When she talked, Catherine was calm and also reassuring. She did surprise me when I woke up in ICU after my surgery. She had flown in just for one night to be with me and had to return to classes the next day. I was so happy and touched to feel her love!

Before I was discharged from the hospital after my staph infection scare, my doctor instructed me to have someone stay with me overnight for one week. I had someone with me for all nights that week, except one night when no one was available for one reason or another. When Catherine learned of my predicament, she offered to be with me. That was quite a surprise, because she was away at a college that was almost 400 miles away and she still had classes to attend. Catherine explained that, even though she couldn't be with me in person, physically, we could still be together via SKYPE (video chats). So, when she got home from class, she contacted me and we "stayed together" online and watched each other sleep. We even woke up with each other online! I had no clue that that was even an option. It touched me so deeply that my beautiful Catherine would even propose that arrangement. How awesome to feel Catherine unselfish love! I'm so very blessed!

Ovarian cancer: When I informed Catherine of my ovarian cancer diagnosis in 2016, she was calm. Well, we were both calm. I gave her the facts again and told her not to worry. I was just going to go through treatment and when it's completed, I'll recover and be done with cancer. By this time, Catherine had graduated from college, but stayed in Southern California where she had a job in Disneyland. Well, in the middle of my chemo treatment, Catherine took two months off from work (FMLA-family medical leave) to take care of me. It was the best feeling to be cared for her and loved by my beautiful daughter Catherine.

ADVICE: How you communicate your diagnosis with your children will dictate how they will react. When they're physically away from you, you want to make sure they don't panic. They need to know you'll be fine, because not being able to physically be with you when you're ill can be really upsetting and serve as a distraction from their schoolwork. Before you speak with your children, take a deep breath and plan how you're just going to inform them of the facts, followed with reassurance that you'll be fine. Even if you aren't completely sure of how your treatment will go, it's important to keep your children from worrying about you.

* Cindy L. *(Kidney cancer)*

My children and I are close, even though we live far from each other. So, it was difficult to share the news of my cancer diagnosis with them. My oldest daughter Ali lives in Royal Oak, Michigan. My oldest son Brennan lives in Tampa, Florida. And my Katie and Harrison both live here. Harrison is married and has four little girls; he's a busy dad and I'm a busy grandma. After some coordination and working through some challenges, we brought everyone together in one town, so that we could all to discuss things together, as a family.

Before I was formally diagnosed, I had already planned to see my daughter Ali in Michigan who kept fainting and, at that time, we didn't know why. At the doctor's office with my husband, I was very emotional, but still kept focus on Ali's situation. So, before my doctor could officially tell me that I had cancer, I said, "Okay. Well, I'll tell you what. I'm leaving tomorrow to go out of town to take care of my daughter. What has been going inside of me didn't just start overnight. It has been here for a long time and it's not going to go anywhere for the week that it's going to take me to see my daughter." For me, I had something more important to do, which was to go take care of my daughter who needed me.

All my children did what they could to take care of me, including helping me out of my chair, tucking me into bed, accompanying me to my appointments and shopping, etc. Even though I usually find it hard to ask anyone for help, I did feel my children's love for me when they came to take care of me. I know that I wasn't the easiest patient to deal with, because there were times I just snapped at them when they didn't read my mind. I'm much better about that now and really appreciate everything they've done for me.

One of my biggest frustrations, during treatment, was not being able to pick up my little granddaughters. At one time, I picked up my 8-month old grandbaby who was 24 lbs. at the time. I paid for that, because I was so sore the next day. Fortunately, I'm healed now and can pick up my granddaughters. Still, I always have to be cautious.

ADVICE: Be honest and open, but be cautious about telling your children that you have a deadly disease. Timing is important. Consider their individual situations. When your children want to support you, let them. It helps to be specific as to what you need for them to do, so they can understand and not have to read your mind. Even though you may be limited physically, you can still support and guide your children in many other ways. Have discussions and share your thoughts and ideas. Take advantage of this opportunity for you to bond with them.

* Hilda K. *(Colon cancer)*

Because I took time off from work for a year, I was able to drop my daughter Adrianna to and from school and her practices. After I dropped her off at school, there was a church nearby where I attended the 8:00 am mass.

When I had enough energy, I made dinner for the family and did everything "normal." I didn't feel much fatigue and I didn't overwork myself. Basically, I didn't try to do more than I could. My family supported me and I allowed myself to go through this experience without any stress.

> **ADVICE:** Yes, take care of your children's needs when you can. However, don't stress yourself about it. Listen to your body and don't try to take on too much. Ask your family or friends to help take your children to/from school or practices, if your body is not up to it.

* Jacki S. *(Breast cancer)*

During treatment, I continued to make sure my daughter was up and dressed for school and I still made her breakfast. I also continued to drive her to the bus stop so she could go to her middle school, after which I would resume my regular routines for the day..

I remained active in Jenise's school, even when I was going through treatment. As a matter of fact, when I found out about my cancer, I was just about set to go on a field trip with her as a chaperone to Disneyland.. The school's orchestra, band and chorus, which my daughter was part of, were going to perform at Disneyland. I let the choir director know that I had cancer and I was going to have surgery. He said that it was up to me if I wanted to go on the trip, or if I felt it wasn't the right thing to do, he would find another chaperone. What I told him was, "I have loved Disneyland from the time I was six years old. I would love to go to Disneyland and won't even think about my cancer the whole time I'm there. Who thinks about cancer when you're in Disneyland?" We were around all the kids. I had a roommate who was another mom. All we did was enjoy the kids, enjoy the performance and their performances. Once I got home, I was booked the next week to have my surgery. I did not let my cancer hold me back from our trip to Disneyland.

* Joan S. *(Rectal cancer)*

I'm very close to my daughters Lori and Shelley and keep in close contact with both of them. They took good care of me when I was ill. I am so blessed and so thankful for them.

* Rachel S. *(Breast cancer: triple negative)*

My children are my hobby and my favorite pastime. I play with them, solve puzzles with them, watch TV with them. We did a lot of singing and laughing at whatever. When I didn't feel good, we would sit down and snuggle and watch minions or whatever my little one's favorite show was. What show we watched didn't even matter, because I couldn't focus on the TV anyway. It just mattered that he was with me.

One weekend, when my daughter visited, we went to Yosemite. It was a really, really hard trip for me, because my muscles hurt and my bones hurt. But, I pushed myself through it, because I wanted to spend the time with the kids and have them have that memory. You know, just doing things for them got me through it. As much as I could, I brought them to school and picked them up from school.

All my children knew what was going on. I didn't keep anything from them. The day I was told I had cancer, I asked my neighbor to pick up my twelve-year old son from school and when my husband returned home from work, he and I talked to our son about it. I also never hid from my children the severity of it. They know there's a risk of it coming back, but only my 20-year old daughter understands how high the risk is.

Everything else from the surgery, the lymphedema to the medications I took ... the cannabis ... they know all of it. I didn't hide anything from them. My twelve-year old didn't ask too many questions. I think it's because I answered them, before he had a chance to ask, most of the time. He didn't shut down, but he kind of changed in that he was turning a lot to music and gaming as a coping mechanism. That was fine; I didn't have an issue with it. He was still doing karate. One day, his sensei came to me and said, "I'm starting to get worried about him. He had a breakdown in class the other day." I said, "Ok." When we got home, I sat him down and told him exactly what his sensei told me and he broke down crying. His question was, "How do you know the treatments are going to work?" I said, "They will". He said "HOW do you know?" And I said, "I don't". I was very honest with him. We have to have faith that it'll work. And so, a lot of it is based around that.

I got criticized for sharing everything with my kids. Some people told me that I gave too much information; that I shouldn't be sharing everything with my kids. But, the way I see it, I think, "How can I expect my children to cope and grow up with a good outcome in their attitudes and their lives if they know I'm lying to them about everything?" It just doesn't work that way.

<u>ADVICE:</u> **Be honest and open in communicating with your children. They are sensitive and can tell what's going on. You are a role model for them. If you show strength and faith, they will pick up on those qualities. If you demonstrate a positive attitude when times are tough, they will grow with the same positive attitude in life, too.**

* Scott M. (*Metastatic Colon cancer to the Prostate & Pancreas*)

My children were in high school and we were very frank and upfront with them. They knew everything as soon as we knew it. At first, they were very quiet. They didn't talk to me too much about it, but I understood that they were fearful. But, because I got up, got dressed, made an effort everyday (and some days I did go out and do things), I showed them that it wasn't going to slow me down and I wasn't fearful. So, they kind of mirror my attitudes.

<u>ADVICE:</u> **Be honest and open when you communication with your children. They will try to deal with your cancer however they can and they'll be watching you, even though they may not say much. Demonstrate strength and courage, no matter how bad you feel. Whatever you do, they will mirror. And you want them to grow up strong and brave. Be a role model for your children.**

* Sondra W. (*Ovarian cancer 3x*)

I have a wonderful relationship with my 50-year old daughter, Dawn, and my 24-year old granddaughter, Kayla. When they learned of my diagnosis, they took the news hard. When I saw how they keyed off of my reaction and how they wanted to protect me, I told them, sort of calmly, what they wanted to know. After they got over the shock and sadness, they started listening to what we were going to do. They wanted to know how they could help and all that; they kind of "kicked in" that way.

<u>ADVICE:</u> **Your children will key off of your behavior and disposition. They're going through the experience with you and may even have great difficulty coping. Talk with them honestly about what you need and be in tuned with their needs as well.**

* Susan M. (*Ovarian cancer, Metastatic Pancreatic cancer to the Lungs*)

Ovarian Cancer: When I was diagnosed with Ovarian Cancer, my daughter was only eighteen months old. Despite my condition, I continued to do what I could for her and participated in all the activities she was involved in before I learned I had cancer. We also spent a lot of time at the park with her.

<u>ADVICE:</u> **It's really important to give your young child some semblance of normalcy, even when you're going through a very serious illness. Somehow it benefits both you and your child, because of the positive energy that you're sharing together. So, focus on the positive. Focus on enjoying times with your children.**

* Yesi L. (*Breast cancer: triple positive*)

My then four-year old daughter Zoe was definitely impacted, because Mommy couldn't run around with her, like I used to. And, I definitely, could not pick her up. However, I did find a way to hold her. I sat in bed and had her sit on my lap. So, that felt like I was picking her up. She would just hold me. And, that was a very deep connection. A very deep connection, which we loved.

When I had more energy, we had tickle fights. When I asked her what she wanted – thinking that she would ask for a toy or ask for something else – she said that she wanted a tickle fight. So, there would be plenty of laughter.

My husband and I were extremely open in communicating with Zoe, as far as everything that was happening to me, because she saw it every day. I believe it's important to prepare your children when you're going to undergo surgery or receive serious medical treatment. We gave Zoe just enough information for her to understand that Mommy is going to go through surgery and will need extra time to rest. Of course, it was important that she knew that, no matter what, Mommy is here for you or Grandma is going to take care of you.

Because I was not working at that time, I was able to take Zoe to school. I was still able to drive. But, I preferred walking to school with her in the mornings. It was only a mile away. And, I would feel accomplished after I walked a mile and back. Besides, she loved it and it was a bonding activity for us. When my energy allowed it, I was able to become very active in her school.

ADVICE: If you cannot physically carry your young child, try sitting down on the bed or chair and have your child sit on your lap. You both can then just hold each other. It creates a beautiful connection.

CLOTHING

* Aaron C. (Prostate cancer, Skin cancer)

All I did was just wear baggy, loose-fitting clothes, like my sweat pants, loose-fitting shorts and stuff like that. It was a pain in the ass doing it. I managed it, but it was painful. Still, I managed it by myself. The hardest time I had with putting my clothes on was when I got released from the hospital. Because they were overbooked, for some reason, nobody was there to initially help me. They didn't even help me put my own pants back on and I couldn't even bend over to get my shoes; the pain was so great. So, I was like, "Hey, can somebody give me a hand here? I can't get my own shoes on." Finally, someone came to help. Yeah, I was miserable.

ADVICE: Make sure you get the help you need when it comes to your clothing. Don't be afraid to ask the nurses or whomever to help you get dressed or changed. Also, make sure you do all the shopping you need (groceries, toiletries, clothing, medications, etc.) to do before the surgery. You don't want to worry about shopping or going anywhere after the surgery. Expect to stay home for the first ten days and do absolutely nothing, except trying to get up every so often.

* Amor T. (Breast cancer, Ovarian cancer)

Breast cancer. When I left the hospital, I remember having a long sleeved front button-down shirt that was easy to wear with my very bruised and sore chest area. I wore a pair of hospital pants with drawstrings, which was difficult to get into given my large abdominal wound. With the help of the hospital aide, I put it on very, very slowly.

After I got home from the hospital, choosing clothes to wear when I had the four surgical drains hanging from my sides after surgery was a challenge, but I learned to be creative. I searched my entire wardrobe and set aside clothes that would work for my situation, i.e. loose dresses or skirts with loose garters or drawstrings, wraps or sarongs and even large scarves that I could use as a wrap. At the time, I couldn't wear pants at all, because of the drains hanging from both sides of my hip.

With the loose wrap dresses or gowns, I used a safety pin to hook the drain bulb with the tube and attached it to one side of the material. When I had to leave my home to visit the doctor, I wore a very loose cardigan or long sleeve top which I used to attach the drain bulbs to with a safety pin. At one time, I had to attend a semi-formal event to receive an award. I wore a long, black halter top gown, over which I covered with a long black cardigan. I attached the surgical drains from my upper torso to the inside of my cardigan and attached the surgical drains from both sides of my hips to the insides of my gown. No one could tell that I had four surgical drains hanging out of my body.

After my surgical drains were removed, I wore tops that opened up in front, like front button-down shirts. When I was at home, I chose to go braless, so my wounds could breathe and heal faster. I preferred wearing dresses, especially tube top dresses, over pants, because of my abdominal incision.

Ovarian cancer. Learning from my breast cancer experience, I already identified loose dresses, tops and drawstring pants I could wear without affecting my abdominal wound. However, this time, I had to also work around my medical port (located below my right clavicle) and the blisters that were created when adhesive tape I was allergic to was used to cover the insertion point of my thoracentesis procedure. This was located below my right shoulder blade. I wore tops and dresses with open necklines that did not cover my port (I did not mind that anyone would see it; it was more important for me to be comfortable). I also chose to wear tops or dresses with low back covers, so that the material wouldn't touch my blisters.

> **ADVICE:** Best clothes to wear after any major surgery, especially when you have surgical drains hanging out of your body, are loose clothes with either drawstring ties or loose garters. Use safety pins to attach the surgical drains to your clothing. If you can, wear clothes (tops or bottoms) that have large pockets for you to place the drainbulbs in. There are actually bras and other accessories that are made specifically for surgical drains.

* Bob G. (Soft Tissue Sarcoma, Skin cancer)

I had no problem getting dressed or choosing what to wear. I buy decent clothes. But, my wife had better taste and got me to wear better clothes.

* Cindy L. (Kidney cancer)

I had a hard time wearing clothes with zippers, because of my abdominal wounds; I still do. Before surgery, I lost weight, but then gained weight after surgery. Fortunately, I kept some of the bigger clothes I had before my weight loss. They're easy on my scars, like my friend's yoga pants. I can wear zippered pants, as long as they are one size too big. Sure, they're too big on the hips, but whatever; who cares?

After my abdominal surgery, I had to wear an abdominal binder that was meant for women who had caesarean sections. It was very soft and washable; it was great.

> **ADVICE:** Wear what makes you comfortable. Even of the clothes are too loose on you, if they're comfortable, then that's what you should wear. If you had abdominal surgery, it helps to use an abdominal binder; the one that they give to women who had caesarean sections. If you're male and you had abdominal surgery, get that binder too. Your gender doesn't matter here. Let your doctor know that you believe the binder will help you and they may get it for you for free.

* Cindy R. (Metastatic Breast cancer to the Stomach)

When I had the double mastectomy, I had to wear a "medical" bra that buttons down the front. It's made like that, so you can pull it from around the back side and then button it down the front, which prevents the tubes from getting in the way. It was given to me by the hospital. I also wore loose, button-down shirts and blouses. As for pants, I wore the loose-fitting ones with the drawstrings. I could just pull them up and get comfortable.

I remember that when I was first diagnosed and after I got out of the hospital, I went crazy and went shopping, buying all kinds of really pretty clothes. I felt so bad that I wanted to look good. So, I just got whatever looked good on me. I did it for myself. I didn't have trouble getting dressed; it was pretty straightforward. I just did it slowly.

(Headwear for Alopecia)

I lost my hair completely when I was going through chemotherapy to treat my breast cancer. I wore a lot of caps and scarves to cover my head, because I didn't like to wear the wig I had. I only wore it on occasion, like the time my sister got married and we went to Hawaii. I was part of the wedding party and I wanted to, at least, look halfway normal. It was so uncomfortable for me. So, I took it off whenever I could and put it back on only when I really needed to. I was more comfortable wearing bandanas, caps and those kinds of things.

My sister and I actually had some fun making our own little hats too. They were almost like babushka hats that you can tie around. We sewed them from different materials and got to be creative. I just wanted to have fun with it.

ADVICE: After mastectomy, you should get a "medical bra" with a front closure. The bra was created in a way where the surgical tubes don't get in the way. Make sure to ask for it, if they don't give you one. It should definitely be covered by insurance also.

Wear loose clothing, especially after surgery, because your body will be swollen from the surgery and medication. You'll want to be comfortable. Button-down blouses and shirts work because then you won't have to raise your arms to pull the overhead tops down through your head. Don't rush to put on your clothes. Be gentle with yourself and just dress yourself slowly.

If you lost some or all of your hair during treatment, there are so many head coverings you can wear, like wigs, caps, turbans, hats, scarves, etc. You can get really creative and have fun with it. Don't worry about what other people will think. They're not going through what you're going through. Just keep it light and have fun. Take care of yourself. Do it for yourself.

By the way, the American Cancer Society has a program that's called "The Look Good, Feel Better" program that helps women with cancer, manage the appearance-related side effects of treatment. There, trained volunteer beauty professionals teach cancer patients simple techniques on skin care, makeup and nail care and give practical tips on hair loss wigs and head coverings (scarves, caps, turbans, etc.). Workshop participants receive a free cosmetic kit and style tips. The workshops are free to women undergoing chemotherapy, radiation or other forms of treatment. I also got a free wig from them. It's a great resource, especially for those patients who learn that treatment will cause them to lose their hair and won't know what to do or where to go when that happens. They're really helpful.

* Glenn M. (Metastatic Colon cancer to the Liver, Lungs & Adrenal Glands)

I'm pretty casual and believe in being comfortable. You can be comfortable and look good at the same time. When I have to go for scans, I make sure I wear clothes that are loose, like sweats. I also make sure my clothes don't have any metal in them, like grommets that the strings pass through or zippers. I have pajamas that I like to wear, but I can't wear those in public.

ADVICE: Whatever you like to wear, just be comfortable. Dress for yourself. If you have to get a scan, wear clothes that are loose (like sweats) and make sure they don't have any metal in them, like grommets that the strings pass through or zippers or metal buttons.

* Hilda K. (Colon cancer)

When I was going through my chemo treatments, I was always cold (hypothermia), especially after each treatment. I also remember my feet and hands tingling and being very sensitive to cold (neuropathy). So, I always wore socks and gloves to keep them warm, as much as I could. Because my whole body was always cold, I basically lived in sweats and kept my entire body covered, as much as possible. When I had to go outside, I bundled up extra, adding a jacket, hat, gloves and a scarf I used to also wrap around my mouth and nose to keep from breathing in the cold air.

I slept in sweatshirts and jackets, adding socks throughout the winter...the six months I went through treatment. Even though I had a comforter to cover me in bed, it was not enough. No matter what, it felt like my body could not get warm enough. What did help was drinking hot or warm liquids.

Since I didn't have to go to work, I wore super casual and comfortable clothes, e.g. sweat pants, t-shirts, jackets, tennis shoes, etc. To strengthen my body and help it heal, I did go to the gym regularly, even when I still had to carry my chemo pump, which was connected to my mediport. It sounds complicated, but it really was easy. With the chemo pump underneath my blouse, no one could tell I was wearing it. It didn't get in the way, at all. I just did my workouts at the gym, washed myself after (holding the chemo pump away from me as I washed) and that was it. It was easy! I'm telling you ... this experience, for me, was really easy!

ADVICE: Wear whatever is comfortable for you, no matter what you look like. Your focus should be your health and your comfort. It really doesn't matter what anyone thinks. If you experience cold, bundle up with sweats, sweaters, jackets, socks, gloves, scarves, hats or beanies/caps. If you have to carry a chemo pump around, it's easy to conceal, because it's small enough to wear underneath your clothes. Also, the chemo pump is easy to manage and shouldn't get in your way. Don't see it as a "burden", because that kind of attitude will create a negative experience for you, which is really unnecessary. See it as an "accessory" like I did. That way, you'll have a positive experience with it.

* Jacki S. *(Breast cancer)*

As far as getting dressed and knowing what to wear, I didn't have any problems getting dressed. Only when I was going in for chemo did I have to make sure I had a short sleeved shirt on, so my left arm was available for the needle. My right arm wasn't available, because I had the lumpectomy on my right side.

ADVICE: Always go for comfort and consider your activity, if necessary.

* Joan S. *(Rectal cancer)*

I had no problems with clothing. I just got elastic pants.

ADVICE: In choosing my clothes, I believe in comfort. Elastic pants worked the best for me.

* J.B. *(Salivary gland cancer)*

I wore normal clothing, like T-shirts and collared shirts. The only time I had to really consider what I had to wear was when I would go to my radiation treatments. If I wore collared shirts, the mask, because it was really big, would come in contact with the collars on my shirt. So, I wore T-shirts to my radiation treatments, instead. It was pretty easy; not a big deal at all.

* Rev. Linda S. *(Pancreatic cancer 3x)*

After my surgery, I dressed for comfort to ensure nothing irritated the healing abdominal incisions. Because my first round of chemo spanned the autumn and winter seasons, I wore berets and scarves to keep my head warm and my hair from scaring people...My head looked like a molting bird! For the last month or so, I wore a human-hair wig when at social functions.

ADVICE: Dress for comfort, especially if you had surgery resulting in incisions that need healing.

* Rachel S. *(Breast cancer: triple negative)*

The majority of the time in the past, I wore the type of T-shirts that had a low neck to them. Since I had the double mastectomy, I could no longer wear them. Also, most of my shirts did not fit anymore, because they were all large; pretty big. So, I wound up having to buy a bunch of new shirts; those that have higher collars. I had a lot of issue with what kind of shirt or top to wear. I coordinated the tops with long skirts or pants.

When the surgical drain bulbs were still attached to me, I hardly left the house. I wore the camisoles (camis) the hospital gave me that had the little pockets you can put the drain bulbs in. Half the time, I didn't wear anything else over the camis, because I was just at home. If I went out, I would wear a really, really loose shirt. This happened in the middle of summer, so I didn't need a sweater.

ADVICE: Be comfortable, especially at home. If you have drain bulbs, there are camisoles with pockets to hold them. Hopefully, your hospital will have them to give you. If you need to go out, just put a loose top on and coordinate with a skirt or pants.

* **Rick S.** (*CLL: Blood & Bone Marrow cancer*)

I had no problems getting dressed. I have no problems choosing what to wear because I'm a male. I did my own laundry and then put on a pair of clean Levis and that was it.

* **Scott M.** (*Metastatic Colon cancer to the Prostate & Pancreas*)

I believe in staying comfortable when it comes to clothing.

ADVICE: Wear what's comfortable for you.

* **Sondra W.** (*Ovarian cancer 3x*)

I always try to wear what's comfortable to me and then dress in layers because sometimes I'm cold even when others around me are not. Getting myself dressed was never an issue.

ADVICE: Dress for yourself and always dress comfortably even if everyone around you is dressed differently. Your comfort is what matters when it comes to clothes.

* **Susan M.** (*Ovarian cancer, Metastatic Pancreatic cancer to the Lungs*)

Pancreatic Cancer: I had a hard time eating during my treatment period and I lost seventeen pounds. Since my clothes were too loose, I had to purchase some new ones.

* **Vida B.A.** (*Breast cancer*)

Before my mastectomy, I went shopping and bought myself some fashionable, loose clothing, like nice blouses with buttons that opened up in front. I also got pretty, loose blouses with wide necklines that I could easily put over my head. Initially, I had to wear the blouses with the buttons that opened up in front, because I had difficulty raising my arms after my mastectomy.

ADVICE: After mastectomy, your arms and your upper body will be really sore. So, it's best to wear tops that are loose and have buttoned openings in front. Later on, when you can lift your arms, you can add loose tops with wide neck openings to your clothing options. By the way, if you have to deal with drain tubes & bulbs, wearing loose clothing is always the way to go.

* **Yesi L.** (*Breast cancer: triple positive*)

Choosing what to wear was not really a focus for me anymore. There were far more important things to focus on. However, on the days where I had a little more energy, wearing beautiful clothes did make me feel beautiful.

I did need help getting dressed and showering, mainly after surgery. My husband and sister-in-law helped me a lot with that. So yes, there are a lot of people I'm extremely grateful to.

Since I had drain bulbs on the sides of my body, we had to get very creative in finding pockets for the drains or hiding them in the clothes I wore. Long sleeved, button shirts were probably the most comfortable for me. We would just pin the drain bulbs to whatever bra I was wearing. Sports bras – the comfortable, stretchy ones; not the very tight ones – were my go-to bras. In fact, I still wear a lot of sports bras.

When it came to headwear, I only wore a wig to go out. I think I used it a total of three times. But, definitely, I wore a lot of scarves and beanies when the weather was cold, because my head would get very, very cold.

COOKING, BAKING

* Amor T. *(Breast cancer, Ovarian cancer)*

Breast cancer. Since I lived alone and couldn't prepare food when I returned from the hospital, my wonderful fellow Foster City Lions organized a "meal train" for me where they took turns bringing food to me; all of them really yummy! I was overwhelmed with gratitude. My refrigerator was full, as was my tummy. After sometime, when my body started feeling stronger, I slowly went to the kitchen to make food or drinks for myself.

Ovarian cancer. My boyfriend took care of my needs and prepared or bought food and drinks for me when I needed them. As I gained more energy and my body felt stronger, I got myself up and about and prepared my own food and drinks and, eventually, meals for both of us again..

ADVICE: When you're recovering from major surgery or cancer treatment, it's really important not to tax yourself unnecessarily. Listen to your body and don't ignore the signals it gives you when it's fatigued and needs rest. Don't try to "be strong" and push yourself ... now is not the time to do so. Your body is fighting a major battle and it's ammunition is rest. In the meantime, ask your support team for help in preparing your meals. You'll be able to return to your cooking and baking when you're stronger and your body tells you it's okay.

* Cindy R. *(Metastatic Breast cancer to the Stomach)*

I love to cook and, when I felt like it, I cooked even during treatment. I live alone. So I do have to fend for myself. I really like to try new recipes too. I would go on Pinterest just to look and find really healthy recipes. Cooking is something I love and I want to continue doing it. Now, when I'm craving enchiladas, my mom would fix them for me.

I enjoy baking too, especially with my mom. Every year at Christmas time, we would schedule one day to bake all day long. Even when I was going through treatment, I was able to bake. Of course, when I got tired, I just said, "Okay guys, I need to sit down a minute and take a break." I also said, "I've got to try all these cookies!" Continuing our annual baking tradition is important. And, yeah, it's great!

ADVICE: If cooking and/or baking is something you enjoy, then you should continue doing it as much as you can, even if your energy is low. Just do it slowly. Of course, adjust when and how you do it, depending on how you feel. The main thing is to not let your sickness get in the way of doing what you enjoy. You'll heal faster when you can do the things you enjoy, even if it's just a little bit.

* Hilda K. *(Colon cancer)*

I took time off from work for a year; I did it for myself. I made my health my priority. Since I had time to take care of myself, rest and stay home, I also cooked and made dinner for my family. I didn't feel much fatigue and I didn't overwork myself. Basically, I did everything "normal" and didn't try to do more than I could.

ADVICE: Your health is your priority, so you should rest when you need to. If you feel you have the energy and you feel like it, then cook for yourself or for your family. The main thing is to not stress about it. Listen to your body and don't take on too much. Ask your family or friends to cook or make the meals, if your body is not up to it.

* Rev. Linda S. *(Pancreatic cancer 3x)*

I love cooking and do so when I have the energy. For several weeks after my surgery, I had neither the energy to cook nor the desire to eat for several weeks. Instead, I drank Boost, ate soups, and nibbled at small portions of meat and vegetables. Unlike some undergoing chemo, I did not have a metallic taste in my mouth when eating.

When I'm too tired to cook, family, friends and even strangers prepare meals for me. Two kind-hearted women I do not know prepared several meals for me. A friend I have known since childhood dropped meals off for me. A dear friend prepared healthful and well-seasoned dinners for me. My heart swells with appreciation and humility.

Also, for the weeks of chemo, when I'm most likely to be exhausted for several days, I made arrangements with an organizer to have prepared meals delivered.

<u>ADVICE:</u> **You can ask family or friends to cook for you. You can also arrange for an organizer to have prepared meals delivered on the days you're unable to cook.**

* Rachel S. *(Breast cancer: triple negative)*

After the mastectomy, my sister set up a Meal Train where people brought me meals every day. I had my surgery on June 14th and they continued bringing me food all the way to July 4th. It was great!

<u>ADVICE:</u> **If you are not able to cook meals, have someone set up a Meal Train. There are many people who would be happy to help and bring food for you and your family.**

* Sondra W. *(Ovarian cancer 3x)*

For a while I couldn't cook or bake because I also had neuropathy in my hands. My sense of hot and cold were so off that I had to be careful that I didn't burn myself. Fortunately, my husband Kenneth got me special gloves to use to protect my hands.

There was another instance when my neuropathy caused pain. One day when I used a knife to crack the shell of an egg, the sharp edges of the broken shell touched my hand, and that was so painful...Oh my! It really was so bad! I couldn't maneuver the eggs with my special gloves, so I had to think of ways to work around them. I figured that I could just crack and open a little part of the egg, enough to get just the egg itself out or do whatever I needed to do because I could eat only the egg whites. Even though eggs were one of the few things I could eat, I didn't want to eat too many, so Kenneth would eat the egg yolks, and I would eat the egg whites.

<u>ADVICE:</u> **If you have neuropathy that causes a tingling or burning sensation in your hands, there are actually special "neuropathy" gloves you can buy on the market.**

* Yesi L. *(Breast cancer: triple positive)*

I was not real big into cooking prior to treatment. But then because I was forced to stay at home, I allowed myself to cook and actually enjoyed it. I somehow had some energy to cook, especially with the diet restrictions. It was good for me to know what I was putting in my body. Now, I totally love it and, as a matter of fact, I found out that I am a great cook! ▯ When I ask my daughter where she wants to go to eat, she would say, "I want Mommy's food." So yes, that makes me feel good.

* Aaron C. (Prostate cancer, Skin cancer)

I was not allowed to drive for ten days after the surgery. It was really uncomfortable. My girlfriend picked me up from the hospital and brought me home. I remember just sitting there in the car, miserable. Since I couldn't drive, I had my ex-wife take my daughters to school or wherever they needed to go. I didn't tell her about my cancer; I didn't want her to know. I try to keep my privacy private. I just told my ex, "Hey, I can't" or whatever excuse I used. The good thing is that most of this happened around July when they were out of school for the summer, so the timing was right.

ADVICE: Just follow the doctor's instructions and don't drive until your groin area has healed enough for you to sit comfortably in the car and drive. If you need something at the store or need to go someplace, ask help from those who support you. Sure, you'll be miserable, because you'll be limited in the things you can do. Still, you've got to tough it out and allow your body time to heal.

* Amor T. (Breast cancer, Ovarian cancer)

Breast cancer. It took almost two months before I felt comfortable enough to drive after my surgery. I definitely had to wait until I no longer depended on my pain medications (opioids) to function. My chest and abdominal wounds were healing, but I remember feeling sensitive about having to strap my seatbelt on, which would apply pressure on the wounds. When I finally did drive, I did so super carefully. I also protected my surgical sites from the straps of the seatbelts by placing a small pillow between my abdomen and the strap and just positioning my left arm over the diagonal part of the seatbelts' strap, so that it wouldn't go over my reconstructed breast. Not a great safety move, I know. But at the time, I was more focused on being able to drive without the threat of pain.

Ovarian cancer. My doctor told me that I should not drive until after six to eight weeks. Fortunately, my boyfriend Bill drove me to wherever I needed to go, even after that period of time passed. A lot had to do with the extreme discomfort I felt from the constipation that just dragged on and on after my hysterectomy, plus the fact that I also started my chemotherapy sessions. I am more than grateful for everything he has done to take care of me. I am truly blessed!

ADVICE: Aside from following your doctor's orders when it comes to when you could drive, follow what your body is telling you too. If you're on opioids, under no condition should you be driving at all. Ask those who support you for help driving you to wherever you need to go. When you're finally able to drive, take the necessary precautions to protect your surgical wounds, e.g. placing a small pillow between your wound and the seatbelt strap if it straps over that area.

* Bob G. (Soft Tissue Sarcoma, Skin cancer)

For my 30 radiation treatments, I drove to the hospital for the first two weeks. For the next two weeks, my wife drove me there. After, I drove myself the rest of the time.

* Cindy L. (Kidney cancer)

Driving was really tricky for me. It was twelve (12) weeks before I was actually allowed to drive. That's quite a long time. Reason for that wasn't only because of my incision, but also because of the clips that tied off the kidney inside my abdomen. Well, what I did for the first two weeks after (and I know it's risky) was had Ed place the seatbelt on me where the part that goes over my chest was behind me. Then, I placed a special small pillow or rolled up towel over my stomach and placed the seatbelt across and on top of that. It gave a little bit of cushion, so the bottom part of the seat belt wasn't pushing into me.

* Cindy R. *(Metastatic Breast cancer to the Stomach)*

Pretty much, through both my breast cancer and stomach cancer treatments, I continued driving. However, there were times when my family or friends would help me, especially with the infusion treatments and the chemo treatments, because I would get so tired after. Of course, if I felt like it, I would get out and drive because I still wanted to feel independent.

After my hysterectomy, there were times when I couldn't drive. Actually, it was interesting, because I've got the smiley face scar and the seat belt goes over it. So my sister and I designed a small pillow that went between the seat belt and my tummy where the scar is. The way it's designed, the pillow keeps the seat belt from rubbing on the scar. We also made one for the upper seat belt too, to keep the strap from rubbing against the area where my medi-port is located.

* Glenn M. *(Metastatic Colon cancer to the Liver, Lungs & Adrenal Glands)*

Yeah, I drove while undergoing treatment. I made sure I was safe and didn't drive when I thought the medication I was taking was going to affect my judgment while driving.

* Joan S. *(Rectal cancer)*

I gauged when I could or couldn't drive. Usually I just drove short distances, like to the doctor's office.

* Rev. Linda S. *(Pancreatic cancer 3x)*

For the few times I had to go to my consultations or radiation treatments at the Cancer Center in St. Louis, MO, I'm behind the wheel for six hours, round trip, for a 30-45 minute appointment. Family and friends accompany me, but I drive unless I have to be sedated. And no, the Cancer Center cannot minimize the number of trips I make down there by scheduling two or three appointments on the same day, because the departments I'm working with all share the same office space and occupy those spaces on different days.

I was able to drive safely again a week after surgery, as long as I did not need opioids for pain management. The one time I took one of those pills, I did not drive.

* Rachel S. *(Breast cancer: triple negative)*

Right after the surgery, I couldn't drive. It was 2 ½ - 3 weeks before I could drive. The Lymphedema I suffered after the surgery prevented my right arm from straightening; it literally felt like I had a metal bar in my arm. I had to work real hard to force it to go straight, because I was getting ready to go back to work.

ADVICE: Wear compression arm sleeves to keep the swelling down.

* Rick S. *(CLL: Blood & Bone Marrow cancer)*

During my treatment period, I drove. Driving was okay for me. They say, "You shouldn't drive", but I'm a maverick, I guess. I just do what I have to do. No one was around to drive me anyway, so I just drove myself. It wasn't problematic, because chemo doesn't affect you in such a way where you can't make decisions. Some chemo treatments may....mine didn't.

Sometimes, I would drive myself to see a good friend of mine in Sunnyvale who always shared with me and never charged me for my food. I'd see him at his Mexican restaurant where he'd sit me down and prepare something special for me. That was nice.

* Scott M. *(Metastatic Colon cancer to the Prostate & Pancreas)*

During treatment, I continued to drive, like when I was just on my normal pain regimen. However, I was always aware of what medications I was on. When I was under the influence of heavy narcotics, of course, I didn't drive. If I had to be somewhere, I asked someone to drive me.

ADVICE: Even if you're a bit uncomfortable, you should still be able to drive. But, if you're taking heavy narcotics, don't drive! Driving while under the influence of heavy narcotics is dangerous, because your judgment and coordination are impaired. If you need to be somewhere, ask someone to drive you.

* Sondra W. *(Ovarian cancer 3x)*

For several months, I didn't have the energy to drive, so I contacted the American Cancer Society for assistance when Kenneth was working and couldn't drive me. They have the "Road to Recovery" program that provides free transportation to and from treatment for people with cancer who do not have a ride or who are unable to drive themselves. During my rides, I met the nicest people. It was really a nice experience. My friends also took me to and from my appointments when I couldn't drive.

ADVICE: When you're not in the condition to drive, ask your family or friends to drive you. You can take advantage of the free transportation service that the American Cancer Society provides to cancer patients called the "Road to Recovery" program, too. NOTE: The service covers only driving you to and from your medical appointments. Also, there are always transportation services from UBER and LYFT that you can use.

* Susan M. *(Ovarian cancer, Metastatic Pancreatic cancer to the Lungs)*

Ovarian Cancer: I couldn't drive for four week after my hysterectomy. My husband drove me to chemo appointments and I drove myself to my doctor appointments.

Pancreatic Cancer: I couldn't drive for three weeks after surgery. After that time, I just drove myself to all eighteen chemotherapy appointments and all follow-up doctor appointments

* Vida B.A. *(Breast cancer)*

I'm a person who loves to drive. But, during my entire treatment, I didn't drive. Fortunately, I was able to hire a driver to take me wherever I needed to go.

* Yesi L. *(Breast cancer: triple positive)*

For the most part, I drove myself, like to regular, follow-up appointments. The only time I didn't drive was after my chemo infusions. My husband would drop me off at the Cancer Center and my best friend would pick me up and drive me home. Most times, because it was late in the day, we would even grab dinner. That was our little ritual.

Definitely after the bilateral mastectomy, I didn't drive for a month. I couldn't really move. It was one of the most painful surgeries I experienced and recovery, for me, was long and slow.

ADVICE: Have your loved ones or friends help drive you when you're not able to, because of your condition. Have patience and just focus on your health. Prepare to not drive for, at least, a few weeks and just allow yourself to be driven to where you need to go.

ENJOYING THE OUTDOORS

* Amor T. *(Breast cancer, Ovarian cancer)*

The "great outdoors" for me when I was healing from both my breast cancer and ovarian cancer treatments was my back-yard. I was (and still am) very fortunate to be able to enjoy the beauty of nature there. I didn't have to do anything, but sit under the sun and take in its vitamin D rays while watching the birds fly around the gardens. Yes, I definitely enjoyed the peace and beauty that comes from being outdoors.

ADVICE: Being amongst nature is healing and peaceful, even if it's a small garden. Taking in the sun's vitamin D rays also helps regulate your immune system, prevents cancer cell growth, stimulates your pancreas to make insulin and strengthens your bones. So, whenever you can, do go and enjoy the outdoors.

* Cindy R. *(Metastatic Breast cancer to the Stomach)*

I enjoy going to concerts a lot. Where I live, there are different festivals during the summer that I like to attend. During treatment, there were times I wanted to go to concerts but couldn't because I just didn't feel good. I told everyone that I had to play it by ear, just in case. Of course, they understood because of what I was going through. It was hard to plan ahead but, at least, there were times then when I was able to go and enjoy outdoor activities.

Before cancer, I also used to go horseback riding, camping and a lot of other outdoor activities. I was really active. The serious car accident I was involved in, between my breast cancer and stomach cancer treatments, changed that. Now, I just like to go out with my dogs to the park. I really enjoy that.

ADVICE: You have to go out, as much you're able to. Don't be a recluse. Don't just stay indoors. It's really import-ant for your overall health to get out there and enjoy the outdoors.

* Glenn M. *(Metastatic Colon cancer to the Liver, Lungs & Adrenal Glands)*

I really enjoy the outdoors, especially around my property where I've got a lot of nature and wildlife. I try to walk the dogs every night to get my exercise in, but sometimes I'm not able to. Does air guitar count as exercise? Also, I do my "gardening" with a 100 HP, six-foot "mower." Well, it's actually a tractor I use for dirt grading. My oncologist didn't have any issues with my "gardening." Being exposed to the UV rays of the sun, however, was a special concern, because of my previous medications.

Free concerts are fun things to do outdoors too and Morgan Hill is great in the summertime; really great. When I was undergoing treatment, I was still able to go to outside concerts. There were also the weekend brunches and dinners with my family. Of course, I had to adjust a little bit, depending on how I felt that day, but not much. Like I said, I tolerated my treatment side effects so well.

ADVICE: Getting outdoors is important, especially when you can go and be with nature or be with your family and friends. It's important to be active, as much as possible; engage with everything! Anyway, when I went outdoors, I was also careful about what I did and how much I did. I was conscious about making sure I didn't overspend my energy and get myself all fatigued. As for gardening, check with your doctor first about any gardening activity you want to get into. Everyone's different.

* Joan S. (Rectal cancer)

I sometimes would go and enjoy outdoor activities. Other times, I wouldn't be able to go, because I didn't feel good. It just would change from day to day.

* Rev. Linda S. (Pancreatic cancer 3x)

While going through treatment for my first bout with cancer, the ordeal spanned the bulk of autumn and winter, when it's cold and snowy here in the Midwest. I was homebound most of the time. In addition, I wanted to limit my exposure to the public to avoid viral infections.

* Rachel S. (Breast cancer: triple negative)

My son had a swim competition on Father's Day weekend; the weekend after my surgery. Since there was a father and son race in the middle of the competition, he really wanted my husband to be there and swim against him. I watched the competition and got really, really sick. The heat mixed with the medications mixed with the surgery I just went through just wasn't a good combination. I strongly advise against doing something like that.

ADVICE: If you just went through major surgery and were given strong medications to take and the weather is hot, then I would strongly advise you to NOT go out at all. Your body is weak and you're supposed to rest in order to heal. So, stay home and rest.

* Rick S. (CLL: Blood & Bone Marrow cancer)

When I had my own home, I did a lot of gardening. Even though I had chemo, I was always out at my garden, making the flowers look better and making the lawn look better. And, my friend helped me with the watering system whenever I had problems with it. I always had a beautiful yard. That's the only thing that kept me going and made me feel good.

* Scott M. (Metastatic Colon cancer to the Prostate & Pancreas)

I love the outdoors and I love riding my horse, Tucson, which is very therapeutic for me. I'm part of the San Mateo County Sheriff's Mounted Search and Rescue Unit. We go for a week every summer, Labor Day weekend, up to the Sierras; 100 guys and their horses. We just ride, live in tents and go "cowboying" for a week. Yes, it's a lot of fun!!

I did it during treatment too. It slowed me down, but we had a couple of doctors in the group. I gave them each a full list of my medications, the contact info for my doctors and where I was the whole time. They were fully aware.

I tried to keep my lifestyle as normal as possible with what I could do and I'm grateful that I was in a financial position where I was able to retire when I did. Because, as you know, there's stress at work. Life is too short.

ADVICE: Do what you can to keep your lifestyle as normal as possible and adjust where necessary. If you have to be outdoors, especially for an extended period of time, you have to inform your doctor. Your doctor should work with you to make sure you don't aggravate your condition and you can still enjoy what you're doing outdoors, even if it's at a slower pace.

* Sondra W. (Ovarian cancer 3x)

I enjoy outdoor activities, like sightseeing, concerts, museums, the movies and the beach. But, during treatment I had diarrhea and fatigue, and my immune system was pretty weak, so it was hard to go anywhere including church. I was away from church for almost a year, so I listened to the services online.

Still, where I went to was actually determined by how fast I could get to the ladies' room. So, if it were someplace where there was going to be a really long line, then I would not go there because it just wouldn't work for me. So, at that time, no big events or concerts or anything like that that I enjoyed outdoors.

ADVICE: Being active and enjoying outdoor activities is wonderful. However, if your condition doesn't allow it, then there are ways to adjust, like listening to church services or watching concerts online. There are ways to protect your immune system while enjoying the outdoors, like wearing a nose mask or staying away from crowded places.

If your condition requires you to be close to the restroom, you'll need to consider the logistics and type of event or activity you're thinking of attending. If long lines to the restrooms are expected, then it probably wouldn't be a good idea to go. You'll also need to consider how your body will manage traveling to and from the event or activity.

* Susan M. (Ovarian cancer, Metastatic Pancreatic cancer to the Lungs)

Pancreatic Cancer: I really enjoy gardening. Unfortunately, I was under doctor's orders to stop any gardening activity, due to mold/mildew in the garden. This restriction continued until a month after my last chemo treatment.

* Vida B.A. (Breast cancer)

I definitely enjoy the outdoors, so whenever I was confined to my house or the hospital, I remember getting so madly bored. When my doctor finally allowed me to go out, I wanted to see the world! Even though I was told to not go to crowded places, I still went. However, I did wear a mask every time I went to the mall or places with a lot of people, because I didn't want to catch any germs or virus.

ADVICE: Being outdoors definitely helps in keeping yourself active. It helps to bring your spirits up too. During treatment, if you want to go out to the mall or places where there are a lot of people, keep in mind that your immune system is weak and vulnerable to catching germs or viruses. If you really need to go out, then protect yourself and wear a mask.

* Yesi L. (Breast cancer: triple positive)

Definitely when time permitted and when my energy permitted, I went to the park or anywhere where I can be in contact with nature. My husband and I enjoyed boating. When I got nauseous, I just took anti-nausea medications, which definitely helped. Water, to me, is very soothing. So going to anyplace that had water was wonderful for me.

I also enjoyed gardening; plants and greenery make me happy. It's very relaxing. I was actually very fatigued most of the time. But, I did have a bit of energy to continue with my gardening.

ADVICE: Do what you enjoy. But, if you are fatigued, listen to your body and rest. If you feel nauseated, take anti-nausea medications. You can continue enjoying the outdoors and your hobbies, etc. when you have more energy.

* Aaron C. (Prostate cancer, Skin cancer)

I started working out at the gym again three months after surgery. But, it was at about the four month mark when I started lifting light weights again, walking around the block and that kind of stuff. When I first lifted weights, I strained and leaked urine, because my bladder wasn't strong enough. I didn't get back into swimming at all, because my bladder was not able to hold water. Also, I didn't want pool water rushing right up into my bladder, since I had no control of holding it. You know what I mean? My bladder is still not 100% at this point, but it's getting better and I don't leak as much. I noticed that my bladder's function improves more like on a month-to-month basis; not day-to-day or week-by-week basis.

It is funny how we take our bladder control for granted, because we've been doing it all our lives. When we were toddlers, we learned how to control our bladders. We go 50 years without even thinking about our bladders; we take all that stuff for granted. And now with this situation, we think about it all the time! When it doesn't work, we're like "Holy sh*t!" But that's normal. It's expected.

ADVICE: Talk to you doctor about when you can exercise again and follow instructions. You need to give your body (and your bladder) time to heal. When you do start working out again, take it slow. Don't be surprised if you leak. It's normal. Accept that progress happens more on a month-to-month basis, than a week-to-week or day-by-day basis.

* Amor T. (Breast cancer, Ovarian cancer)

Breast cancer: Initially, it was tough for me to exercise, as I was quite bruised and swollen from multiple surgeries. After the swelling decreased, I was able to move around, slowly but surely. When my doctor stressed to me the importance of moving around (however slowly) to help my body heal, I walked around the house when I had the energy and continued until I got tired..

Ovarian cancer: Walking was my go-to exercise during treatment. Aside from energy-depleting fatigue, I experienced so many side effects that made me hesitate, like neuropathy in my feet. Still, I knew I had to push myself to walk when I had the energy. Bill also helped to encourage me and provide me support when I didn't feel stable. We had daily walks around the neighborhood, which I feel was key to my recovery.

Less than a month after my last chemotherapy session, I started back on my personal training with Chris of My Core Balance. I was super weak, bent and definitely out of alignment. Chris patiently guided me through core and muscle strengthening moves that definitely made me grow in energy and stability.

ADVICE: According to the American Cancer Society, "exercise is not only safe and possible during cancer treatment, it can improve how well you function physically and your quality of life. Too much rest can lead to loss of body function, muscle weakness, and reduced range of motion." Very true! So please do what you can to exercise, even a walking or moving about slowly. You'll reap the rewards of strength and energy sooner than later.

* Bob G. (Soft Tissue Sarcoma, Skin cancer)

For exercise, I go swimming and also do the bicycle for 30 minutes for my legs. I actually went back to swimming three days after my surgery. Because I swam 3-4 days a week and I was in great shape before I had cancer, I recovered quickly. Even during treatment, I swam. I swam slower and not as long, but I still swam. I also have 5 lb. weights at home. I just want to keep alive and be usable. While I'm watching television, I use my weights and I do a regular routine. If I feel a strain, I don't do it. I don't go fast. This routine is just to keep fit. It keeps me alive.

ADVICE: Exercise is really important for your health. Find a way to exercise, even if you don't do it fast. Just exercise to keep fit. It'll help you recover quicker and keep you alive.

* Cindy L. (Kidney cancer)

I exercise, not only to lose weight, but also to strengthen my overall health so that my remaining kidney can be strong to do what it needs to. Also, exercise is one of the best ways to control the high blood pressure that I have. For exercise, I looked for workouts to strengthen my lower abdominal muscles. That's because with my weakened abdominal muscles, I was not able to pick up my granddaughters, even the 8-month old baby who weighs 24 lbs. Yes, I did try to pick her up, but I paid for it. I was really sore the next day.

At eight weeks, I saw my nephrologist. My daughter, Ali, was with me. I asked him, "Hey, can I start doing some workouts to strengthen my abdominal muscles?" He looked at me and said, "No!" The way he said it, it was like, "I can't even believe you asked me that!" I said, "Okay." That was the end of that for a while. In the meantime, I enjoyed doing Pilates, some yoga, walking and riding on my stationary bike at home. I used the resistance bands too; they really help the arthritis I have on my back.

When my nephrologist finally allowed me to work on my abdominal muscles, I found a video online that went through all the basics. Also, I wore an abdominal binder that was meant for women who had given birth by caesarian section. It was great and very soft and washable too.

I'm past the basics now and am looking for something that's really going to strengthen my core and my abdominal muscles. I have an exercise room in the house where I have weights, a bicycle, and elliptical and a treadmill. I'm not as religious about using my exercise room, because I let everything else be the excuse not to get in there. Before I had the surgery, I was in there every day. Also, before my surgery, Ed and I would walk three miles a night on the beach. Body resistance; keeps the bones stronger.

Now, to strengthen my lower abdominal muscles, I do pelvic tilts. There are also certain Pilates movements that are effective. I like riding on my stationary bike and walking, which are both very good. I'm still trying to find more exercises to really target the lower abdominal muscles. I'm getting back in shape slowly; not as much as I would like, but I'm getting there. And I'm definitely feeling stronger every time I do it.

> **ADVICE:** If you had abdominal or other major surgeries, you should check with your doctor first before you do any exercise. You want to make sure your body is healed enough to where you can perform certain movements. Start slow and easy with activities like, daily walks, yoga and riding the stationary bike.
>
> When your doctor allows you to do abdominal exercises, again, you should start slow and easy. Keep in mind that when the surgeon cut into your abdominal muscles during surgery, those muscles were weakened. So, while you're focusing on exercises to strengthen those muscles, make sure to wear a comfortable abdominal binder to protect your abdomen. Don't overdo it. Find a beginners abdominal workout online video or class. Go for the basics first. After time has passed and your body has gotten stronger, then you can progress to the next stage.
>
> Pelvic tilts and certain Pilates movements are effective in strengthening the lower abdominal muscles. Continue walking and using bodyweight exercises that help strengthen the bones. Main thing is to keep active every day.

* Cindy R. (Metastatic Breast cancer to the Stomach)

For exercise, I have a treadmill at home that I use everyday for about half an hour. Also, I love to dance. Just put on the eighties and I'll be dancing around, just having fun. When I went through both treatments for breast cancer and stomach cancer, I pretty much had to play exercising or any physical activity by ear. Still, I didn't want to just sit there. So when I felt like exercising or dancing, I did it. But I made sure I didn't overdo it.

> **ADVICE:** Moving your body is really important for your overall health. Even if you don't feel good or are low in energy, you can still do something to move your body. Walking is the simplest exercise. Even it's slowly, your moving around will help your body heal. Dancing is also something that can be really simple. You don't have to follow any dance steps; just move your body any way you want. Whatever you choose to do, listen to your body and don't overdo it.

* Glenn M. (Metastatic Colon cancer to the Liver, Lungs & Adrenal Glands)

To strengthen my muscles, I try to lift some weights and do some crunches with the bar. The bar has a pulley, a built-in pillow and padded handles. I do a set of 25 crunches with the bar, but I used to do three sets of 25. I do this in the living room with the dogs. I have a little gym at home with weights and a bench press. I also do a little bit of push-ups. I need to do more. I need to get into a regular routine. Sometimes, I'll go to a gym outside and use the inversion table to stretch my back out. I don't want my muscles to atrophy, so I do what I can to work out.

For exercise, I also ride my bike once in a while for about a little over half a mile. I walk my dogs too probably four nights a week. They have their way of getting me to walk them. When I get home from work and come in the door, they jump at me; their faces looking at me as if to say, "We love you! We're glad you're home! Feed us! Walk us!"

Sometimes, I'll ride my bike and walk my two dogs at the same time... safely ~ you know, with the helmet, elbow pads and knee pads – because my dogs conspire. They talk to each other. I can hear them thinking, "Okay, when we get to the pole, you charge left and I'll charge right and we'll SLAM him into the pole and then, we'll tie him up!"

ADVICE: It's important to exercise, if you have the energy. If you only have a small amount of energy, meter it out. Don't waste it all in one place (just one exercise), because you may get fatigued. Like right now when I take a shower, I need to lie down for a few minutes after, because it just takes too much work. Staying clean is hard work.

Just exercise slowly and do what you can. Exercising helps you gain strength, which your body really needs when it's trying to heal. Oh yeah, if you have a pet you can walk, it's a good way to get your exercise in too.

* Hilda K. (Colon cancer)

To strengthen my body and help it heal, I did go to the gym regularly, even when I still had to carry my chemo pump, which was connected to my mediport. It sounds complicated, but it really was easy. With the chemo pump underneath my blouse, no one could tell I was wearing it. It didn't get in the way, at all.

I also participated in a program at the YMCA called "Live Strong". As a cancer patient, they gave me a six-month membership to work with a special rehab trainer who knew how to help all types of patients in different stages of cancer and recovery. The trainer taught me how to build my strength and how to use the machines there. I also got to meet a lot of people there with various cancers and who were in different stages of treatment. Together, we helped each other through the program and through our treatment experiences. It was definitely a positive experience for me.

ADVICE: Exercise is important to your health and recovery. Even if you don't feel like exercising, you need to get your body moving, even slowly. With exercise, your strength will grow and you'll heal faster. Find a gym nearby or ask your doctor if there's a program (like Livestrong) you can participate in that helps those with cancer.

* Jacki S. (Breast cancer)

Being an ice skating coach, I'm quite active and fit. Skating was exercise enough for me.

* Joan S. (Rectal cancer)

My exercise was housework, laundry, picking up five things and putting them away.

ADVICE: Moving around is important, even if you move slowly. It helps the body heal. Doing housework and laundry are good and practical exercises. I get my exercise in and I help my body heal.

* J.B. (Salivary gland cancer)

Exercise really did help me feel stronger and recover quicker. For exercise, I did a lot of walking on the school campus. I even took longer routes, just to make sure I walked more throughout the day. During treatment, I was still able to go boxing, just not as often.

* *Rachel S.* (*Breast cancer: triple negative*)

I didn't really exercise; I was constantly way too tired. Besides, I was trying to save whatever bit of energy I had for my boys. That's "exercise as it is". So, yes, whatever energy I had (after work), I had to conserve it for my boys when I got home at night.

* *Rick S.* (*CLL: Blood & Bone Marrow cancer*)

When I could, I'd try to get, at least, a 30-minute combination of the bicycle, stair-stepper and treadmill machines at the gym. I also lifted weights, something I enjoy. I would lift weights for two or three hours, sometimes four hours. I couldn't swim, so I never swam. I also can't do Yoga, so I didn't do Yoga. However, I know that it's one of the better exercises. If I could advise anybody about any exercise, it's to do Yoga.

* *Scott M.* (*Metastatic Colon cancer to the Prostate & Pancreas*)

With the Livestrong program (http://www.livestrong.com/), I was told to avoid public swimming pools, because of the germs and the bacteria, so I didn't get my exercise through swimming. But, I did join a gym and I took yoga. Also, I've since equipped my house with some gym equipment. I know that there are a lot of free programs out there for cancer patients.

I ride my horse, not every day, but I probably ride two to three times a week in the good weather. Then, I also do Whole Body Vibration. It's a platform you stand on, and at different speeds, and it vibrates your body, and you can do movements and curls with two or three pound weights, and the G-forces actually make the weight stronger as your body is vibrating. You might get 1,800 involuntary contractions in a minute. You're working the muscles, and there's ways to do it for stretching and relaxation. I used to do whole body vibration for strength. You're supposed to limit it to 12 minute sessions, one in the morning, one at night. It works! After doing it for a while, I could feel my abs just really tightening up. It's something that NASA had designed for their astronauts when they came back to earth, and their bone density and circulation was poor because of being in zero gravity for so long. The whole body vibration machine stimulates the muscles, which helps them strengthen the bones. It also gets your circulation going, which also strengthens bones and the lymphatic system. I do whole body vibration, because of my neuropathy. I usually don't take walks away from home. I stand on a treadmill and I walk on a treadmill. I have an exercycle too that I will get on and ride a few miles; again, just to get the heart pumping and the aerobic stuff.

* *Sondra W.* (*Ovarian cancer 3x*)

Once I got out of chemo, I did the Living Strong, Living Well strength and fitness training program for adult cancer survivors. That was really good, and I'm glad I was able to do it. They had exercises and all kinds of creative movements to make you use your muscles. When I went through the program, it was at my own pace; what I could do because I actually was behind everybody in the class, energy-wise. I was so worn down. The instructors didn't mind that. They always told me how I could do things to adjust. They were also aware that I had my knee issues, and I had really bad neuropathy, which threw off my balance as well. So, they showed me how to adjust. Because of the extent of my condition, I could not use any equipment. I had a little exercise routine that I did down the hall while all the rest were doing the weight training part of the regular program. I learned a lot and built up some stamina, and that's a really good thing.

* Susan M. *(Ovarian cancer, Metastatic Pancreatic cancer to the Lungs)*

After each surgery, whether for Ovarian Cancer or Pancreatic Cancer, I did a lot of walking. I knew walking would help me recover faster from my surgeries. Three months into my chemo treatments for pancreatic cancer, I started attending yoga classes twice a week, as well as, attending meditation classes.

* Vida B.A. *(Breast cancer)*

Before treatment, my exercise was swimming and badminton, which I really enjoyed. Unfortunately, with all the bacteria in pools, I stopped swimming because I'm afraid of getting an infection.

For exercise now, I enjoy walking and stretching. Even when I was going through treatment, I tried to walk as much as my body allowed me, because I knew it would help me heal faster. I also got a good workout climbing up and down the stairs of my 3-story townhouse, which included an attic and a basement. Although I felt fatigued, when I walked around, I felt that I was healing too.

* Yesi L. *(Breast cancer: triple positive)*

I did not have the energy to exercise throughout the entire treatment. I was just extremely fatigued. I guess I could say that my exercise was walking, dropping off my daughter to and from school. Walking was the only exercise I was able to do without suffering and depleting myself of energy.

Yoga was a form of exercise I always liked too. However, I had to stop during treatment, because of the wounds; stretching the areas operated on was painful. My skin was also so delicate from treatment, which made it hard to work with my arms. I actually did go back to Yoga after treatment. Now, I also power-walk for my exercise.

FAMILY / SIGNIFICANT OTHERS / FRIENDS

---

* Aaron C. *(Prostate cancer, Skin cancer)*

My girlfriend is wonderful and has been very, very supportive from the very beginning. We hang out together and support each other. I remember how her mom cried when she found out that I had cancer. She was very supportive too. I have a healthy relationship with my daughters and I'm very honest with them. I didn't get into too many details, because they're young. I, basically, said that I had prostate cancer and I'm going to be okay. When they heard that, they got worried and thought I was going to die. I told them, "No, I'm not going to die. I'm going to have surgery." Then I said, "I'm going to be a little bit out-of-commission for a while, but your dad's going to be fine."

When my kids came over to be with me, we just hung out and watched movies and stuff. There were a few things I couldn't do, like run and chase them for a few months, like I used to. One day, they saw the bag attached to my leg. So, I had to explain to them that I had to urinate into the bag. Then I told them, "I need you to help me do this and this…" At first, they got grossed out by it. But then after, they were totally cool with it, because they wanted to help me. You know, help their daddy.

The first ten days after surgery, when I couldn't do anything because of my catheter, I had my ex-wife take our kids to school or wherever they needed to go. I didn't tell her about my cancer; I didn't want her to know. I try to keep my privacy private. I just told my ex, "Hey, I can't" or whatever excuse I used. The good thing is that most of this happened around July when they were out of school for the summer, so the timing was right. Now, I'm able to have fun with my daughters and chase after them, like I used to.

ADVICE: I am fortunate that I have the love and support of my daughters and my girlfriend. It's important to be honest with them and to let them know when you need help. Going through the cancer experience together has brought us closer.

* Amor T. (Breast cancer, Ovarian cancer)

I am blessed with the best daughter, the best siblings and the best boyfriend! When times were toughest, I could count on them to, not only love and support me, but also to bring me up. Even though my beautiful daughter, Catherine, was away at college in Southern California, my big brother, Roman, was in Taiwan and my sisters Joy and Melody were in the Philippines, they made sure I felt how close they were to me in thought and in spirit. They checked on me and sent prayers out all the time and brought me so much laughter and comfort during our conference calls and video chats. It really seemed like they were right there with me!

Even though Catherine was away at college when I was diagnosed with breast cancer, she made a special trip to visit me. When I awoke in the ICU after surgery, she surprised me coming through the door. I was ecstatic to see her, even though I was pretty doped up from the pain meds. Catherine was able to stay with me overnight in ICU. Although I was really sad that she could only take one day off from school and work, I was so very grateful and blessed that we were able to spend precious time together. Seeing her strengthened my resolve to get better and beat cancer!

And then, there was the one night she "stayed" with me overnight via Skype video chat. When I was discharged from the hospital after my staph infection scare, I was instructed to have someone stay with me each night for a week. My awesome girlfriends and fellow Foster City Lions were able to stay with me every night, except for that one night. When she learned of my predicament, that's when Catherine offered to spend the night overnight with me…thank God for the internet! So, we actually watched each other fall asleep and saw each other when we woke up. It was a really awesome experience that makes my heart melt every time I think of how Catherine thought of that idea, so she could be with me when I needed her.

The wretchedness of cancer treatment would've been magnified, if not for the love and support of my significant other, Bill. He accompanied me to every one of my appointments and made himself available, no matter what, when I was going through treatment. Any instability I felt, he was there to support me. When I felt miserable, he was there to comfort me. He motivated me to move around and walk, assuring me that he would be there to help stabilize me, when I needed it. He, unselfishly, helped me get back on my feet and regain my strength. I truly couldn't have asked to be with a better man than Bill, my rock.

Throughout both my cancer journeys, my friends and relatives were the absolute best! It was overwhelming to know and feel their love and support. I felt so valued, something I don't think many of us realize, until we experience a hardship. I know that their positive thoughts, prayers and energy accelerated my healing.

By the way, even though I felt the man I was dating at the time of my breast cancer diagnosis didn't really care for me, I was still thankful for his assistance then.

ADVICE: When it comes to family relationships, love relationships and true friendships, think of this quote from American spiritual teacher and author, Gary Zukav: "Eventually, you will come to understand that love heals everything, and love is all there is." No matter how we're connected, we're all different. The key to happiness and healing is celebrating and respecting, without judgment or expectation, those differences. Love is really all there is.

* Bob G. *(Soft Tissue Sarcoma, Skin cancer)*

Because recovery after radiation treatments was slow, my family and I stayed home a lot. We did go out to a movie once.

* Cindy L. *(Kidney cancer)*

Our family is close, even though we live far from each other. So, it was difficult to share the news of my cancer diagnosis with my children, because they were all over the place. My oldest daughter Ali lived in Royal Oak, Michigan. My oldest son Brennan lives in Tampa, Florida. And my Katie and Harrison both live here. Harrison is married and has four little girls; he's a busy dad and I'm a busy grandma. After some coordination and working through some challenges, we brought everyone together in one town, so that we could all discuss things together, as a family.

My cancer was just one of the things I had to tackle during this period. My husband who needed a double hip replacement, put aside his surgery to take care of me. My daughter Ali kept fainting and, at that time, we didn't know why. So, I was beside myself thinking about how I much wanted to take care of them, but couldn't do it because of my limitations.

During my first ten days home from the hospital, I slept on a chair in the living room. I could not get up on my own. I had to be pulled up out of the chair with, literally, one person on each arm. I couldn't go to the bathroom by myself without help. My husband, for the first several days, had to shower me on a shower chair and wash my hair, because I couldn't physically do it. When I was finally able to sleep in my bed, my family had to tuck me in a certain way where I couldn't move, I couldn't roll and I couldn't lie on my side. I was so dependent on a lot of people and it was really tough for me.

Asking for support is something I have a hard time with. I'm used to being the one supporting others; not the other way around. Anyway, I'm getting better about not expecting my family to read my mind and know what I need. I learned how to keep myself from just snapping at them when they didn't read my mind to know what I need. I'm getting better about that and, as time goes by and my body is getting stronger, I'm doing more and more for myself.

> **ADVICE:** Having your loved ones together in one location is ideal, so you can share and discuss things together. However, if your loved ones live in different states or are far away, you'll have to carefully consider each individual's situations. Be honest. That way, everything is out in the open and you can all better support each other.
>
> When your body is weak and you're in pain, this is the time for you to lean on your family and loved ones for support. Just remember that you would do the same for your loved ones if they were weak or in pain. It's understandable when you're frustrated, because of your limitations. Let your family know specifically what you need; they cannot read your mind. And then, take a deep breath and allow yourself to be cared for.

* Cindy R. *(Metastatic Breast cancer to the Stomach)*

I've been so blessed to have my wonderful family and so many friends support me throughout both my cancers, as well as all those people all over the world who prayed for me. I believed that that really helped, especially knowing that people do care, even if they haven't met you; they still care so much and want you to do good. So, having that kind of support was really great, especially when I didn't have to ask for it. That has just been such a blessing.

Even now, my two aunts, who live about an hour and half away from me, check on me, asking me stuff like, "So, is your mom taking you to do this treatment? If so, I'm taking you to the next one." My other aunt then would say that she'll take me to the following one. They would drive out, take me to my treatments, stay the night or do whatever I needed. They would do that without my asking. It's like what do you need and we're just going to set it up and we're just going to do it...whether I like it or not. I'm so blessed!

Shortly after my breast cancer treatment, I had to take care of my mom, because she, actually, received her breast cancer diagnosis and had to go through treatment, like I just did. It was my turn to support her, taking her to treatments and helping her with whatever she needed help with.

And then, there's my Disneyland story; a great family story. It was my 40th birthday and I had just had my surgery and I was going to start my chemo treatment. Since I already had my Disney vacation planned before my diagnosis, I said, "Well, we're going to go to Disneyland anyways and it's just going to be me and my mom." So, we went down there and my sister called and said she was coming. Because it was my 40th birthday and I was going through cancer treatment, the staff at the Disneyland Hotel told us, "Oh, we're upgrading you and oh, it's a fabulous room." I just said, "Okay." But then, when we walked into the room, I said, "Wait..wait...wait... This can't be right. This is the Honeymoon Suite." They said, it was right.

And so, I called my sister and told her, "Oh my God, I can't believe you did this. Thank you so much!" She cried and I cried too and then I heard a knock on the door... And, my two sisters, my brother-in-law, my cousin ... everybody came up and joined us! Oh, my God, it was so touching! It was so wonderful! It was the best birthday ever! I just love my family so much and feel so very blessed to know that they love me too!

ADVICE: Having a family is such a treasure, even if there are differences and even if you're not blood-related. When your friends support you and give you love, they're family too. Show your family and friends your appreciation for what they do for you. With them, you have been blessed.

* Glenn M. (Metastatic Colon cancer to the Liver, Lungs & Adrenal Glands)

My wife Barbara also had cancer and we supported each other. It was kind of good we didn't have to go through treatment at the same time or else we would have been in trouble. Unfortunately, her cancer was much more advanced than mine. I took care of Barbara for about five months before she passed. But, she took care of me before. I didn't do anything she wouldn't have done for me double. I also had help from others too. It was so sad to watch her get so weak. I could tell it was very hard for her.

There is a lot I wish I could've done better, like be a better cook for her. I wish I knew how to make something tasty that she could enjoy and not have to just take four bites. Even if I were way up there with my cooking skills and creativity with food, her taste buds changed with all the medication and stuff. I don't know for sure if having better cooking skills would've helped. Maybe it would've; maybe no difference. I also wish that I had paid more attention to the training they gave me in caring for her, like giving her the injections for her osteoporosis. I just wish I could've done more to help her.

Most of the time, I handle her demise intelligently and sensibly and like an adult. But I also have my "train wreck moments," I call it. When she was still alive, I had this "train wreck moment" when I laid beside her and soaked my pillow with tears. I was pretty sure she was asleep, but she knew exactly what was going on. She pulled herself up next to me and said, "You're going to be okay." There she was on her deathbed and she's worried about me.

We have four children, but they live far away. They did visit with their mother before she passed and tried to take care of her too when they could. They also visit with me from time to time. Like I said, I enjoy the weekend brunch and dinners with my family, although I had to adjust some things when I was going through treatment.

So, I'm basically self-sufficient for the most part. I do have a live-in guy on site (Tim) who assists me. He's good in technology and computers and so helps me with my computer issues. Since he eats at Safeway every night, I just give him my grocery list and he gets my groceries for me. He puts them away in my refrigerator too, which helps me.

ADVICE: If you're the spouse or partner, make sure you're familiar with how your spouse or partner does things in the house. I couldn't cook well. I didn't know where stuff was. As far as laundry, I worked it out. I've got my systems so different from my wife's, but somehow they work. Well, the only thing is my house is a mess.

* Hilda K. (Colon cancer)

There is no doubt that my family totally supported me. There were times, however, when they showed me how scared they were that it started to scare me too. It was crazy; just crazy. Anyway, because I didn't want to be scared, I just focused on keeping myself positive and didn't let their fears affect me.

One thing I want to mention is how my family and friends wanted to make things "normal" for me. It was interesting, because they made like things were "normal", but they treated me very delicately, because they knew that what I was experiencing was really serious. Well, in their attempts to keep things "normal", they wanted to celebrate my 50th birthday with a big party, which happened to be the day I came home from the hospital. It was a big deal, but I was not in a 50-year old mode to celebrate. Still my family held the party for me, because it was a milestone birthday, and it was held at my house. At the party, I basically said "hello" to the people who came and then went to my bed to lay down. I went back and forth doing that. It really was nice to have my family there; I felt so much love. They didn't expect me to do anything, but show my face and go to my room to lay down in bed, then show my face when I was ready again...and back and forth, which is what I did.

When I had the energy, I did what I could to take care of my family. I drove my children to and from school and their practices. And, I also made dinner for my family when I could. I didn't feel much fatigue and I didn't overwork myself. Basically, I did everything "normal" and didn't try to do more than I could.

ADVICE: It is wonderful to have the love and support of family. Even though you may want to take care of your family's needs, you must make your health your priority. Listen to your body and don't take on too much. Do keep in mind, however, that if your family, friends or anyone, gets really emotional, worried and fearful about your cancer, you should focus on keeping yourself positive about your health and recovery. Feeding into their worries or fears will not help you at all. So, stay positive. Do it for yourself.

* Jacki S. (Breast cancer)

My family was always checking up on me. My mom had passed away, so I didn't have my best support there. I had gotten my cancer 6 months after my mom passed away, which I attribute to stress which probably could've brought that on. The other thing I was thinking about that could've given me this cancer was the fact that I am an ice skater. I was always a competitor. I was always brought up in ice arenas. And out on the ice after the machines ~ the Zambonis ~ would make some new ice, I'd have to go back on the ice and train. So, whatever fumes were left on the rink from the Zambonis is what I was breathing in. So I have a feeling that could've been a little bit of what I was just breathing … those toxins going into my body from the machine. We had no family history of cancer.

So I didn't have anybody from my family to turn to, to find out what it was like. But my husband was so supportive. In fact, he liked the way I looked when I lost my hair from the chemo, because he said I looked like Cleopatra. I had a good-looking head without hair on it, which I guess doesn't happen for everybody. So, my family was very supportive and my husband gave me compliments on how I looked.

* Joan S. (Rectal cancer)

My family was with me through all my challenges and I am so grateful for their wonderful support. Even though they were supporting me when things got tough, I could see that it was really hard on my family too. They wanted to do everything to help me, but sometimes really didn't know what to do.

ADVICE: Even though you're not feeling good, make sure to appreciate your family and friends who are supporting you. It can be really hard on them too.

* J.B. (Salivary gland cancer)

My family knows me as someone who doesn't really seek emotional support. So, I had to process things first, before I opened up and asked my girlfriend and family for support. When I did, I learned a lot about myself in an intimate, emotional setting with my family. Surprisingly, I found it pleasant, even though it wasn't something I was really used to. My family and I got together regularly and they were very helpful to me.

ADVICE: People like me aren't used to intimate or emotional settings with family members. It's not a bad thing; it's just the way it is. However, when you're in a health crisis that affects your family, then it's important to open up to them. I advise that you just go for it, even if you're not the type to open up.

* Rev. Linda S. (Pancreatic cancer 3x)

When I was first diagnosed, one of the things I feared most was leaving my elderly mother (Ma Mere), for whom I am primary caregiver. My family helped me cope, especially my sister, Sam, who is a retired nurse. She put her life in San Diego on hold to be here for as long as she needs to be; she dropped everything and rushed over for me.

After sharing with her the upsetting news about the return of my cancer, I remember saying that we would have to hire someone to move in with Mama (Ma Mere), because I could not take care of her while undergoing more radical treatment.

In reply, Sam said, "Well, I've been praying about that". Then she laid out her well-thought plan. Turns out, my little sister has shown herself to be adept and efficient at coordinating the appointment calendars for the three of us: Ma Mere, me and herself, juggling multiple tasks, making sure Ma Mere stays engaged and active and resting when she needs to, taking her medications on time, bathing and dressing well, taking walks, and eating well.

Besides taking care of all the household chores, Sam picks up my prescription refills when I can't. She informs me regularly of all the things I need to know to ensure our mother's physical, emotional, mental, spiritual, legal, and financial welfare. She takes care of her elderly cat. And she somehow manages to maintain her own social life, take an online class and write a school paper. Plus, she is FUNNY! Sam amazes me constantly and I love her to pieces!

* Rachel S. *(Breast cancer: triple negative)*

During treatment, I still put my baby to bed every night, even though at times I felt weak. I kept the routine as normal as I could, minus reading books, because I couldn't see the words. My twelve-year old, he has a lunch card, so I don't have to make his lunches. I just tried to keep the routine as normal as possible. My mother-in-law was with us for about five months. She helped some with the housework. Thank God!

ADVICE: Try to keep your daily routine with your family as normal as you can, especially if you have young children. It will strengthen your bond and even allow them to take care of you.

* Rick S. *(CLL: Blood & Bone Marrow cancer)*

I didn't have any regular family activities and I didn't watch TV. If I did anything, I read. I never asked my family for support; it's actually the other way around. My kids ask me for support. I took care of my oldest daughter. My youngest daughter was pretty independent. But, if she needed help, I'd take care of her too.

That's a valuable point: If you have somebody you really care about, go ahead and care about them more than anything in the world. It'll help you get your mind off of yourself. You take good care of them and you make sure they're okay. You love them and that helps you lose yourself in them (have a sense of purpose). When they're not there, then you're happy you sent them off feeling loved and doing well.

* Scott M. *(Metastatic Colon cancer to the Prostate & Pancreas)*

Yes, I felt like I was at someone's mercy the whole time. So, I really don't see how anybody could do this alone. I don't think it's possible.

ADVICE: Sure you feel like you're at someone's mercy. But, you are really sick and you need people to help you! So, don't hesitate to ask for support.

* Sondra W. *(Ovarian cancer 3x)*

At the time I was informed I had cancer, I was caregiving for my 95-year old mother who was wheelchair-bound. I had to make arrangements to send her to my brother in Ohio, so she can be placed in a facility there. When I told my doctor that I was going to be gone for two weeks to take care of family matters, he said, "You do need to get your mother taken care of by other family members, because you will not be able to do anything for her care." He continued, "But, you only have one week. You need to be back here in a week, because we need to be doing the surgery." That stepped me up a little bit more into the urgency of my situation. First, I had the reality. Then, I had the urgency.

Fortunately, my daughter was able to take off from work and go with me to Ohio because we had to deal with my mother being wheelchair-bound. On the flight, everything went smoothly. However, things did not go smoothly getting her into the facility. It was very stressful. Eventually, I felt the tiredness and the stress of all that I had to do before I could even go in for my surgery. I was there for a week.

In the meantime, my doctor scheduled the surgery. I felt like I was in a whirlwind. Things were just happening left and right. We were busy with my mother and then the surgery was scheduled. I flew back to California on my birthday, of all days. And then, I had to get ready and get some tests and do this and that. I had anxieties because of all I had to do; it was just overwhelming! Finally, I learned how to allow others do things I used to do, and I also learned how to help people help me, like telling them exactly what I needed. When we had that understanding, things got better.

For family in the Bay Area where I live, it was only my daughter and my husband and my granddaughter with me. They gave me all the support that they could, and I feel so, so blessed and thankful for all they did to take care of me, especially when I needed it the most.

Not too much happened when it came to regular family activity. What we did was change some things. For example, instead of cooking Thanksgiving dinner or Christmas dinner (especially since my daughter was working and trying to help me at the same time), we ordered from Pluto's because they serve healthy food. So, for the year I was dealing with my treatments, we just ordered in for big occasions or holidays, and it worked out great.

ADVICE: Your family and loved ones are also having to make adjustments to the changes you're going through. It can be really emotional and even overwhelming for everyone involved; not only you. Help others help you, by communicating exactly what you need, only when you really need it. Also, don't take on too much or try to fix everything. Stay positive, focus on your health and save all your energy to fight cancer.

Family activities don't have to be complicated. Instead of worrying about cooking dinner and serving others, like you used to do before your illness, order in for your family celebrations and get-togethers.

* Susan M. (Ovarian cancer, Metastatic Pancreatic cancer to the Lungs)

Ovarian Cancer: My family means the world to me and I fought hard to heal from my illness. During my first three chemo appointments in the hospital, I had a friend or family member stay at the house to help with our daughter. Even when I was undergoing treatment, I tried to still take care of my family, especially my baby daughter who was only eighteen months old. I continued participating in activities with my daughter that she as involved in before I learned I had cancer and we took many trips to the park as a family.

ADVICE: If you can muster the strength to spend time with your family, especially if you have young children, it will somehow energize you and help you heal. It will also help your children and your family grow stronger.

* Vida B.A. (Breast cancer)

I only have one sister here in the Philippines with me. She was with me when my doctor informed me that I had breast cancer. I informed my children and my other siblings about my diagnosis right away and they immediately showed me their support. All of my children live in the United States, so yeah, we use "Viber" (international instant messaging and voice over application) all the time. We're a close-knit family.

My eldest daughter, Michelle, worked as an oncology nurse in the City of Hope in Pasadena, CA. Early in the morning, while I was on the hospital bed waiting to get my mastectomy done, she called me on Viber. As I continued talking to her, the door to my room opened and, there she was, in person! She said, "Surprise! I'm here!" I was really surprised! Then she said, "You know, mama, I take care of all kinds of cancer patients. Why shouldn't I take care of you?" Yes, my wonderful daughter took some vacation time off from her work in the States to be with me. She was able to stay for only four days. So short, but I enjoyed every moment of it.

When my family or friends visited me at my house, I required them to wear a mask to make sure I'm protected from any outside germs. I kept a box of masks here at home.

ADVICE #1: When you share your situation with your family, it enables them to support you, even from a distance. Even if the time you physically have together is brief, treasure every moment. Feeling their love and support will help you through your challenges more than you know and set you on your healing journey.

I shared news of my diagnosis with my close friends and they immediately expressed their love and support. My very best friend who, herself, had experienced breast cancer and a mastectomy several years back, knew what I was going through and supported me throughout my journey. We continue to share everything with each other, unconditionally.

ADVICE #2: There are several points I would like to share: (1) Having cancer is not something you should be embarrassed or ashamed about. When you inform your friends who love you, you'll enable them to support you and you'll all benefit from the experience. (2) Love makes everything more colorful. At the lowest point in your life, when everything looks black and white, love will add color to your life. If you emphasize love, it will make you so happy that your sickness will become secondary. The love you feel from those who care for you, support you and pray for you; that's love that is so strong and powerful. So, open yourself more to loving and being loved. (3) Forgive your past and those who hurt you. You have to get out of your system everything that is negative because they just cause you stress, which is what contributes to cancer. Just be positive and forgive, as much as you can. If you cannot forgive a person, just don't think about them at all. Just keep all the good thoughts, good energy and positivity.

* Yesi L. *(Breast cancer: triple positive)*

I was definitely not ashamed to ask my family for support. I allowed myself to be vulnerable and asked for their help whenever I needed it. I was so blessed that my then fiance/now husband was around. Definitely, my parents too. They definitely helped with my daughter.

As for family activities, they were definitely impacted. Still I did what I could and my family adjusted. My daughter and I enjoyed our walks to school and the park together. They weren't as frequent, but we still enjoyed them and my daughter and I bonded together that way. Besides, it was good exercise!

ADVICE: Be kind to yourself and allow yourself to be taken care of. Definitely ask for support from anybody anytime you need it. There are a lot of people who feel happy when people ask them for help. So ask and reach out. Every contact is an opportunity that you can benefit from and they can benefit from, as well. So, ask for support whenever possible. I think that it's very important, especially if you have children.

FINANCES / HEALTH INSURANCE

* Aaron C. *(Prostate cancer, Skin cancer)*

I was in an HMO (Health Maintenance Organization), so there were no financial issues. I paid only $100.00 for the Robotic Prostatectomy, which is actually a $60,000 surgery. And, I did have a $10.00 copay for each of my doctor visits. Having HMO insurance is a good thing, because I was treated with the most modern technology for surgery and just paid minimum out-of-pocket.

ADVICE: Good thing about HMO insurance is that you get treated with the most modern technology for surgery and you pay minimum out-of-pocket. Of course, you have to do your research on what works best for you to keep your expenses to the minimum, while getting the best care.

* Amor T. *(Breast cancer, Ovarian cancer)*

Breast cancer: When I was diagnosed with breast cancer, I had COBRA healthcare coverage with United Healthcare. I paid all my premiums on time, but later learned that I got caught in a technical snag. During my second week in the hospital, suffering from my staph infection, a social worker visited and started to tell me about how she could help me get financial aid to pay for my hospital bills, which I would get a discount for, because I have no insurance. And the "discounted rate" was a little over $100,000, which I could pay in installments. I exclaimed, "What?!!!" Since I still had a high fever and was still fighting my staph infection, I was shivering. However, when she told me I had no insurance coverage, I got fired up (still shivering though) and my mind started going 100 mph! I told her that I have proof at home that I paid all my premiums on time and that I should be fully covered by insurance. When I got home, despite still being weak, I organized all the documented proof I had in my records, contacted United Healthcare and sent them copies of the proof they needed. I was a caught in a technical error on their end and they apologized for the inconvenience.

Ovarian cancer: Since I was not working, I had both Medicaid and Medi-Cal coverage, which was confusing. Medicaid was used to cover my cancer treatments and Medi-Cal covered my regular (non-cancer related) doctor visits. I had subsidized Anthem Blue Cross and kept very detailed paperwork, which came in handy when the hospital where I had my hysterectomy sent me a bill for the full cost of my procedure and two-day stay and then called a week later to ask for payment. When I told the caller from accounts receivable that they should get payment from my insurance company, she said that it was the hospital's practice to first get payment from the patient and then collect from the insurance company after. They will reimburse the patient whatever is deemed to be double payment after they review payment received from the insurance company. I was stunned, but kept calm and told her I was going to look into it further.

I contacted Anthem Blue Cross via the patient portal and wrote them what the hospital's representative told me. The Anthem agent said that the hospital actually has the right to ask for payment first from the patient. However, the patient is not obligated to pay before the insurance company does. So, I waited until I saw the Anthem Statement of Benefits online showing the hospital's charge, what Anthem paid and the amount that I (the patient) am responsible for. With that, I wrote a note on the invoice the hospital gave me, encircling the actual amount there that I was responsible for and sent them check for only that amount. I did not hear back from them again.

Another incident happened when I noted that the doctor's office charged me for a procedure that Anthem Blue Cross denied. In my Anthem Explanation of Benefits, Anthem had placed a denial code next to the procedure they were charged for. I asked the Anthem agent (again, via site messaging) what the code was and why charges for the procedure was declined. He said that code the doctor's office used was not applicable and didn't make sense. Anthem had already informed the doctor's office about their need to correct the code, but hadn't yet received the adjustment. I sent the invoice back to the doctor's office with a written explanation as to why I wasn't going to pay the bill; basically, based on the information I received from Anthem. I didn't hear back from them and was not charged for the procedure.

ADVICE: Because health insurance can be complicated, it's really important to keep track of all your dealings with them. Be sure to use the patient portals that you have access to on the internet. They can provide you the information you need. Communicating with the insurance agents via the portal is the wisest thing to do, because your communication with them is documented and they can provide you with information, e.g. insurance codes and legal verbiage to defend yourself when you're being unfairly charged.

It is also critical to keep records of billings from hospitals, doctors' office, imaging centers, etc. Again, sometimes the wires between them and the insurance companies get crossed and you can get caught in between. The representatives are just doing their jobs, so it's not a personal thing. You just have to look out for yourself and keep good records, so that you're ready, just in case.

Here's a small sample of the spreadsheet I created to track my medical insurance and expenses. By the way, this information was very useful when it came to deducting the amount for my taxes.

Anthem Claim Number in EOB	Service Date	Doctor/Facility	Total Charges	Member Responsibility per Blue Cross	Amor Charged &/or Paid	NOTE/Comments
2016316CJ5378	11/9/2016	Radiology Services	$268.00	$0.00	$0.00	Dexa Bone Density Axial
201631CJ5625	11/9/2016	Radiology Services	$417.00	$0.00	$0.00	Mammogram
2016285CL9491	10/6/2016	Oncologist Appt	$410.68	$410.68	$410.68	Dr. Dormady follow-up
2016281CT2009	10/4/2016	Radiology Services	$3,609.00	$0.00	$0.00	Full-body scan
2016279CW4060	9/12/2016	Hospital Lab Services	$6,225.41	$0.00	$0.00	Port Draw/125
'2016249BR2514'	8/2/2016	Hospital's Cancer Center	$11,745.50	$0.00	$0.00	Chemo 8/02 & 23
2016215CM8198	7/28/2016	Hospital of Port Surgery	$30,920.00	$0.00	$0.00	PORT surgery
2016215CZ3097	7/28/2016	Radiology Services	$37.00	$37.00	$37.00	Chest X-ray
201628CA1715	7/28/2016	Anesthesia for Port Surgery	$1,080.00	$0.00	$0.00	Anesthesiologist
201622CD4538	7/21/2016	Labs	$142.00	$0.00	$0.00	Lab Pathology
201622CD4539	7/21/2016	Labs	$260.00	$0.00	$0.00	Lab Cytopathology
2016209CR8650'	7/21/2016	Hospital Biopsy Services	$19,717.00	$0.00	$0.00	CT Guided Biopsy V-cuff/R armpit
2016204CT7128'	7/20/2016	Radiology Services	$4,300.00	$0.00	$256.75	PET Scan
2016200CJ9543'	7/13/2016	Labs	$128.00	$0.00	$0.00	Regular CA 125/CBC
'2016200BP0426'	7/12/2016	Gynecologist Appt	$150.00	$0.00	$0.00	Dr. Tae Noh
'2016181CS2614'	6/23/2016	Radiology Services	$3,604.00	$0.00	$256.75	CT Scan
'2016168CX5512'	6/13/2016	Radiology Services	$409.00	$0.00	$157.34	Ultrasound
'2016086BE9476'	3/17/2016	[Hospital Services]	$82,002.00	$2,427.60	$556.00	Hysterectomy
		1st adjusted bill received	$83,214.00	>>>>	>>>>	$3,081.6 charged
		Final adjusted bill received	$84,032.00	>>>>	$1,871.60	PAID!
'2016098CJ4595'	3/17/2016	[Pathology services]	$5,400.00	$0.00	$0.00	Pathology for hysterectomy
'2016112BQ6696'	3/17/2016	Hysterectomy Surgeon (Onc Gyn)	$14,100.00	$11,830.88	$2,000.00	Dr. Jeff Lin
'2016112CJ7794'	3/17/2016	Hysterectomy Services	$6,000.00	$0.00	$0.00	Dr. Tae Noh
'2016153BJ3905'	3/17/2016	Hysterectomy Anesthesia	$1,425.00	$21.65	21.65	Anesthesiologist

* **Bob G**. (*Soft Tissue Sarcoma, Skin cancer*)

While I bought and sold property, my wife Elizabeth handled the paperwork aspect of the business. She was very methodical. With the success of our business, we "never had to worry about a nickel" since.

* **Cindy L**. (*Kidney cancer*)

I have Tricare Prime insurance coverage and wasn't billed one thing. I have not paid one dime. I did not receive any hospital bills, doctor bills or bills for my surgery or aftercare. The only bills that I saw were bills for MRI and other procedures done out in the civilian community. But, those were also taken care of by Tricare. It also helps that I was a Tricare liaison when I lived in California back in the '90s. I was familiar with the process. I feel extremely fortunate and blessed, because I know so many people don't have the same excellent coverage I have.

ADVICE: It helps to become familiar with whatever insurance coverage you have and the process.

* **Cindy R.** (*Metastatic Breast cancer to the Stomach*)

Thankfully, my mind was well enough to keep track of financial things, like expenses, paying bills, etc. I've got binders to organize my medical files, bills, insurance. etc. I also have my mom on my account. There were times when I could take care of things and then there were times when she would have to take over. I'm so thankful for my mom! There were times I thought, "Gosh, what if I were really, really sick and didn't have somebody with me. That would just be devastating."

Unfortunately, there are so many people who take advantage of those who are sick. I've seen cases where really sick people were double charged and taken advantage of, which is just terrible!

When I first had breast cancer, I was insured through my employer, which was really good coverage. Since my car accident, I'm now on permanent disability. I'm on Medicare and then I have my secondary insurance with Blue Shield. So, fortunately, I'm all covered.

For one of the medicines I'm taking right now, there's a huge deductible or copay: $2,900 a month. So, I went through the process and got a grant for that. I'm going through a specialty pharmacy now and they were able to help me with the financial assistance. How I got that was a little complicated. Basically, I gave them a call and asked for it.

I also have a wonderful doctor and medical team. The first time around, they gave me a huge binder containing information about financial aid and how to deal with all the different things that are going to come up. Then they gave me the name and phone number of someone I could talk to, if I had questions or needed anything. That was very helpful.

ADVICE: Since you'll be receiving a lot of medical statements, records, invoices and various other paperwork related to your condition and treatment, you really need to keep all your paperwork organized. You want to make sure you're being charged correctly and paying for services you actually received. Unfortunately, there are terrible people out there who take advantage of those who are sick. Don't let them take advantage of you. Organize your files, so you can find the information you need. It's also important to have someone you trust have access to your files and be able to work with you on them.

* Glenn M. (Metastatic Colon cancer to the Liver, Lungs & Adrenal Glands)

Don't get sick until you have Medicare. I wish they could teach Anthem what insurance is supposed to be like, you know. With Medicare, I don't have to do anything. Since I don't have to pay the bills, I don't have to keep track of expenses. Well, not much anyway. The lady in accounting at the hospital took care of most of them for me. I have my secondary insurance through AARP (American Association of Retired Persons). So by the time both Medicare and AARP contribute, there's almost nothing left for me to pay.

When I get the bill, I don't pay right away. I want to make sure both Medicare and AARP chipped in. Sometimes, I get a bill and am told I have to pay it ahead of time and I'll get reimbursed after Medicare and AARP pay. Well, I don't listen to them, because if I pay the bill ahead of time, I'm just not going to be reimbursed. I already got burned before. I went to see an Endocrinologist that was fed up with Medicare and the wait times. He told me that I had to pay up front and Medicare was going to reimburse me. Well, I did pay him and I still haven't been reimbursed by Medicare.

ADVICE: Get to know the bookkeeper at your hospital. Bring them chocolates. Get them nice pens. That's important. Also, as much as possible, don't pay charges for doctor visits until after your insurance pays. If they tell you that you'll be reimbursed after, don't believe them. They should get their payment first from your insurance company.

* Hilda K. (Colon cancer)

Financially, everything was good because I got to use my SDI (State Disability Insurance) the whole time, which means I had medical coverage for the entire year I was off work.

God is good. If it could've happened, it happened when I was working full-time, which gave me full healthcare coverage. I also had a lot of accrued vacation time saved up. So, all those things made my taking a year off financially easier. Also, because I had healthcare coverage, emotionally, I was less stressed.

Through my work, I was still able to have my family's health benefits covered for a year too, even though I wasn't working per se. Because of SDI and our plan, I was able to supplement every pay period, every month. I supplemented 30 hours a pay period, which allowed for the healthcare coverage for us to continue.

The year before I found out I had cancer, I had saved up all the vacation benefits I had accrued at work (around 300 hours), because my family and I had planned to go on a big vacation in the summer to Croatia and stay there for a month. Those benefits paid for our trip! When I returned to work, I had no accounts receivable; I didn't owe anyone anything. I really couldn't have asked for a better set-up!

So, yeah, I had cancer that year and I went through it. I was set back for one year. But, God works His ways into making sure you have something. I know that even if I didn't have medical benefits to cover me and my family, I would've found my way through it. Basically, everything was fine.

* Jacki S. *(Breast cancer)*

I had an HMO insurance that basically covered all the bills. There was a $10 or $15 co-pay when I went in for an office visit. Other than that, my HMO covered everything else.

* J.B. *(Salivary gland cancer)*

I'm fortunate enough to be covered under my dad's insurance. So, I didn't have any problems with insurance, paying bills, money concerns or stuff like that.

* Rev. Linda S. *(Pancreatic cancer 3x)*

I had no problems whatsoever in this area. I was able to handle all financial matters with no difficulty. I knew not to pay bills or balance my checkbook the day of or the day after chemo because of chemo brain fog.

* Rachel S. *(Breast cancer: triple negative)*

Fortunately, we have double insurance coverage because my husband and I both have jobs. We had no co-pays; absolutely nothing to pay out of pocket. So, we had nothing to worry about when it came to that. As far as State Disability benefits, it took them about 1½ - 2 months before they started sending me my disability check. We wound up dipping into our savings account initially, in order to pay the bills. But, as soon as that money started coming in, I was able to replenish it. So, it wasn't too bad. It was just the wait time.

> **ADVICE:** **If you had to stop work because of your illness, make sure to apply for State Disability benefits. It definitely helps to pay the bills.**

* Rick S. *(CLL: Blood & Bone Marrow cancer)*

In terms of budgeting, I'm pretty successful. I'm pretty blessed, because my Department of Defense Medical Blue Shield Blue Cross and my Medicare B covered my expenses totally. I didn't have to pay any co-payment at all. All I had to do was come in and say, "I'm here". And they'd say "Good. Go in there and we'll torture you ... I mean ... TREAT you. [laughter followed] And, they did. And so, I was pretty fortunate with finances. I never did pay.

Regarding paying bills, once my problem with the DOD (Department of Defense) got fixed, there were no longer problems. My pay would be in the bank on the first of every month. And so, I didn't have any trouble with insurance coverage because God blessed me with the ability to pick Blue Cross Blue Shield and Medicare B and I didn't know that when I was signing up. I didn't know what was in my future.

I didn't have to keep track of expenses because there were none for me. I had no money concerns. I lived in my mom's house and all I had to be concerned about was paying the taxes. When my brother was alive, taxes were low enough to not be concerned with money.

* Scott M. *(Metastatic Colon cancer to the Prostate & Pancreas)*

Everyone's circumstances are different. Ours was in good shape. I was able to retire the day I was diagnosed. And then, having really good insurance really saved us too. So, we never really had to stress any bills for the chemotherapy, which can be just out-of-this-world expensive. When it comes to paying the bills, I continued to do that; it was something that allowed me to feel like I was still contributing to the family.

When it comes to keeping track of expenses, I tried to deal with the invoices as soon as they came in, so they didn't start piling up. Once they pile up, it would probably take a whole day just to play catch up. So I would take a day I felt good and work fifteen to twenty minutes a day on the billings. I took advantage of the times I felt good to work on them.

ADVICE: Hopefully you have good insurance and can budget around paying the bills. If not, there is financial assistance for those that need it. I have a bunch of friends that work at Stanford organizations that do grants for folks in need and also for research purposes and things like that.

* Sondra W. (Ovarian cancer 3x)

The subject of finances was kind of tricky because I did all the budgeting and paying bills and everything before I was diagnosed with cancer. Now all of a sudden, I couldn't do it. That taught me the importance of teaching my husband Kenneth where everything is, how my system works, and how to take care of the different things in our budget, especially those that need action.

On top of that, we're actually still working on organizing and finding the right places for things in our new home. We moved twice, and this time had to downsize our space. It's definitely a work in progress.

ADVICE: If you took care of the finances before, you need to pass on your knowledge of the budget, paying bills, etc. to your spouse or partner or children...anyone you could pass on the responsibility to. With all you've got going on physically, mentally and emotionally, you certainly don't need to worry about your finances. Identify where all your important financial and legal papers are maintained.

* Susan M. (Ovarian cancer, Metastatic Pancreatic cancer to the Lungs)

I have always handled the finances in our family and continued with no problems during both my ovarian cancer and pancreatic cancer experiences.

When I was diagnosed with ovarian cancer, I had full coverage with an HMO plan. When I was diagnosed with pancreatic cancer, I had the Senior Advantage Plan with the HMO. So, I had to pay $1,900 of the hospital expenses and also had co-pays for X-rays, PET & CT scans.

* Tet M. (Colon cancer 3x)

I was fortunate enough to have a good job with great benefits, so I was in good shape financially.

ADVICE: Depending on where you live, there may be government assistance you can avail of, if needed. There may also be caregiving assistance offered by some government agencies, especially if you live by yourself. Start by talking to your doctor or social worker. They may know what resources may be available to you. If you work for a company that provides private insurance, talk to Human Resources about your coverage.

* Vida B.A. (Breast cancer)

I was so blessed to be able to afford my treatment. Several years before my cancer diagnosis, I purchased a medical protection plan for women called "Eve". It's a plan that covers women who get major diseases like breast cancer. The insurance company has a similar protection plan for men called "Adam."

At one time, I was tempted to stop paying the premiums, because the plan didn't cover the total hysterectomy procedure I went through; they stated that it was a pre-existing condition. This really upset me. My friend who sold me the insurance, however, convinced me to continue paying the premiums. I'm glad I did, because when I informed them of my breast cancer diagnosis, they gave me ⏦ 1.3 million (Philippine Pesos), which covered my treatment. In addition to that, one of my best friends offered to shoulder all costs for my chemotherapy treatments. Her generosity is such a blessing!

* Yesi L. *(Breast cancer: triple positive)*

I must say that I'm blessed to have a supporting husband. So from that aspect, I didn't have to worry financially because he took care of us. But definitely, paying bills, insurance coverage, keeping track of expenses, money concerns... Yeah, we had to have a lot of communication with the insurance company. There were times we were told some procedures weren't covered. For the most part, my husband and I worked on those issues together with the hospital's accounting department. They were amazing, because they sent me my bills via email, instead of having me pay co-payments when I visited the hospital. When I received the bills, I would just call and discuss what the bills covered and then simply pay, using my credit card. It was simple and fast.

ADVICE: Try to find someone to help work out the financial issues with you at home and in the billing office (at the hospital or doctor's office). If not, the process can become overwhelming.

GROOMING

---

* Aaron C. *(Prostate cancer, Skin cancer)*

I didn't take any baths after surgery; I had to wait a few days. I was able to wash my hair, but I had to be careful. To get my body clean, I just used baby wipes. I had to be very careful, because (here's the other thing too) I still had all the staples in and I couldn't get my sutures wet. After ten days, when I went in to get the catheter removed, they removed the staples, they removed the tube that was draining and they did it all in one shot. They took it all out.

The staples they removed from me were metal staples. So, I thought, "My God, I'm going to be scarred up." But, the scarring ended up being just minor. I thought it would be worse. But, I used ScarAway and it worked.

ADVICE: Be very careful about getting your sutures wet. Baby wipes are easy to use and will do the job to keep your body clean when you can't take a shower. The scar diminishing gel, ScarAway, really works in lightening your scars or making them disappear altogether.

* Amor T. *(Breast cancer, Ovarian cancer)*

Breast cancer: After a week in the hospital, I was sent home with four JP (Jackson-Pratt) surgical drain bulbs hanging from my body: one by each breast and one by each side of my hip. The drains removed the fluid that had built up in my body after surgery. I was instructed to clean the wounds in those areas and also measure and record the fluid collected in the bulbs every day. Since showering with the four drain bulbs hanging from me was a bit awkward, I chose to just give myself daily sponge baths. I also used baby wipes, occasionally. My drain bulbs were finally removed after three weeks.

Ovarian cancer: While the large abdominal wound from my hysterectomy was still healing, I chose to just give myself sponge baths. It was just too tough for my body to move around in a regular shower. When I had alopecia due to chemo, it was actually easier to clean myself, because I had no hair whatsoever. All other grooming activities were easy.

ADVICE: You can groom yourself without having to take a full bath or even shower. When you're still not stable on your feet, sponge baths are the way to go. Baby wipes are pretty handy too.

* Cindy L. *(Kidney cancer)*

The first night after surgery, I remember experiencing a lot of discomfort. I wanted to brush my teeth. So, the tech stood behind me, because I was pretty unsteady. Obviously, a tall person made the sink, because I couldn't get high enough to reach over to spit into the sink. I'm 5'1" and a half. I'm very long-waisted and my legs and arms are shorter than a person who is the same height as me. Anyway, I remember getting so frustrated, the tech grabbed me a little basin to spit into. It was the small basin the hospital has for patients to vomit into when in bed. Good thing the tech was swift-thinking, because I was about to gag and just couldn't reach the sink. After, I said, "Boy, this sucks. I can't even reach the sink in here!"

The first several days home, I couldn't even get up out of the chair and go to the bathroom by myself without help. So, my husband had to shower me on a shower chair and wash my hair. I just couldn't do it on my own; I wasn't physically able to. Bathing on my own was hard, at first. I used a shower chair and a hand-held nozzle spray to shower with. That made it easy to bathe myself and wash my hair.

ADVICE: After major surgery, you'll most probably need help bathing and washing your hair, because you're just physically not able to. Don't hesitate to ask others for support. When you feel your energy returning and you're able to bathe on your own, use a shower chair and hand-held nozzle to shower with. Also, if you're short in stature and cannot reach a tall sink to brush your teeth and wash your face, use a step-stool. If you don't have a step-stool available, grab a small basin you can spit into when brushing your teeth.

* Cindy R. (Metastatic Breast cancer to the Stomach)

I didn't have any issues with grooming. I moved slower, but other than that, my grooming activities were pretty straightforward. I was able to shower with my chemo pump on me. However, I couldn't get it wet. They instructed me to place the chemo pump outside the shower, cover my port with saran wrap (the press-n-seal type) and then put a little tape around it. That will keep it dry and it did.

ADVICE: If you have a chemo pump, you can still take a shower with it on you. Since you can't get it wet, place the chemo pump outside the shower (hang it somewhere), cover your port with saran wrap (the press-n-seal type, as much as possible) and then put a little tape around it. That will keep the important parts of your chemo pump dry when you shower.

* Glenn M. (Metastatic Colon cancer to the Liver, Lungs & Adrenal Glands)

Bathing was exhausting while I was going through treatment. I needed to take like a ten-minute nap after taking a shower, because it felt like "hard work." My hair is kind of crummy. I don't have good hair and I think that my chemo drug Xeloda was the culprit. Anyway, I try to keep oil out of it, so that it's a little fluffy. It looks like I have a little more hair than I really do.

When it comes to caring for my teeth, I don't let the dentist do x-rays. I've refused them for two years now. They recently told me that they needed the x-rays because it's been a long time and they want to make sure nothing's hiding in my teeth. Well, I think their x-rays are probably a low enough dose, it won't hurt. Besides, I'm not going to go through another radiation treatment, other than a scan. So, I'm probably okay and will just let the dentist do his thing.

ADVICE: Grooming is really important to feeling better about yourself and your health. Even if taking a shower or combing your hair is tiring, just do it slowly. Also, be aware of how much exposure you're getting to radiation, including dental x-rays. Too much radiation will weaken you.

* Hilda K. (Colon cancer)

The fact that I didn't have to go to work helped tremendously. I mean, I lived in sweatpants, t-shirt, jackets and tennis shoes. I was really comfortable and I know that contributed to my recovery. When I had to go out, I kept myself warm by wearing a sweater, jacket, socks, gloves, a scarf and a hat or cap.

Connection of the mediport to my chemo pump was underneath my blouse. So, whenever I had to change my clothes, it was easy. I just had to remove the clothes that were over my mediport and chemo pump.

When it came to showering, I was prepared. I made sure I showered the day before my chemo infusion at the cancer center, because I knew I would have to wear the chemo pump home. During the two to three days I had the pump on me, I decided not to shower. I mean, I could've taken a shower with the pump, by just holding it out with one hand (like an IV), but I just chose not to. When I worked out at the gym, I cleaned myself by washing myself, holding the pump away from me.

> **ADVICE:** You can continue to keep yourself clean and groomed; just be prepared. If you have to wear a pump, just plan ahead and take a shower before your chemo infusion. You can choose to shower with the pump, but you don't have to. If you choose to, just hold out the pump with one hand (like an IV) and then shower. Or, you could just manually wash yourself down.

* Jacki S. (Breast cancer)

During treatment, I was able to take regular showers without a problem. Actually, it was easier, because I didn't have any hair to shampoo. I also opted to wear a wig versus head scarves. For me, head scarves are very noticeable on cancer patients and so, they would draw more attention to me than if I wore a wig. But then, that was my personal preference.

Since I also lost my facial hair (eyebrows, eyelashes), I went with a group of cancer patients and survivors at the hospital in a program called "Color Me Beautiful." In that program, we were shown how to apply makeup, how to make our eyebrows again, how to put the eyeliner on (because we didn't have eyelashes), how to put blush on our face and how to give ourselves a little more of a bright lipstick, because it can enhance our face a little bit more. After the program, we all got a box of our own cosmetics to take home. That was a special treat.

And then the other real fun thing I experienced when I had no hair was getting the free hats when I went in for radiation. Because there are so many patients that go in for radiation and don't have their hair yet, there's a special group of women (I don't know who they are; they're just angels) who make hats for patients who need them. What they do is they put these hats in a basket right inside the office. Before you go in for your radiation and, if you feel like you need a new hat or you would like to have a hat for another occasion, the hats are in the basket for you to take, free of charge! So, that was very nice. I did have a bunch of them. But then, I brought some back to the radiation department and some I took to the Salvation Army, because there is always someone who could use them.

I also went out once in a while for a professional manicure or pedicure. But, I typically do my own manicures and pedicures. I didn't have any issues with my teeth from the chemo or the radiation. And, I continue to go to my regular dentist every six months.

* Joan S. (Rectal cancer)

I was still able to take showers and even get manicures & pedicures.

* J.B. (Salivary gland cancer)

Oral hygiene was very important to me because, for the most part during radiation treatment, the radioactive beam kept hitting my back teeth. So, I made sure to really go double time on my oral hygiene. The medical team told me that oral hygiene was especially important, because radiation therapy around the area of my mouth definitely weakens my teeth, which will then make my teeth susceptible to bacteria. Here is a mouthwash formula they gave me to use every day.

Combine one (1) tablespoon of salt with one (1) tablespoon of baking soda
Mix the salt and baking soda solution into water to make a mouthwash

To this day, I continue the practice.

* Rachel S. (Breast cancer: triple negative)

Right after the mastectomy, my husband had to give me sponge baths and then, eventually I was able to start washing myself, making sure to stay away from the area I was operated on. I have a shower in my bathroom and my kids' bathroom has a tub. So then, we'd go into the kids' bathroom where I would lean over for my husband to wash my hair for me. When my husband wasn't home, my twelve-year old would wash my hair for me. We had to do this for a couple of weeks after the double mastectomy. After that, I was able to wash my own hair. We did have to do it again, for seven to ten days, after I had the port put in.

I had issues with my nails, so I didn't have pedicures or manicures. In fact, my doctor told me that I can never again have a pedicure or manicure. When it comes to my teeth, I have cavities I need to get filled. However, I need to wait until the chemo wears off, because I still have dry mouth.

* Rick S. (CLL: Blood & Bone Marrow cancer)

I've always bathed, no problem. I've always combed my hair. I felt like, the neater you were, the better you feel. I never had any manicures or pedicures, because I am a man, thank God! ☺ I just kept my nails clipped and my daughters would come over and take care of my toes, because I couldn't reach that far. I always brushed my teeth and flossed. It is important to keep up those grooming habits. It makes you feel better and gives you a better prospect to your day. It makes you feel a whole lot better, like working out does.

* Scott M. (Metastatic Colon cancer to the Prostate & Pancreas)

I definitely had to adjust when it came to shampooing my hair and bathing, especially since I had to make sure to keep the wound areas dry. I had help with sponge baths and that kind of stuff. There were times, even in the hospital, my hair would be so nasty and those shampoo caps that they give you just don't do the right thing for my hair. So, with some help, I would sneak into the nurses' bathroom, where they had a hair-washing sink, and then have my hair washed. All the nurses knew we were in there. So, after a while it was, "Can I have the key?" Having my hair washed just made me feel like a real person again.

* Sondra W. (Ovarian cancer 3x)

There was about a month period of time when I got so weak and the neuropathy was so bad that I had to have a home health aide come in and help me take my shower since Kenneth was still working at the time. We knew I could not be in the shower alone, with no one around, just in case. So, that arrangement lasted about four weeks and then I got better.

Now, I can shower and wash my hair; I'm thrilled! Some people don't know how BIG that is. It was like, "Oh, I'm just THRILLED to death!" I go to the bathroom and there's no bleeding. I'm just THRILLED … My goodness, this is so much FUN!

They're specially trained to assist patients with all their physical needs, including bathing, showering or shampooing your hair.

* Susan M. *(Ovarian cancer, Metastatic Pancreatic cancer to the Lungs)*

I had no problems bathing, shampooing my hair or with manicures and pedicures. The only thing I could not do was dye or perm my hair until a month after my last chemo treatment.

* Tet M. *(Colon cancer 3x)*

Taking a shower was a challenge because, at the time I was being treated with the chemo drug Fluorouracil, water would come out smelling metallic and somewhat similar to onions. Strange, huh? The smell was so off-putting for me. So, I took quick (but still thorough) showers and, while doing so, I tried to inhale and exhale through my mouth.

ADVICE: If water comes out smelling like something you don't want to have contact with (like showering), just do what you have to do with it quickly. Inhaling and exhaling through your mouth (vs. smelling it with your nose) should help too.

* Vida B.A. *(Breast cancer)*

I enjoyed taking showers, even when I had my drain bulbs. What made it easier was the fact that I didn't have hair in my body, including "down there."
    There was a time when I smelled something coming out through the pores of my skin; like the smell of medicine. It wasn't body odor. It was a funky kind of smell and it irritated me. So I took a shower twice a day and, eventually, the strange smell went away.

ADVICE: Do what you can to keep your body clean, so that you don't catch germs. If you have drain bulbs, get instructions from your doctor on how to keep them clean. If you can shower with them, that's great. Showering can be therapeutic too.

* Yesi L. *(Breast cancer: triple positive)*

Since I didn't have to worry about hair, I took the fastest showers ever! Looking at the positive side, I was happy that I was not using a lot of product and I was conserving water. I also wasn't spending an hour blow-drying and styling my hair. I felt that I was also helping the planet!
    The only time I needed assistance bathing was after my surgeries. My sister-in-law helped me bathe. Other times, I didn't need assistance; I was fine.

ADVICE: Ask for assistance in bathing, especially after surgery. If your treatment caused you to lose your hair, look at the positive side and how much you're helping to save water, electricity, hair products, your energy and the planet!

LAUNDRY

* Amor T. *(Breast cancer, Ovarian cancer)*

When I couldn't move around much, I was fortunate to have my family and friends help me with household chores, including laundry. I didn't have much laundry anyway, because I basically wore a lot of the same loose clothes, so there wasn't much to wash.

* Cindy L. (Kidney cancer)

I wasn't able to do laundry for several weeks. And then, when I felt strong enough to do laundry again, I had my husband Ed, my daughter Katie, or whoever was at home with me, carry the laundry basket out to the laundry room for me. I did the laundry, but I didn't cart the clean laundry back to the bedrooms, hang the clothes or anything like that. Everyone had to put away their own clean laundry.

* Jacki S. (Breast cancer)

I continued taking care of the laundry throughout my treatment. I may have done it slower, but I still took care of all our laundry.

* Joan S. (Rectal cancer)

Doing laundry was part of my exercise routine.

* Rachel S. (Breast cancer: triple negative)

I still did the laundry, but had to adjust, because of my lymphedema. I couldn't carry the laundry basket. So, I just put it down and shuffled it across the floor with my feet. It definitely took a lot longer to do laundry than it normally did.

* Rick S. (CLL: Blood & Bone Marrow cancer)

I've always done my own laundry. I didn't need anyone to do it for me. I just put my dirty clothes in the washer and then, after, I put them in the dryer. Then, I folded them up. It didn't have to be perfect. I always thought laundry is important.

* Yesi L. (Breast cancer: triple positive)

Fortunately, my husband and mother helped with the laundry. My mother also helped clean and organize the house, while I went through treatment.

* Aaron C. (*Prostate cancer, Skin cancer*)

Yeah, I have my two or three medications to take daily, but it was no problem.

* Amor T. (*Breast cancer, Ovarian cancer*)

To this day,. I keep my medications and supplements organized. I have all my prescription and OTC (over-the-counter) medications and my supplements my medicine cabinet. I have a weekly (7-day, Sunday through Saturday) pill organizer to help me remember what to take daily and I also have a large container of L-Glutamine powder on the counter with a measuring spoon inside.

During active treatment, the pills I had to take on specific days and times, I set to one side of the cabinet. Then, I arranged my pill bottles by category, e.g. nausea, allergies, pre-chemo, fever, gas, constipation. Also, with the L-Glutamine powder, I just remembered to take that three times a day (10 grams each time) with water-diluted 100% juice.

ADVICE: It critical to have a system for managing your medications, especially when they vary in how and when they should be taken, e.g. daily, every other day, once a week, with or without food, etc. Having a pill organizer or two will definitely help. Just make sure to fill them ahead of time and refill when necessary. Don't hesitate to refer to your doctor's written instructions or call, if you're not sure.

* Bob G. (*Soft Tissue Sarcoma, Skin cancer*)

I have one of those weekly Monday through Sunday organizers even though I have only two prescriptions: Losartan for blood pressure and Lovastatin for cholesterol. I never had the high blood pressure. I would walk the halls like mad; I liked it. When I go to see the doctor, I would have to wait a while. And so, I'd walk just far enough from earshot of the door to hear my name. Well, I found that because of all my walking while I'm waiting, my blood pressure would show as high.

Because I can't stay out in the sun, I had to compensate and take a Vitamin D supplement. I also take half Baby Aspirin once a day.

* Cindy L. (*Kidney cancer*)

My husband Ed helped me manage my medications and even administered them to me. He made sure he had all the written instructions and followed them, including using a daily organizer.

ADVICE: My biggest suggestion is to get yourself a little pad of paper and write down everything you need to remember when it comes to your medication. There's a reason why nurses write down when people are given medication, what they were given, the date, time...everything. Even if you're administering it to somebody, write it down. Don't count on your memory to remember what you took and when. It's so easy to get confused, especially if you have a bunch of medications to take. Use those plastic pill containers that have multiple days (representing the days of the week). They actually help.

It's one of the things that we nurses do for the elderly, because they can get very forgetful. They would say, "Oh boy, did I take my blood pressure medicine? Oh boy, I think I just took two of them!" That sort of thing. Also, I lost a friend who accidentally mixed a pain medication with another medication, after breast cancer surgery. It was a total accident and it was terrible she lost her life because of it.

* Cindy R. (*Metastatic Breast cancer to the Stomach*)

To treat my stomach cancer, I got this organizer from my doctor, because I had to start taking the pill Ibrance, which is targeted therapy; not traditional chemotherapy. I have to follow a very specific schedule with Ibrance, i.e. three weeks on and one week off. Although the pills are color coded, having the pill organizer is really invaluable. Otherwise, it would be confusing.

Aside from Ibrance, I had to take a daily pill. So I programmed an alert on my cell phone to remind me to take it. The pill organizer and alarm really make a difference. They're so great, because once I get started on my day, I'll tend to forget if I didn't have those tools.

ADVICE: When you're sick, you need to take it easy and not worry about anything, as much as possible. You definitely don't want to worry about when to take your medication or if you took your medication, right? So, the best thing to do is to get a pill organizer; the 7-days per week, Monday - Sunday one. There are so many kinds for so many situations or schedules. Just choose the one that will help for your medication schedule.

* Glenn M. *(Metastatic Colon cancer to the Liver, Lungs & Adrenal Glands)*

I've got a big pill organizer with AM and PM sections. I load it up once a week. That's six pills a day: three in the morning (AM) and three in the afternoon (PM). It helps me keep track since I'm on a lot of meds.

ADVICE: Get a pill organizer and use it carefully, making sure you know what day of the week it is. Otherwise, you might mess up and miss a day, or double up on your dose. And neither one is good, especially if you're on oral chemo. So, the pill organizers are necessary to make sure you take your meds when you should.

* Hilda K. *(Colon cancer)*

I didn't have a lot of medications to take; just the basic stuff. I did have to take a stool softener when I needed it, because chemotherapy made me constipated. Other than that, I didn't have to think about managing medications.

ADVICE: Try not to stress or overthink things. Take the medications you need and use a schedule, if necessary. The main thing is to keep it simple, as much as possible.

* Jacki S. *(Breast cancer)*

My doctor gave me the anti-nausea drugs for the chemo, just in case I got nauseated. I don't think I was given anything for my radiation treatments. Once my treatments were done, I started taking Tamoxifen, as part of ongoing treatment for my breast cancer. Originally, when I started on the Tamoxifen back in 2011, it was just going to be a 5-year plan. As I got closer to that five year mark and with more testing, the doctors got together and said, "Well, maybe we can make this work a little bit longer. I then found out that I could go for ten years on the Tamoxifen. So, I decided to do that.

During that time, my doctor wanted me to try another drug called Arimidex (Anastrozole). So, I went ahead and started that. I took it for a while and then noticed that all my bodily fluids dried up. It was painful for me when I had any kind of contact with my husband. I also noticed with the medication that I had a little more tingling on my feet than I had before; something to do with the nerves. I discussed my concerns with my oncologist who then decided to have me stop taking the Arimidex (Anastrozole) and return to taking the Tamoxifen until I reach the maximum 10 years. When I switched back to the Tamoxifen, there were no problems.

* Joan S. *(Rectal cancer)*

I did get a daily pill organizer to manage my medications.

ADVICE: A daily pill organizer helps me remember what medication to take and when, which is really important. You should definitely get one to manage your daily medications.

* **Rachel S.** (*Breast cancer: triple negative*)

The way I saw it, I had a whole lot of medications to take. For some people, it's probably not a lot, but for me it was. I had four nausea medications, two pain medications, sleeping pill medications and constipation medications. In my mind, it's a lot because I don't take medication on a day-to-day basis. Like right now, I'm not on anything. So, to me, that's a lot, but it depends on your perspective.

* **Rick S.** (*CLL: Blood & Bone Marrow cancer*)

I never had a problem managing my medication. I didn't have the organizer, because I didn't need it. I just knew what to take or what the doctor wanted me to take and I took it. But it is a good idea to have the little box or organizer with the weekdays marked Monday, Tuesday, Wednesday, Thursday, Friday, Saturday and Sunday. It takes a bit of work, but it's better than forgetting. That's a good way to do it.

* **Scott M.** (*Metastatic Colon cancer to the Prostate & Pancreas*)

If the narcotics I had to take were such that they were pretty heavy duty, I wouldn't remember the last time I had them. So, I got help with administration of the meds and we'd write down the time I took them, what I took and how much I took, so that we'd know if I was taking too much or too little.

> **ADVICE:** Notice if you're having difficulty remembering what meds to take, when and how much. If you're unsure, it's important to have someone to administer your meds for you. You need to make sure you're following directions when it comes to your meds.

* **Sondra W.** (*Ovarian cancer 3x*)

I have to be a little careful with managing my medications. I have a pill box organizer that I use and it helps. Still, I need to be careful, because my medications could still be easily messed up. For example, I had to take the blood thinner Xarelto at the exact same time every day. I also have to take my blood pressure medication Amlodipine at the exact same time every day too. The schedule is a bit tricky. That's why I have to be careful.

During my current phase of treatment, my medications are constantly changing, and we are experimenting to find the right combination of meds. The reason we're doing it is to eliminate the edema in my lower body, and also lower my heart rate. To keep from getting confused, I post the changing medications on the door inside the cabinet where I keep my meds.

> **ADVICE:** You need to be extra careful with your medications because directions on how and when to take them vary, e.g. with or without meals, first thing in the morning or before you go to bed, whether or not you can take them with other medications, etc. Definitely use a pill organizer. There are a lot of different types to help make sure you take your medications on schedule. It also helps to post your medications and instructions - like whether it must be taken with food or an empty stomach - on the door inside the cabinet where you keep your meds. Using colorful highlighters, pens or markers, you can write important notes on the medicine bottles themselves.

* **Vida B.A.** (*Breast cancer*)

With so many medications to take, I had to be organized. After my chemotherapy sessions, I would be given prescriptions for medications I had to take. Before returning home, I would pass by the drugstore to have the prescriptions filled. And then I would take them, following a specific schedule. I had a method; a routine, which was important because I wanted to make sure I was on the right track in taking care of my health.

> **ADVICE:** If you have different medications to take, you must be organized. Having cancer and going through treatment can cause confusion. You can't depend on your memory and you definitely don't want to miss taking

your medications or take the wrong ones. So, it really helps to keep notes or keep your medication in a medicine organizer.

* Yesi L. *(Breast cancer: triple positive)*

I had such a big collection of medicine bottles; I have never had to take so much medicine before! My husband picked up most of my medications. Then, I was pretty much in control and knew what I had to take and when to take them. I didn't have to use organizers.

MOVING AROUND THE HOUSE / APARTMENT

---

* Aaron C. *(Prostate cancer, Skin cancer)*

Generally, I wasn't in that bad of a shape. When I had the catheter on, moving was painful for a while, but I was still able to move. When I came home from the hospital, I remember that I was light-headed, at first, and all I could do was lay down all day long. I was able to walk around the house a little bit, but I was really limited to what I could do, at that point. When I moved around the house, I had to cling to the banister and be really careful when I walked.

We did have a dog in the house who liked to jump up on people. I had to keep her away from me while I was trying to recover; I was so unsteady then. So, I just yelled at her to stay away and she knew to stay away from me.

ADVICE: Don't rush to move around. Move slowly, one step at a time, and give your body enough time to recover. When you move around, be careful where you walk. Make sure you don't trip on things, including your pets. Cling to the wall, banister, couch or whatever you can hold onto to keep you steady.

* Amor T. *(Breast cancer, Ovarian cancer)*

Since I went through major abdominal surgeries during both my breast cancer/DIEP flap breast reconstruction and ovarian cancer experiences, I practiced the same safe methods in moving around the house.

Throughout my first two months home, I pretty much lived in my living room. I slept on my long couch at night and also rested there, propped up by many pillows, during the day, while I watched TV, worked on my laptop or read books or magazines. Whenever I had to get up from the couch, I used the backrest or armrest to stabilize myself. Then, I held on to the walls and nearby furniture to get to wherever I needed to go in the house. I moved very, very slowly. I also decided not to use a walker, because I was strongly advised against it by one survivor. She stated that using the walker would make my abdominal muscles heal in the "bent" position and I would have difficulty standing up and walking straight after recovery. That made sense to me.

Of course, it was really tough moving around when the wounds were fresh. Fortunately, in taking my painkiller (oxycodone or hydrocodone)), I felt strong enough to move around. Still, I moved very, very slowly and didn't walk normally, to start. I actually shuffled my feet. During the times I needed help walking around, like when I was fatigued or severely constipated or in pain, I always had someone there to support me.

ADVICE: It can't be stressed enough how physical activity benefits the healing patient. However, when wounds are fresh, caution must be taken. Start just one step at a time, day by day, and listen to signals from your body. Yes, rest is important, but so is activity. You need to find a balance between the two, which you'll be able to find as time passes and your body starts to heal. In the meantime, don't worry about hugging the walls or your furniture for support. Don't worry if you're shuffling your feet or leaning on someone for support. Just do what you need to do to move around the house one step and one day at a time.

* Cindy L. (Kidney cancer)

The first several days home, I couldn't even get up out of the chair and go to the bathroom by myself without help. So, my husband had to shower me on a shower chair and wash my hair. I just couldn't do it on my own; I wasn't physically able to. It was also, initially, hard for me to walk around. But I had to do it more and more to gain strength. I didn't have to use a walker or a cane. I just walked very, very slowly. I worked on getting better hard enough to see my granddaughters on Halloween. They came over. And of course, that was just three days after surgery.

Since I had abdominal surgery, I used a pillow, at first, for a splint. If I had to cough or sneeze or get up, I used that. After a while, I found that a rolled-up towel also worked. I would place the rolled-up towel inside a soft pillowcase. It was faster and it kept the towel rolled up too. I would have one on either side, as a splint, to get up from a chair, when I walked around or when I moved from the bed at night. It just helped to splint everything.

At eight weeks, I saw my nephrologist. My daughter, Ali, was with me. I asked him, "Hey, can I start doing some workouts to strengthen my abdominal muscles?" He had looked at me and said, "No!" The way he said it, it was like, "I can't even believe you asked me that!" I said, "Okay." That was the end of that for a while. In the meantime, I enjoyed doing Pilates, some yoga, walking and riding on my stationary bike at home. I used the resistance bands too; they really help the arthritis I have on my back.

I also had to move around the house when I started doing laundry again. However, this time whoever was at home with me had to help me carry the laundry basket out to the laundry room for me. Also, even though I did the laundry, I didn't cart the clean laundry back to the bedrooms, hang the clothes or anything like that. Everyone had to put away their own clean laundry.

> **ADVICE:** Your body is weak when you come home from the hospital. So, you need as much support as you can get from those around you. Don't try to push yourself to do anything. You must rest. Nevertheless, it is important for you to move around when you're able to. Moving around is necessary for you to gain strength. Just do it very, very slowly and gently, when you start.
>
> When you have abdominal surgery, your abdominal muscles will be weak and you'll feel pain when you do anything that requires movement in your abdomen, like coughing, sneezing, getting up from a chair or bed, etc. A pillow or a rolled-up towel in a soft pillowcase works great as a splint! All you have to do, when you feel you need to cough, sneeze, get up from your chair or bed, etc., is to place the splint on your abdomen and press gently, but firmly, against it right before you cough, sneeze, get up from your chair or bed, etc. This action will keep your injured muscles from moving, as much as possible, which helps curb the pain.
>
> Take it easy when it comes to laundry, especially when you have others in your household. Have whoever lives with you help in the process, including putting away their own clean laundry. When you need help carrying the laundry basket to the laundry room, ask for help. Don't do it on your own, especially when your energy is low or your body hasn't completely healed.

* Cindy R. (Metastatic Breast cancer to the Stomach)

I live in a one-story home. The only stairs I have to deal with are the ones that go outside. I actually had difficulties walking around my house, because of a car accident I was involved in. So, I have a cane and a walker too. During treatment, there were a couple of times where I actually, in the middle of the night, went to the restroom, went back to my bed and then passed out. That was pretty scary. That was a time when I should have had somebody with me. But, I was stubborn and just thought, "Oh, I can just take care of myself." Yeah, that was not smart, at all!

> **ADVICE:** If you pass out once, you're going to do it again. So, make sure someone's with you and always keep your cell phone with you, just in case you fall or something. Make sure you can get a hold of someone immediately. And just be really careful. Make sure your walking path is clear and there aren't things you can trip on or fall on.

* Hilda K. (Colon cancer)

People helped me when I came home; they were waiting for me. My daughter's godfather and my husband had already put in the handrail to help me walk up and down the stairs. They wanted to have it ready for me to use when I got home.

Those kinds of things, I didn't have to ask for help. My family and friends were prepared for me to be at my worse. But really, nobody had to babysit me, because I was able to function on my own.

Because I was going to be off of work for a year (and I had never taken a year off before), I had all these great plans of the many things I was going to be able to do, like organize my photos. Instead, I just got up, hung out at home and mostly watched TV all day. Basically, I didn't accomplish much. I must say, though, that I did take Adriana to and from school, I did the laundry, I cooked dinner and other small things. The days just went by so fast. So, for a full year, I didn't accomplish the projects I planned to finish. However, I did take care of myself and I did make a full recovery. And that is a HUGE accomplishment!

> **ADVICE:** Getting yourself to move around, no matter how fatigued you feel, is what helps you get stronger. Even though I had a lot of support from family and friends, I didn't want to depend on them all the time. I knew I had to find that strength within me to heal. If you have stairs in your house, it would help to get handrails put in. If you don't have handrails, you can still move around by holding the walls and going slowly and carefully. Whatever you do, it is important to keep in mind that moving your body will help make you stronger and get your body to heal faster.

* Joan S. *(Rectal cancer)*

I had a cane and, sometimes, a walker to use when moving around the house.

> **ADVICE:** In order to heal, you need to move around. Even if you're slow, just move. It really is important to the recovery process.

* Rev. Linda S. *(Pancreatic cancer 3x)*

There were days when I was too fatigued to do anything. But, I remember my doctor telling me that my moving and being active, as much as possible, is critical to my recovery and health. For example, on a good day, I would sit outside on my shade-filled deck, comfortable in my nightgown and bathrobe, sip wild raspberry tea, listen to the soothing sounds of the birds, crickets and cicadas and watch my playful dog Murphy romp around the backyard, discovering new smells and reconnecting with familiar ones. Ah, the simple pleasures of life! Then, I'll do laundry, make potato salad to bring to Ma Mere and my sister Sam, make quiche and marinade chicken to oven barbeque for dinner, swap lamps in the house to update the family room look and, in between chores, cuddle with Murphy, who has been such a devoted and amazing companion to me.

> **ADVICE:** Moving around and being active, as much as possible, is critical to your recovery and health. So try to move, even if it's slow.

* Rachel S. *(Breast cancer: triple negative)*

There were times, I had to walk along the walls to hold myself up. With a double mastectomy, I would also sleep on the couch versus the bed, because I could hoist myself up using the back of the couch. Still it was really difficult, because you're using your chest plus your stomach muscles.

> **ADVICE:** Use the walls for balance when you need to move around the house. A couch could be easier to sleep on than a bed, because you would have the back of the couch to hoist yourself up, if you need to.

* Rick S. *(CLL: Blood & Bone Marrow cancer)*

I never had a problem moving around the house. I always vacuumed the floor myself and I always cleaned the bathroom myself. Yes, I like to keep active. It's important.

ADVICE: Don't just sit in a chair or lay on the bed. You have to keep active, even if you're slow. You have to keep active. It's important.

* Scott M. *(Metastatic Colon cancer to the Prostate & Pancreas)*

I try hard to stay active, even if I don't feel good. And I've found that the more I move, the better I feel. Even when I didn't feel good, every day, I would get up from bed, walk slowly to the other end of the house and sit or lay on the couch. Even if that was the only thing I did all day, at least I moved around.

ADVICE: Try to stay active, if you can. Once you get moving (even slowly), you'll feel better.

* Sondra W. *(Ovarian cancer 3x)*

In moving around my home, I just made sure that there weren't things I could trip over. I also watched out for loose, unsecured, frayed rugs with curled edges. I didn't want to get caught on them and trip. Other than that, I had grab bars installed in my shower, just in case I slip.

ADVICE: Move slowly and carefully. Be aware of where you're walking and hold on to the walls or furniture, if your footing is not stable. Have grab bars installed in your shower; they'll definitely help keep you from falling when you're in the shower.

* Vida B.A. *(Breast cancer)*

My bedroom is on the third floor of my 3-story house and my living room is right outside my bedroom. Even though there were times I didn't go downstairs for two weeks, I still tried to maneuver up and down the stairs as much as I could. I knew that it was good exercise for me; good for my healing. If I needed assistance moving around, I just called my helper to help. She has been such an angel to me.

ADVICE: Moving around your house or apartment is a good form of exercise. Even if you move slowly, as long as you move, it will help your body heal. Ask someone for assistance or cling to the furniture or walls around you to help you with your balance. The main thing is to move.

PETS

---

* Aaron C. *(Prostate cancer, Skin cancer)*

We have a dog who stays indoors with us. She likes to jump up on people. I had to keep her away from me while I was trying to recover because I was so unsteady then. So, I just yelled at her to stay away and she knew to stay away from me.

ADVICE: If you have a dog or some pet that you can trip over and be knocked down by, make sure you keep them away while you're trying to recover. Have someone take care of your pet, if necessary.

* Cindy L. *(Kidney cancer)*

My daughter Katie brought her dog with her when she came to stay with us. So now, we have Rocco who is 75 pounds. We have our dog, Roxy, who was rescued from our other son who lives with us; she is about 75 pounds. And, we have an 11-year-old tiny little cat who rules the rest. At first, everybody took care of their own pet. But then, of course, everybody pitches in with pet care, no matter whose pet. So, that obviously helped.

* Cindy R. (Metastatic Breast cancer to the Stomach)

During the time of my breast cancer diagnosis, I had a couple of dogs, different from the ones I have now. Anway, I was actually training one of the dogs to be in a show. I had a trainer who was able to come to my house, whenever I was feeling really bad, and help me train her. And then, when I felt better, I'd go to his place or I'd go to the park and train her there with a group. So, I adjusted the scheduling of the training, depending on how I was feeling at the time.

Unfortunately, I couldn't continue with her training, because I got so sick to the point where I just couldn't do it, no matter how hard I tried. The worst part was when I was in bed all the time, thinking that this might be the end. I watched a lot of TV, which helped me get my mind off things. I tried to watch a lot of comedies so that I could laugh. My dogs would climb in bed and snuggle up with me, while I pet them. At the time, that was all I could do with them. I also had my aunt who lived right around the corner from me. She would come over and help me walk around the block with my dogs a couple of times. That was really nice.

I now have two "new" dogs: Harley (12) and Shelby (6) who are the sweetest things. They inspire and motivate me to go out and exercise with them. They also are such comforting companions for me. Harley is my little follower. He makes sure and gives me expressions that seem to ask, "Are you okay? What are you doing?"

When I was going through my stomach cancer treatment, I did need help taking care of them. I got Shelby just a couple of months before I was diagnosed. When I received my diagnosis, I thought, "oh, my gosh, what am I going to do?" When I sat down with my mom to discuss the situation, she asked me, "Do you want to give her back?" I said "Absolutely not. She's my little girl and I'm going to keep her. But, if anything happens to me, please make sure and take care of her." Before my diagnosis, I actually gave them both baths in the bathtub. Thankfully, there's a new place that opened up down the street that is reasonably priced. So, I just take them in and bathe them there.

There were also ladies I called to take care of my dogs whenever I was going to go on vacation or somewhere where I couldn't take care of them. When they found out I was going through cancer treatment, they said, "Just let us know what you need us to take care of your dogs." They also offered to help me with anything and at no charge too! It's so fabulous just to have people who are there and who want help.

I play with my dogs all the time and they're really great companions for me. I have to take care of them. So, I can't be sick. That was my mindset in dealing with my sickness. My life had purpose and, even though I was dealing with cancer, I was living my life with purpose.

* Glenn M. (Metastatic Colon cancer to the Liver, Lungs & Adrenal Glands)

I've got hens and my dogs, Maggie and Molly. Maggie is a Pomeranian and picks fights with big dogs. Molly is a rescue who loves to roam around and explore. They don't get their walks as often as they should and they sure give me such guilt about it too! They know how to work the guilt trip. They say to me, "Hey, what's up? Where's our walk?" Molly's nickname is "flight risk." At one time, she was gone four days and nights; we went nuts! It was agony, like losing a child. It psychologically ripped open my heart, especially because she's a black dog out at night. We found her that time. However, she's done it again, at least three times! I figured I must do something. So, I contracted with a company called Whistle (formerly Tagg) and they sell GPS (global positioning system) collars and tracking services for pets, in case they get lost. It costs me $10.00 per month for the service, which is nothing when it gives me peace of mind and a way to get my roamer dog back home safely.

I have a good relationship with my dogs. They definitely keep me on my toes. They also constantly demand my attention and question me. I used to eat ice cream, but I stopped. One time, my dogs looked at me as if to say, "Where's our ice cream?" Well, I decided to put ice cream in their respective bowls. When I did that, they looked at me as if to say, "You mean dinner is ice cream?" I then looked at the clock and noticed that it was 11:00pm and we hadn't had dinner. So anyway, I fed the dogs and then put them to bed.

For exercise, I ride my bike once in a while for about a little over half a mile. I walk my dogs too probably four nights a week. They have their way of getting me to walk them. When I get home from work and come in the door, they jump at me; their faces looking at me as if to say, "We love you! We're glad you're home! Feed us! Walk us!"

Sometimes, I'll ride my bike and walk my two dogs at the same time... safely ~ you know, with the helmet, elbow pads and knee pads ~ because my dogs conspire. They talk to each other. I can hear them thinking, "Okay, when we get to the pole, you charge left and I'll charge right and we'll SLAM him into the pole and then, we'll tie him up!"

ADVICE: Pets are great companions and can give you a lot of comfort. Of course, they can also demand a lot of your attention and energy. So, choose wisely. If you've got a "roamer" dog or pet, get a GPS collar for it. I recommend getting it from the company "Whistle." When your pet decides to go out and explore without your permission, all you have to do is click on the Whistle app that you download on your phone. It'll draw a map with the address of where your pet currently is AND the path he/she took to get there.

* J.B. (Salivary gland cancer)

I have one cat. I didn't have to take care of him. He's very independent.

* Rev. Linda S. (Pancreatic cancer 3x)

My handsome black mini schnauzer, named Murphy, helps me in the healing process and takes my mind off cancer. When I'm physically and emotionally drained, he stays with me. On some of the days when I'm physically and emotionally drained, I cling to him as if he were a comforting teddy bear. And he lovingly lets me, licking me in the process. Thank God for him and his unconditional love and unending sweetness!

* Rachel S. (Breast cancer: triple negative)

We had two cats, three dogs and a fish. We all kind of took care of them. Unfortunately, I kind of didn't pay attention to them while I was going through my chemo treatment. My sister would joke, "Awww... Misha's so neglected." And I would say, "Yes, I know. She'll go find love somewhere else".

ADVICE: If you're too tired or just cannot take care of your pets, don't worry. They'll find someone who will.

* Rick S. (CLL: Blood & Bone Marrow cancer)

I never had pets, because I was always on the go and I didn't want them to just sit there all alone at home while I'm gone. They're living organisms too and they need love and attention. So, I would like to give my advice about pets.

ADVICE: Pets are good to have. If you can't give your pets love and attention, then no use having them. That's a shame. But if you're home all the time and have a nice pet, God bless you. If you have a nice dog or a nice cat, it always helps you, especially when you're alone.

* Scott M. (Metastatic Colon cancer to the Prostate & Pancreas)

I have four dogs, seven cats, five chickens and two horses and they're a huge part of my life. It was interesting to observe how they had a sixth sense knowing that I was ailing; they were much, more gentle with me.

ADVICE: Animals have a sixth sense, especially around those ailing. Your pet would be able to sense your illness. Just let them be around. Not only is it interesting; it can be therapeutic too.

* **Susan M.** (*Ovarian cancer, Metastatic Pancreatic cancer to the Lungs*)

We have a dog and, throughout treatment, I walked our dog every day.

SCHOOL

---

* **Aaron C.** (*Prostate cancer, Skin cancer*)

The first ten days after surgery, when I couldn't do anything because of my catheter, I had my ex-wife take our kids to school or wherever they needed to go. I didn't tell her about my cancer; I didn't want her to know. I try to keep my privacy private. I just told my ex, "Hey, I can't" or whatever excuse I used. The good thing is that most of this happened around July when they were out of school for the summer, so the timing was right.

> **ADVICE:** If you're unable to drive your child or children to school, ask help from those who support you. It's best to ask them ahead of time, i.e. before surgery or treatment, so they can plan their schedules too.

* **Hilda K.** (*Colon cancer*)

Because I took time off from work for a year, I was able to drop my daughter Adrianna to and from school and her practices. When I had enough energy, I tried to continue doing everything "normal." I didn't feel much fatigue, I didn't overwork myself and I didn't try to do more than I could.

> **ADVICE:** Yes, take care of your children's needs when you can. However, don't stress yourself about it. Listen to your body and don't try to take on too much. Ask your family or friends to help take your children to/from school or practices, if your body is not up to it.

* **Jacki S.** (*Breast cancer*)

During treatment, I continued to make sure my daughter was up and dressed for school and I still made her breakfast. I also continued to drive her to the bus stop so she could go to her middle school, after which I would resume my regular routines for the day..

* **J.B.** (*Salivary gland cancer*)

Nothing really changed in my school schedule, so I didn't have to inform my school about my cancer. I just planned my treatment schedule around my class schedule, because the semester was actually ending when I got my surgery. I had time to prepare for my classes around the daily radiation therapy.

There were a few times when my treatment schedule conflicted with my class schedule. When that happened, I just told my professors individually. They were all very understanding of it. If and when I had to miss classes, I would e-mail my professors, tell them what I had to do and request to be excused. My professors were aware that I had cancer and kept it confidential.

* **Scott M.** (*Metastatic Colon cancer to the Prostate & Pancreas*)

We did notify the school for my kids to keep an eye on them for any behavioral issues they may demonstrate at school, but not at home.

> **ADVICE:** If you have school-aged children, inform their school/s that you have cancer, so that the school may keep an eye out for any behavioral issues they may demonstrate at school, which may stem from your having cancer

* *Yesi L.* (*Breast cancer: triple positive*)

I was fortunate to be able to walk my daughter to and from her school. When I couldn't do it, I had the help of family and friends to do that.

SEXUAL INTIMACY

[**Note:** **For privacy reasons, the names of the contributors in this chapter are not included.**]

I'm not bashful about sexual intimacy or any of that. I was a birth doula and a nurse. So, I had to be able to openly talk about it. Besides, a normal, healthy sex life is part of overall health for every human being. When I was a birth doula, a lot of dads asked me, "When can we have sex again?" I would answer them honestly and elaborate if needed or they had questions. Since I had to be able to talk to the moms and dads about natural ways to get labor started ... and having sex if the doctor says it's ok is one of those ways, I just learned quickly to get over any discomfort about the subject.

For pleasure, my husband and I use good lubrication. I've found lately, going into menopause, that it's necessary. There are some good lubricants in the market, like Sliquid Satin (totally organic, flavorless and tasteless), Good Clean Love (vegan) or Bare Naked (really clear). The vegan lubricant Good Clean Love comes in a tiny, little tube (3 oz.) and costs around $12.00. You can order it from Amazon or find it at adult stores too. I also like the one called Bare Naked, which is really clear. These are the most organic ones I've found. But, everyone has to find what works for them. Astroglide is one of the better lubricants, but I react to it.

After my surgery, my husband and I had to wait before we could have sex again. We resumed after about five weeks, when I felt that I could tolerate movement while having sex. Of course, my husband was very gentle and sensitive and we were both very careful.

ADVICE: Be open and honest with your partner about your comfort level in resuming sex, as well as, what would feel good or not feel good. You should also feel free to talk with your doctor about sex; ask any questions you may have. Don't be shy or ashamed. They've heard it all and, in their profession, they're trained to know when the body is ready to resume sexual intimacy. They can provide you the guidance you need.

After cancer our sexuality may change in many ways... both physically and emotionally. Explore these changes as a couple or individually but understand that it's most likely still an important part of your life...even if it has been on the back burner for quite some time. Don't expect your partner to read your mind or hopefully they're not expecting you to read theirs. Good, open communication is vital in regards to this subject.

If you feel you or your partner are dry, don't hesitate to use lubrication. There are some good lubricants in the market, like Sliquid Satin... my favorite and found in adult stores (totally organic, flavorless and tasteless), Good Clean Love (vegan), Bare Naked (really clear) or Astroglide. The vegan lubricant Good Clean Love comes in a tiny, little tube (3 oz.) and costs around $12.00. You can get it at Target or find it at adult stores too. These are the most organic ones I've found. But, everyone has to find what works for them.

*****

I was fortunate that my doctor, who is a gynecologic oncology specialist, brought up the subject of sexual intimacy. I understood that so much was removed during my surgery, but I didn't know that he placed a "wall" there, so I would basically be protected. When he said that I would have an issue with dryness, I told him that I had that issue before. So, he suggested that we use the lubricant called Glide. When I expressed hesitation, he said, "You should be on top. That way, you can control how deep things go, and what's happening." And he said, "Everything should be good."

Because I really didn't know what to think or how I should do this and that to take care of myself, I decided that I would go to my gynecologic oncologist for female medical matters. I just go to him and see him every four months for check-ups. He would then check to feel lumps and bumps or if there's any tumor or anything like that. Then, he goes by the PET scan to see whether there's anything lighting up.

On the same sexual intimacy topic, the hospital had a speaker give a presentation to us about all aspects of cancer and sexual intimacy. At first, I thought it was a woman, but it turned out to be a man. He echoed what my doctor had said, i.e. the woman should be on top to avoid getting hurt. In the end, he concluded his talk by saying, "Now go and have a normal life."

ADVICE: Have an open conversation with your doctor about how and when you can return to sexual activity. Don't be embarrassed because your doctor is a professional and is the one who can give you the medical advice that you need. If you are a woman, then you should be on top of your male partner. That way, you can control the depth of penetration and avoid getting hurt. Also, if you had a hysterectomy, expect vaginal dryness. The lubricant Glide can help with this issue. It is available for purchase in many stores.

*****

Because of my hormonal imbalance, my sex drive declined. Sexual intimacy was definitely impacted. Since it's essential to have open communications with your partner, I talked with my husband about it. I also knew that it was temporary. I did discuss the issue with my doctor a lot of times, because I knew my hormonal imbalance was a side effect of the treatments I was getting at the time.

During my treatment period, dryness was my biggest problem. But, I had the solution right in my kitchen cabinet. Coconut Oil. Coconut oil saved my sexual life!

ADVICE: If your sex drive changed, it is possible that it is a side effect of your treatments. When that happens, it is essential that you have open communications with your partner and also openly discuss your issues with your medical professionals (doctors, nurse practitioner, nurses, etc.). Don't be ashamed. Ask questions and reach out for help. Because, more often than not, they will have the solutions. Just think that you are not the first to ask questions about how your treatment affects your sex drive. Also, for vaginal dryness, try using coconut oil. It may save your sexual life!

*****

How did I know it was okay to have contact with my husband? Well, it depended on how I felt. But, I kept up with my husband all the time. We had our regular sexual things. However, when I started taking the anti-cancer drug Arimidex, all my personal bodily fluids actually dried out. When we had sexual relations, it was very painful for me. So, we tried using different types of lubricants. Then, I developed a latex allergy. So, we had to use condoms that were made out of animal skin, which were very expensive. It was tough for us, because what we knew to be an enjoyable activity actually became more of a task. I expressed my concerns to my oncologist who then put me back on Tamoxifen and my body responded really well to that. We got back into having sexual relations without too many problems and my husband and I felt much happier.

ADVICE: First, be open and honest with your partner about how you feel about sexual relations. If you notice a change in your body, especially when you've been taking various chemo medications, discuss it with your doctor. You need to let your doctor know, so your concerns can be addressed and you can enjoy your sexual relations again.

*****

I had a really tough experience going through sex after my mastectomy and reconstructive surgery. The man I was with at the time was clearly repulsed by how I looked. He did not have to say it in words, but he did so in his actions and expressions. When we had sex, I had to wear a top to cover myself. I felt "broken" and even repulsive. I felt I was being used for sex, but I did not complain, because I was just trying to focus on being thankful that I, at least, had a sexual partner and, maybe, he did care for me, despite how he treated me. Yes, I know. My self-esteem was really low back then. Looking back, it would've been better for me to not have a sexual partner at all, because it was just a meaningless act. Unfortunately, going through that experience took an emotional toll on me. So, I learned that if my partner doesn't respect me, then he doesn't deserve to be with me at all. Period.

ADVICE: First and foremost, respect yourself! Don't feel you have to have sex with someone who doesn't honor you or love you. You're better off on your own. Let your experience with cancer remind you of what's really important in life. Aside from your health, it's your self respect. Life is way too short to waste it on someone who doesn't make you happy or someone who just uses you. You deserve to be taken care of. No ands, ifs or buts. And don't settle either.

*****

It's tough if one partner wants to be intimate and the other one doesn't. For sure, you know you've got a problem there whether you're a cancer survivor or not. With the age difference between my wife and me, and then her condition, I couldn't expect her to still want to fool around.

ADVICE: If it really gets to you or your partner and there's a mismatch, then you should probably get some kind of counseling. If neither of you wants sex or you both do, then there isn't a mismatch. Now, if there's a physical issue...and God knows He did enough digging around in me and in her too...then let love and respect guide you.

*****

This took a huge hit, especially with the prostate cancer, depending on the surgeries. And, the radiation changed it where I can still perform and my body can still orgasm, but without ejaculating the semen. I'm not shy about sharing my challenges when it comes to sexual intimacy, because I want to let people know what happens and be up front and honest and real with it. And maybe, my experience will help somebody else without going into it.

ADVICE: Always be honest with your partner and consider what he or she is going through. Discuss how the treatment or drugs will affect your sex life, e.g. libido, performance, etc. Keep your expectations realistic and be open in your communications, so that you both can support each other.

*****

As soon as we got the diagnosis, my husband kind of started backing off, because he was afraid of hurting me. And it was quite some time before we did anything. It was actually more me initiating it, because I felt bad for him. It's like I said, "I need to take care of you". And he said, "But you're not feeling good." And I would say, "I know, but ..." Even today, it's not where it used to be. He's so afraid of hurting me.

ADVICE: Having sex is important for a couple to share. And the fact is, men need sex more than women.

*****

Before the surgery, they told me that I might have a problem getting an erection and stuff, after the procedure, and that I'll have to take Viagra. Fortunately, when they removed my prostate, they also did a nerve-sparing surgery where they avoided cutting the bundle of nerves that go right around the prostate gland and right up to the penile shaft. Those are the nerves that are critical for erections. Although the surgeon couldn't exactly see the nerves, he knew where they were, because he's done so many similar surgeries before.

The first time we had sex after my surgery was after four months. We tried to have a little bit of fun, but I was sore just getting an erection. So, we had to play it by ear. Initially, I leaked urine when I orgasmed, so we had to be careful. It was messy and I was like, "Ugh, I don't feel like doing this." That was the worst part of the whole thing. Fortunately, my girlfriend was very understanding throughout the entire ordeal.

Now, there's another thing I had to get used to as a man. I had to get used to a dry orgasm, which meant I couldn't ejaculate anymore. When I reach sexual climax, there is no fluid released anymore. Nothing. But the pleasure is still the same!

I still have to take Viagra. Sometimes it takes a year or more to be back to full "normal" function. But, I noticed a difference already. I'm still not 100%, but yeah, I can actually have sex again, which I couldn't do before. So, that's like a major marker; a milestone marker.

Viagra's an amazing drug, man. Luckily, I'm at a time in my life when this stuff is around because 20 years ago, Viagra wasn't even an option. And, it's part of the treatment too. The doctor actually made me take the Viagra to keep the blood flow going.

ADVICE: When you first have sex, remind yourself that you just had serious prostate removal surgery and it'll take time to get an erection. Just take it slow and expect some leakage. Things will get better. You also won't be able to have a normal ejaculation (with fluid), but you'll still be able to reach a sexual climax. The pleasure stays the same. Also, take Viagra; it's an amazing drug!

*****

Our intimacy wasn't particularly affected by my surgery. I had one less breast but there wasn't any other impact on our sex life.

ADVICE: Honest and open communication with your partner is vital for your relationship. You can be creative in finding new ways of enjoying sex together.

*****

It was, I won't say normal. I think it was due to fatigue and weakness. But, overall, it was about the same. We were in tune with each other and communicated our needs.

*****

When I was first diagnosed with breast cancer, I was 39 years old and I was divorced. But, I still considered myself a young woman and thought, "Wow, now I'll have no breasts." And then I had a hysterectomy and thought, "Yeah, no one's ever going to care about me again. Yuck, I'm all scarred up and it's all gross." But, then I realized that when I find the right person, it's going to be great because he'll just accept me for who I am. We'll be meant for each other, because I've got all this stuff going on and he still loves me, regardless. So, it'll be great. It's not something I'm going to worry about, because there's a lot of life to live and that's what I'm focused on.

ADVICE: You may have no breast because of mastectomy or you may be missing some of your female parts from hysterectomy, but you're still you and that's something no one can take from you. You deserve a partner who'll love you for you, no matter what. Focus on all the many positives in life and be thankful that you're alive to enjoy them.

*****

My sexual experience with my boyfriend after my hysterectomy, was nothing short of beautiful. I felt loved, very loved, and respected. He was very sensitive to my needs and very gentle. We had sex slowly and communicated our needs. We were very open with one another. We did not immediately have sex. I felt strongly that we had to check with my doctor first to make sure that it was okay. Even though we were told beforehand that we could resume sex after six weeks from the hysterectomy, we still were nervous and needed reassurance. I felt conscious about asking my doctor (male), but I put that aside because, honestly, I couldn't wait to have sex again. When I called for an appointment, I was told that I was not due another visit with him until two weeks later. I begged the clinical coordinator to please adjust the calendar, which she did, thankfully. With my boyfriend present, my doctor performed a manual pelvic exam and gave us the "go" signal. Of course, we were excited!.

At first, we were awkward with our movements, since we were very conscious of my wounds. After we finished, I felt strong cramping in my lower abdomen. So, while placing my hands on my abdomen to comfort it, I worked to relax my breathing. Eventually the cramping went away.

The position that created discomfort and pain was when I was on my knees, because then I had to hold my abdomen during sex, because it would be hanging down.

The two positions that were enjoyable and worked best were when I was on the bottom, because my abdomen was protected, and when I was on top, because there I had more control over my movements. Of course, my boyfriend gently helped me throughout our intercourse.

ADVICE: If you had a hysterectomy, talk with your doctor about when you can resume sexual activity. If it would make you more comfortable, ask for a manual examination to make sure your body has healed enough. Because of your abdominal wound, you may want to be either on the top, where you have more control over your movements or on the bottom, where your abdomen can be protected. Avoid being on your knees, since your abdomen won't be supported in this position..

SHOPPING

* Amor T. (Breast cancer, Ovarian cancer)

I didn't shop that much during both my cancer experiences. I tried to avoid places where there were many people to keep from getting sick, since my immune system was not strong. If I had to shop, it would be for needed groceries or the pharmacy to get my meds and, even then, I would avoid the "rush hour" times, like lunchtime, after work hours or during the weekends.

When I was going through chemo, the only time I could go shopping was during my third week aka my "happy week", because it was the time I had the most energy. Of course, the following week, we'd start the 3-week chemo cycle again where fatigue and other side effects would keep me home. When I did go out, I wore my colorful, knitted beanies or colorful scarves. Wearing color just made me feel more energetic.

ADVICE: When you're going through active chemo treatments, you really need to protect yourself, because of your weakened immune system. If you need to go out and shop, do so during the hours when there's the least amount of people, i.e. outside of the rush hours of lunchtime, after work and weekends.

* Cindy L. (Kidney cancer)

Oh yeah, I'm a shopaholic; I love shopping! At first, I couldn't go grocery shopping or do any other shopping, like run around a mall, because of my condition. That was difficult for me, because I'm in a small area and sometimes shopping is all there is to do. So, when I got stronger, I returned to shopping and was very careful. I walked slow and made sure I had a cart to hold on to. I was good.

I did, however, feel a bit of shame when I had to use one of the little electric scooters at Walmart while I shopped. This happened the first couple of weeks after surgery. It seemed that people looked at me and I felt I needed to explain why I was using the scooter. I also felt that I was taking the scooter from someone who actually needed it. But then, I realized that I actually needed it because our Walmart is huge and I physically couldn't walk around without assistance from the electric scooter.

ADVICE: You do need to be careful about shopping after surgery. Make sure you're physically well enough to go and deal with all the activity and people. Walk slowly and find a cart to hold onto. If your body is still recovering from surgery, don't feel ashamed about using the electric scooter in the store, if they're available. Because of your condition, you have a valid reason to use it.

* Cindy R. (Metastatic Breast cancer to the Stomach)

I love shopping! Actually, the first time around, it was so funny because right after I got my treatment shots, I got a "high" like I had a lot of energy. The nurses had told me to make sure I walked around for about half an hour so that the medicine could run through me and I didn't get a knot from the shot. Since the shot was a really thick liquid, they had to inject it into me really slow. If I didn't move around after, like if I just sat down after, the liquid would've bunched up right where I was injected and I would've felt really blah. So, I said, "Okay, got half an hour. Let's go shopping real quick! Let's go!"

We usually go to Costco or Sprouts or Trader Joe's or someplace like that. So, yeah, I wanted to take advantage and get some shopping done while I could. After a half hour of shopping, I was low on energy. At least, I had the energy to shop for half an hour and that was fun!

ADVICE: If shopping is what you enjoy and you have the energy to go shopping, you should go. You just have to be careful about overdoing it, because when your energy runs low, you don't want to be completely wiped out and feel really blah, which will happen if you overdo it.

* Hilda K. (Colon cancer)

Since I wanted to keep everything "normal" as much as possible, I did go to the store to buy groceries and I did shop for other things too. Of course, I listened to my body and didn't try to do more than I could, because I wanted to heal properly. I am fortunate that I didn't experience much fatigue, so I had some energy to do some shopping.

ADVICE: I think that you should try to keep your life as "normal" as possible, doing the things you used to do ... of course, always considering your energy and how you feel. If shopping is what you used to do and, especially, enjoy doing, then you should continue shopping. Just always keep in mind that your body needs to heal. So, don't overdo it. Listen to your body and don't' try to take on too much.

* Jacki S. (Breast cancer)

I love to shop! I was always finding fun things to go shopping for, even when I was going through treatment. I didn't feel my shopping schedule had to depend on whether it was crowded or not. I had my good wig on and I had no problem going shopping. What I did find though, going through cancer ... all of a sudden, I'm attracted to the color pink more – because that's the breast cancer color.

* Joan S. (Rectal cancer)

I tried to shop, but did only if it was necessary and only if I felt well enough to do so.

ADVICE: If you need to shop for something and you're unable to, don't hesitate to call on your family or friends to help, especially if it's something you really need.

* J.B. (Salivary gland cancer)

I shop online. We get everything on Amazon Prime, especially when it's free shipping.

* Rev. Linda S. (Pancreatic cancer 3x)

On my good days when I have a bit of energy, I muster up the strength to run errands, keeping them brief and, thus, minimally taxing.

* Rachel S. (Breast cancer: triple negative)

I usually had someone go with me, because I couldn't lift anything during the whole trip. The big thing that my sister, my daughter and I always did since my daughter was eight years old, was the Day-after-Thanksgiving shopping. I was not giving it up. I didn't care if we just went to one store; we were going! And I had chemo that day, too. First, we left the house at midnight and did our shopping. We took it very slow. If I needed to rest, we sat down and rested. We didn't go to as many places as we normally did, but we had an amazing time. When we returned home from shopping, I rested. Later that day,

I went in to get my chemo. There's actually a Facebook picture of me and my daughter when we went to Target and I got $800+ worth of merchandise for free! I'm not going to let cancer control me. I make my choice.

> **ADVICE:** Go shopping if you really want to, but take it slow. The main thing is you can still do what you enjoy, especially if it's important to you. Just pay attention to what your body is telling you, and adjust what you're doing when you need to. Don't let cancer control you.

* Rick S. (CLL: Blood & Bone Marrow cancer)

During the time I was going through the intravenous chemo treatment at the oncology lab, I was living in my own home. So if I needed something, I would go shopping for it outside of my chemo treatment time. I basically shopped whenever I needed. I tried to be selective of the time, but it didn't bother me. If I needed something, I went ahead and got it. I don't have to shop now that I live in a retirement community. And, I'm now taking the pills, which are a lot better.

* Sondra W. (Ovarian cancer 3x)

I used to have stamina for shopping, but I got tired easily and wasn't so good with shopping anymore. So, I just shopped online when I needed something. Initially, I got overwhelmed with everything that was happening. Aside from my treatments, I also had to continue dealing with the residual-effects of my move, which was like boom...boom...boom.... It was really a struggle.

But now, I'm better at shopping online and am exploring options to have groceries and other local products delivered to my home.

> **ADVICE:** Going through treatment is draining. So, you won't have much energy to do anything else, including shopping. Shopping online is the easiest way to get whatever shopping you need done. Or, you can ask someone to shop for you. In any case, just choose to do things that are really necessary, so you don't get overwhelmed. And, ask your loved ones or friends for help, when you need it.

* Vida B.A. (Breast cancer)

During treatment, I didn't do a lot of shopping for fear I would catch a virus when I'm in a crowd of people. Christmas shopping, however, was an exception, so I allowed myself to go out one time and do a bit of shopping. I wore a mask to make sure I didn't catch anything. I chose to shop at places that were not too crowded and I shopped in the afternoon of a weekday, when most people were at work.

> **ADVICE:** Your immune system is really weak when you're going through treatment. So you have to be really, really careful about going to places where you'll be in contact with a lot of people. If you have to shop, choose the days and times when the stores are not crowded, like weekday afternoons. Also, you should wear a mask, just to make sure you protect yourself.

* Yesi L. (Breast cancer: triple positive)

I shopped when I felt I could. When I felt I couldn't and needed to buy something, I had the help of family and friends to shop for me.

SLEEPING / NAPPING

---

* Amor T. *(Breast cancer, Ovarian cancer)*

Breast cancer: It was quite awkward trying to sleep with the four surgical drains I had hanging out from my body, after my mastectomy and breast reconstruction (DIEP flap) surgery. I had them on for three weeks and, for the entire time, I had to sleep upright.

Best place for me to sleep was on the long couch in my living room, which was in front of the TV. Even after the surgical drains were removed and I was able to lay down to sleep, the couch remained my "bed." The firmness of the seat cushions with the support from the arm rests and the back pillows were perfect. I used those supports to push up from every time I needed to get up. They really helped because, as in any abdominal surgery, the tissues (muscles, skin and other connective tissues) were cut, thereby rendering my abdominal muscles quite weak. Additionally, using my arms to push myself up versus using my abdominal muscles was the only way for me to get up, at that time.

Ovarian cancer: I did have problems sleeping when I suffered serious constipation after my radical hysterectomy. I tried sleeping with my bottom up, so I could let out some gas. Sometimes that worked, but sometimes it didn't. What did work most times was placing a firm pillow between my knees and sleeping on my left side in the "fetal" (curled up with your knees to your chest) position. The left side was the most comfortable for me. I also had a large wedge pillow to use whenever I had a tough time laying down. Even though it wasn't the most comfortable position, it did help me to sleep.

> **ADVICE:** Trying to get into a comfortable sleeping position when you come home after surgery can be really tricky ... and painful. Here are some tips I hope will help:
> 1. If you have surgical drains hanging out from your upper torso, it's best to sleep in an upright position. Use a wedge pillow to lay on or, if you prefer the couch, use a bunch of cushions and pillows to prop you upright.
> 2. If you have serious and painful constipation, it may help to:
>   a. sleep on an incline, using a wedge pillow,
>   b. sleep with your bottom up, so you can let go of trapped gas, or
>   c. try placing a firm pillow between your knees and sleep on your left side in the "fetal" (curled up with your knees to your chest) position.
> 3. If you have any abdominal surgery, sleeping on a regular bed may not work for you, because most times, it's too soft and/or it doesn't have the proper support. Ideal is a long couch with firm, yet comfortable seat cushions. The firmness of the seat cushions with the support from the arm rests and the back pillows will be perfect. Use the arm rests or back pillows to support yourself by pushing up from them every time you need to get up. They'll really help because, as in any abdominal surgery, the tissues (muscles, skin and other connective tissues) were cut, thereby rendering your abdominal muscles quite weak and sore. Use your arms to push yourself up versus your abdominal muscles. That'll save you from from more pain.

* Bob G. *(Soft Tissue Sarcoma, Skin cancer)*

I did have trouble sleeping or getting back to sleep when I woke up in the middle of the night. Sometimes it was because of night fears and other times there was no reason; I just couldn't sleep. I tried taking one to two sleeping pills, but then I couldn't wake up in the morning. I did also play solitaire when I couldn't sleep.

What I did to deal with the night fears was think good thoughts. My good thoughts? Well, some of the nurses! I always say, "God's greatest gift to man is woman!" That's one of my favorite sayings! Also, for men, I recommend finding a good woman. It just makes staying awake a little bit nicer!

> **ADVICE:** The best medication for recovery is a good night's sleep. If you have night fears, think good thoughts only. If you have a hard time sleeping or getting back to sleep, try some activity, like playing solitaire. It does help to have someone stay awake with you.

* Cindy L. *(Kidney cancer)*

During treatment, I went to sleep when I needed to and when I needed to take a nap, I took a nap. I didn't feel guilty about it, because I knew that it was part of my body's healing.

> **ADVICE:** Sleep and nap whenever you need to. Don't worry about the time of day or night your body feels like napping or sleeping. When you're going through treatment, your body will tell you when it needs rest and you have to follow its lead. It's part of your healing process.

* Cindy R. *(Metastatic Breast cancer to the Stomach)*

The port didn't really bother me when I slept. However, the chemo pump did, because it was on my side and hooked up to my port. So, when I wanted to turn, I had to adjust and do it carefully. I didn't have to use extra pillows; just a small pillow that kind of protected the area my pump was in. I placed it there, so that I wouldn't roll over on top of my pump.

Thankfully, my chemo pump didn't hum or make noise or even vibrate. However, I could definitely tell it was there, because of all the tubing. I still had to wear the fanny pack with the pump when I slept. Even though it didn't make any sound, I could tell when it was working, because of the liquid that I could see running through the tube. It just did its thing quietly.

> **ADVICE:** Figure out what you need to do to adjust to changes in your sleeping arrangements. You can be really creative. For support, extra pillows are great. If you have to sleep with a chemo pump, use a pillow as a barrier to keep you from rolling over your pump. Hopefully, your chemo pump doesn't disturb you. If it does, you need to just relax and deal with it. In time, you'll get used to it.

* Hilda K. *(Colon cancer)*

Because I had a chemo pump, I had to adjust how I slept. I slept with my pump next to me and made sure I didn't turn while sleeping by placing pillows next to me. So, basically, I slept on my back and was able to be comfortable and sleep regularly.

Getting up from bed, initially, was tough. Fortunately, I had a little pillow that the hospital gave me to use as support when I had to pull myself up. All I had to do was place the pillow on my tummy and continue holding it there while I pulled myself up, so that my midsection wouldn't have to strain as much. I saved that pillow for two years after treatment ended, because it was such a positive reminder of how that little thing helped me get out of bed.

I was kind to myself and listened to my body. I napped when I felt I needed to, but didn't have to do that often, because I still had energy to do things around the house.

> **ADVICE:** If you have to sleep with a chemo pump, just place the pump next to you and place several pillows around you, so you don't roll over the pump. Sleeping on your back would be best. If you had surgery around your abdominal area and you need to get up from your bed or couch or any place low, get a little pillow to use. Then, with one hand, place the little pillow on your tummy and hold it in place while you pull yourself up with your other hand. That will definitely prevent your midsection from straining. Be kind to yourself and listen to your body.

* Joan S. *(Rectal cancer)*

I absolutely slept and napped whenever I felt the need.

> **ADVICE:** When your body is tired and needs rest, it will tell you. So, listen to your body and sleep or nap when you feel the need. It is part of the healing process.

* Rev. Linda S. (Pancreatic cancer 3x)

I sleep well at night and nap during the day when my body demands it. My puppy Murphy is often curled up beside me for naps, as well. When I have to have the chemo pump with me, I strategically place bed pillows around me to keep Murphy from harming me or the chemo pump. This works well.

* Rachel S. (Breast cancer: triple negative)

I have a hard time sleeping, because of my Lymphedema. I had to learn to sleep with my right arm elevated. To sleep on my back, I learned to put pillows on either side of me, so that I can keep my right arm elevated. If I wanted to sleep on my left side, I still had to keep my right arm elevated. Of course, I couldn't sleep on my right side, because of my Lymphedema. It's taken a while to get used to, but this is how I'll have to sleep for the rest of my life. Unfortunately, that means that I can't curl up next to my husband.

The hospital gave me these heart-shaped pillows that I used after my mastectomy to cushion my arm away from my body. When I couldn't move my neck, because the veins in my neck were messed up, I used the same pillows to support my neck when I needed to lay down. Those were the best things ever!

ADVICE: Get good pillows that can support you. See if the hospital can give you support pillows too.

* Rick S. (CLL: Blood & Bone Marrow cancer)

I had trouble sleeping. Napping? I did have trouble napping, because, first, I never was a napper. I'd feel guilty about laying down to take a nap when the sun was shining, because I should be outside, if I could.

* Scott M. (Metastatic Colon cancer to the Prostate & Pancreas)

I joke around that I'm a professional napper. If I'm tired, I go rest. And usually, when I close my eyes, I'm out for two hours. My body's saying, I need to rest; I need to recover. And, I listen.

ADVICE: Your body is trying to heal. So, if your body is telling you it needs to sleep or nap, follow what your body is telling you and sleep or nap.

* Sondra W. (Ovarian cancer 3x)

I learned how to take naps later during my treatment period. It's something I wish I knew how to do way back when I first started treatment instead of coming home and working because I thought I had energy, which I realized later I didn't really have. But now, I know, so I've gotten into the good habit of napping.

ADVICE: You need naps to enable your body to rest and heal. Make sure you take a good nap after you return from your treatments even if you feel you have energy or don't need a nap. The energy you're feeling won't last long, and your body definitely needs to rest after going through treatment which is really hard on your body.

* Susan M. (Ovarian cancer, Metastatic Pancreatic cancer to the Lungs)

There were many times I felt tired or fatigued. So, I took naps whenever I felt I needed to.

ADVICE: Listen to your body. If you are feeling tired or fatigued, REST. Sleep or just lay in bed or the couch and REST. Your body needs it to recoup from surgery and medication.

* Vida B.A. *(Breast cancer)*

Because I wanted to heal right away, I was a good girl and went to bed early, even if I wanted to stay up. I understood that sleep will, not only help my body heal, but it will also protect it from infection. Sleep will help boost my immune system and strengthen my body too.

ADVICE: During treatment, your body will be going through a tough battle. That's when you'll feel fatigue. Pay attention to your body and sleep or rest whenever you feel fatigued. Even when you feel you have energy and want to stay up, you have to be conscious of how much sleep you're getting. Sleep is critical to your healing and strength, so make sure you give your body enough sleep.

* Yesi L. *(Breast cancer: triple positive)*

Whenever I felt fatigued, no matter what time of day, I just slept or napped. I did not feel any shame and I didn't judge myself, because I knew my body needed the rest.

ADVICE: When you feel fatigued, just sleep or take a nap. Your body needs the rest. There is no need to judge yourself and feel ashamed. Allow yourself to rest.

SOCIAL, FAMILY AND/OR RELIGIOUS GATHERINGS

* Aaron C. *(Prostate cancer, Skin cancer)*

I didn't go out very much, because for one, I couldn't sit down for long periods of time. Going through treatment, I was so uncomfortable. I didn't do a lot of socializing for, at least, the first month or so after my surgery.

ADVICE: There's no need to rush going out to socialize. Give your body enough time to heal. You can return to your social (and other) activities after you recover.

* Amor T. *(Breast cancer, Ovarian cancer)*

While I was going through my breast cancer experience, it was difficult for me to get around. So, instead of me going out for gatherings, my family and friends visited me at home. There were a couple of times I really wanted to attend an event at my beloved Foster City Lions Club. I was so fortunate to have friends accompany me and help me through the event. Both times, my body was weak, but my spirit was strong. I did notice that I had to be careful about how much energy I expended, especially in talking with others in my excitement. Because, both times, I started to get a bit dizzy and nauseated. Nevertheless, I really enjoyed myself. Having been a member of the amazing Foster City Lion Club was truly a blessing and an honor.

Going to Sunday mass every week is an activity that is very important and dear to my heart. When I was finally strong enough to attend Sunday masses, after recovering my surgeries or during my chemo "happy" week when my energy was at its highest, I was still aware that my immune system was still fragile. So I made sure to attend the masses that had the least attendance. That turned out to be the latest (evening) mass and it worked out beautifully.

ADVICE: It's wonderful to be amongst family and friends or go to events you enjoy. However, when you do, make sure you pace yourself. Conversing with people will require extra breathing and energy from you. If general anesthesia was administered during your surgery, your lungs were definitely weakened. Also, when your body is still trying to recover, your immune system needs rest to be able to regain its strength.

If you have to attend gatherings where there are a lot of people, e.g. church services, choose to attend one that isn't crowded. You want to make sure you protect your weakened immune system, as much as possible.

* Cindy R. *(Metastatic Breast cancer to the Stomach)*

For the most part, I tried to stay positive and got involved in ladies' groups, even though I was sick. I belonged to four or five different ladies' groups. With the different ladies' groups, I would go to luncheons. We have monthly luncheons and people would help me out with that. I was actually on the board with one of them, but had to step back at one time, because I got so sick. Now that I'm feeling better, I'm back on the board and doing more; getting more involved.

And then there was the time with my family in Disneyland. Actually, it's a great story because it was my 40th birthday and I had just had my surgery and it was before I was going to start my chemo treatment. Since my Disney vacation was planned before I received my diagnosis, I said, "Well, we're going to go anyways and it's just going to be me and my mom." So, we went down there and my sister called and said she was coming.

It was my 40th birthday and I was going through cancer treatment. When we arrived at the Disneyland Hotel, the staff told us, "Oh, we're upgrading you and oh, it's a fabulous room!" I just said, "Okay." But then, when we walked into the room, I said, "Wait..wait...wait... This can't be right. This is the Honeymoon Suite!" They said, it was right. And so, I called my sister and told her, "Oh my God, I can't believe you did this. Thank you so much!" She cried and I cried too and then I heard a knock on the door... and my two sisters, my brother-in-law, my cousin ... everybody came up and joined us! Oh, my God, it was so touching! It was so wonderful! It was the best birthday ever!

ADVICE: Even though you have cancer, it's important to stay positive and be active with groups that interest you, as much as possible. Having a positive attitude and being active will really help you become stronger, physically, emotionally and mentally. Spending time with family is valuable too. When you surround yourself with love, your health will definitely benefit and there will be a lot of joy to share with loved ones.

* Joan S. *(Rectal cancer)*

I enjoy being with my family tremendously. Time with them is so wonderful and precious. When I was going through treatment, my daughters went with me to whatever gatherings I wanted to attend. I'm an active member of the Lions Club (a community organization) where I live and I'm also active with my sorority. Even when I was going through treatment, I tried to attend our meetings. Of course, when I didn't feel well, I didn't go.

ADVICE: It's important to still go out and do things you enjoy, as much as possible. Just take it slow and don't tire yourself.

* J.B. *(Salivary gland cancer)*

I attend service every Sunday at the United Methodist Church and accompany the choir with my guitar. I didn't miss any of the services during treatment. I was pretty consistent. It was really obvious that I had treatment on my face, but I just let it be. It didn't bother me.

* Rev. Linda S. *(Pancreatic cancer 3x)*

To this day, I continue my attempts to normalize my life and stay in the present moment, while my subconscious continues to work on my concerns. Still, I go on. Again, I have no choice. I go out with my mother (Ma Mere) who has Alzheimer's, attend church on Sundays and meet and chat with friends. Every so often, there are times I don't feel well and would prefer to remain at home rather than go to church. But that still, small voice urges me to go and when I do, the Sunday lesson turns out to be what I just needed to hear.

* Rick S. *(CLL: Blood & Bone Marrow cancer)*

I always went to church; that's important. I went to prayer meetings on Monday nights and service on Wednesdays. If I felt bad and couldn't drive myself, I'd ask someone to come by and get me. And then, I'd lay on the back pew. I laid on the back pew on Easter Sunday, because I felt so bad. When I was weak and needed to go to the bathroom, I would just get myself there, open the door and hold the little handles on the wall. After I was done, I would then work myself back to my pew and lay down again.

* Scott M. (Metastatic Colon cancer to the Prostate & Pancreas)

I tried to keep my life as normal as possible, as if I didn't have cancer. So, when it came to going to family get-togethers, church services or activities like that, I tried to go, even if it was for a little while.

> ADVICE: If you can muster the strength to go, with no commitments on how long you're going to stay, because you might be there ten minutes and all of a sudden feel nauseous or whatever, TRY ... make an attempt to live your life, as if you didn't have cancer, as normal as possible.

* Sondra W. (Ovarian cancer 3x)

For family in the Bay Area where I live, it was only my daughter, my husband and my granddaughter with me. They gave me all the support that they could and I feel so, so blessed and thankful for all they did to take care of me, especially when I needed it the most.

Not too much happened when it came to regular family activity. What we did was change some things. For example, instead of cooking Thanksgiving dinner or Christmas dinner (especially since my daughter was working and trying to help me at the same time), we ordered from Pluto's, because they serve healthy food. So, for the year I was dealing with my treatments, we just ordered in for big occasions or holidays, and it worked out great.

> ADVICE: Your family and loved ones are also having to make adjustments to the changes you're going through. It can be really emotional and even overwhelming for everyone involved; not only you. Help others help you, by communicating exactly what you need, only when you really need it. Also, don't take on too much or try to fix everything. Stay positive, focus on your health, and save all your energy to fight cancer.

I went back to church after a long hiatus which was due to my being constantly fatigued and having to deal with my diarrhea. So, for almost a year, I just listened to the services online.

When I did eventually return to church, I sometimes found it hard because the people there were so sad for me and their sadness made me sad. I remember that I would be doing fine, and then I would see them and they would be so sad for me, saying they would pray for me ... it just overwhelmed me sometimes. I realized that I was just caught off guard when I first went back to church. I hadn't expected all of that ... kind of like being in the ocean. So I just learned to prepare myself, and now I can better handle all that when I go to church.

> ADVICE: If your condition doesn't allow you to participate in certain activities you enjoy, there may be ways to still participate that don't require you to physically be there. Check for similar online activities, like for religious services or video chats with the family.

* Susan M. (Ovarian cancer, Metastatic Pancreatic cancer to the Lungs)

Going through treatments for both my cancers didn't stop me much. So, I participated in all family and social gatherings we were invited to.

* Tet M. (Colon cancer 3x)

There were times when I wasn't feeling up to attending social gatherings, but my friends insisted it would be good for me to enjoy a night out. And they were right!

> ADVICE: Depending on the severity of your illness and treatment, plan for worse case scenarios. If you're worried about feeling nauseated during the gathering/event, be sure to bring your medication kit with you, as well as a

change of clothes. Be prepared for an outpouring of concern and well wishes from people who know what you're going through.

There may also be instances where the person you're talking to may be naïve or unintentionally tactless or even rude. So, be prepared for anything. However, try not to take any negative comments personally. They don't benefit you. Instead, brush them off and ignore them.

Be ready to answer questions, and if you can, try to sound positive, so as not to make the interaction uncomfortable. Whenever I discussed my condition with people, even to this day, I'd make light of the situation and would go as far as joke about it. It helps to create positive interactions. Above all, think that you're there to accomplish a mission, i.e. to enjoy yourself, because you truly deserve it.

* Yesi L. *(Breast cancer: triple positive)*

When time and my energy permitted, I went to mass with my mother on Sundays. It was one of the ways for me to get the best connection with God. Being there with the community, I poured my heart out every time, just singing. It recharged me and re-energized me so much that I just kept on going.

Being that Spanish is my first language, I went to Spanish mass where I felt the most connection. It wasn't really packed when I went, so I wasn't really concerned that my immune system might be weakened there. Being in church, I just felt such a positive vibe, I was refueled every time. So, I looked forward to attending mass.

SPORTS

---

* Cindy R. *(Metastatic Breast cancer to the Stomach)*

I'm a season ticket holder for the Oakland Raiders and have been a fan for 17 years now. It was really fabulous and I went to a lot of games. Even if I wasn't feeling good, I would just bring my cane and walk in there and do what I could. Cancer can't stop me from going to the games.

During my cancer treatments and everything, there was another really special thing that happened. The first time around (breast cancer), my sister called them (the Oakland Raiders), told them what was going on and they sent me all kinds of Oakland Raiders goodies. The second time around (stomach cancer), my niece who is close friends with an actual Oakland Raider told them, "My aunt's going through all this stuff..." Then, I got a message on Facebook from the Raiders' quarterback and a couple of other players. They said, "Cindy, we love you. Hang in there. We're supporting you. You're going to make this!" Oh, my gosh, I was just in tears! I was like, "Oh, my God, I can't believe it. How amazing!"

ADVICE: If you enjoy going to sporting events, go when you have the energy to. Of course, make sure you have someone with you for support. Even if you're not feeling good, doing things you enjoy will actually change that. Of course, don't overdo it and listen to your body. Rest is super important when your body is trying to heal. But, being active and continuing to do things you enjoy will make a positive difference in your recovery process. It's a matter of balance. Give it a try and adjust when you need to.

* J.B. *(Salivary gland cancer)*

A month after surgery and while I was still undergoing radiation treatment, I actually went with my girlfriend to the boxing gym. It's the same one that world boxing champion Manny Pacquiao trained at. Anyway, my parents were not happy about my decision and I understand how they felt at that time, i.e. they thought I should just rest. Anyway, I did take it slow and was really cautious. I really wasn't in too bad of a condition, but I definitely couldn't spar.

ADVICE: If you really want to participate in sports or some physical activity, first listen to your body and take it slow.

* Rachel S. *(Breast cancer: triple negative)*

During the time I was diagnosed, my twelve-year old son, Ryan, was doing his first season of swim. After the surgery, I wasn't really able to go to many of his events, because I couldn't sit in the sun; it would make me sick. So, a friend of mine took Ryan to his practices and competitions. Ryan is also a black belt in karate. When I could, I took him to karate with my baby, Sawyer. But then, there were times I got too weak and couldn't lift Sawyer or handle it. I had another friend who went with me to help out. And, when it got to be too much for me, she just took over taking Ryan to karate for me, altogether. Sometimes, she still does that for me when Ryan has his later classes on Tuesday nights.

> **ADVICE:** It's important to be with your children in their sporting events, when you can. If you're feeling weak or tired, ask friends or family to help.

* Scott M. *(Metastatic Colon cancer to the Prostate & Pancreas)*

While I was going through treatment, I still attended sporting events. I was a season ticket holder to San Francisco Forty-Niner football games, before they moved. I enjoyed the games, but there were a couple of times when I had to have somebody else drive me up to the stadium, because I didn't feel too good.

> **ADVICE:** Don't give up what you enjoy, as much as possible. Just adjust as you go along, like asking someone to drive you to and from the game, if necessary.

TRAVELING

* Aaron C. *(Prostate cancer, Skin cancer)*

I planned ahead and did my traveling before surgery, because I knew that I wouldn't be able to travel anywhere after. So, I went on a cruise with my girlfriend and really enjoyed it.

> **ADVICE:** Think ahead. Make travel plans before your surgery and treatment period. That way, you can really enjoy your travels without pain or worry.

* Amor T. *(Breast cancer, Ovarian cancer)*

When I was going through my later chemo treatments, I traveled with Bill to our new home in Penn Valley, which was a 3.5 hour drive from our home in Santa Clara. Those were short 2-3 weekdays or weekend trips and we scheduled them during my "happy" weeks when my energy was at its highest after chemo. Although I didn't feel strong, it was still good to be able to go out and have an adventure, especially after many days of being cooped up at home.

> **ADVICE:** Time your traveling to when you have the most energy. If you're on a road trip that takes several hours, make sure to take stretch breaks. As much as possible, try not to use public toilets along the way, because with your weakened immune system, you want to avoid all the germs and bacteria usually found in public toilets. If you absolutely must use them, then try not to touch any of the surfaces, especially the door knobs, without a paper towel or shield for your bare hands.

* Cindy L. *(Kidney cancer)*

On New Year's Eve 2016, ten weeks after my surgery, I packed a few things in my suitcases and drove off, on my own, fifteen hours one way from Florida to Ohio. I did make one stop in Kentucky to spend the night before continuing on the road the next day. My husband, I know, was totally freaked out with me making that trip so fresh from my surgery. But, I had to go there to see my dying aunt who had Alzheimer's. Something told me to "Get up there" and I believe it was the guardian angels, because I was able to see her before she passed away.

When I arrived, I found out that my mother was suffering from bacterial pneumonia, which she got directly from my aunt who eventually died from it. So yeah, that was a mess and I ended up taking care of my mother too. I had no choice but to drive for the trip, because I couldn't fly at that point. Being so fresh from my surgery, there was still the risk of blood clots that flying could cause. And I had no one to go with me. So, I had to go by myself. I was very cautious while driving. I used my pillow across my stomach and I stopped every hour to get out and walk. I drank a lot of fluid and tried to eat as healthy of fast food as I could. The most important thing was for me to make sure that I did everything I could to keep blood clots from forming after my abdominal surgery.

ADVICE: If you have to drive and you had abdominal surgery, place a pillow across your stomach to protect it. Stop and walk every hour, drink a lot of fluid and try to eat as healthy of fast food as you could. The main important thing is that you keep your body physically active to prevent the risk of blood clots that tend to form after abdominal surgery.

* Cindy R. (*Metastatic Breast cancer to the Stomach*)

I actually went to Disneyland and got a scooter there. Yup, it was really fun! In fact, I was like, "Okay. Look out, everybody... Coming through! beep...beep!" Actually, it's a great story because it was my 40th birthday and I had just had my surgery and it was before I was going to start my chemo treatment. Since I already had my Disneyland vacation planned before my diagnosis, I said, "Well, we're going to go anyways and it's just going to be me and my mom." So, we went down there and my sister called and said she was coming.

Because it was my 40th birthday and I was going through cancer treatment, the staff at the Disneyland Hotel told us, "Oh, we're upgrading you and oh, it's a fabulous room." I just said, "Okay." But then, when we walked into the room, I said, "Wait..wait...wait... This can't be right. This is the Honeymoon Suite." They said, it was right. And so, I called my sister and told her, "Oh my God, I can't believe you did this. Thank you so much!" She cried and I cried too and then I heard a knock on the door... And, my two sisters, my brother-in-law, my cousin ... everybody came up and joined us! Oh, my God, it was so touching! It was so wonderful! It was the best birthday ever!

I also traveled to Walt Disney World in Florida. Then, after I was just diagnosed the second time, we went on a Disney cruise to the Panama Canal. I don't know if I told my doctors. My family and friends said that I needed to plan it. But I said, "I'm turning 50. I'm going. Sorry." It was really cool experience, because since I had started my asparagus regimen (four tablespoons of pureed asparagus twice a day), my mom told the ship's crew what I was going through and asked if they could help provide me the asparagus puree I had been taking daily. They accommodated our request and even followed up with me everyday, asking, "Did you eat your asparagus today? You sure you got it? You're all good?" And each time, I answered, "Yes, I'm good." It was really neat.

ADVICE: When you have cancer, life doesn't have to be dull and boring. Sure, you're sick. But, you don't have to be down all the time. Even with your sickness, there is a lot you can do for yourself to enjoy what you have. Traveling is one of those things that can be a really fun adventure for you to enjoy. Just communicate what you need and things will work out.

* Hilda K. (*Colon cancer*)

Before I was diagnosed, my family and I had some great plans to travel to Europe. When we were ready to go, I informed my oncologist. When I told her that I was going to be gone for a week, she asked, "Where are you going to?" I told her, "Europe." She then told me firmly, "You are not going anywhere." So, I had to cancel my trip and I lost money for that. Even though I cancelled for medical reasons, I couldn't get my money back. Anyway, my oncologist explained to me that I could travel anywhere in the United States, because there was medical access. However, to travel out-of-country just would not be good for me.

As soon as I was done with my chemotherapy treatments and I felt ready, I did travel to Hawaii with my daughter Adriana and visited my mom there. We stayed there for a week or two. Even though my hair felt funky, I went anyway. Still, I tried to stay out of the sun, because my entire body with the chemo chemicals was still super sensitive. I know that it was crazy to travel then, but I really wanted to go. And before I knew it, the year was over and I had to get back to work. Still, I got to see my mom in Hawaii and I was glad I did.

> **ADVICE:** Let your doctor know if you have travel plans. Since your doctor knows your condition and treatment plan, getting their approval is necessary. Traveling is good for the spirit. However, if you get sick during your travels, you need to get proper guidance and treatment. Your doctor will know best when you're strong enough to travel and where you can or cannot travel.

* Jacki S. *(Breast cancer)*

I remained active in Jenise's school, even when I was going through treatment. As a matter of fact, when I found out about my cancer, I was just about set to go on a field trip with her as a chaperone to Disneyland.. The school's orchestra, band and chorus, which my daughter was part of, were going to perform at Disneyland. I let the choir director know that I had cancer and I was going to have surgery. He said that it was up to me if I wanted to go on the trip, or if I felt it wasn't the right thing to do, he would find another chaperone. What I told him was, "I have loved Disneyland from the time I was six years old. I would love to go to Disneyland and won't even think about my cancer the whole time I'm there. Who thinks about cancer when you're in Disneyland?" We were around all the kids. I had a roommate who was another mom. All we did was enjoy the kids, enjoy the performance and their performances. Once I got home, I was booked the next week to have my surgery. I did not let my cancer hold me back from our trip to Disneyland.

> **ADVICE:** If you enjoy traveling, find ways to do it with approval from your doctor. If you're not allowed to travel yet, then adjust your thinking. Plan what travel you'll do after treatment is complete. In the meantime, focus on getting stronger.

* Rachel S. *(Breast cancer: triple negative)*

We drove to Disneyland a week after I started chemo. It went really well, actually. I got my doctor's permission; talked to him first. Initially, he did not want me to go. But when I mentioned that my dad rented me an electric scooter, he was totally fine with it. So, my family and I went down and we stayed at my dad's house. My dad got the electric scooter from where he worked, and I just rode that all over Disneyland and it worked out great! In the car trip to Disneyland, I was sick part of the time. But it wasn't too bad. It could've been worse. I had just started treatment, so at the time, I wasn't dealing with the bone pain and everything yet.

When we went to Yosemite in November, that trip was a lot harder, because I had the bone pain and I couldn't sit still. No matter what I did, I was hurting. I just took pain meds to get through it. No, I would not recommend going. But if I had to do it over again, I would definitely do it, because it was something that I did with all my kids; my daughter was on vacation.

> **ADVICE:** If you need to travel, always let your doctor know. Do what's important to you, but adjust where you can and let whoever you're with know what you need.

* Scott M. *(Metastatic Colon cancer to the Prostate & Pancreas)*

Traveling can be difficult with medications, because so many of the medications I'm on are narcotics. The prescriptions are for only a 30-day supply and they'll only be re-filled, if I'm within two or three days from the end of the 30-days. So, I haven't done a ton of traveling, since I've been diagnosed. But, I did a lot of traveling in my Air Force life, as well as, in my civilian job, when I traveled around the country.

> **ADVICE:** Check with your doctor, if you have plans to travel. You may have to keep it short, if you're on narcotics, given the strict rules about prescribing them.

* Sondra W. *(Ovarian cancer 3x)*

Fortunately, before I started treatment, I was able to travel a bit with Kenneth. Of course, after treatment started, where I went to was actually determined by how fast I could get to the ladies' room. So, if it was someplace where there was going to be a long line, then I would not go there because it just wouldn't work for me. I also had to consider how my body would manage the travel time and conditions.

As I'm getting stronger now, I'm thinking of going on some short trips, like going back to Yosemite and places like that. I'll figure out how to make that work. I might start with an even shorter trip than that. We do get over to the beach and to the coast, and that's really nice. I really enjoy that. Now, we're trying to see how I can manage a little bit longer travel and work through that.

> **ADVICE:** If your condition requires you to be close to the restroom, you'll need to consider the logistics and how long it would take for you to get to your destination. You'll also need to consider how your body will manage travel conditions. Do get approval from your doctor before you go.

* Susan M. *(Ovarian cancer, Metastatic Pancreatic cancer to the Lungs)*

Ovarian Cancer: Although my treatment schedule was for six chemo sessions, we took a short trip to Maui after my fifth chemo treatment. Of course, I informed my doctor and I was very careful. I had a wonderful time!

* Vida B.A. *(Breast cancer)*

After the completion of my chemo and radiation treatments, I travelled to New Zealand to celebrate. It was perfect timing, because I actually booked the trip one year prior; even before I knew that I had cancer. So it came in handy.

Since I had lymphedema in my left arm and I knew that the cabin pressure on the flight to New Zealand would cause my arm to swell, I bought a compression sleeve to wear on the plane. The purpose was to apply pressure on my arm to prevent lymphatic fluid from building up. Unfortunately, my arm swelled up as the plane was making its steep climb up to cruising altitude. It was so painful. So I ended up removing it, which was a relief. For the rest of the flight, I tried to relax my swollen arm and lightly massage it.

> **ADVICE:** If you have lymphedema and you have to travel by airplane to your destination, let your doctor know so that you can get instructions on what to do when your lymphedema kicks in during the flight. Compression sleeves (for the arms) are necessary to prevent lymphatic fluid from building up. Ask your doctor what to do if your lymphedema acts up and you don't have a compression garment.

* Yesi L. *(Breast cancer: triple positive)*

I love traveling. But, definitely, the cancer treatments changed a lot of my travel plans. In fact, when my husband won a trip to Hawaii from his company, we didn't go. It was a good thing we didn't go, because that was the weekend I ended up hospitalized for Neutropenic Fever. My doctor told me "I won't allow you to travel, because if you do, you're going to be traveling with practically no immune system." I just thought of all the passengers in the airplane and the airports and told myself that Hawaii was always going to be there. So, we didn't go then, but we did eventually go afterwards.

> **ADVICE:** If your doctor says you're not allowed to travel, listen to your doctor, even if the trip is free. Your life is far more important. You can travel after your treatment is done.

* Aaron C. *(Prostate cancer, Skin cancer)*

When I returned home from surgery, I just walked slowly around the house, holding the banister and furniture nearby when I had to. Three months after surgery, when I returned to working out at the gym, I also made a point of walking around the block. Walking is important, because it improves blood flow and also speeds wound healing.

ADVICE: After surgery, it's really important to move your body, so you can get your blood circulation going to promote healing and grow stronger. Walking is a great way to do that, because you don't have to move fast. Just walk, even if it's slow. And hold on to something to support you and keep you steady when you do.

* Amor T. *(Breast cancer, Ovarian cancer)*

I tried to walk as much as I could. At first, I walked slowly around the house, clinging to the furniture and hugging the walls for stability. Then, when I felt stronger, I walked outside with Bill's encourage and support. The only difference between my post-mastectomy/breast reconstruction surgery and post-chemotherapy walks was that, during the latter, neuropathy affected my feet, causing me to lose the feeling of my feet on the ground. It was really unnerving. Also, the strong chemo drugs in my system created a lot of angst for me and I was fatigued much of the time. When I did have the energy to walk, I'm so thankful that Bill was there to support and encourage me. Having him by my side made a huge difference in my recovery.

ADVICE: Walking after surgery is one of the most important things you can do after having a procedure. It may seem like a simple thing, but a quick walk every hour or two, even if it's around your room, around your apartment or house, can help prevent serious complications. Walking is a gentle way to return to physical activity and can help promote a return to regular activities.

* Cindy L. *(Kidney cancer)*

The biggest prevention of blood clots and post-surgery complications is walking. So, I walked as much as my body would allow me to after surgery. Initially, it was hard for me to get in and out of the car or to walk around a store very much. But I had to do it more and more to gain strength. I didn't have use a walker or a cane. I just walked very, very slowly.

Walking also helped me cope with my anxiety. I went for walks and changed whatever activity I was doing when I got anxious to try something else, like getting back out to nature, going for walks on the beach or taking pictures. I physically changed the activity I was doing. That helped me with my anxiety.

When I got down in the dump, feeling sorry for myself, thinking – "Why me? Why did this happen to me?" and realizing, "Well, it just did and lying down in the dump isn't going to change it." – I would go out for a walk and it would take me right out of that kind of thinking. Also, when I walked around, like through Walmart or wherever I saw people much worse off than myself, I would get that reality check and straighten that little self-pity attitude for me. I always tell my kids, "When you feel sorry for yourself; when you think you got life bad, take a look around you. Because there's always somebody there much worse off than you are."

ADVICE: You need to walk in order to get your body to heal. Start slow or very very slow, if necessary. The main thing is to start walking. Walking gets your guts moving again and it's really good for you. "A body in motion stays in motion."

Walking is a great way to release your negative feelings of anxiety and self-pity. Not only will it lift up your spirits or distract you from feeling down, it will also help you realize, when you look around at people much worse off than you are, that you still have it a lot better than many others.

* Cindy R. (*Metastatic Breast cancer to the Stomach*)

During my breast cancer treatment, I tried to walk with my dogs (different from the ones I have now), but when I couldn't, my aunt would come over and help me walk them. She lived right around the corner from me. So, we were able to just walk around the block a couple of times, which was really nice.

Unfortunately, that changed when I had the car accident. Now, because of physical limitations, I walk on my treadmill at home.

ADVICE: You have to exercise to heal and become stronger. Walking is one of the best and easiest forms of exercise. You don't have to walk fast. Walk slow, if necessary. Just walk. It's really important and really good for you too.

* Glenn M. (*Metastatic Colon cancer to the Liver, Lungs & Adrenal Glands*)

Walking, for me, is a gauge of how I feel. In the winter, or if it's lousy weather, I'd suit up in rain gear if I felt okay. But the dogs didn't have rain gear and after their walk, they'd mess up the car. So, you know, it's a lot of work. I know I don't do it as much as I should. I'll try harder.

ADVICE: I think walking is good for everything, if you can do it. And I see people who are obviously in pain doing it, but they're muscling through. So I feel like a wimp, if I can't muscle through.

* J.B. (*Salivary gland cancer*)

I'd say I walked about an hour every day. That's probably because I had to go to a lot of classes at school. In between classes, I also walked back and forth to the library. Typically, I walked around three miles a day. I also drank plenty of water and carried my water and protein drink with me wherever I went.

* Rev. Linda S. (*Pancreatic cancer 3x*)

I have no problems walking per se. But, I have to be careful about my rambunctious puppy tripping me. Being told that a high risk factor for Pancreatic Cancer is a sedentary lifestyle is driving me to tell everyone, "If you aren't doing so, get off your tushes and MOVE for at least 30 minutes a day." Conscious of what the doctor told me, I try to walk and move and be active, even while I'm going through treatment. Nevertheless, there are days when my body is fatigued and tells me to rest....and I listen.

During chemo week, I can barely walk around the house. Although I can drive, I find it hard walking from the parking lots to medical buildings and stores. Now having gone through so much chemotherapy, which has undoubtedly caused me terrible joint pain, I was able to get a permanent disabled driver placard. Now, I can park closer to building entrances, especially when my joints ache.

ADVICE: It is really critical to your health that you be active and WALK, for at least 30 minutes a day, even if slowly. Do apply for a temporary or permanent disabled placard with the DMV, if you have difficulty walking from your car to the stores, hospitals, etc.

* Rachel S. (*Breast cancer: triple negative*)

During treatment, I was too fatigued to walk. My shortness of breath would get to me. When I returned to work, they made a special parking spot for me, so I didn't have to walk that far. After that, the bone pain was too intense, it just hurt. So, unfortunately, I didn't walk that much.

* Rick S. (*CLL: Blood & Bone Marrow cancer*)

Whenever I felt bad, I'd try to walk around the block. And if I felt really bad, then I'd walk around the block twice just to show my body that I "ain't gonna give up"!

* Scott M. *(Metastatic Colon cancer to the Prostate & Pancreas)*

I feared that I would walk too far and my feet would start hurting. Now I'm a mile and a half from home and because of my feet, I'm in so much pain. So, I bought a treadmill. I could walk as far as I want and once my feet start hurting, I'm already home. So, I walk on a treadmill.

> **ADVICE:** Walking is one of the best things you can do for yourself. Just get out and walk, if you can, even if you have neuropathy. You can still go a little bit and come back. If you have the same fear I have, get a treadmill.

* Sondra W. *(Ovarian cancer 3x)*

I'm going to get back into walking. I have to get some new shoes as my feet have changed. When I had really bad neuropathy, I got some really good shoes that had comfortable inserts. Unfortunately, they're not working now, so I'm going to get a new pair of shoes. I'm also going to get a nice walking stick; it doesn't have to be a cane. There are a lot of nice walking sticks out there to choose from.

> **ADVICE:** Walking is a really important physical activity that will help strengthen your body. Start slow and go very short distances if you have to, but just start. When you get stronger, increase the distance. Get a good pair of walking shoes and a nice walking stick (or cane) for balance.

* Susan M. *(Ovarian cancer, Metastatic Pancreatic cancer to the Lungs)*

I did a lot of walking while trying to recover from both my cancers. I really believe that walking contributes to faster healing.

* Vida B.A. *(Breast cancer)*

During treatment, if I had energy, I walked as much as I could. I knew that walking was a really important part of my healing process.

> **ADVICE:** After chemotherapy, you're likely to get side effects like fatigue and nausea. This is because the toxic chemo drugs in your body are working with your immune system to kill the cancer cells. Walking is an easy exercise to keep your body moving to help boost your immune system, so try to walk as much as you can.

* Yesi L. *(Breast cancer: triple positive)*

Right after my chemo infusions, I felt like a defenseless little baby. I took baby steps. So, my best friend gave me a little turtle, because she said I took "turtle steps". Yes. Turtle steps. I took one step at a time and got to where I wanted to go, eventually. Patience was definitely needed. I cannot emphasize patience enough.

> **ADVICE:** If you have a hard time walking or walk slow, be patient with yourself. You'll get to where you need to go, eventually. Be good to yourself. Be patient.

WORK (YOUR JOB)

---

* Aaron C. *(Prostate cancer, Skin cancer)*

Since my job required a lot of travel and dealings with people, I knew I had to put it on hold while I went through surgery and treatment. I cancelled a whole bunch of appointments and told all my clients that I was not going to be available to monitor anything for two or three months. Of course, after treatment, I returned to work.

* *Amor T.* (*Breast cancer, Ovarian cancer*)

I wasn't employed during both cancer journeys. However ... having worked in human resources management for over 20 years, I'd like to provide some tips on how to work with your employer, what options you have, as well as, what your rights (in the United States) are.

ADVICE:

FEDERAL LAWS that PROTECT YOU:
1. ADA (Americans with Disabilities Act) of 1990 with its amendment, ADAAA (Americans with Disabilities Amendments Act) of 2008 ...... applies to employers with 15 or more employees 2. FMLA (Family Medical Leave Act) of 1993 ....applies to employers with 50 or more employees
• According to the ADA, individuals with disabilities include those who have impairments that substantially limit a major life activity, have a record (or history) of a substantially limiting impairment, or are regarded as having a disability.
• As a result of changes made by the ADAAA, people who <u>currently have cancer, or have cancer that is in remission, have a disability</u> under the ADA's definition of disability because they are substantially limited in the major life activity of normal cell growth or would be so limited if cancer currently in remission was to recur. <u>https://www.eeoc.gov/laws/types/cancer.cfm</u>
• Given the above, your employer cannot discriminate against you for having cancer, going through active cancer treatment or taking time off for follow-up appointments. For appointments, it helps to have proof of your appointments, if not your schedule..
• When your cancer is in remission and you're needing to take time off to deal with delayed or permanent treatment side effects that keep you from performing your job, e.g. lymphedema, osteoporosis, etc. your employer cannot discriminate against you.
• If you're going through active cancer treatment and want to continue working, they must provide with you with <u>reasonable accommodations</u>. A reasonable accommodation is a modification to a job, work environment or the way work is performed that allows an individual with a disability to apply for a job, perform the essential functions of the job, and enjoy equal access to benefits available to other individuals in the workplace.
3. Discuss your request with your manager and human resources (HR), who should provide you with the documentation that you and your treating physician need to complete. Your doctor must identify the specifics on what you can and cannot do, as it relates to your work. From that, HR and your manager will determine what the company can accommodate and what they need to do to accommodate you, e.g. adjust schedules, purchase a special ergonomic chair, etc. If your employer can prove that your request for accommodation poses an undue hardship for the business, then they don't have to accommodate you. <u>Note:</u> This rarely happens.

Work During Treatment

If you decide to work through treatment, first let your doctor know so that he or she may be able to schedule treatments around your working hours or give you suggestions on how to deal with work stress while in treatment. Also, ask your doctor about possible treatment side effects that could affect your daily routine, e.g. nausea, fatigue, chemo brain, etc. and ask for guidelines on how to manage them.

If you're experiencing chemo brain or other treatment-related cognitive problem, e.g. memory loss and lack of concentration, try keeping a work journal to do the following:

- Record meetings and appointments on paper with time and date, who the appointment was with, and what was discussed. You can keep track of work meetings and doctor's appointments;
- Jot down important conversations. Make notes that include ideas you want to remember and decisions made during the conversation. If you have regular meetings at work, bring your journal for note-taking.
- Track deadlines. List when things are due, and keep a timeline of goals met along the way.
- Make a to-do list and add to it each time you think of something new. Check off items as you complete them.
- Set realistic goals for tasks to be completed. Try to stick to your goals as much as you can..
- Keep a written schedule to help you remember your work days and days off.

Telling Your Boss and Co-Workers

Sharing news of your illness depends on you how you feel. You can keep it private or you can share it with your co-workers. Do what feels right for you; whatever makes you comfortable.

If you notice your energy waning and your co-workers noticed that you haven't been "yourself," you may want to inform them, or at least your supervisor and/or a trusted select few. Not informing others means they will expect you to perform your job as usual, without regard to your health condition.

When you share your health condition with others, discuss it in a comfortable and private area. Don't be afraid to ask for their help and understanding, for some flexibility in your schedule and support in some projects. Assure them of your commitment to your job and that you will do your best to get well. In the meantime, prepare them for possible changes in your appearance, e.g. hair loss, weight loss, etc.

Plan on talking with your supervisor or co-workers about what needs to be done with your workload when you go on leave. This will make it easier for them, as well as, for yourself when you return. One of your co-workers could even act as a "go-to" person, answering questions or making decisions for you in your absence. Provide them with a "cheat-sheet" of information to refer to, e.g. passwords, codes, location of files, projects you're working on, contact list, etc.

Now, if you're not comfortable talking with your co-workers, inform your supervisor and HR. If you wish, you can ask them to keep your having cancer private; your co-workers do not need to know specifics. Make sure you complete all the necessary paperwork and establish regular communications and updates with your supervisor and HR, as much as you're able.

Taking Time Off from Work

If you decide to take time off from work to concentrate on your cancer treatment, inform your human resources (HR) representative who should provide you with the FMLA paperwork that you and your doctor need to complete. They should also walk you through your rights, responsibility, the timeline you need to work with and your options.

FMLA allows you to take up to twelve (12) weeks of unpaid leave (continuously or intermittently) to take care of your serious health condition while keeping any benefits you may have (vacation leave, sick leave, PTO "paid time off", ESL "extended sick leave", or seniority) and maintaining your position with the company. To be eligible for FMLA, you should have worked at least 12 months and a minimum of 1,250 hours at the company in those 12 months..

Since you won't be earning regular income for hours worked, you can draw from different sources. For example:

- Any vacation leave, PTO "paid time off", sick leave or ESL "extended sick leave" benefits that you have accrued. Your paycheck should reflect how many days/hours you have accrued to date. If not, have HR or Payroll provide you with the numbers.
- State short-term disability programs (California, Hawaii, New Jersey, New York, and Rhode Island only) that provide you with a percentage of your income in the event of an injury or illness covering three to six months.
- Employer-sponsored short-term disability program. Check with your HR representative.
- Employer-sponsored long-term disability program. Check with your HR representative.

Returning to Work

Deciding on when and how to return to work will bring about a lot of questions. I suggest gradually easing your way back. Work part-time and/or shorter hours. You will want to pace yourself, so your body and mind can adjust in order to avoid getting overwhelmed. Remember that, with cancer treatment, your body just took a brutal beating and is different from the body and mind you had before treatment.

After you make your decision, discuss it with HR and your supervisor. If you need to work full-time in order to be keep your health insurance, ask about taking rest breaks throughout the day, keeping in mind that this is a gradual re-entry into your work environment.

Sometimes, no matter what, returning to work is harder to adjust to than earlier thought. To make your transition easier, make your workspace a little more comfortable. You could:

- Listen to soft, relaxing music. Classical piano is a favorite.
- If you have a personal cubicle or an office, hang some inspirational pictures or quotations.
- Bring in live plants to give a "homey" feel. Some great, easy-to-care-for office plants are: Peace Lily, English Ivy, Spider Plant, Chinese Ivory and Gerber Daisy.
- Decorate your work space with pictures of family and friends.
- Try relaxation techniques such as meditation, mindfulness, taking slow, deep breaths, etc.

Legal Assistance

- If you feel it necessary to seek legal assistance, you'll need an attorney that specializes in employment law and has experience working with people who have had cancer.
- If you cannot afford legal fees, there are non-profit organizations that provide pro bono legal assistance. Check out your county's legal aid or legal services office for contact information. .

A Few Legal Information Websites

- Cancer Horizons: https://www.cancerhorizons.com/free-stuff/legal-assistance/
- Probono.net: https://www.probono.net/oppsguide/organization.66518-Legal_Information_Network_for_Cancer
- Cancer Legal Resources Center: https://thedrlc.org/cancer/
- National Coalition for Cancer Survivorship: https://www.canceradvocacy.org/news/new-website-helps-national-cancer-community-locate-free-legal-assistance/
- CancerCare.org: https://www.cancercare.org/tagged/legal_assistance

There are many similar websites and resources for free legal aid. Just google "free legal aid for cancer patients" and watch what pops up!

* Bob G. (Soft Tissue Sarcoma, Skin cancer)

I continued working while I was going through my cancer treatment. Eventually, I gave up the office because I wasn't quite feeling up to par. I was just losing energy. Still, I did the swimming; I just scaled back....adjusted as necessary. I scaled back some more, lessened my work hours and my efforts and gradually phased myself out. I didn't even try to sell anything. I went with the flow, especially during treatment. The funny thing is I make more money now just sitting back than when I did the real estate business. When you get old, you have to be careful; not take risks. You can afford not to have a whole lot of money, but you can't afford to lose what you have.

* Cindy L. (Kidney cancer)

I resigned my nursing position at the place where I worked and started my website. I was offered a fun job as a nurse at a pediatric office, but unfortunately, the commute was too long and the pay wasn't enough. So, I had to decline the offer.

ADVICE: If you have a job during the time of your diagnosis, you'll need to consider a lot of things. Top priority should be your health. Give yourself time to process your diagnosis and treatment, before you make any decisions. The main thing is to make sure your job does not get in the way of your health.

* Cindy R. (Metastatic Breast cancer to the Stomach)

I was an underwriter in a mortgage company before I was first diagnosed with cancer. When I had breast cancer, I ended up taking medical leave for nine months to cover my treatment period. I was blessed, because my company told me, "Do what you need to do. You just get well." From the beginning, my doctor informed me that I was going to get four treatments of this and four treatments of that and then the radiation. So it was pretty straightforward. Once I was approved, it was done. When I returned to work after treatment, they put me right back to work as usual.

ADVICE: Just let your company know how much time you need off and make sure to provide them with your paperwork from your doctor to support your request for time off. It shouldn't be a problem and they should accommodate you. This is your time to focus on your health; not on your job.

* Glenn M. (Metastatic Colon cancer to the Liver, Lungs & Adrenal Glands)

I owned my own business and basically did a 180 from being interested and focused and concentrating on work efforts to being completely away from the business and focused on my health and treatment.

Before my diagnosis, I was the one double-checking my employees' work. After my diagnosis, I just lost interest and wasn't very passionate about the work anymore. It was a challenge to do invoices and focus on work when I was foggy in the head. Extra communication was needed, and for a change, someone actually had to double-check my work. It took extra effort on the part of my employees to adjust to my change in disposition. Fortunately, I was able to sell my business and retire. Now, I can really focus on my health.

ADVICE: If you're the boss, have meetings and delegate. Communication is super important too. And, if you can, retire.

* Hilda K. (Colon cancer)

As soon as I was told that I had colon cancer and was scheduled for immediate surgery, I informed my manager and office mates. I had given it careful thought. I thought of how people at work have demands and how those demands cannot be controlled. I reminded myself of how I had been working a lot of hours, how committed I had been and how I refused to be stressed out by anything. My health takes priority over my job.

So, I told them that I was going to be out and that I was going to take a whole year off. At that point, I also told them that I saw no reason for me to come back to work. However, I reassured them that I was going to keep them up-to-date.

* *Jacki S.* (Breast cancer)

I work part-time in two jobs. One job is as an ice skating instructor at the Ice Arena and the other job is at our local Elementary School, where I'm a chaperone and yard supervisor in the morning, with a stop sign. I didn't have to worry about job security. Everybody at the Ice Arena and the school knew what I was going through and I never had to ask for time off, other than the day of the surgery and two days afterward for rest and recovery. I went back to work, as usual, and made it through.

Throughout treatment, I still took care of getting my 12 year old daughter up and ready for school. I also made her breakfast and drove her to the bus stop to go to her middle school. Then, I continued my routine, which was based on a schedule I coordinated between my job as an ice-skating instructor and my radiation and chemotherapy appointments. There were times when I had to give lessons on the days I had my radiation treatment. I didn't have any side effects or anything. So, I went on with my regular day.

* *Rachel S.* (Breast cancer: triple negative)

At work, I was extremely open with my boss and with human resources (HR). Some people might say that I was too open about it, but I believe in being very open, because I think that it imparts a lot more compassion for what you're going through. With that, they were extremely accommodating to me. They made a parking spot, very close to the building for me. I could pick out whichever spot I wanted. They put a sign out there, so no one else could park there, except me.

It wasn't handicapped parking; it was specialized parking. And even if I had a handicapped placard from the doctor (you can get a handicapped placard when you're going through treatment), I didn't want to use it, in case somebody else needed the space. My specialized parking spot was a little bit farther than the handicapped, obviously, but it was so much closer than the rest. During my breaks, I would go out to the car and take naps, trying to get through the day.

My company did not have a "work-from-home" policy. However, because I was very open with them and I was very trustworthy, they adopted a "work-from-home" policy for me. So, if I couldn't go into work, I would just email my boss, "I'm not going to be able to make it in today, but I am working from home." I logged everything I did, so he knew. And, if I didn't feel like working, I would just let him know: "I don't feel like working today." And, they were completely okay with that.

Each time I had a doctor's appointment, I'd give work an update from the appointment. I'd show it to my boss and I'd give a copy to HR. Even when I was on leave, I called them every couple of weeks to update them on what was happening.

Also, HR explained to me, "You've got three months of FMLA [*Family Medical Leave Act*]" leave and they were literally marking it down by the hour. When I left for my doctor's appointment, they marked it down by the hour and deducted it from the three months FMLA leave I was allowed. They told me that my leave would run out by December 2nd and "once you run out of leave, you might not have a job. Or, if we let you keep your job, then you may be without benefits" ... all kinds of stuff. But, there wasn't anything I could do. I've worked there for 18½ years. If they were going to fire me, then fire me. It's not like I could do anything about it. Before December 2nd came, I got a letter from them saying, not only did they approve for me to continue with my job, they were also going to continue paying for my benefits, until I returned on January 3rd. They cited something about ADA [*Americans with Disabilities Act*] laws in regards to my keeping my job.

beyond what they're required to do by law. It is also important to know your legal rights; what laws cover you when you're out on disability leave. Check out the FMLA and the ADA laws.

* Scott M. (Metastatic Colon cancer to the Prostate & Pancreas)

I know some people can still work while going through treatment. When I was diagnosed with cancer, I was already retired from the Air Force and I decided to retire from my civilian job too. I went on disability and then long term disability. Then, once I was on social security disability for two years, I was placed on Medicare, even though I'm not yet 65 years old. They placed me on Medicare when I was 56 ... almost ten years early. And, it's been really good.

* Susan M. (Ovarian cancer, Metastatic Pancreatic cancer to the Lungs)

When I was diagnosed with ovarian cancer, I was working full-time and continued work, even during my chemo treatment period. My employer was very accommodating of my time off needs. My job was secure.

* Tet M. (Colon cancer 3x)

I was fortunate enough that the company I worked for had an exceptionally convenient work hour structure put in place shortly before I was diagnosed with cancer. The timing was impeccable. We would put in extra time from Monday through Thursday, which enabled us to leave early on Fridays. My weekly Chemo sessions fell perfectly into place on Friday afternoons, which gave me the weekend to deal with possible side effects.

ADVICE: Don't hesitate to ask your manager or Human Resources Department for contingency plans. You'd be surprised how some companies will go above and beyond to help you out, especially if they feel you're a huge asset to the company.

* Vida B.A. (Breast cancer)

I'm an artist and I design glass art. At the time of my diagnosis, I owned an art glass and interiors design business. Designing was therapeutic for me, but sometimes, it wore me out; it was a lot of work. So, after all my cancer treatments, I decided to close shop. I needed to get rid of the stress of owning a business, so I sold it to my ex-husband who's still my friend. The company bears his last name, so he's the perfect person to buy it.

ADVICE: Stress definitely contributes to cancer and also affects your immune system. You need to do everything you can to remove the stressors in your life. If your job stresses you out, it may no longer be the right job for you. Your health should take higher priority over your job.

* Yesi L. (Breast cancer: triple positive)

I was fortunate that I was not working when I was told I had cancer. So, I had the luxury to be able to stay home. However, there was a downside. Since I was used to working in a job and there was not enough at home to keep me busy, I fell into a depression.

ADVICE: If you have the luxury to be able to stay home, consider it. But, make sure you have something to keep yourself busy. Otherwise, you'll fall into a depression

~ 0 ~

RELATING WITH YOUR MEDICAL TEAM

Medical teams are comprised of different medical professionals who are members of their respective medical organizations. As they are in all other organizations, work cultures are varied in medical institutions. How each medical professional relates to their patients varies. You can say that success of the patient-medical professional relationship is based on the individuals concerned. However, much of it is truly based on the organization's work culture and how they practice (or not) the mission and values they espouse.

In this chapter, you will hear about the experiences we had relating with our respective medical teams: some excellent; some unfortunate. No matter what our experiences were, it is the wisdom borne from our them that we would like to share with you. Hopefully, it will help you have a positive and healthy relationship with your medical team.

----

* **Aaron C.** (*Prostate cancer, Skin cancer*)

My doctor had a nurse I could call anytime I had questions. Also, my doctor was good at calling me back when I needed to talk with him. We also communicated through the hospital's e-mail system. Whenever I emailed my doctor with questions, he always responded within two days. I also had nurses I could talk with and ask, "Hey, this is what's going on." And, they would tell me, "Oh, that's normal. Don't worry." Even when I was worried about the bit of blood in my urine, after surgery, they took time to look into it, asking, "Did you strain yourself at all?" I said, "Well I may have." Then, they said, "Okay, that's normal. You're still healing." So, they were good about reassuring me.

The only time I had a challenge with the medical team was when I was in the hospital. Unfortunately, for some reason, the hospital was overbooked and I didn't get a chance to sleep in a regular, private room. I was given a bed in the outpatient (or whatever it's called) area, like the recovery area they wheel you into after surgery. There was a lot of noise going on all night and the nurses kept me up with their chatter. So I said, "Can you guys turn the emergency alarms off here so I can sleep?" Then, I had the hardest time putting my clothes on when I got released from the hospital. Again, because they were overbooked, nobody was there initially to help me. They didn't even help me put my own pants back on and I couldn't even bend over to get my shoes on; the pain was so great, so I was like, "Hey, can somebody give me a hand here? I can't get my own shoes on." Finally, someone came to help. Yeah, I was miserable then.

Researching on my own was how I happened to find my doctors. During one of my researches, I found a guy who was a urologist in Arizona. He recommended the current doctor I now use. I remember him asking, "Have you gone to so and so in Riverside?" I said, "No, I never knew he was out there." He goes, "Yeah, this guy's a great surgeon." So I contacted and interviewed this doctor in Riverside and he ended up being the doctor who trained the other doctors on Robotic Prostatectomies, like the one he performed on me.

ADVICE: Open communications with your doctor and nurses. Don't be afraid to ask personal questions of your doctor, about sex, erections and all that kind of stuff. Your doctor has seen a lot of cases similar to yours and so would tell you. Before meeting your doctor, write down your questions so you don't forget to ask them. Ask questions like: "What is normal?" "What isn't normal?" And keep on asking questions throughout your treatment, so you know what's going on. Take notes, if it'll help you remember the doctor's answers to your questions. Research on your cancer and your options, so you're aware.

Also, research doctors you'd want to work with. Don't settle. As much as possible, you want the best doctors and surgeons working to take care of you. You won't know until you ask around.

Your medical team also needs to know when you need help, especially when they've got other patients to take care of too. Ask when you have questions. Express your concerns when you have them. Let them know what you need when you need it, so they can properly attend to you.

* *Amor T.* (Breast cancer, Ovarian cancer)

Breast cancer: Because I believe that having a healthy, open and respectful relationship with my doctors and the rest of my medical team (including the receptionists, technicians, hospital aides, etc.) is critical to the success of my treatment. I made it a point to engage with them and be assertive, yet flexible, whenever I needed information and assistance. I researched the background and experiences of the doctors and surgeons who treated me. I was very keen on how they engaged with me themselves. Were they dismissive and robotic or were they down-to-earth and honest with me? For me, trust is of critical importance in a patient-doctor relationship. My life is in his or her hands and I must be comfortable in their care. Otherwise, I look elsewhere.

One night in the wee hours of the morning (around 2am, I think), I was alone in my hospital room, connected to seemingly "everything" there was to be connected to in that room. I couldn't sleep and thought of my physical circumstances. I felt awful and didn't feel like watching TV, much less read a book; I didn't really have many options as I was very restricted in movements. All I had to occupy my mind was ... my mind! Okay, so I could daydream. Well, I actually didn't feel like daydreaming. At that time, I was in a bit of a loss. So, I prayed, which does give me peace and makes me happy. Next thing I knew, someone (a nurse or a phlebotomist) quietly came in to take my blood for testing. He quickly introduced himself and told me that he was going to draw some of my blood for testing. I said, "ok" and then proceeded to ask him questions, like "How long have you worked here?" "What's your ethnic background?" "What made you decide to be a phlebotomist?" "Are you single or married?" "Do you have any pets?""What is the name of your pet?" "How many siblings do you have?" etc.

I found that I enjoyed my short conversation with that phlebotomist. There was a positive energy that I had created. I realized that although I didn't have control over my physical circumstances, I actually had control over my spirit. I can create positive energy by engaging with others, so as much as I was able (like if I was awake enough), I engaged with everyone who came into my room. I asked them their name, what they were doing, what medication they were giving me, purpose, side effects, how long they worked at the hospital, were they single of married, any pets, pet's name/s, siblings, their names, parent's names, where they came from, what hobbies they had, what they enjoyed doing for leisure, etc. etc.

After I got to know everyone who came into my room, I no longer felt like I was in a cold hospital room, being cared for by strangers. Knowing everyone's names (even though I would sometimes forget) made my stay more comfortable and even pleasant. If the hospital employee initially came in to see me, all formal or without a smile, that all changed after we got to know each other's personal backgrounds. There were things we shared in common that we wouldn't have learned about had I not asked. I enjoyed joking with them too. My medical team became like "family" to me while I was there. We had developed a rapport; a wonderful energy that I know contributed to my strength and ability to recover.

Ovarian cancer: I couldn't have asked for a better team of medical professionals than the doctors and oncology nurses who took care of me when I was going through my ovarian cancer experience. Even the admin staff and the volunteers were wonderful and very receptive to my needs. I made it a point to know everyone's name, as much as possible, and develop a healthy rapport with them. In return, every time I visited the Cancer Center, whether for appointment, treatment or just to visit, they treated me like I was family and took really good care of me.

I felt very comfortable to ask questions and express myself. Their expressions of love, giving heartfelt hugs to those of us who needed it, sure went a very long way. I really believe that their abundance of positive energy and genuine desire to help patients like me fight cancer contributed to my healing and strength.

* Bob G. *(Soft Tissue Sarcoma, Skin cancer)*

When I saw the surgeon, I could tell something was wrong. By the look in his eyes, I could tell that I wasn't out of it; something was still wrong. But he and the other doctors weren't telling me. Nobody ever told me that I had cancer. But, the way they described what they were going to do, I had a strong feeling that it was cancer. One day, going to the hospital, I told my wife, "They haven't told me what it is, but I'm going to have surgery and I just want you all to be prepared, because it's real bad.....very bad." But, the doctors then never officially told me. I guess everyone thought that someone else told me.

I was doing fine going around the hospital and reached a glass door with a sign that said "Tumor Institute". I told the medical staff there, "You should be ashamed, calling it the "Tumor Institute." When they asked, "Why?" I said, "Well, all these people coming in, they're afraid they're going to die when they come here." Then they asked, "What would you call it?" And, I said, "The House of Love. Yeah, call it, The House of Love." Unfortunately, they didn't get a chance to change that name because the hospital was bought out.

The doctors in the Radiation department were all UC doctors. My doctor was one of them and was very, very good. One time, they had a visiting lady doctor from Israel and one of the doctors pointed to me and said, "He's been rearranged!" When they asked me where things were, I just said "I don't know, but they still work!" At that hospital, we had a good relationship.

Unfortunately, I had a couple of bad experiences with the medical team at another hospital. The first incident was regarding the nurses who brought me painkillers. Whenever I saw the bottle, I asked them, "What's in that little bottle?" They would take out two white pills and say, "They're painkillers." I told them that I didn't need them. I have no pain. But, they insisted that the doctor said I had to take them. So, I said, "Well then, give them to the doctor. I'm not going to take the painkillers." When they still argued, I said, "Don't argue. The message I'm getting is, you want to give me pain pills, so I will have pain for the doctor?" After that, they stopped bringing the painkillers to me. Interestingly, the same thing happened when I went to rehab. They wanted to give me painkillers. I have a high threshold for pain and really don't need painkillers.

The second incident also happened during my stay at that hospital. I was hooked up to a machine with the IV going through that had a cocktail of drugs, which included morphine. So, I had no choice; I had to take it. One time, my early morning nurse didn't show at 4:00am and the IV meds went dry. That was my sustenance, my medicine....all in one. So then, I made a lot of noise. Another nurse ran in and said, "This is not my station, but I'm going to take care of you." And I said to her, "I don't want to see that nurse who was assigned to take care of me ever again! I could've died! I don't want to ever see her again!"

* Cindy L. (Kidney cancer)

Since I'm a registered nurse, I can easily talk with doctors and the rest of my medical team. I'm direct in asking them questions and letting them know what I need. I think it's really important to have that open communication, including challenging them if I don't agree. That's because I need to be informed and understand what's going on. So, a whole eight months went by since this thing grew and the first radiologist said, "Don't worry about it." Even though I am one, I often wonder how many people just listen to medical professionals and don't know to question the stuff.

One of my nurses was a male nurse who would visit and watch Christmas movies with me. He was wonderful company and attended to my needs. After my surgery, I couldn't stomach much. One day, when he saw that I was so hungry, but just couldn't get myself to eat any of the food that was brought to me on the tray, he said, "I want to know what sounds good to you." I said, "Vanilla pudding." And, he said, "You got it!" Then he went out to get vanilla pudding for me. He kept me in supply of vanilla pudding the whole time I was there, because I could eat it. He modeled what all nurses should do, which is: Relate to your patients and find out what they need. It's so important for the patient's state of mind and healing process.

> **ADVICE:** Create an open and honest relationship with your medical team by communicating with them. Ask them questions and let them know of your concerns, if any. When you tell them what you need, you actually give them the opportunity to take better care of you.

* Cindy R. (Metastatic Breast cancer to the Stomach)

I have a wonderful doctor and medical team. The first time around, they gave me a huge binder containing information about financial aid and how to deal with all the different things that are going to come up. Then they gave me the name and phone number of someone I could talk to, if I had questions or needed anything. That was very helpful. I think that how comfortable you feel during treatment will depend on how well your medical team takes care of you. Trusting them is huge in your getting your health back. I really felt that my medical team was on my side and they were going to help me beat cancer.

I was open in communicating with my doctors and nurses. I showed them my mind and told them that I wanted to know what was going on, how the treatment was going to affect me, etc. So, I kept an open dialogue. I would say something simple like, "Hey, what's going on?" For example, when my sister was getting married in Hawaii, I just told my doctor "Okay, look doctor, I need to go to Hawaii. So can you fix me and make sure that I'm okay while I'm over there?" So, he gave me enough medication to last for three weeks. And I told him, "Perfect! I'll send you a postcard!"

> **ADVICE:** When you meet your medical team (doctors, nurses, technicians, receptionists, etc.), make sure they're on your side. Make sure you're comfortable with your doctor and nurses. Make sure they're listening to you, understanding what YOU are going through. They should focus on your personal situation and not treat you like everyone else. Because, we're all different.

* Glenn M. (Metastatic Colon cancer to the Liver, Lungs & Adrenal Glands)

I have a great relationship with my doctors and my nurses. They really do a fantastic job to take care of me and all their patients. Because I engage with them and ask them questions and show them how much I appreciate them, our relationship is stronger.

> **ADVICE:** Ask questions and take notes when you meet with your doctors and nurses. Because of your condition, you may forget half of what they told you. So, it's good to write things down. Also, ask questions; don't be shy. Shy doesn't get you very far.

* Hilda K. (Colon cancer)

I was very fortunate to have a great medical team! I started with my head nurse who I happened to know personally. She was the mother of my daughter's best friend. Because I knew her and I knew that she, in her profession, would keep everything confidential, I confided in her and looked to her for guidance. Having her there, really helped me maneuver through this experience.

She told me what to expect, who I was going to see, who my surgeon was going to be and who my oncologist was going to be. Before my meeting with each of the doctors, I remember asking her what I should say to my doctors. She said, "Tell them that you are healthy and that you want them to be aggressive. Tell them that you want them to take your situation seriously." And so I did. I remember how my surgeon described how the colon is all twirled up, how there's the big and small colon and if you stretch it out straight, it will be so long that having half of it taken out wouldn't really make a difference. Basically, it's not a big deal. It was his way of saying, "Don't worry." He informed me that I had Colon Cancer and described the four stages to me...and I was at stage III. After he explained the procedure and everything to me, I told me, "All I can say is please be aggressive and don't hesitate to take extra out, because I don't want it to come back. So, take out as much as you want. And, if you find that it spread to other parts of my body, then while you're in there, take them out too! Take out the uterus...whatever you have to take out. Take it out, because I want to live and I want to see my children get old!" He was really nice and I felt a good connection with him. My oncologist was just as nice and knowledgeable.

I was given an opportunity to get a second opinion if I wanted it, but I chose not to, because I felt good about both doctors. I saw my medical team so much during my first six months of treatment and I could see that their hearts were in the right place; I didn't need to second guess them. My oncologist, especially, was very thorough. At the same time, I felt like she asked me the right questions, checked my whole body: my ankles, my toes, my fingers, etc. I am so lucky to have her. Since I've passed the five years since I was first diagnosed with Colon cancer, I now see her once a year. That's where I am now.

ADVICE: Having doctors you can trust and who make you feel comfortable is ideal. It's really important, no matter what, to communicate your thoughts and let them know what you need. Have them explain everything to you, so that you're aware of what to expect. When it comes to meeting with doctors you don't know, keep in mind that your input is going to affect how they interact with you. Stress to them your need to be taken seriously and why it's critical that they do everything they can to remove your cancer and get you on the road to recovery. Here are some pointers my head nurse and friend gave me that really helped:

1. Tell them that you are, otherwise, healthy and that you want them to be aggressive in removing your cancer.
2. Tell them that you want them to take your situation seriously.

* Jacki S. (Breast cancer)

My doctors at the hospital were excellent, except for the first doctor I saw about my cancer. I did not feel comfortable with him, because he just didn't seem personable. He was very serious about everything and suggested that I have a double mastectomy, even though I didn't really need it.

I ended up having a lumpectomy only on my right breast after I got a second opinion, at the advice of my friends. When I got the second opinion, the doctor I saw was actually the head of the department. He was wonderful! I found out that he's a fisherman, like my husband. He had children. He was very personable, asking me about my life and my family. I just felt really comfortable with this doctor. He took a look at the lump and said that he felt I could just go with the lumpectomy. He respectfully asked if that would be my choice and if I would be okay with that. And, I said, "Yes!"

Also, all the nurses and everybody that I worked with at the hospital were so amazing, especially the radiologist and my second doctor/surgeon. Everyone was so welcoming, helpful, personable and friendly. They put me at ease.

ADVICE: Your cancer treatment is serious and so you need to be with a doctor who you trust and who you are comfortable with. If you are not comfortable with your doctor, don't hesitate to get a second, or even, a third opinion. You are the patient that the doctors are supposed to support, not the other way around. And, if the doctor you're seeing just wants to force his opinion on you, then you should change doctors and go with one who respects you and your feelings.

* Joan S. (Rectal cancer)

During my chemo treatment period, I got really sick several times for different reasons. At one time, my friend Mary picked me up to take me to the hospital. By the time we arrived at the hospital, I could not walk. I just could not walk! When we got to my doctor's office there, we learned that he was on vacation and so we, instead, met with another doctor. That doctor, unfortunately, kind of blew me off. He told me to "go home for a few days." Well, I said to him, "You could send me home with every registered nurse in here, there's something wrong with me!" I was really adamant. So, he reconsidered and they admitted me into the hospital. They gave me a CT scan and, sure enough, I had a hernia in my rectal tract. The hernia had wrapped around my bowel system; I was unable to move my legs.

For the most part, I had a wonderful relationship with my medical team (except for that one doctor). My visiting nurse, Melissa, who took care of me for several months was amazing! I am very thankful for my medical team.

> **ADVICE:** Always get a second opinion, if you're not happy about your diagnosis or care. However, be careful. While you're asking for a second opinion and you're given a second opinion, don't put any of your doctors down, even if you're unhappy with them.

* J.B. (Salivary gland cancer)

I had a really good relationship with my doctors and nurses; I really appreciate what they did to support me. They were open to answering my many questions, whether online or in person, and they also tried to reassure and encourage me when I had doubts about my future. During treatment, their guidance, especially when it came to coping with my side effects (fatigue, loss of appetite, teeth changes and skin changes), really helped me stay strong and recover quickly.

In person, I communicated a lot with the nurses who conducted every treatment. I saw them every day and they were very nice to me. I didn't relate with the doctors in person as much. I communicated more with them online. My primary doctor, who was a Radiation Oncologist, just saw me very briefly (about 30 seconds) every week. He would just ask me how I was doing. If nothing was wrong, then nothing more followed.

* Rev. Linda S. (Pancreatic cancer 3x)

For two years, I had been going to a highly-rated and prestigious cancer center in St. Louis, Missouri for my first two rounds of treatment to battle pancreatic cancer. The doctors, nurses, technicians, aids, food service staff and receptionists were wonderful. My surgeon and his team were quite open and clear about the surgery procedure and expected outcome. Everyone answered my questions clearly, most of the time. Even when inevitable delays occurred, the medical team apologized and did what they could to make things better for me. Most of all, they were genuinely warm, compassionate, and caring. They felt like my friends, and I guess they were for that time.

Never once did I detect professional detachment, until ... I received a call from the hospital's radiation oncology department, saying they had "done all that they could for me and were now turning my total care over to my local oncologist." The caller then ended the phone conversation with, "Good luck!" Needless to say, that call was very unsettling. It seemed cold, routine, insensitive and dismissive; it pissed me off! I was both livid and hurt. The sloppy, insensitive way the the St. Louis team ended our relationship was the only negative incident I experienced.

> **ADVICE:** I hope it never happens to anyone. But if it does, do not hesitate to speak up! Push for more training rather than for disciplinary action. Sometimes, people in the medical field get into a rut and fail to feel empathy for the patient. Medical teams would benefit from being sensitive to how their words land on others.

* Rachel S. (Breast cancer: triple negative)

I don't know that I necessarily "related" to my medical team. I actually trusted my clinical trial nurse more than I trusted my doctor. And I don't even know if "trust" is the right word for it. I communicated better with her than I did with my doctor. I think it's more of just "don't be afraid to mention how you feel, even though you think it's weird, because it just might not be" kind of thing. There were a couple of times I brought something up, like the first time I was in radiation, and they kind of made me feel stupid for bringing it up. Because it was my first appointment, I said, "This is what I'm noticing" and they said, "Yeah, that should be happening; don't worry about it." I learned to just speak up and not worry about what they would think.

ADVICE: Just bring everything up, even if you don't know how to question them. Your speaking up might just be something important they wouldn't have known, if you didn't ask.

Have somebody with you to take notes for the important appointments. If it's for general check-ups, when it's pretty much going to be the same information as before, then I wouldn't bother bringing somebody, because then you'll just be wasting their time, which would make you feel bad. That's how I felt when I brought my sister with me a couple of times and nothing happened. All they did was check my heart rate and everything, but no additional information was given. So, just judge which ones are the important appointments and ask for help for those appointments only. It will make you feel better and a bit more in control.

* Rick S. (CLL: Blood & Bone Marrow cancer)

I related well to my medical team just fine. They were outstanding! We just kidded and joked around. That's very important. To have an outstanding team to be a part of. There, you, the patient, are a part of the team. You're not there to be the center of attention. You're the most valuable part of the team.

* Scott M. (Metastatic Colon cancer to the Prostate & Pancreas)

All I can say is that in seven years at the Cancer Center, I have yet to have a complaint. They have a lady on staff who is incredible. Early on, I got a PET scan and my insurance company refused to pay for it. When I told her about it, she said, "Oh, give me all the paperwork." Two months later, I received a check from my insurance company, refunding me the amount I had paid them. I realized this wonderful lady was fighting my battles for me. When I asked her, "Why do you do that?" She said, "Because we don't' want you guys to stress." How wonderful is that!

Then there was a time I had a blood infection. We were over the hill in Santa Cruz driving home, when it really kind of hit me hard. I called up the Cancer Center and told them I was coming in. I said, "I'm coming in, whether you have space for me or not. You can put me in the closet, but I need treatment; I need help." Well, the lady on the phone asked me, "Are you the guy who always says this is your '*spa day'?" I said, "Yes". And she said, "Yes, come right on in." By the time we got me there, I was completely slumped over, completely white as a sheet of paper. They wheeled me in and the nurses took one look at me and said, "Over here!" and right away, I had a team of four or five oncology nurses. I have a special place in my heart for all nurses; for all the care that they do. But, oncology nurses are a step above that. So many of who they deal with are in such critical, dire need of care. And, many of these oncology nurses are former ICU nurses, ER nurses or OR nurses and there's not a lot that phases them. And they know exactly what to do in time of emergency. They're very much pillars of strength. And now, I look forward to my chemo sessions. So, how messed up is that?

[*Note: I used to joke with the staff there that my chemo sessions were my "spa day", because where else can a guy go, be welcomed by beautiful women, put in a recliner, have warm blankets put over him and be cared for and have a food cart wheeled up to you.... I mean it was like a spa; it was great! And I'd get to nap and they didn't bug me. So, I would always walk in and say, "I'm here for my spa day!"]

ADVICE: Make yourself known to your nurses and the rest of the staff. Don't be quiet. Get to know them all, because there may be a time when you're going to have to do an unannounced drop in, like I did.

* Sondra W. (Ovarian cancer 3x)

I have a great relationship with my medical team. And, the way I did that is just by openly telling them how I was feeling, what things I was experiencing, asking the questions that I wanted to ask and getting information from them. They were really good in explaining anything that I didn't understand about the tests and talking about options.

ADVICE: Be proactive in communicating with your medical team. Don't hesitate to ask them questions or ask them to repeat their explanations or ask them to help you with anything, any information you need. They are there to make you comfortable and help you regain your health. I suggest keeping notes~ questions to ask and answers you receive. That way, you have a better chance of knowing and understanding what's going on and what to expect.

* *Susan M.* (Ovarian cancer, Metastatic Pancreatic cancer to the Lungs)

I received great care for both my ovarian cancer and pancreatic cancer experiences. It was easy to talk to all my doctors, nurses and technicians. During my 22-day stay in the hospital for the pancreatic cancer surgery, my nurses were outstanding. The lead nurses on the floor were always checking to make sure I was comfortable and when I did express concern, they were quick to act on them.

ADVICE: It's really important to have a positive relationship with those who care for you. It'll help make your experience a positive one from which you will benefit.

* *Tet M.* (Colon cancer 3x)

I'm very thankful for my medical team, from the doctors and nurses to the technicians. They treated me with kindness and respect and attended to my needs, as best they could.

ADVICE: I understand how debilitating cancer and its treatments can get. But, if there's one suggestion I can make, it's this: Talk to your health care providers with respect and friendliness. This starts with the hospital or medical office front desk all the way to the doctor or nurse who will treat you. They're aware of the discomfort or anxiety you're going through. So, let's not lose sight of the fact that they're human too. There's no guarantee, but chances are, it will be amazing how they will reciprocate the gesture.

* *Yesi L.* (Breast cancer: triple positive)

The medical team at the Cancer Center saved my life. I was completely open with them in my communications, no matter what. We discussed everything, e.g. my treatments, sex drive...everything. I felt absolutely no shame in communicating with them. I just thought that they weren't going to judge me and they were working with me to save my life. So, I was very open in my communications with them.

ADVICE: Be as open as possible in communicating with your medical team. Just think that they are there to save your life and you are not the only patient with questions or concerns, even about private subject matters. Think that they've probably heard the same questions or concerns a million times. So be open when you communicate with your medical team. It will really help you cope better.

~ 0 ~

Chapter 11

YOUR MEDICAL RECORDS

Practices vary when it comes to keeping medical records at home, especially since hospitals & doctors' offices should always keep record of your visits. When home medical records are kept, how they should be organized, what should be included, how much should be kept, etc. are all personal.

————————————————

* **Amor T.** (*Breast cancer, Ovarian cancer*)

I keep my home medical records as complete as possible. This includes my doctors reports, summaries of visit, prescriptions, lab results, imaging results, operative report, post-op reports, etc. Since there is so much information surrounding both my cancers and their respective treatments, I found it essential to keep as much information as I could. That way, I could access the information whenever I wanted to without having to wait for the doctor's office or hospitals to search for it and get back to me. I also learned that they actually don't always have all the information, especially when I had to change doctors and/or had several doctors working on my case.

Regarding patient electronic records kept by the hospitals or medical systems, I found that I couldn't depend on them too. I understand that electronic records are dependent on the person who enters them into the system, like what they believe is necessary to keep on record. Therefore, details that I may think are important are missed by the data entry persons who don't think they are. C'est la vie.

I have several big binders that hold all of my medical records. They contain lab results, imaging (PET scans, MRIs, CT scans, ultrasounds, DEXA scans, mammograms) results, all medical paperwork received from the doctors, reports, referrals, visit summaries, hospital stay information, instructions, calendars, authorizations, consents and other information like, description of treatment, surgical drain output record, etc.

I also keep a large binder that contains medical insurance and billing information. Keeping complete records here has, literally, saved me thousands of dollars!

ADVICE: As you may already know, navigating through treatment when you have cancer can be really confusing. Keeping strong records for yourself is key. You can follow my lead in creating binders for medical, insurance and billing records or you can gather whatever paperwork you have and file them chronologically in a folder or box. Whatever you choose to do, try to have a system that you will understand. Being able to retrieve the files you need in a timely manner will help you process information and, especially, challenge erroneous billing demands that may come your way.

* Cindy R. (*Metastatic Breast cancer to the Stomach*)

I have a wonderful doctor and medical team. The first time around, they gave me a huge binder containing information about financial aid and how to deal with all the different things that are going to come up. Then they gave me the name and phone number of someone I could talk to, if I had questions or needed anything. That was very helpful.

ADVICE: Since you'll be receiving a lot of medical statements, records, invoices and various other paperwork related to your condition and treatment, you really need to keep all your paperwork organized. Arrange your files, so you can find the information you need when you need it. It's also important to have someone you trust have access to your files and be able to work with you on them.

* Glenn M. (*Metastatic Colon cancer to the Liver, Lungs & Adrenal Glands*)

My medical records aren't organized and I know they should be. I wish I could've managed my medical records better.

ADVICE: Looking back, getting a two or three-inch binder to arrange your records chronologically would be best. To make it easy to find things, attach tabs on the documents. Use the same binder; don't deviate. My brother taught me that. Don't deviate. If this item lives here, it lives here. Don't move it. Don't move its domicile. Don't deviate. It's there, because you put it there for a reason. I've been gauging for a long time the quality of the day by how much time I spend looking for stuff I misplaced. And sometimes it's very aggravating because it's important stuff, like my medical records.

* Rev. Linda S. (*Pancreatic cancer 3x*)

I kept my medical records simple. Everything is in one file folder organized chronologically by date.

* Sondra W. (*Ovarian cancer 3x*)

I was informed by one of the volunteers at the Cancer Center that the American Cancer Society gives out free medical record organizer kits to cancer patients to help keep track of medical information and records. She said that I would need that organizer because I was going to have so much to keep track of. I told her, "Yes, I would like to have that." So, she arranged to have that sent to me. I now have my pre-diagnosis medical records in one file and my cancer treatment records in the organizer I got from the American Cancer Society. I separated them only because they're different systems.

ADVICE: It is really important to keep your cancer treatment medical records organized because there's so much that you'll have to track throughout your treatment period (and even after) like test results, medications, billings, etc. Contact the American Cancer Society to request the free Personal Health Manager they have for cancer patients. Their system is really helpful, so it would be a good idea to get one.

* Tet M. (*Colon cancer 3x*)

I have one file box that contains all my medical records from the beginning to present. I'm thinking of storing a second set of copies at a friend's house, in case of an emergency, when my records are needed and the doctor's office is closed.

ADVICE: It's good practice to organize your medical records, because there are times either you or your doctor will need to refer to them. Have a second copy made and stored at the place of a trusted family member or friend, in case of emergency.

* *Vida B.A.* (*Breast cancer*)

I have a file with all the medical records relating to my breast cancer treatment, including the test results, various reports and, even, the bills too. Any document I received from my doctors and the hospital, I placed them in that file. After every chemo infusion, they gave me a white folder with the updated information. I just wrote the dates on top of the folder and filed it with the rest of my medical records.

> **ADVICE:** Keep a copy of your medical records, including your bills and receipts. That way, you can keep track of your health and all the treatments and procedures you went through, including progress and expenses.

~ o ~

PART FOUR

Chapter 12

GOOD STUFF TO HELP GET YOU THROUGH

Amidst the difficult challenges in our respective cancer journeys, there was good stuff that raised our spirits and helped us cope. In this chapter, we share what inspired us, made us laugh, distracted us from our suffering, lifted us up and/or kept us strong. Although every cancer patient and survivor's journey is personal, the battle is shared; you are not alone! Yes, there are many times when the bad stuff seems overwhelming, but in reality, there is actually good stuff there too! We all just need help in finding them.

So read on, and see what good stuff helped us through our trials and tribulations. We hope that you will find some good material here that will point you in the direction of what personally raises your spirit and strengthens you, if not immediately lift you up!

THOUGHTS TO PONDER

★ **Amor T.** (*Breast cancer, Ovarian cancer*)

- "I choose to be thankful and focus on the positive, because doing so lifts my spirits and enables me to feel peace and be happy. I find absolutely no reason to focus on the negative, which does the opposite."
- "I may not be able to control my circumstances, but I can create my own positive energy to lift myself above them."
- "My trust and thankfulness are the portals through which I receive God's Peace."

★ **Bob G.** (*Soft Tissue Sarcoma, Skin cancer*)

- "I may never ever work again, but I will never retire!"
- "If it rains, you have to enjoy the rain! If it's foggy, you have to enjoy the fog!
- Because we don't have time to wait for the future!"
- "God's greatest gift to man is woman!"
- "There is no room in this world for both me and cancer!"

★ **Cindy L.** (*Kidney cancer*)

- "You'll never know how strong you are until strong is all you have."
- "Sure, you can't be happy 24/7. So, yes, go ahead and feel your sadness, frustration, anger, etc. Feel it, own it and then move on. Just don't unpack and live there."

- "The biggest prevention of blood clots and post-surgery complications is walking. It gets all your guts moving again and it's just good for you. A body in motion stays in motion."
- "Amazing how strength is drawn from depths you didn't know existed."
- "Don't take peeing for granted."

★ Cindy R. (*Metastatic Breast cancer to the Stomach*)

(On being told she had three months to live)

- "Well, it's not 100% guaranteed. Okay wait…I only have today really. Whether or not I have cancer, I have today. So what I'm going to do is make it good for me and make it good for others too, as much as I can!"
- "When you're given a serious diagnosis, ask yourself, 'What do I want to do? What have I always wanted to do?' And then, just do it, because life is short. It is. But, we can make it also just a BLAST! "

★ Glenn M. (*Metastatic Colon cancer to the Liver, Lungs & Adrenal Glands*)

- "Teach your kids how to take pills. It's very important, because medications they need when they become adults will, more often than not, come in solid form, e.g. pills, capsules, caplets or tablets. Some are large and hard to swallow. If your kids grow up to be adults and they're gaggers, then it will really affect their health tremendously if they can't get their pills down when they need to."
- "Learn to cough up phlegm. Boys are better at coughing up phlegm than girls who were taught that it's not lady-like. But, being able to eject phlegm when it accumulates in your throat is important to your health. If you don't, then the phlegm in your throat will accumulate and cause health issues."

★ Rev. Linda S. (*Pancreatic cancer 3x*)

- "And so I wait to see what is next. I'm not so great at waiting, but I am being reminded constantly that I control nothing about this process - nada."
- "I realize that I tend to focus more on death during chemo week and on life during the following week of recovery. And then, we start the cycle again."

★ Rachel S. (*Breast cancer: triple negative*)

- "When I asked "why me?" I would tell myself of others who have it worse and then would stop feeling sorry for myself. I began to want to help others, I began to thrive on the idea of helping others, I began to live for it. This made me stronger."
- "Everyone has a different road to take. Every diagnosis, every treatment, every side effect will not affect everyone in the same way. Don't compare yourself to others."
- "Learn to be comfortable with the "New you". Life will never be the same as it was before. And that's ok. You will come out stronger than you ever knew was possible!"
- "It's ok to ask for help. This was something that was very difficult for me. But, I learned that friends and family, and even strangers at times, want to help. You just have to let them know how."
- "Remember, the sickness, the pain is only temporary. A small blip in the page of your life. Before you know, that page will turn and this will all be a bad memory."
- "If I'm spending all my time stressing on how I look, that's what I'm going to worry about. Is my wig going sideways? I need to freshen up my make-up….. Why stress yourself out with that?"
- "People who go through cancer become part of a club no one ever wants to belong to. But, when they get into that club, they're met with nothing, but love and compassion."

★ **Sondra Williams** (*Ovarian cancer 3x*)

- "A huge lesson I also learned and that I want to make sure to pass on to every woman is this: "If you think that you may possibly have cancer, then you need to have the CA 125 blood marker test for ovarian cancer done. If necessary, insist on it. Also, get an ultrasound done too."
- "Feeling the outpouring of love and prayers for me is beautiful beyond words. It only goes to show that there is no place for cancer, where God and love are present."

★ **Susan M.** (*Ovarian cancer, Metastatic Pancreatic cancer to the Lungs*)

- "Having cancer is life-altering. It turns your life upside down. It is okay to have anxiety, to be scared or to cry. This is normal. But, remember FIRST to take care of yourself....before family and friends. The best way to heal is to put yourself FIRST. You can't take care of others, if you are not well. If people offer to help, i.e. cooking a meal, driving you to the doctor/appointments, visiting, taking you out....take it! "
- "Research your cancer. But, remember that too much research can be frustrating and depressing. Talk over your concerns with your doctor. I remember what my nurse advocate said: "Googling can be dangerous." Things can be taken out of context."
- "Today, I just want to thank God for the gift of life. No requests, no complains; just thankful to be alive."

★ **Tet M.** (*Colon cancer 3x*)

- "If you're a religious person, now would be a great time to double up on prayers. Next to prayers, laughter has been known to be the best medicine. Laugh your worries away!"
- "During the darkest times, there's always hope to pull you through. You'll realize that you have inner strength that you didn't know you had until your back is shoved against the wall."

★ **Vicda BA** (*Breast cancer*)

- #1. Having cancer is not something you should be embarrassed or ashamed about. When you inform your family and friends who love you, you'll enable them to support you and you'll all benefit from the experience.
- #2. Love makes everything more colorful. At the lowest point in your life, when everything looks black and white, love will add color to your life. If you emphasize love, it will make you so happy that your sickness will become secondary. The love you feel from those who care for you, support you and pray for you; that's love that is so strong and powerful. So, open yourself more to loving and being loved.
- #3. Forgive your past and those who hurt you. You have to get out of your system everything that is negative because they just cause you stress, which is what contributes to cancer. Just be positive and forgive, as much as you can. If you cannot forgive a person, just don't think about them at all. Just keep all the good thoughts, good energy and positivity.

★ **Yesi L.** (*Breast cancer: triple positive*)

- "Cancer and everything that goes with it does not define you. When you accept yourself for who you are, then those around you owill do the same."

SURVIVORS' COLLECTION OF QUOTES

★ **Amor T.** (*Breast cancer, Ovarian cancer*)

- "The good Lord gave you a body that can stand most anything. It's your mind you have to convince." ~ *Vince Lombardi*"

- If you must look back, do so forgivingly. If you must look forward, do so prayerfully. However, the wisest thing to do is to be present ... gratefully." ~ *Maya Angelou*"
- Be miserable. Or motivate yourself. Whatever has to be done, it's always your choice." *Wayne Dyer*
- "If you change the way you look at things, the things you look at change." *Wayne Dyer*
- "You can't let fear cripple you. It's harder being miserable than it is to be happy." ~ *Fatima Ali*
- "Life is not the way it's supposed to be. It is the way it is. The way you cope with it is what makes the difference." ~ *Virginia Satir*
- "The only disability in life is a bad attitude." ~ *Scott Hamilton*
- "What lies behind us and what lies before us are tiny matters compared to what lies within us." ~ *Ralph Waldo Emerson*
- "I learned that courage was not the absence of fear, but the triumph over it. The brave man is not he who does not feel afraid, but he who conquers that fear." ~ *Nelson Mandela*
- "I can be changed by what happens to me. But I refuse to be reduced by it." ~ *Maya Angelou*
- "We either make ourselves miserable or we make ourselves strong. The amount of work is the same." ~ *Carlos Castaneda*
- "Whether you think you can or you can't, you're right." ~ *Henry Ford*
- "Choose to be optimistic. It feels better." ~ *Dalai Lama XIV*

★ Cindy L. (*Kidney cancer*)

- "Just chuck it in the f*ck it bucket and move on!" A. *Wise Person*
- "You never know how strong you are, until being strong is your only choice." *Bob Marley*

★ Rev. Linda S. (*Pancreatic cancer 3x*)

"Many times during difficulties I want to cling to structures of knowing with every fiber of my being. I tightly clench certainties and principles that I believe will be my salvation from the suffering of grief, anger, depression, and shame. But if I don't also have space for the mystery, for dancing with the discomfort in order to learn what is unfolding for my growth, I will never know the wholeness of this life I live." *Rev. Kelly Isola*

"For me, cancer never felt like a war. cancer wasn't something I "had," but a process my body was going through. Brutal but effective medical treatment paused that process, as far as I know today. By the grace of science and God, I'm alive with no evidence of active disease as I share these words. It's as close to "cured" or "winning" as I get, one day at a time. And I'll take it, with gratitude." ~ *Xeni Jardin*

"I love when people that have been through hell walk out of the flames carrying buckets of water for those still consumed by the fire." ~ *Stephanie Sparkles*

"You do not need to know precisely what is happening, or exactly where it is all going. What you need is to recognize the possibilities and challenges offered by the present moment, and to embrace them with courage, faith, and hope." ~ *Thomas Merton*

"Unease, anxiety, tension, stress, worry — all forms of fear — are caused by too much future, and not enough presence." ~ *Eckhart Tolle*

"A sacred illness is one that educates us and alters us from the inside out, provides experiences and therefore knowledge that we could not possibly achieve in any other way." ~ *Deena Metzger*

★ Joan S. *(Rectal cancer)*

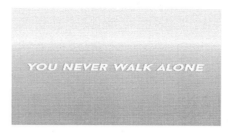

SONGS

★ Cindy L. *(Kidney cancer)*

A song that I listened to and still listen to when I am full of doubt, worry, or extreme stress is Eric Clapton's "Holy Mother" which he wrote after the death of Prince in April 2016. When depression hit me hard and I was unconsolable before my surgery, this song somehow, strangely, brought me peace. It still does. I was certainly not a Debbie Downer all the time. But, when I needed to wallow in it, this song provided me the ability to do so and to be able to crawl back out of my hole again.

HOLY MOTHER *by Eric Clapton*

Holy Mother, where are you? / Tonight I feel broken in two.
I've seen the stars fall from the sky. / Holy mother, can't keep from crying.
Oh I need your help this time, / Get me through this lonely night.
Tell me please which way to turn / To find myself again.
Holy mother, hear my prayer, / Somehow I know you're still there.
Send me please some peace of mind; / Take away this pain.

I can't wait, I can't wait, I can't wait any longer. / I can't wait, I can't wait, I can't wait for you.

Holy mother, hear my cry, / I've cursed your name a thousand times.
I've felt the anger running through my soul; / All I need is a hand to hold.
Oh I feel the end has come, / No longer my legs will run.
You know I would rather be / In your arms tonight.
When my hands no longer play, / My voice is still, I fade away.
Holy mother, then I'll be / Lying in, safe within your arms."

★ **Amor T.** (*Breast cancer, Ovarian cancer*)

Not only is my short-term memory horrible, but so is my short-term memory.

Have you ever just sat and thought...

Damn, I've been through a lot of shit...

★ **Rev. Linda S.** (*Pancreatic cancer 3x*)

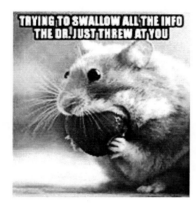

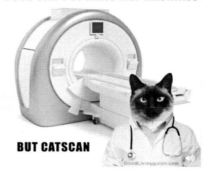

★ **Scott M.** (*Metastatic Colon cancer to the Prostate & Pancreas*)

"I always tell people, the best thing about getting a colonoscopy is they take pictures. So, for guys, they can take those pictures home and prove to their wife that their head isn't up there!"

I Like It Like That

We've got wild turkeys in the front yard
Black tail deer in the back
No one dares harm them
And I like it like that

Oh, the deer munch the landscaping
And the turkeys unevenly trim the lawn
But sometimes we get lucky enough
To see a new born fawn

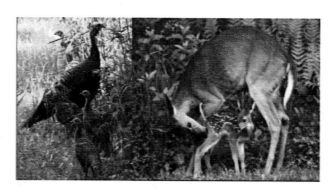

Through the window we watch the
show
As we lay here in the sack
The blue jays stealing the food
From our spoiled lazy cats

The Jacuzzi's hot and ready
To sooth our aching backs
My mate's right here beside me
And I like it like that

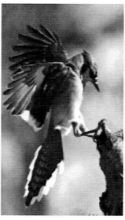

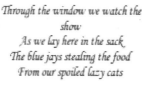

The mockingbirds mock
While the hummingbirds hover
I'm so lucky to share this day
With such a wonderful lover

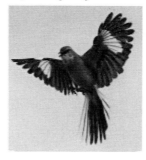

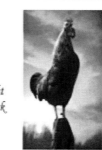

Wish each morning could start this way
Makes goin' to work almost ok
But if I had designed the weekends
They'd have at least one more day

Every place has it's annoyances
Like when our roaster crows at night
He makes me want to adjust his clock
But I've forgiven him by daylight

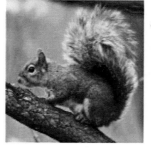

Down by the creek the squirrels bark
It's fun to watch them play
If it weren't for all the guilt
I could lie around all day

When it comes to decision making
A dog's vote has equal weight
When figuring out where we go
And who we're going take

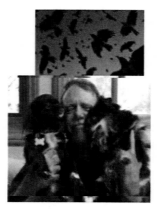

Crows are flying over head
I like to hear them "Caw"
It reminds me of my Grandma's place
And how I miss Grandpa

There's always a lot to do around here
At times I only take up the slack
But she's here doing it all with me
And I like it, just like that

Glenn Maaty

Heaven

Don't we wish that Heaven had email
So we could stay in touch
With our dearly departed
That we miss so much

Just think, if Heaven had email
And we wanted to chat with someone that's gone
We could just type in their name
At Heaven, dot.com

We could attach our pictures
And even video clips
And keep them right up to date
With all of our trips

And if we had a Scientific question
Like, "When did the world begin?"
We could just type in "Albert Einstein"
Or maybe "Carl Sagan"

Think of the advice we could get
And the mistakes we could avoid
And how happy we would be
If we could fill that void

But how would we ever get to work?
Or even go outside?
If we could connect with our computers
To the other side

And who better than they
To bring us down to earth?
And remind us what to be thankful for
They'd be way better than church

Glenn Mooty

Manteca, California Relay for Life Speech by Cancer Survivor Rachel Salinas

Friday, May 27, 2016 is a day I will never forget; the day my life would be changed forever. I was home alone with my baby when I received a phone call from the doctor with the words: "You have cancer, but not just in the lump that was found, but in the lymph nodes as well.

Suddenly my world came crashing down around me. As if hearing that I had breast cancer wasn't enough, in my head, once cancer hit the lymph nodes, life was over.

My friends and family rushed home from where they were to be by my side. We tried to make sense of all of this, because there was no cancer in my family ... None! How could this happen? I was confused. I was devastated. I was heartbroken. I was angry. We all were.

That first weekend was spent with many unanswered questions and a lot of tears. I was surrounded by loved ones and yet felt so very alone. I felt like I had been handed a death sentence.

I remember crying as I watched my baby sleep one night. In my tears, I asked my husband to please not to let him forget me. Then, I felt a different type of anger. A defiant anger. I would FIGHT with everything I had! If cancer wanted me, it was going to have a HELL of a time getting me! I would do everything possible to ensure I was with my babies as they got older and they would not have to "remember" me.

The next several days were spent attending numerous doctors' appointments. At one of the appointments, I learned that I had the type of breast cancer that was the most aggressive and difficult to treat; a cancer that was more likely to spread and recur. I had stage III triple negative breast cancer.

I learned that the cancer had invaded all the lymph nodes in my right arm and that this was the only type of cancer that does not have a treatment beyond chemotherapy and radiation. I was told that it was not a matter of whether the cancer comes back, but when. I felt so defeated and heartbroken. With all the research and studies that go into cancer, how could this be?

Again, I decided I would FIGHT! This time, I decided I would not only fight, but I would also be on a mission to bring awareness to triple negative breast cancer. I never want another woman to be told she does not have hope, because there is no treatment.

On June 14th I had a double mastectomy and on July 15th began chemotherapy. The doctors kept trying to tell me all the side effects that could happen. I stopped each one of them and asked two simple question: "Will I be alive? Will this procedure help me survive?" I told them, "If this treatment/surgery will help me live, then I don't care about the side effects, **because I will be alive to deal with them!**"

During this time, I decided to take to Facebook and post updates of my fight. I had some people tell me I should be quiet during this time; that this is not something that should be shared. They did not understand. I have been using the Facebook platform to bring attention to our fight against breast cancer, including helping women everywhere learn about the different types of breast cancer. Most of all, I used Facebook to help me get through the difficult challenge of living with cancer. When upset, I would read back through my posts and the messages and comments my Facebook family and friends leave would lift me up. I realize I have so much support; there was NO WAY I am going to let my family and friends down!

In addition to using Facebook for support, I focused a lot on my kids: my two-year old Sawyer, my twelve-year old Ryan and my 20-year old Kaitlyn.

During treatment, my husband, Eusebio, did whatever he could to make sure I was comfortable. Ryan, my twelve-year old, helped me with whatever I needed when my husband was not there. Sawyer, my two-year old, helped me focus on something besides me. I tried very hard not to let them see me cry. It was because of them that I stayed so strong.

I thought, if this thing DID beat me, then they would remember me as happy and strong mother; a FIGHTER! When the pain was so unbearable, I felt like I was going to die, I would keep repeating in my head, "This is only temporary. This is only temporary. You won't die from the pain!" And you know what? IT WORKED! This mentality is what got me through a lot of bad days. I spent a lot of time just being silly with my kids. I would use whatever energy I had to do silly dances to the Wiggles, or any other music, and just dance and laugh. I was weak, exhausted, sick....but DAMMIT, I was ALIVE!

I am not one to ask for help nor have I ever been. I learned quickly that I had to put that sense of self-reliance aside. This was not the time for me to be on my own.

The weekend I was diagnosed, my sister had already put together a meal train, so that my family would be taken care of while I recovered from surgery. I had a group of amazing women get together to help ensure my kids had a memorable

Christmas. I had my mom come out from Iowa and my mother-in-law come from Mexico to help. SO many people came forward to help. I had people come help me clean, play with my kids, take my son to karate, spend time with me, and pray with me. I will NEVER be able to fully express my gratitude to EVERYONE who helped me. All I can do now is PAY IT FORWARD by helping others in this situation, which is EXACTLY what I am doing.

When I completed my radiation treatments on February 7th, 2017, I was told that my cancer is in remission. I am now participating in three trial studies with Kaiser in hopes of finding a treatment for triple negative breast cancer patients. I was interviewed by an author who is writing a book about the cancer experience. In that interview, I shared my story which, when published, will further my efforts to bring awareness to breast cancer.

Cancer gave me a LOT of heartache, lymphedema, a lot of pain, and a fear that will NEVER go away. BUT it also gave me a new purpose in life; a STRENGTH I never knew I had; a CONFIDENCE in who I am and what I stand for. I am a warrior, a fighter and a survivor.

My fight will NEVER be over. I know the risk of it returning is great, but my will to survive is GREATER!

We are all here for the same purpose. We have all been afflicted by this horrible disease in one way or another. Once you are diagnosed, you become part of a club nobody wants to be in. HOWEVER, once you are here, you are met with love, understanding, and encouragement!

Whether we are survivors, caregivers, family members or friends, our fight will NEVER be over. I believe we CAN win and we WILL win!...TOGETHER! WE ARE WARRIORS! FIGHTERS! WE...ARE...SURVIVORS!!

Thank you.

RACHEL

SOCIAL MEDIA ACTIVITIES

★ *Amor T. (Breast cancer, Ovarian cancer)*

Facebook https://www.facebook.com/: I have found that sharing my cancer journeys on Facebook not only kept my family and friends in the loop, it also served to lift my spirits, no matter what time of day or night. I posted pictures of how I was losing my hair and videos of my fun head shaving party. I also posted pictures before and after my surgeries, including pictures with my doctors, nurses, hospital aides, and family and friends who cared for me. During the times I felt blah or couldn't sleep, I remember looking through my Facebook profile and continuously seeing all the wonderful posts and comments of love and support from my family and friends around the world. I remember reading the prayers and feeling the positive energies they sent my way. They lifted my spirits. Sharing through Facebook has been therapeutic for me and I'm grateful for the access to my family and friends around the world that it has enabled me to have.

WhatNext.com https://www.whatnext.com/home is a cancer support network community where we all share our experiences with various diagnoses, treatments, drugs, etc. with each other. Although I've survived two cancers, I still have survivorship issues, e.g. "canceritis", "scanxiety" that only those who've been through cancer can understand.

It's a pretty cool community to join, because everyone there has empathy for you. Many understand what you're going through, because they either have or had the same diagnosis or have received the same treatment or drugs and experienced their effectiveness or side effects too. It's great to have found an online community I can discuss my cancer survivorship issues with openly. They have welcomed me and really want to hear what I have to say. We have an unspoken bond. Yes, they're virtual strangers, but they're also my cancer survivor sisters and brothers.

Nalie Agustin https://www.nalie.ca/about-me/ When I was researching how to cope with my impending hair loss in 2016 due to chemotherapy to treat my ovarian cancer, I happened upon Nalie's story and was immediately inspired by the then 24-year old breast cancer survivor. Her blogs and YouTube videos were really interesting and informative. Even though her cancer metastasized to her lungs in 2017, Nalie continues to thrive and inspire me and so many others..

★ *Cindy L. (Kidney cancer)*

I'm part of midlife communities now. My friend Michelle and I started a Facebook group called "Midlife at the Cabana." It's a perimenopause and menopause support group page where anyone who wants to stay awesome through midlife and beyond can join. It's a closed group site where members share their midlife experiences, have fun and make friends. Those who want to join and add to the conversation just have to promise to be polite and respectful, even if they do not agree with someone's position. No medical advice is given and no promotion of products for sale is allowed. Search for us on Facebook: Midlife at the Cabana - Perimenopause and Menopause Support

I also used Facebook to share my experiences during treatment and received so much support from my friends and family on Facebook. If you were to look at my Facebook page, you'd probably see me say, at least, a couple of times, "I need to practice to pause" which is one of the ways that has helped me emotionally cope with my circumstances.

> **ADVICE:** Social media has many advantages. It brings together people and enables you to communicate with your social media friends at any time of day or night. It also allows them to express their support of you; something which you can read, also, at any time of day or night. It's therapeutic and fun. I highly recommend joining an online support group to help you through your challenges before, during and after treatment.

★ Rev. Linda S. *(Pancreatic cancer 3x)*

I use Facebook to share my thoughts, feelings and observations with my family and friends. Sometimes, it's a distraction. However, it helps me keep in touch with those in my personal community. It also allows my family and friends to reach out and share their thoughts and feelings. I have found it profoundly comforting to know that my Facebook family is with me in thought, prayers and spirit, despite time or distance, especially when I'm physically, emotionally and spiritually drained.

★ Rachel S. *(Breast cancer: triple negative)*

During this time, I decided to take to Facebook and post updates of my fight. I had some people tell me I should be quiet during this time; that this is not something that should be shared. They did not understand. I have been using the Facebook platform to bring attention to our fight against breast cancer, including helping women everywhere learn about the different types of breast cancer. Most of all, I used Facebook to help me get through the difficult challenge of living with cancer. When upset, I would read back through my posts and the messages and comments my Facebook family and friends leave would lift me up. I realize I have so much support; there was NO WAY I am going to let my family and friends down! I did a lot on Facebook. That was basically my "counselling." That was my "support group."

★ Vida BA *(Breast cancer)*

I really enjoyed going on Facebook to share and exchange thoughts, ideas, picture, updates, etc. with my family and friends. It was a fun activity and therapeutic for me. Reading words of encouragement and support from my family and friends on Facebook really helped lift up my spirits.

SPIRITUAL HEALING

Spiritual Healing is the activity of making a person or one's own self healthy without using medicines or other physical methods, sometimes as part of a religious ceremony. It has an ancient pedigree, with much evidence of success.

Following is a compilation of the prayers, songs and quotes that have comforted and inspired us in our cancer journeys. They have helped to lift up our spirits without which, we believe, we would not have found the strength to survive as we did.

★ Amor T. *(Breast cancer, Ovarian cancer)*

Throughout both my cancer experiences, prayer kept me strong and calm. However, it was during my ovarian cancer journey when I finally understood the amazing benefits of praying the rosary and spending quiet time in thoughtful and active communication with God. I found a deeper sense of peace and joy that really transported me out of my physical circumstances and strengthened me in more ways that I thought it could.

When I was in physical pain, I learned to focus my energy to praying for strength, at the same time, thanking God for all the blessings He's given me.

"ANGELA'S PRAYER"
Lord, bless this day. Help us give it back to You."

"THE SERENITY PRAYER

God grant me the serenity to accept the things I cannot change, courage to change the things I can and the wisdom to know the difference." ~ *Reinhold Niebuhr*

"PSALM 23
The Lord is my Shepherd, I shall not want.
He maketh me to lie down in green pastures.
He leadeth me beside the still waters.
He restoreth my soul. He leadeth me in paths of righteous for His name's sake.
Yea, though I walk in the valley of the shadow of death, I will fear no evil;
For Thou art with me; Thy rod and Thy staff, They comfort me
Thou preparest a table for me in the presence of mine enemies
Thou anointest my head with oil; my cup runneth over
Surely goodness and mercy shall follow me all the days of my life
And I will dwell in the house of the Lord forever."

"THE LORD BLESS YOU AND KEEP YOU"
Composed by John Rutter
"The Lord bless you and keep you
The Lord lift His countenance upon you
and give you peace and give you peace
The Lord make His face to shine upon you
and be gracious unto you
The Lord be gracious, gracious unto you
Amen Amen Amen Amen Amen."

"BE NOT AFRAID"
You shall cross the barren desert, but you shall not die of thirst
You shall wander far in safety though you do not know the way.
You shall speak your words in foreign lands and all will understand
You shall see the face of God and live.

(Refrain)
Be not afraid. I go before you always. Come follow Me. And I shall give you rest.

If you pass through raging waters in the sea, you shall not drown
If you walk amidst the burning flames, you shall not be harmed.
If you stand before the pow'r of hell and death is at your side
Know that I am with you, through it all. *(refrain)*

Blessed are your poor for the Kingdom shall be theirs
Blest are you that weep and mourn for one day you shall laugh.

And if wicked men insult and hate you all because of Me
Blessed, blessed are you! *(refrain)*

★ **Joan S.** *(Rectal cancer)*

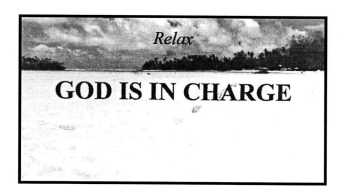

★ **Rev. Linda S.** *(Pancreatic cancer 3x)*

"GOD IS MY COMFORT.

If I desire freedom from anxiety and worry, I need to take a break from any tendency to ponder "what could go wrong" scenarios. Clearing my mind, I turn within to my one true source of all comfort and overcoming. I relax into the shelter of Divine Presence.
Any frazzled nerves are soothed. Anxiety from what seems lost or unavailable to me dissipates. Nothing can interfere with the assurance from my Creator that the unknown cannot disturb the peace of my soul. I receive the enrichment that strengthens me to the very core of my being."

"I am prepared to live wholly today and each new day. The presence of God is within me and everywhere present to comfort me." *August 24, 2017 Daily Word: A Unity Publication*

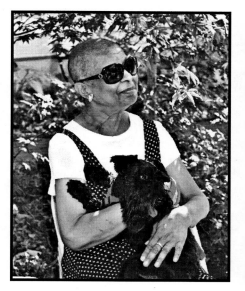

"I CHOOSE JOY.

I may feel sadness, impatience, or even anger because of my life's circumstances. But I recognize that these emotions are temporary, for my spirit will always naturally seek to express joy. True joy is not about outside circumstances. Rather, it is an inner awareness, developed through consciousness.

Inner joy is about my connection with God, with the truth of my being, with nature, and with all life. Undeterred by the opinions of others or even by difficult circumstances, the peace I feel is the result of an inner decision to live my life in joy."

Peace fills me, and a sense of purpose directs me. Because of my decision to choose joy in my life, I make a positive difference in the world." *July 7, 2017 Daily Word: A Unity Publication*

"The power in committing something to prayer comes not when I make a request, but when I release my attachment to the outcome and accept what unfolds. What I'm seeing with my human understanding is just a small piece of the overall picture. The path I travel comes together like a divine puzzle; perfect pieces from expected and unexpected sources fall into place as I go.

As I open to the energy of prayer, I relax into the awareness that I may not yet have every answer, every piece to complete the puzzle. I have faith that everything is in divine order and then release it all to my Source. I no longer try to dictate a specific solution and instead trust that each outcome is for the best. With confidence and faith, **I let go and let God.**"

I AM THERE (by James Dillet Freeman)

Do you need Me? I am there.
You cannot see Me, yet I am the light you see by.
You cannot hear Me, yet I speak through your voice.
You cannot feel Me, yet I am the power at work in your hands.
I am at work, though you do not understand My ways.
I am at work, though you do not recognize My works.
I am not strange visions. I am not mysteries.
Only in absolute stillness, beyond self, can you know Me as I am,
and then but as a feeling and a faith.
Yet I am there. Yet I hear. Yet I ianswer.

When you need Me, I am there.
Even if you deny Me, I am there.
Even in your feel most alone, I am there.
Even in your fears, I am there.
Even in your pain, I am there.
I am there when you pray and when you do not opray.
I am in you, and you are in Me.
Only in your mind can you feel separate from Me, for only in
your mind are the mists of "yours" and "mine."
Yet only with your mind can you know Me and experience Me.

Empty your heart of empty fears.
When you get yourself out of the way, I am there.
You can of yourself do nothing, but I can do all.
And I am in all.

Though you may not see the good, good is there, for I am there.
I am there because I have to be, because I am.
Only in Me does the world have meaning; only in Me does the world take form;
only because of Me does the world go forward.

I am the law on which the movement of the stars
and the growth of living cells are founded.
I am the love that is the law's fulfilling. I am assurance. I am peace.
I am one with you. I am.

Though you fail to find Me, I do not fail you.
Though your faith in Me is unsure, My faith in your never waivers,
because I know you, because I love you.
Beloved, I am there."

★ Rick S. (CLL: Blood & Bone Marrow cancer)

"I can do all things through Christ who strengthens me." Philippians 4-13
(*Painting given to Rick by the pastors of Garden City Church. Their notes were written on the back of the painting.*)

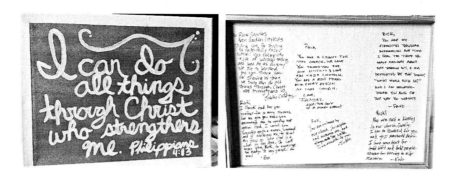

★ Susan M. (*Ovarian cancer. Metastatic Pancreatic cancer to Lungs*)

"God grant me the Serenity to accept the things I cannot change...the Courage to change the things I can....and the Wisdom to know the difference."

"Today I just want to thank God for the gift of life. No requests, no complaints, just thankful to be alive."

This sign hangs in my kitchen: "Good Morning, this is God. I will be handling all your problems today."

★ Vida BA (*Breast cancer*)

I have some prayers that have helped me through my challenges. In one of my favorite prayers, I say:

> **"Jesus, cover me; please cover me in your blood. Protect me and take
> all the bad cells away from my body and renew me with good cells."**

In another favorite prayer, I say, **"Lord, if you're going to take me, let me be with you."** Yes, I'm prepared. I'm prepared to be with the Lord.

★ Yesi L. (*Breast cancer: triple positive*)

Spirituality helped me during treatment. I completely just gave myself to God. I said, "I'm here, Lord. I'm yours. Do with me as you wish." I had so much faith and so much hope. I never had such a beautiful connection that felt so deep. That definitely helped me and kept me going.

~ o ~

Chapter 13

INTEGRATIVE HEALTHCARE COORDINATING CONVENTIONAL AND COMPLEMENTARY APPROACHES

Integrative healthcare utilizes the best therapeutic options from conventional Western medicine, as well as holistic practices, also known as complementary therapies and healing practices. It emphasizes a holistic, patient-focused approach to health care and wellness (mental, emotional, functional, spiritual and community aspects), thereby treating the whole person rather than one organ or system.

Complementary medicine refers to healing modalities that are used to complement allopathic or conventional approaches. It is not the same as "alternative" medicine, which refers to an approach to healing that is utilized in place of conventional or complementary medicine. Integrative healthcare is based on good science.

COMPLEMENTARY MIND & BODY PRACTICES

ACUPUNCTURE

Acupuncture is a Chinese medicine technique that involves the the insertion of very thin needles through the skin at strategic points on the body. It balances the flow of energy or life force ("chi") believed to flow through pathways (meridians) in our body. It is used to treat pain and promote overall wellness and stress management.

* *Amor T.* (Breast cancer, Ovarian cancer)

I have received acupuncture treatments to reduce inflammation in my knees from the osteoarthritis I got from my chemo and hormone treatments.. They have not only enabled me to climb two steps up and down without pain (something I wasn't able to do before), they have also helped me relax ... I mean, really, really relax.

EFT* TAPPING THERAPY

Tapping, also known as EFT (Emotional Freedom Technique), is a powerful holistic healing technique. It has been proven to effectively resolve a wide range of emotional issues by tapping with the fingers specific Chinese acupressure median endpoints of the body while reciting "setup statements," followed by unconditional affirmations of yourself as a person.

* Sondra W. *(Ovarian cancer 3x)*

Tapping, for me, is a really good technique to learn when having to deal with our negative emotions, because ~ and this is HUGE! ~ it gives us the affirmation we need to cope. The instructor showed us the points and explained how everything works in opening up these energy points. In the practice session, I thought, "Okay, let me go right to the heart of my thing."

So what I recited as I tapped (and you only speak in terms of how you feel; not who you are) was:

"Right now, I'm feeling sad, because I might not live as long as I expected.
But, for today, right now, I am here and I'm fine."

That really made a big difference for me when I kept saying it, while going through all my tapping points. It just put me in a different frame of mind while using these energy channels. And that was really good.

MASSAGE / CHI NEI TSANG / LYMPHATIC DRAINAGE MASSAGE

- Massage is the rubbing and kneading of muscles and joints of the body with the hands, especially to relieve tension or pain. Massage may also help with nausea, anxiety, depression and mood disorders for cancer patients. Light, relaxing massage may be performed on patients at all stages of cancer. However, tumor or treatment sites should be avoided.
- Chi Nei Tsang is an ancient Chinese healing touch therapy that focuses on deep, gentle abdominal massage in order to "train" the internal abdominal organs to work more efficiently, which in turn is said to improve physical and emotional health.
- Lymphatic Drainage Massage is a specialized massage type that gently assists the lymphatic system in maintaining the body's fluid balance, blood circulation, and immune mechanisms.

* Amor T. *(Breast cancer, Ovarian cancer)*

I was informed by my integrative health doctor that Chi Nei Tsang abdominal massage can help clear my liver of the simple cysts that had formed there, the largest being 10.5cm. The four sessions I experienced were truly eye-opening! The Chi Nei Tsang practitioner (Anya Devi) walked me through the process and then performed slow, deep yet gentle, meditative massage throughout my entire abdomen. She told me beforehand that I shouldn't worry at all about burping or farting, because expelling air and gas is expected and, actually, a good thing; I shouldn't hold it in at all. So, with her gently pressing down and massaging my small intestines, colon, and other organs in my abdomen, I burped and pass gas multiple times. And, each time, Anya said, "Good!"

Not only did I learn about how our bodies can reabsorb simple (fluid-filled) cysts, I also learned how the 18-20 feet of small intestine we have all coiled up and folded in our abdominal cavity plays a huge role in our digestion of food, yet we don't really think much to take care of it! How true!

Using various Chi Nei Tsang techniques, Anya was able to release a lot of my built-up gas, loosen the complex web of tough abdominal adhesions I had collected from my many abdominal surgeries and, also help me sleep and breathe better.

* Sondra W. *(Ovarian cancer 3x)*

Once, after my PET scan was completed earlier in the day, I went to my massage appointment. The masseuse is Swiss and had been a nurse before. She had also survived cancer, as well. I described all my health issues to her and she listened to everything I had to say. I even forewarned her that I have digestive issues and may have to jump off the table at the last minute to use the restroom. She said, "Not a problem. What I don't want you to do is be uncomfortable here on the table." She then added, "I've been there myself. It's fine." She taught me how to massage my lymph areas and what to do, because they need to move.

On the following day, I went to the hospital for my regular visit. I had so much energy; it was the best I've felt in three years. Really! I'm definitely going to go back to her. Her massage helped me so much ... so much!

When the nurses up at the Cancer Center noticed my energy, they were excited and even took a picture of her card. What she did made such a difference for me that my oncologist included it in his report. They said that they don't always know who is good enough to recommend, until a patient tells them of their positive experience. And that information, they want to share with other patients. Boy, did she help!

MEDITATION

Meditation is a practice where an individual uses a technique – such as focusing their mind on a particular object, thought or activity – to train attention and awareness, and achieve a mentally clear and emotionally calm and stable state.

* Amor T. (Breast cancer, Ovarian cancer)

Before I say my daily prayers and rosary, I find a quiet place ~ preferably where I can view nature ~ and clear my mind. I focus on the sky, trees, grass ... the beauty of nature and just clear my mind. It's such a peaceful, calming exercise.

* Scott M. (Metastatic Colon cancer to the Prostate & Pancreas)

Life is too valuable. It's too precious. I just can't imagine giving up on it, no matter how tough. There are days when I think, "Oh, I can't do this anymore." But then, I remind myself that I can; I just have to. That's where meditation and mindfulness comes in. I spend 10-15 minutes per day meditating; just having nothing on my mind; letting it go blank. If a thought comes to me, I acknowledge it, then push it aside.

MINDFULNESS

Meditation is a mental state achieved by focusing one's awareness on the present moment, while calmly acknowledging and accepting one's feelings, thoughts, and bodily sensations.

* Amor T. (Breast cancer, Ovarian cancer)

When I felt really awful (physically and emotionally), I tried to look around me and focus on being grateful for everything. I learned this practice from the Dominican nuns I was raised with in Taiwan. They told me that whenever darkness comes to my thoughts, all I have to do is thank God for every single thing I see. So, I learned to look around and say, "Thank you" for everything my eyes landed on.

I remember a time when I was really fatigued and didn't feel like watching TV or talking with anyone; I just felt miserable. I remembered the practice of being present and being thankful for everything. So, I looked around me and started saying, "Thank you, Lord, for the table. Thank you for the chair. Thank you for the lamp. Thank you for the blanket. Thank you for the couch. Thank you for the trees. Thank you for the sun. Thank you for the TV. Thank you for the electrical outlets. Thank you for the plugs. Thank you for the dust ... and then I smiled and started to get amused, because I was checking out every minute thing and getting silly.

The nuns were right. When I break away from negativity and focus on gratitude, the darkness fades away and is replaced by positive thoughts and energy!

* Cindy R. (Metastatic Breast cancer to the Stomach)

Although I'm Catholic, I don't practice it. I'm into nature and see good in everything. I'm also spiritual and I talk to the cells in my body. I was into Taekwondo before and read this interesting book about a Taekwondo Master that greatly influenced me.

In the book, the Master talked about how he healed himself. What he did at night was concentrate on whatever injuries he had. He would pretend like these little guys went in and did work on this particular part of his body that wasn't good. And then, when he wakes up, things would be better.

Even though it sounded silly to me, I told myself I was going to do it too. So at night, I have the little guys going down into my stomach and they're chipping away at the cancer and vacuuming it up. It's like an exercise in positivity. It's mindfulness and it works.

* Scott M. (Metastatic Colon cancer to the Prostate & Pancreas)

Life is too valuable. It's too precious. I just can't imagine giving up on it, no matter how tough. There are days when I think, "Oh, I can't do this anymore." But then, I remind myself that I can; I just have to. That's where meditation and mindfulness comes in. I spend 10-15 minutes per day meditating; just having nothing on my mind; letting it go blank. If a thought comes to me, I acknowledge it, then push it aside.

Same with mindfulness. I'll sit and I'll think how I want to be ... think positive reinforcements; those kinds of things. You are your primary thought. If I think that I don't have cancer, then I don't "have" it. I read something where it said, "Every cell in your body eavesdrops on your mind every moment." If you say you're sick, all of body cells are going to say, "Hey guys, we're supposed to be sick, so..." But if you say, "I'm perfectly healthy," then all your body's cells are going to say, "Okay, guys, we're all supposed to be really healthy. So, if any of you are not healthy right now, let's get you fixed. Immune system, kick in over here..." That kind of thing. That's why I envision it.

YOGA (CHAIR)

A Hindu spiritual and ascetic discipline, a part of which, including breath control, simple meditation, and the adoption of specific bodily postures, is widely practiced for health and relaxation. Chair yoga is a gentle form of yoga that is practiced sitting on a chair, or standing using a chair for support.

* Rev. Linda S. (Pancreatic cancer 3x)

To help with my aching hip, knee and ankle joints, as well as to improve my overall health, I take chair yoga classes. Chair yoga is a gentle form of yoga that can be done sitting on a chair or standing on the ground while using the chair for support. Despite my aching bones, I go my chair yoga classes, because they help me. Besides, I have a wonderful instructor who motivates me. That's really important.

COMPLEMENTARY NATURAL PRODUCTS

DIETARY SUPPLEMENTS & ESSENTIAL OILS

These complementary natural products include vitamins, minerals, herbals, probiotics as well as essential oils that we survivors use to enhance our health.

* Amor T. (Breast cancer, Ovarian cancer)

Vitamins & Minerals: Along with my daily intake of multivitamins and iron, I take "elemental" calcium (600 mg), vitamin D (4,000 IU), vitamin K (165 mcg) and magnesium (180 mg) for my bones, vitamin C (1,000) and zinc (18.5 mg) to boost my immune system, copper (1.9 mg) to support both healthy bones and immune system and manganese (3.3 mg) to strengthen brain and nerve function, aside from having great antioxidant properties for strength..

Frankincense (Boswellia essential oil): I heard so much about the immune-enhancing abilities of frankincense and was told that it is known as one of the "most prized and precious essential oils" because of its extraordinary health benefits. I bought a bottle for that reason, but didn't really believe it until I had to use it. One day, I woke up in the middle of the night and felt a cold coming on. I immediately dabbed some Frankincense on my thumb and applied it to the roof of my mouth (fleshy soft palate in the back called the "velum") and went back to bed. When I awoke, there was no longer any signs of a cold. I have since experienced many cold or sick feelings trying to sneak up on me and have applied Frankincense every time. And, every time, the cold or sick feeling disappeared, like magic!.

When I researched more about frankincense, I learned that it has immune-enhancing abilities that help destroy dangerous bacteria, viruses and even cancers. It can prevent germs from forming on the skin, mouth or in your home. It has the ability to eliminate cold and flu germs naturally and its antiseptic qualities help to prevent gingivitis, bad breath, cavities, toothaches, mouth sores and other infections from occurring. I highly recommend getting one for yourself and your family. Even though it isn't cheap at $90 for a 15 mL bottle, I bought mine over a year ago and, after many uses, I have almost a full bottle left.

L-Glutamine: During treatment, the one supplement I was told to take 3x a day (10g each time), every day was L-GLUTAMINE. According to my wonderful oncologist, I needed to take L-Glutamine to boost my immune system and bone health, especially during chemotherapy. [NOTE: L-Glutamine is a "free form" supplement of Glutamine.] So, I researched the benefits of Glutamine / L-Glutamine for better understanding. Here's what I learned:

What is Glutamine, where does it come from and what is its function in our body?

- Glutamine is an important *amino acid with many functions in our body. [*Amino acids are the building blocks of protein and a critical part of our immune system.]
- Glutamine helps gut function, the immune system, and other essential processes in the body, especially in times of stress. It is also important for providing "fuel" (nitrogen and carbon) to many different cells in the body.
- It is produced in our muscles and distributed by the blood to the organs that need it.
- Around 60% of our skeletal muscle is made up of Glutamine – and supplementing with this amino acid can aid protein synthesis and help naturally balance our pH levels.
- It acts as the primary fuel for rapidly growing cells (immune system and intestinal cells).
- Glutamine is also a major nitrogen transporter and helps to regulate our body's acid-base balance.

When should we take Glutamine supplements aka L-Glutamine?

- We should take L-Glutamine when our body may require more Glutamine that it can produce, i.e. when our body is facing disease or other muscle-wasting conditions or when going through treatment (e.g. chemotherapy) that challenge our overall immune system.
- Although Glutamine can be found in both animal and plant proteins, most of us don't get enough Glutamine from food alone. So, we need to supplement our diet with L-Glutamine in order to boost our immune system and improve our ability to fight infection and diseases.

How does Glutamine work in the body?

- After surgery or traumatic injury, nitrogen is necessary to repair the wounds and keep the vital organs functioning. About one third of this nitrogen comes from Glutamine.
- If the body uses more Glutamine than the muscles can make (i.e., during times of stress, disease), muscle wasting can occur. This can occur in people with cancer, HIV/AIDS, etc. Taking Glutamine supplements keep the body's Glutamine stores up.
- Some types of chemotherapy can reduce the levels of Glutamine in the body. Glutamine treatment is thought to help prevent chemotherapy-related damage by maintaining the life of the affected tissues.

7 Proven L-Glutamine Benefits

1. Improves gastrointestinal health
2. Helps leaky gut and ulcers
3. Boosts brain health
4. Improves IBS and diarrhea
5. Promotes muscle growth and decreases muscle wasting

6. Improves athletic performance and recovery from endurance exercise
7. Burns fat and improves diabetes

Foods with L-Glutamine Benefits

- Asparagus
- Bone Broth
- Broccoli Rabe
- Chinese Cabbage
- Cottage Cheese
- Grass-fed Beef
- Spirulina (*supplement made from blue-green algae, is touted as a "superfood*)
- Turkey
- Venison
- Wild-Caught Fish (cod & salmon)

(<u>NOTE</u>: There is no real difference between Glutamine & L-Glutamine in supplementation. Whether it says "L-Glutamine" on the container or just "Glutamine", supplements always use L-Glutamine.)

* *Cindy L. (Kidney cancer)*

My vitamin D level was so low after surgery. So, my doctor instructed me to take 50,000 IUs of vitamin D daily for eight weeks. Since it's a high dose, I had to get a prescription from him. Now, I take 3,000 IUs a day. My vitamin D deficiency was also responsible for my foot cramps. I still have them, but not as often. So, I'm staying on the vitamin D therapy and eating Greek yogurt that has a good amount of vitamin D in it about three to four times a week.

I take a good quality probiotic daily. My doctor started me back on those while I was still in the hospital. I also take Nordic Naturals Fish Oil supplements (great source of healthy omega-3 fats and vitamin D), a multivitamin (Zincovit) and Atenolol for my high blood pressure every day. And that's really all I take.

> **ADVICE:** Make sure your doctor checks your vitamin D level to make sure it's sufficient. More so if you're a kidney cancer patient. Vitamin D is responsible for your immune system and your bones. It helps in the absorption of magnesium. Studies have proven that vitamin D deficiency plays a big role in chronic kidney disease. Since you cannot get high doses of vitamin D in the market, get a prescription from your doctor. Also, eat Greek yogurt that has a good amount of vitamin D in it for about three to four times a week.

Because of the fact that I only have one kidney, I have to protect it. For pain, I can take Tylenol or anything with acetaminophen in it. But, I can no longer take any NSAIDs (non-steroidal anti-inflammatory drugs) like Motrin or Naproxen. When it comes to antibiotics, I have to be careful, because I have a lot of antibiotic allergies. As much as possible, I need to avoid any medication that is excreted by the kidney, because it puts a strain on my remaining kidney.

Levels of creatinine in my blood reflects my kidney function. My creatinine levels have fluctuated between 0.8 mg/dL (pre-surgery) to 1.13 mg/dL (post-surgery). Normal creatinine levels for women should be between 0.5 to 1.1 mg/dL. So, I have been keeping a close watch on my creatinine levels. I'm also watching the sodium intake in my diet, because sodium is the all-important electrolyte in the blood that helps to maintain adequate blood volume, which is needed for proper kidney function. As you can see, I'm taking extra care to protect my remaining kidney, because it's already struggling. I have been seeing my doctors for follow-ups to make sure I'm on the right path and getting stronger every day.

> **ADVICE:** You want to make sure you're on the right path to full recovery, right? So, learn what you can about your health and ask your doctors and nurses whatever questions comes to mind. Also, see a nutritionist or dietitian to make sure you're eating the right foods your body needs to heal and become stronger.

* Hilda K. *(Colon cancer)*

I was never prescribed any anti-cancer medication to take. However, I was strongly advised by my oncologist to take certain supplements. I started by taking Baby Aspirin and then Vitamin D, both for preventative measures.

What also helped with my healing was taking a year off from work. If you can financially afford to, then just do it. Give yourself time to accept your diagnosis and go through treatment, without other things to think about. Be with your family, but don't be stressed about them either. Any kind of stress from your life, stay away from. Just be normal and be at peace with whatever you're going through. Taking time off from work was definitely the best thing I could've done for myself!

* Rick S. *(CLL: Blood & Bone Marrow cancer)*

I couldn't take supplements while I was going through my chemo treatments. The supplements I took for weightlifting were contrary to the treatment plan that I was given. Before my chemo, I was taking one aspirin a day as a blood thinner. I learned that I couldn't take aspirin while taking chemo, because the type of chemo I was getting was already in itself a blood thinner. In fact, I couldn't have any surgeries and be on the chemo, because of the chemo drug being a blood thinner.

Before chemo, I used to take soy supplements for my prostate, fish oil supplements, because it's good for the heart and aspirin. When my doctor found out about my supplements, he took me off of everything, except the soy supplement for my prostate. Soy is good for the tissues of the prostate; it protects the prostate.

* Sondra W. *(Ovarian cancer 3x)*

I take three medications. The rest are supplements, like: B6, B12, CoQ10, D3, Omega3, L-Glutamine, a multivitamin and a probiotic. I like Turmeric, which helps fight cancer. But, I was told that I couldn't take it, as well as all herbs, while being treated with chemotherapy, because they could get in the way. So, until I get to a "better place", I'm staying away from them.

* Susan M. *(Ovarian cancer, Metastatic Pancreatic cancer to the Lungs)*

After surviving both Ovarian Cancer and Pancreatic Cancer, I became more diligent in taking my vitamins and I found that I had more energy! I take a Women's Multivitamin, B12 and Calcium with D3. I found the gummy vitamins were easier for me to take; almost like having a treat. This is my personal preference.

* Tet M. *(Colon cancer 3x)*

Vitamins like A, C, D, E, Beta Carotene, Selenium and Turmeric are staples. PLEASE BE SURE TO CONSULT YOUR DOCTOR before taking supplements.

MEDICAL MARIJUANA

Medical marijuana uses the marijuana plant or chemicals in it to treat diseases or conditions. It's basically the same product as recreational marijuana, but it's taken for medical purposes. The marijuana plant contains more than 100 different chemicals called cannabinoids. Each one has a different effect on the body. (CBD) cannabidiol and (THC) Delta-9-tetrahydrocannabinol are the main chemicals used in medicine.

THC can increase appetite and reduce nausea. THC may also decrease pain, inflammation (swelling and redness), and muscle control problems. Unlike THC, CBD is a cannabinoid that doesn't make people "high." These drugs aren't popular for recreational use because they aren't intoxicating. It may be useful in reducing pain and inflammation. To date, the FDA has approved two man-made cannabinoid medicines ~ dronabinol (Marinol, Syndros) and nabilone (Cesamet) ~ to treat nausea and vomiting from chemotherapy. Sources: 12/15/2018 *WebMD Article Reviewed by Neil Lava, MD and https://www.drugabuse.gov/publications/drugfacts/marijuana-medicine*

* Glenn M. (*Metastatic Colon cancer to the Liver, Lungs & Adrenal Glands*)

When I got nauseated and needed relief, I turned to one of my favorite meds, Marinol. I didn't really take it that much. One doctor told me, "If you're using Marinol for nausea, take two 5mg capsules." Well, two 5mg capsules gives me a nice three-to-four hour high. Very nice. It's not like smoking marijuana or weed, because it's synthetic and they pull all the bad stuff out, so it's tuned. I think it shows promise for appetite too.

In fact, we're giving it to my 97-year old mother and it's helping her. It helps her mood and her appetite; it's something else! We talked to her doctor and he's on board with giving her 5mgs. Also, my brother and I figured out how to split the capsules: Freeze them solid. Then, put them in the pill-splitter, split them and take it. You might have to take them with some food. We were able to reduce her dose, so she didn't notice she was high.

ADVICE: **Marinol is great medicine for nausea. If you decide to take it, it'll not just take your nausea away, it'll also give you a nice high. It helps for appetite too. One to two 5mg capsules should do the trick. Talk with your doctor first before taking Marinol.**

* Scott M. (*Metastatic Colon cancer to the Prostate & Pancreas*)

The nausea I experienced was a side effect of my taking the chemo drug, Xeloda. When I was nauseous, I didn't feel like doing anything. I did have a couple of anti-nausea drugs I could take. One was Reglan and the other was Ondansetron. I gave each one an hour to work and they didn't. So, at that point, I smoked a little pot (marijuana) and it worked almost immediately. I got it from a neighbor, so it wasn't the medical one. I personally didn't like the "high" it gave me, but it did work to get rid of my nausea.

ADVICE: **There are anti-nausea drugs you can take, if you get nausea. If for some reason they don't work, don't be afraid to experiment with marijuana. I would recommend taking medical marijuana versus the one you can get off the streets.**

~ 0 ~

Chapter 14

CANCER FIGHTING NUTRITION

"Every time you eat or drink, you are
either feeding disease or fighting it."
~ Heather Morgan, MS, NLC

We now know that to be healthy, we need to eat healthy. But, aside from the obvious, "avoid junk food", how do we determine what we should be eating based on our individual set of circumstances? There is no "one-size-fits all" answer. There are, however, various approaches to eating healthy to fight cancer, as you will see from what we share with you here in this chapter.

CANCER FIGHTING FOOD & DRINKS

* **Aaron C.** (*Prostate cancer, Skin cancer*)

Well, I've always been fairly healthy. I occasionally splurge on a hot dog or have some salami. I don't overdo it. Moderation is the key, you know. But, you've got to enjoy life a little bit too. My cancer experience hasn't turned me into a fanatic. I did have to adjust and lessen my salt intake, however, because I get a reaction now to it. I've always taken vitamins. I'm eating more broccoli, more greens. Good thing I like broccoli!

* **Amor T.** (*Breast cancer, Ovarian cancer*)

Cancer has taught me that I can no longer take my health for granted and that I must choose wisely whatever I put into my body. I've done a ton of research and learned a variety of ways to prepare and cook healthy foods. I focus on both cancer-fighting and anti-inflammatory foods and avoid those that cause cancer and trigger inflammation.

Cancer cells enter our body where our immune system is weakest. And, because the immune system is weak at the entry point, it doesn't recognize the cancer cells to be a problem worth fighting. So, I believe that the focus should be on eating foods that will strengthen my immune system.

I also believe in eating foods that reduce inflammation (anti-inflammatory), because it has been scientifically proven that many cancers arise from sites of infection, chronic irritation and inflammation, and inflammation is a critical component of tumor progression.

Cancer-fighting & Anti-inflammatory foods that are staples for me	RULES *of* THUMB to follow:	AVOID! Cancer-Causing & Top Inflammation Triggers
1. Avocados 2. Beans 3. Beets 4. Bone Broth 5. Broccoli 6. Carrots 7. Citrus Fruits 8. Coconut / Coconut Oil 9. Fatty Fish 10. Garlic 11. Ginger 12. Green, leafy vegetables 13. Mushrooms 14. Olive Oil 15. Tofu 16. Tomatoes 17. Turmeric 18. Walnuts	**VEGETABLES & FRUITS** Should be the bulk of dietary emphasis. Enjoy them in abundance. Strive for locally-grown or organic **MEATS** Strive for local organic, pasture-raised, grass-fed beef, chicken, lamb, turkey or pork **EGGS** The best are organic eggs from "pasture-raised, free-range" chicken **FISH/SEAFOOD** Strive for "wild-caught", not farmed **GROCERY SHOPPING** Buy fresh, as much as possible. Read ingredients of packaged beverage and food items. Avoid those that contain added sugars or sugar substitutes and additives like preservatives, benzoates, sulfites ... basically, any unnatural ingredient and those you cannot pronounce.	• "3 Ps": Processed, packaged or prepared foods • Alcohol • Artificial sweeteners (Splenda, Equal, Sweet & Low, Truvia) • Dairy products (except kefir & greek yogurt) • "Diet" Foods (with saccharin, artificial colors, flavors, etc.) • Food additives (sulfites, preservatives, benzoates, etc.) • Farmed Fish • Fried foods - Fries, potato chips, nachos, etc. • GMOs (genetically-modified organisms / Glyphosate • Hydrogenated & Trans Fats (margarine, shortening) • Hydrogenated Oils - soybean, sunflower, corn, vegetable oil • Microwave popcorn • Processed meats • White flour (refined) • Wheat products • White sugar & sweets

Stevia & Sugar: Although it has been proven that sugar does NOT cause cancer to grow or spread more quickly and that our body's cells actually need sugar to keep our vital organs functioning, I have chosen to limit my pure sugar intake to those found in fruits and vegetables. When I want to sweeten anything, I use either pure 100% STEVIA extract, honey, maple syrup, agave syrup or molasses. With my coffee or tea, I add a dash of Turmeric and a pinch of STEVIA.

Carbohydrates & Gluten-Free Products: I try to stay away from carbohydrates or food with gluten. However, if I feel like eating rice, I'll choose brown, red or black (emperor's or "forbidden") rice. If I feel like eating breads, I'll choose sourdough bread. For pasta, I'll get those that are made with gluten-free flour. Of course, I eat these foods in moderation, e.g. one slice of bread or a cup of rice or pasta.

Interestingly, I've found that there are a variety of gluten-free flours I can use, e.g. sweet potato flour, rice flour, buckwheat flour, green banana flour, etc. I did have to learn that how my baked good comes out is dependent on the type of gluten-free flour I used.

Keeping it Alkaline: Cancer cells thrive in acidic (low pH) environments. So, I try to keep my diet high in alkaline (high pH) foods. Basically, alkaline foods are vegetables, beans and grains, gluten-free bread, grasses, sprouts and good oils (avocado, coconut, flax and olive) and certain nuts and seeds, i.e. almonds, coconut, flax seeds, pumpkin seeds, sesame seeds and sunflower seeds.

I keep away from acid (low pH) foods, like meats, seafood, dairy, eggs, fruit, sweeteners, alcohol, colas, energy drinks, sweet fruits (dates, peach, strawberries, orange, honeydew, pineapple, plum, etc.) and certain nuts and seeds, i.e. cashew, peanuts, pecans, pistachios, brazil nuts, hazelnuts, macadamia nuts. When I do any of the above, I do so in moderation.

Water: I try to drink, at least, three 16-oz glasses of water in the morning and two 16-oz glasses of water in the afternoon/ evening. To be properly hydrated, the general rule is "drink between half an ounce and an ounce of water for each pound you weigh, every day." Water maintains the balance of fluids in our body and ensures proper digestion, absorption, circulation, creation of saliva, transportation of nutrients and maintenance of body temperature.

Body Detox: To remove toxins from my body and strengthen my liver, I occasionally down a combination of one teaspoon apple cider vinegar with the juice of half a lemon, which I drink first thing in the morning, on an empty stomach. I don't do it daily, because it has affected my teeth. I also learned it best to sip the liquid detox with a straw placed on my tongue towards the back of my mouth, to avoid the it affecting my teeth.

Bean Puree: I found a creative way to use beans. Aside from eating it whole on a dish, I found that pureeing the beans with some liquid (water, broth) and adding some salt, granulated garlic and chopped onions made for a nutritious, savory and healthy salad dressing. Try it,. It's nutritious and delicious!

* *Cindy L. (Kidney cancer)*

I was the typical kidney cancer patient with a very low vitamin D level. So, after surgery, my doctor put me on 50,000 international units (IUs) of vitamin D daily for eight weeks. Aside from the supplements, I also ate Greek yogurt with a good amount of vitamin D three to four times a week.

ADVICE: Make sure your doctor checks your vitamin D level to make sure it's sufficient; more so if you're a kidney cancer patient. Vitamin D is responsible for your immune system and your bones. It helps in the absorption of magnesium. Studies have proven that vitamin D deficiency plays a big role in chronic kidney disease. Since you cannot buy high doses of vitamin D in the market, get a prescription from your doctor. Also, eat Greek yogurt that has a good amount of vitamin D in it for about three to four times a week.

* *Cindy R. (Metastatic Breast cancer to the Stomach)*

For my treatment, I didn't really do anything that was holistic. I just thought, "I've been getting conventional medical treatment, I might as well stick to that." However, I did some serious research on nutritional healing and learned everything I could about food, how it affects our bodies and what people have found that has helped them. In my research, I discovered that foods like turmeric, asparagus, greens … just tons and tons and tons of greens strengthen our bodies and prevent sickness. So, I've juiced them; I've "smoothied" them; I've had them in soups; I've just eaten them in a salad, everything. Even though I eat them everyday, I couldn't go completely vegan.

I also heard about the sugar controversy. At first, it was like, "Don't eat sugar; it's really bad for you. Cancer eats sugar." And then I heard, "Well, it might not be as bad, because our bodies do need some sugar." Anyway, I really cut back on sugar by just not eating desserts and really trying to watch how much sugar I consume.

ADVICE: Nutrition is super important for the strength and healing of your body. Even if you're receiving medication from your doctor, you need to eat the right foods to take care of your body, so that you don't get sick or get a recurrence of your cancer. Turmeric, asparagus and greens, in any form, are best. Eat plenty of those everyday. Cut back on sugar, as much as you can, especially those in desserts. Yes, your body needs sugar, but you can get it from fruits and some vegetables, like carrots and beets.

Here are stuff I believe helped me get well (I like to do natural things)
- Cut back on sugar a lot; no more than 26 grams per day. Cancer feeds on sugar. So, it makes sense to cut way back, if not eliminate it altogether.
- Eat kale and spinach daily in a salad

- Eat cooked Asparagus! Canned can be used - preferably the brands Giant or Stokley, because they contain no pesticides or preservatives.
- According to the US National Cancer Institute, asparagus is the highest tested food containing "Glutathione", which is considered one of the body's most potent anticarcinogens and antioxidants.

* Hilda K. (Colon cancer)

During my treatment period, I remember eating less meat, because I didn't want to be constipated (one of my chemotherapy side effects). I also ate more soups because I needed everything warm, due to my hypothermia, another chemotherapy side effect I experienced. Other than that, I kind of ate regular food; nothing really different. I still drank coffee and I still drank wine, but not as much as I used to. I definitely stopped smoking, though I wasn't a big smoker to start with. Smoking just scared me. I was really trying to be good to myself.

* Rev. Linda S. (Pancreatic cancer 3x)

I am not a believer in "cancer-fighting food and drinks." Instead, I eat wisely, choosing more vegetables, less meat, and mostly avoiding white foods that convert to sugar. As I have always done, I drink three 16.9 bottles of water a day and sometimes a cup of tea during the day. I have always avoided coffee and sodas because I do not care for them. I also still enjoy a glass of wine with dinner two or three times a week.

I have not changed my diet that much, since I had cancer. I'm close to being a Vegetarian; I use meat, fish, and poultry as side dishes. I enjoy enchiladas, mini-barbeque turkey loaves, baked sweet potatoes, baked chicken breasts, whole-grain macaroni and cheese, collard greens and hot and sour soup.

I think that healthful food can be nutritious AND delicious and not taste like sawdust and look like bird droppings. For example, I was thrilled to see that the October/November issue of Fine Cooking Magazine has tantalizing photos and dishes that everyone would enjoy, like: Butternut Squash and Swiss Chard Lasagne, Heirloom Bean and Potato Cassoulet, Potato and Leek Galette with Rosemary and Sea-Salt Crust, Pasta with Roasted Fennel and Tomatoes, Shaved Fennel Salad with Oranges, Black Olives and Pistachios.

* Scott M. (Metastatic Colon cancer to the Prostate & Pancreas)

We're learning a lot about eating healthy and preventive nutrition. I try to eat organic, natural foods, farm-fresh, grass-fed, fresh fish, however I can. And, I've gone back to eating real food, not processed food.

In my house, we've gone back to eating real butter and not margarine or anything that's been processed. Just use a little bit. Also, there's good fats and there's bad fats. We try to eat more vegetables and fruits. I personally try and limit myself to no more than eight ounces of red meat in a month. I belong to a men's group where we have dinners twice a month and they always have the best London Broils or New York strips. When I go, I'll say, "Just cut me a piece that's maybe three or four bites. That's all I need." Then I put it in my mouth. I chew it and I savor it. That's all I really need. I'm not eating a full 16 ounce steak or I don't go for that 72 ounce steak that you get for free, if you can eat the whole thing, like that restaurant in Arizona does.

Is Turmeric really the anti-inflammatory miracle drug that everybody says? Well, I don't know. But, I do know that I put Turmeric on my eggs now, rather than pepper. So, maybe there's something to it.

Pretty much every cancer center that I know of has a dietitian and easy-to-follow recipes that are cancer-friendly. And, at the hospital cafeteria, they have a cancer-friendly, heart-friendly main course item at lunch.

ADVICE: Learn about eating healthy and preventive nutrition. Try to eat organic, natural foods, farm-fresh, grass-fed, fresh fish, however you can. Go back to eating real food, not processed food. There are several different shows that talk about nutrition and juicing and all those kinds of things. Find what works for you. Watch "Knives over Forks" (on Netflix).

Sondra W. (*Ovarian cancer 3x*)

There was a time when I couldn't eat very much and was on a low fiber eating plan. I could only eat egg salad with egg whites. I ate that and peanut butter and cheese. Normally, I'm not a big cheese person. But, when I got down to not having hardly anything to eat, I was able to tolerate them. I was allowed to have just about any cheese; just nothing spicy, like jalapeno jack pepper cheese. So, I ate Swiss, provolone or parmesan cheese and added them to my dish.

Unfortunately, I'm not able to drink the Boost or Ensure high protein nutrition shakes, because of my lactose intolerance. The same for yogurt or yogurt-based foods. And then, because I'm diabetic, I can't eat a lot of fruit and have to stay away from drinking fruit juices altogether. So, we have to play around with the limited foods that could eat, at that time. So, that made a smoothie not something that I could have.

Now that I'm better, I can have apples, bananas, beets, berries, carrots, green beans, kiwi and potatoes, but I can't eat much at one time. I can also eat broccoli, although they sort of said I shouldn't. What I've always had trouble with – and this is not a cancer thing – are beans, which is unfortunate, because that's something I enjoy eating. The good thing is I can have hummus. I can't eat a lot of soups, because many are cream-based, but I can do chicken noodle and some vegetable soups because they're cooked down. I have a banana every day for the potassium, because if I don't, I'll get leg cramps. As long as I have a half of a banana every day, I'm good.

Also, I bought two anti-cancer recipe books and someone gave me another anti-cancer recipe book called *Clean Soups*. In that book, they have some really good recipes that I'm trying out. I had to modify some recipes, because they add a lot of healthy elements that I'm unable to eat, especially the sugar content. So I'll cut down the sugar and do things differently. Fortunately, I have the energy to try some of the recipes. I wish I could have more greens, but because of my digestive issues, my body cannot tolerate them, at this point.

ADVICE: Have a good discussion with the nutritionist at your cancer center or hospital. They are trained specifically on your cancer and what foods and supplements will work to strengthen you and what won't. They will also take into consideration your other health conditions. Knowing what to eat, when you're going through treatment and taking different medications, can be a really confusing thing, if you try to figure it out yourself. So save yourself the confusion and get help and clarity from your nutritionist.

Susan M. (*Ovarian cancer, Metastatic Pancreatic cancer to the Lungs*)

I also began buying more organic food, especially fruits, vegetables, eggs, crackers, meat and poultry. If I can't get organic, I wash my produce/fruit in vinegar and water and buy products that are as natural as possible. I try (which is hard for me) not to eat a lot of sweets because of the sugar.

Tet M. (*Colon cancer 3x*)

Depending on the type of cancer you're fighting, dark, rich colored vegetables, like broccoli, carrots, squash and dark, leafy greens, are recommended. A nutritionist or your doctor will be able to help you determine what will benefit you the most. Low fat, high fiber diet is almost always the right way to go. Vitamins like A, C, D, E, Beta Carotene, Selenium were my staples back then. PLEASE BE SURE TO CONSULT YOUR DOCTOR before taking supplements.

You definitely must avoid the following:

- Alcohol and tobacco (sorry, but it may interact with your Chemo drugs)
- Cured and/or smoked food like bacon, ham, sausage (again, my apologies)
- Fatty foods
- Red meat, i.e., beef: I found that eliminating beef from my diet helped reduce the number of polyps in my colon by as much as 50%. While it may have been a fluke, there's still no harm in at least cutting down on beef products.

Intermittent fasting is an umbrella term for various eating patterns where you cycle between periods of eating and fasting. It offers benefits for cleansing, detoxification, metabolic health, cognitive function and overall healing from cancer and other chronic illnesses.

It allows the immune system to become more efficient in fighting cancer that is already present and reduces levels of systemic inflammation. When fasting, you'll enter into a state of cleansing and autophagy ("self-eating") where your body will eat and recycle old, dead and damaged cells and then concentrate on building new ones.

Most popular intermittent fasting plans are:

- **The 16/8 Method**: Fast for 16 hours each day, for example by only eating between noon and 8pm;
- **Eat-Stop-Eat:** Once or twice a week, don't eat anything from dinner one day, until dinner the next day (a 24 hour fast), and
- **The 5:2 Diet**: During 2 days of the week, eat only about 500–600 calories.

———————————————

* Amor T. (Breast cancer, Ovarian cancer)

After I completed treatment, I found myself getting tired a lot and losing energy. I knew I had to make some changes to increase my energy. So, I walked for 30 minutes every day and changed my eating habits. I looked into intermittent fasting and gave it a try. I followed the 16/8 schedule where I stopped eating at 8:00 pm and resumed eating at 12:00 noon the following day. It was easy, because I was actually asleep for eight of the sixteen hours. I, basically, skipped breakfast and just had lunch as my first meal of the day.

After the second day, I felt more energized. I found that as long as I didn't stuff myself with carbohydrates (rice, bread, potatoes) before 8:00 pm, I didn't feel any hunger pangs. I did this for three weeks and, actually, lost some weight, aside from gaining more energy. When the three weeks was over, I just resumed my regular eating, which was already pretty healthy, i.e. organic food, no sugar, very low carb intake, and lots of vegetables. When I feel low on energy, I'll return to intermittent fasting, which does help in perking me up again!

ADVICE: Intermittent fasting is a great and proven way to increase your energy and brain function, lose weight and, most of all, boost your immune system. You can try the 16/8 method where you fast for 16 hours and then eat for 8 hours. Best part of about this schedule is that you're asleep for most of the 16-hour period. Or, if you prefer breakfast over dinner, you can stop eating at 4:00 pm and resume eating at 9:00 am the next day. Not only will you feel more energized, you'll find that you've lost some weight too. Just make sure to eat healthy foods and keep foods with sugar, bad fats, GMO or artificial ingredients away.

IMPORTANT: If you're interested in intermittent fasting and you are diabetic, please check with your doctor first..

HEALTHY, EASY-TO-FOLLOW RECIPES

* Amor T. (Breast cancer, Ovarian cancer)

- **ABC Juice**

  Blend together one of each: Apples, Bananas and Carrots. Enjoy a sweet, refreshing & healthy shake!

- **Julio's Tuna Salad**

  In a large bowl, mix together the following. Measurements are based on what you like. Just play around with the ingredients and taste the mixture often to see what you need to add.

• Canned tuna or salmon (make sure it's labeled "wild-caught"	• Raisins
• Pickle relish (3 tablespoons or more)	• Chopped dill
• Malt or balsamic vinegar	• Chopped or granulated garlic
• Onions, chopped	• Mayonnaise (I use vegenaise)
• Bell pepper, chopped	

- **Dutch Baby Pancakes**

    Preheat oven to 375 F degrees & place a 8-10" cast iron skillet into oven. Mix dry ingredients and wet ingredients separately.

(dry)	½ cup gluten-free flour	(wet)	2 eggs
	½ tsp salt		1 tablespoon oil for mixture
	1 tablespoon hemp seeds (optional)		2 tablespoons maple syrup or raw honey
			½ cup cashew, soy or other nut or seed milk

Pour wet ingredients into bowl with dry ingredients & mix well.
Remove cast iron skillet from oven and coat with 1 tablespoon oil
Gently pour batter into hot pan and bake on top shelf for 38 minutes or until golden brown and puffy.
[NOTE: My favorite gluten-free flour to use is sweet potato flour.]

- **T.A.O. (a great, nutritious snack!)**

    Just mix together a can of Tuna, ½ Avocado in chunks and chopped Olives

- **Easy, Flavorful Fish**

    30 oz - 1 lb. of wild caught cod, sole or salmon
    ½ large onion, chopped
    1 leek, sliced thinly
    1 tbsp fresh ginger, chopped
    2 tbsp avocado oil, then 1 tbsp avocado oil (you can use other healthy oils of your choice)

    In 2 tbsp avocado oil, saute chopped onions, leeks and ginger, then set aside
    Salt & pepper fish and cook in 1 tbsp avocado oil
    When done, pour in sauteed onion, leek & ginger mixture.

    Extra Tip: Puree canned organic beans (red, garbanzo, white, split peas, etc.) and add salt and garlic powder, taste. Heat up the pureed beans, put it in a plate and place the above cooked fish on top. Mix as you eat the dish. Yummy and full of nutrients!

* *Cindy R. (Metastatic Breast cancer to the Stomach)*

- **Asparagus Puree**
  - Liquify cooked or canned asparagus in a blender to make a puree
  - Store in the refrigerator
  - It can be diluted with water and taken as a cold drink or a hot drink
  - Take 4 full tablespoons 2x a day (morning & evening)
  - You can also add the puree to your rice or anything you'd like to mix it with.
  - Taking it straight, however, allows the nutrients to get into your system quicker and fight the bad out.
  - You could add a pinch of salt. It's not the best tasting thing in the world, but it works.

- **Cancer-fighting Tea:**

Boil together in water for 20 minutes the following:
- ○ Turmeric Root, chopped
- ○ Ginger, sliced
- ○ Black Peppercorns

- **Cancer-fighting "Purple Drink"**

Mix together in a blender the following:
- ○ 1/3 cup organic cottage cheese (recommend Nonas from Raleys), grind to a cream
- ○ 3 Tbsp flax seed oil
- ○ Frozen blueberries
- ○ Fresh strawberries

* *Rev. Linda S.* (*Pancreatic cancer 3x*)

Here's a fun recipe for Cheese Enchiladas made from scratch. I serve them with a small iceberg lettuce wedge dressed with Italian vinaigrette. I never measure anything; I just eyeball ingredients.

- **Rev. Linda's Cheese Enchiladas**

Directions:

Preheat oven to 350 degrees Fahrenheit

Lay out six (6) small corn tortillas + finely chop a small Visalia onion and a few black olives.

Grate equal portions of the following:
- Tillamook Extra-Sharp Cheddar cheese, Tillamook Pepper Jack cheese & Nuestro Queso Quesadilla cheese.

Place all, but the tortillas, in a mixing bowl and sprinkle in the following:
- Cumin. Oregano. Smoked Paprika. Black Pepper (freshly grated)

Mix above ingredients with a fork

Pour a bit of Old El Paso Red Enchilada Sauce (10 oz. can) in the bottom of a small casserole dish that will hold the Enchiladas snugly

Pour the remaining sauce in a skillet

Dip each tortilla into the sauce before adding the cheese filling

Roll each tortilla tightly and place seam down into the dish

Pour the remaining sauce over all and top with grated cheddar

Cover lightly with foil and bake for 25 minutes until bubbly.

ENJOY!

~ 0 ~

Chapter 15

EFFECTIVE CANCER-FIGHTING WORKOUTS

Whether we're still going through treatment or we've completed treatment, the fact still remains that exercise benefits us all in so many ways. With our predisposition to cancer and our physical circumstances, the question is "how?" Before we delve into the answer, we need to address the question, "Why don't we exercise?"

We now know, more than ever, that taking care of our health should be a priority and one of the best ways to take care of our health is through exercise. However, many of us (I'm definitely including myself here) will find various reasons to <u>not</u> exercise, e.g. I don't have time, it's too hard, I'm too weak, it's boring, etc. For the most part, these are not valid reasons; they are excuses. There is actually a REAL reason behind our excuses to not exercise.

We don't exercise because we want to avoid any experience of discomfort, and exercise is uncomfortable ... compared to our expected reality of comfort. When we exercise, our muscles strain and hurt and we struggle to breathe normally. In short, exercise is hard ... again, compared to our expected reality of comfort. So, what can we do to resolve this?

Well, for one, we can purposefully do simple things everyday that make our bodies "uncomfortable", like get our heart rates up and get out of breath by doing jumping jacks, dancing continuously or even lifting each of our legs or arms alternately while we're sitting down. Merely moving our bodies more than we have in the past is a good start. Then, we can build up from there. When we consistently do these "uncomfortable" movements, we will eventually realize that what was uncomfortable before no longer is. With repeated discomfort comes resilience. When we power through our initial discomfort, we will feel a huge sense of accomplishment and our health will strengthen.

Finally, to answer the question, "How?", my personal trainer Chris Janke-Bueno has provided us here in this chapter, his Effective Cancer-Fighting Workouts. Although the movements are "basic," they have been proven highly effective. I know, because when I came to work out with Chris after my many cancer treatments, my body was bent, extremely out-of-balance and very weak. With these workouts, I gradually gained strength and balance, all of which have helped me to grow healthier every day.

Thanks, Chris!

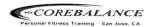

EFFECTIVE CANCER-FIGHTING WORKOUTS

Any type of disease, injury, or illness can wreak havoc on the body. As a cancer patient or survivor, you know that sometimes the treatment can be equally taxing. Recovering from this barrage of invaders might seem like a huge uphill battle. So I encourage you to take small steps, be happy with progress no matter how small, and think of the long term.

You may not be ready to just leap into your local gym and sign up for a membership just yet. That's why each of these exercises is designed with **zero equipment needed**.

It's really important to keep in mind that you will not be doing these exercises perfectly at first. That's OK. In fact, that's how it is designed. If you could do these exercises perfectly from day one, I would say you are ready to progress to a harder exercise program.

So, keeping in mind that progress comes in many forms, here's what you want to keep in mind about simple progressions.

FIRST, get the form down 100%. If you can't do the form exactly like the picture shows, make a modification that feels good. For example, bending the knees, softening the shoulders, or not moving as big of a range of motion.

SECOND, make sure that you feel the muscles that you are supposed to be feeling. Focus on them while you're doing the exercise; close your eyes if it helps to focus. If you don't feel your muscles, you might need to modify a little bit more.

THIRD, once you have the form down and it feels good, now you can begin a time progression. When you start out, 10 seconds might be all you can do. As you progress, start to add more time, e.g. add another 5 seconds, to challenge yourself. Be sure to stay within a time range that feels good.

ULTIMATELY, as with any fitness program, you are walking a fine line. You want to be able to push yourself hard enough to get results, but not so hard that you risk injury. Be extra cautious at this early stage of your recovery. Take it one day at a time, and try not to compare yourself to anybody else (not even to the past version of yourself!

I commend you for your tenacity, and wish you all the best in your mission to become stronger, fitter, and healthier. Let me know how I can help.

In health,

Chris Janke-Bueno
Personal Trainer and Owner, My Core Balance
http://www.mycorebalance.com/

LOWER BODY MOVEMENTS

Bridges

- Lie on your back with you knees bent and your feet flat on the floor.
- Relax your arms out to the side.
- Engage your glutes and lift your hips up off the floor.
- Slowly lower yourself back down. Repeat.

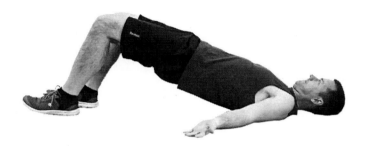

Donkey Kicks

- Begin on your hands and knees.
- Keeping the knees bent at a 90-degree angle, lift one leg behind you so that the foot points up to the ceiling.
- Slowly lower back down. Repeat.

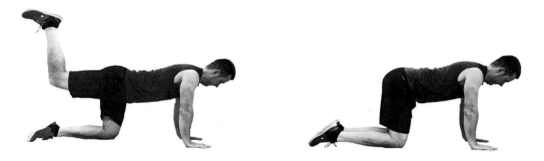

Leg Raises

- Lie on your back with one knee bent and one leg straight.
- Lift the straight leg up until the knees are the same height.
- Slowly lower back down.

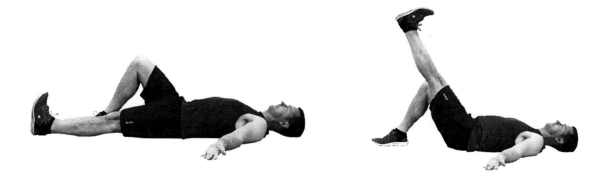

Static Wall

- Lie on your back with your legs up the wall.
- Tighten your thighs, and pull your toes down toward you.
- Make sure that your hips are flat on the floor.
- If your hips come up, move off the wall until they lie flat. Hold for 1 minute.

Foot Circles

- Lie on back with one leg extended and the other leg bent and toward chest.
- Clasp your hands behind the bent knee while you circle that foot.
- Reverse and circle the other way.
- Make sure the knee stays absolutely still with movement coming from the ankle and not the knee.
- For the point/flexes, bring the toes back toward the shin to flex, then reverse the direction to point the foot.
- Switch legs and repeat.

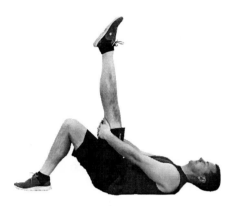

UPPER BODY MOVEMENTS

Elbow Curls

- Get on your hands and knees.
- Bring the knuckles of one hand to your temples with your thumbs pointed toward your shoulders.
- Next, pull your elbows back, and then bring it forward toward the other elbow.
- As you lift the elbow up, simultaneously lift the opposite leg out to the side.

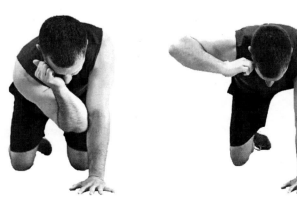

Floor Glides

- Lie on your back with your knees bent over a chair.
- Bring your arms to the floor, so your elbows are at shoulder level and your hands are on the floor.
- Next, slide your arms on the floor so your arms go overhead.
- Lower back down to the starting position.

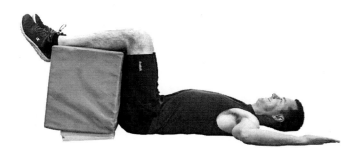

Pullovers

- Lie on your back with your knees bent and your feet flat on the floor.
- Interlace your fingers out in front of your chest, keeping your elbows straight and your palms touching each other.
- Next, bring your arms over your head.
- Perform this motion with very little effort, in fact you're going to let gravity bring you down.
- Once you get to the limit of your range of motion (without forcing yourself down), then return to the starting position.
- Halfway through the set, switch the grip of your hands so that the opposite thumb is on top.

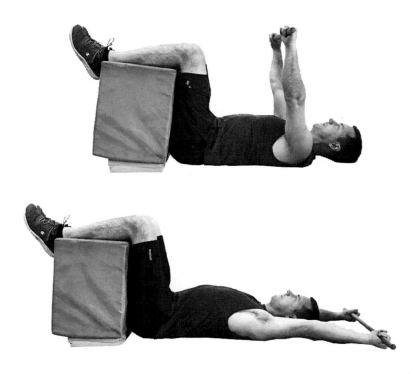

Bird-Dog

- Begin on your hands and knees.
- Next, point one arm forward and the opposite leg back.
- You want to create a straight line from your fingertip all the way to your toes.
- Hold this position for one minute.
- Then repeat on the other side.

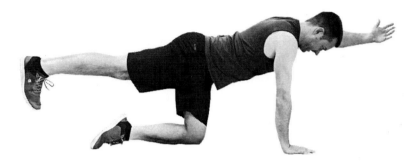

Cats and Dogs

- Start on your hands and knees.
- Roll your hips forward, put an arch in your back, and look up.
- Then switch positions, so that your hips tuck under, your back rounds, and you look down.
- Focus more on the movement than you do on the endpoints of the movement. Repeat for 1 minute.

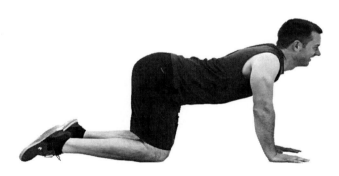

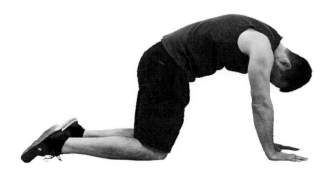

PART FIVE

Chapter 16

SURVIVORSHIP: DURING & AFTER CANCER TREATMENT

A cancer survivor is a person with cancer of any type who is still living. According to the National Cancer Institute, a person is considered a "survivor" on the day they are diagnosed with cancer and throughout the rest of their life. It does not only refer to those who have completed cancer treatment.

When it comes to cancer, survivorship focuses on the health and life of a person with cancer post treatment until the end of life. It covers the physical, psychosocial, and economic issues of cancer, beyond the diagnosis and treatment phases. Survivorship includes issues related to the ability to get health care and follow-up treatment, the late effects of treatment, second cancers, and quality of life. Family members, friends, and caregivers are also considered part of the survivorship experience.

As you will note in this chapter, each of us are dealing with survivorship is our own ways. Post treatment, we are now on another journey in our lives. Truth is, the cancer experience doesn't end when treatment does. Read on to learn how we're navigating our survivorship, making the most of life after treatment, and how you can too.

FACING SURVIVORSHIP

* Aaron C. (Prostate cancer, Skin cancer)

I just realized that if I live another 30 years, a year and a half is going to mean nothing, in the big scheme of things. I figured that I would give myself a year and a half to be out of commission, so to speak. In the big scheme of life, I've already been retired for over five years. So, time goes by fast. It's already been over a year since surgery; it went by really quick. So another six months? You know, it's a blip. It's just a short time and it goes by quick.

You've got to think of all the positive things you have. For me, I think, one: I'm alive. So, that's good, although, I'm not afraid of death. I'm just not afraid of it; I'm not afraid of dying. You've just got to think of all the good things you have in your life and focus on them.

* Amor T. (Breast cancer, Ovarian cancer)

Moving forward after surviving two cancers has been interesting and unexpected. After I went into remission from breast cancer in 2013, I actually put everything behind me and moved forward. However, I didn't really change my lifestyle in being a workaholic, which I now know contributed to my getting breast cancer in the first place. After I went into remission from ovarian cancer in 2016, I had a clearer understanding of how my health must be a priority but, similar to what I did after breast cancer, I put everything behind me and moved forward. However, the BIG difference this time was how I changed my outlook on life and my health.

With the help of my boyfriend Bill I learned how to cook and eat "clean" (non GMO, organic, low carb, no sugar, etc.) as well as strengthen my body through regular exercise. I experienced a lot of side effects from treatment, some of which still remain. Nevertheless, I adjusted and just work with them in my life. My faith and trust in God, which deepened so much while I was going through treatment was the BIGGEST eye-opener for me. The pure peace and joy I found continues in my life; mere words cannot express my immense gratitude!

Having had to face my mortality, I developed something called "canceritis" or fear of recurrence after a cancer diagnosis. When I had a headache, I immediately thought "brain tumor." When any part of my body hurt or felt "off", I thought cancer had returned, and I spent a lot of time researching symptoms and treatments...too much time.

I also experienced "scanxiety" which is the anxiety or worry that accompanies the period of time before undergoing or receiving the results of a medical exam, e.g. MRI or CT scan.

Sometimes, the canceritis and scanxiety still grip me, but I try to push them aside. Prayer continues to help in calming my fears. I don't know if the canceritis or the scanxiety will stop. I just know that everytime they appear, God will provide me with the peace and joy I need. All I have to do is ask ... and trust in His ways. I truly am so blessed!

* *Cindy L.* (Kidney cancer)

There is so much information out there about cancer, but not much about "life after cancer." I've experienced profound changes on so many levels as those closest to me can attest to. Each of us who go through cancer and survive come out a totally different person after the journey.

I have a "new normal" for sure, but always in the back recesses of my mind is the thought that the journey may not be over. And so, that pushes me to live more in the moment instead of 10 or 20 years down the road. With more people surviving cancer, it's important to recognize that there can be a very serious emotional fallout and the need for a psychosocial care plan for survivors is real. There are ways to help survivors like me face the fear of recurrence, learn to channel that fear into something else and move on with living life. That fear can lead to paralysis, so learning how to face it is critical.

My husband talked with me about his military training, and how in the military, they train the soldiers on how to survive. And, it's not a physical thing. It's how they look at certain things and focus on a goal. They take little steps at a time towards that goal, so they feel a little accomplishment here and there. And that strengthens them. I can definitely learn from them because these soldiers, are out on the battlefields and have seen things that would cause me to immediately crumble onto the ground. Yet, they don't talk about it. Yes, I can definitely learn a whole lot from them.

The first thing I learned to do was recognize it for what it was: fear of recurrence based on my experience. Even though I knew the fear was in my head, it still felt real. I had anxiety where I couldn't separate reality from my fear and it was paralyzing. In time, and with the help of my psychologist, I learned that I can't be happy 24/7. Whenever I'm unhappy, I should just go ahead and feel it, own it and then move on. I just shouldn't unpack and live there in my unhappiness.

Right now, I'm more concerned about the actual kidney function of my remaining kidney than I am about there being cancer somewhere. That's the biggest thing for me right now. So, I have a few of my thoughts in pictures, and I also have positive thoughts and prayers to keep kicking cancers ass!!! In the middle of it all, I am always reminded of this passage from the Bible *Isaiah 43:2:* "When you go through deep waters, I will be with you."

ADVICE: If you find yourself afraid, feeling anxious or getting depressed about the possibility of cancer returning, first know that it's normal to feel that way. For many survivors, cancer is a traumatic experience that does not end with the last medical treatment and going into remission. Let yourself have those feelings. You can also have your little pity party with them. Get it out of your system. But then, pull yourself up by your bootstraps and move on.

Find a way to channel your fear into something else. Focus on a goal, like finishing a project or going out with friends or family. After you identified that goal, then take little steps at a time towards that goal. Even little simple steps like getting up from your chair or physically picking up a book or walking to the window one step at a time to look at the activity outside or just pet your dog or cat ... any activity that gets you moving, not just staying in your negative thoughts. Follow each little step with another little step towards your goal. When you take those little steps, one at a time, you'll feel a sense of accomplishment here and there. Don't be hard on yourself if you're not unable to take a certain step. Be kind to yourself and take a deep breath. The main thing is to focus on your goal to take your mind off of those anxious thoughts and keep yourself moving.

Also, remember that nobody wants to be around a Debbie or Danny Downer all the time. Of course, you can't be happy 24/7. When you feel unhappy, go ahead and feel it, own it, and then move on. Just don't unpack and live there in your unhappiness.

I believe that every cancer patient who has completed cancer treatment should go through a psychosocial care plan to understand their survivorship. Such plans are not actively promoted or are simply non-existent at some treatment facilities. This is so unfortunate because with more people surviving cancer, that means that there are more of us trying to pick up the pieces of our lives after suffering through cancer.

People can say that as a survivor, I'm just afraid to die. Well, not that that isn't true. There's a whole snowball effect that comes with having experienced a deadly disease, like hearing the phone ring after completing a test or scan. The reason I dreaded hearing the phone ring was because when I heard the phone ring before, I got the news that I had cancer. Some people may think, "Oh, that's silly." To them, I say, "Walk a mile in my moccasins."

I'm now more aware of time. I have a sense of urgency in life where I can't see my future. Of course, no one can actually see the future. However, having gone through cancer and facing possible mortality, I can say that I really can't see my future.

ADVICE: Ask your doctor about the psychosocial care plan offered at the cancer facility you are being treated at. Even though you may not think you need it, you should avail of it because you'll learn critical information about life after cancer that you didn't know existed. You really need to be aware and be prepared. If for some reason, your cancer facility does not offer a psychosocial care plan or something similar, then ask them where one is offered. You need to pursue this for you, not for them, so please speak up.

If you feel that you're struggling with your life after cancer, especially in feeling incomplete or weaker than you were before treatment, seek help from a psychologist. Don't try to wing it yourself, because you can easily get lost in the negativity and fear. A trained professional has the experience and knowledge you need to guide you out of your struggles.

* Cindy R. (Metastatic Breast cancer to the Stomach)

My first time around (with breast cancer), they said that after five years, I can stop taking the breast cancer prevention pill Tamoxifen. So, at that time, I was in that frame of mind, thinking of how the years will pass without cancer. Then, I hit my ten-year anniversary mark. To celebrate, my sister (also a survivor) and I did the Relay for Life through the American Cancer Society. We walked on the track as survivors, and each got t-shirts and a medal. I got the medal for surviving the first five years cancer-free.

Then we both trained for and walked the Avon Breast Cancer Walk. That was, oh my gosh, that was crazy hard. Still, we both did it. It was really exciting because when survivors like us reached the end, they had us walk through all these people on both sides cheering us on. The tears were just flowing, and they led us right up to the front of the stage, and they celebrated the survivors. So, my sister and I did that, and we celebrated our survivorship.

All throughout my experience, I tried to stay positive. Even though I went through a tough time with the last diagnosis (metastatic breast cancer in the stomach) and treatment, I remained positive. Going through it twice, I really tried not to think so much about surviving and living with cancer. I just tried to focus on living with a purpose and living the best life I can, in the most positive way I can. One thing I do want to do, and thankfully with your help, is get information out to everybody about how to cope with cancer. So, if anyone asks me, I'm more than happy to talk with them about it and share my experience, so that they can learn and, hopefully, benefit from my help.

ADVICE: After treatment, you should definitely celebrate your survivorship as much as you can. It's really quite an achievement and something you should be very proud of. Of course, you may have anxieties about getting cancer again. Well, you have to push those anxieties out and replace them with positivity and everything you want to do to enjoy life. Focus on living with a purpose and living the best lifei you can in the most positive way you can. Don't have the attitude of a victim. Have the attitude of a winner, and be proud of it. Let that thinking energize you!

* J.B. (Salivary gland cancer)

My last treatment was over a year ago, and I feel relief. Before my radiation treatment, my case went before the Tumor Board. Because radiation therapy actually adds risk for me developing a separate type of cancer, this group of oncologists had to discuss whether radiation treatment would benefit me in both the short term and the long run.

Since I'm so young, they determined that the radiation therapy would be the best option for me. Psychologically, I have to worry about recurrence, but I was told my odds are good, considering my age and health. If my cancer were to recur, then it may happen in 10 or 20 years. So, this possible recurrence causes me anxiety. However, I'm learning everyday how to cope with it.

* Rev. Linda S. (Pancreatic cancer 3x)

I have gone through a lot of emotions and soul-searching since I was first diagnosed. My cancer is my cancer and side effects are side effects. I have high-energy days, and I have low-energy days. Most of my days aren't dark even though those days are often brutal. Much of the time, I enjoy my family, friends, my handsome dog Murphy, daily spiritual practices, church, spiritual direction practice, shopping, cooking, dining out, reading, watching excellent movies and television shows, sitting in silence and reminiscing or talking to God, enjoying my house - just appreciating the things I have, in spite of living with a life-limiting illness. I am thankful.

* Rick S. (CLL: Blood & Bone Marrow cancer)

There are cancer support groups where people who've gone through similar experiences with cancer understand each other and share together. I just didn't attend because I didn't want to dwell on my cancer. I have a tendency to dwell. So, I just wanted to move on to other things.

The Leukemia Society is a good resource for CLL. They sent me a big folder that contained all the written pamphlets about leukemia.

* Scott M. (Metastatic Colon cancer to the Prostate & Pancreas)

So, I've survived cancer. I'm now helping others with cancer. That makes me feel really good.

As far as emotions go, you're going to go through the full gamut, and I'm sure the psychologist will tell you. You're going to go through anger and depression, and then you're going to be sad and you're going to say, "Why me?" and all that. Hopefully, after you process it all in time, you'll end up in a happy place.

* Susan M. (Ovarian cancer, Metastatic Pancreatic cancer to the Lungs)

After completion of treatment, it's a great time to celebrate and be grateful. As time goes by, however, it can sometimes be a struggle to return to "normalcy" and keep positive. There are times with thoughts of recurrence appear out of nowhere, and I get upset.

I found that the more I read about cancer the more upset I became. So I stopped reading and began to stay focused on being a more positive person. I put the negative thoughts in the back of my head and prioritized what really matters. When something upsets me, I ask myself, "Is it worth my energy to fret over?" If the answer is "No", then I move away from it. I'm not always positive, but I try to be. Also, I can still get depressed. When that happens, I use meditation, which helps considerably.

* Tet M. (Colon cancer 3x)

Focus on one main thing: Cancer can AND will be beaten. Fighting and surviving is the best reward you can get and the best gift you can give to your loved ones who stood by you during the darkest times.

* Vida B.A. *(Breast cancer)*

When I was told that I was in remission, that I was as normal as I could be, of course, I was happy. My dark times of dealing with chemo and radiation treatments are in the past and now, I'm free! I can go around with no problems, and I can drive. I even brought my sister to provinces we've never been to before. I'm just loving life right now!

However, for me there is a negative part. That part is not knowing what to do next. In my case, I really didn't want to stress anymore, so I closed my store and sold my business. I didn't have to deal with the employee or client issues anymore. I'm done with all that. So the questions are: What's next? How will I earn a living? Thank God, I have some savings, but I do need to do something to have income.

> **ADVICE:** It is such a blessing to be able to survive cancer. Even though the next step on what to do next is a reality check, keep a focus on your blessing and enjoy your second chance with life. Enjoy it, and don't panic. Think positively of your options and what you can do; not what you can't do. This is your opportunity for new beginnings.

* Yesi L. *(Breast cancer: triple positive)*

Facing life immediately after cancer treatment was probably one of the most difficult experiences for me. There was no one guiding me anymore. I had a nurse navigator before who guided me through my entire cancer treatment. But now, in remission, I was expected to return to normal. However, I didn't feel "normal". I had to find my new "normal". My life had been impacted in so many ways psychologically, emotionally and physically, which meant I had absolutely changed! I did not know what to do.

So, I lived in a void for almost a year, trying to get myself to a "new normal". However, since I didn't have professional help at the time, I was in a lot of denial. I thought I was okay, but I really wasn't. I was alive, but I wasn't happy. I felt very agitated, upset, resentful ... and I didn't have any happy feelings. That was the sign. I just beat cancer's ass and I didn't have happy feelings. There was definitely a problem that was beyond my control.

Looking back, it was absolutely a sign of PTSD (Post Traumatic Stress Disorder). At that time, I wasn't aware it was a problem because I just thought I was trying my best to move on even though deep down, I wasn't happy. I was all negative. Unfortunately, my daughter noticed it too. She noticed that I was sad, very agitated and she felt sad along with me. So, she was definitely affected.

It took my very patient husband about a year of dealing with my negative state to understand that there was something going on inside of me that was stuck. We had a very, very serious conversation about my negative condition and a harsh decision that had to be made. Looking back, I'm glad we had that serious conversation and made that hard decision because then I snapped out of it.

I went to see a psychologist who explained to me how various cancer treatments can affect the brain. In my case, my treatments sucked my brain dry of serotonin. Unfortunately, my body cannot produce serotonin; it is only produced within the brain and does not go beyond the blood-brain barrier. So, it was definitely out of my control. He gave me a prescription of antidepressants, which have been a lifesaver for me. Now, I definitely understand that I was given a second chance in life. I am very happy and it's one of the most amazing feelings!

> **ADVICE:** Check your emotions. You just beat cancer's ass. That is a major accomplishment! However, if you don't feel any happiness, if you feel very agitated, upset or resentful, then you have a problem. Ask yourself, "Am I really happy?" "Am I really enjoying getting the second chance at life?" If the answer is "No", then there is definitely some psychological issue, and you must seek professional help, like reach out to a psychological therapist.
>
> Also, it's important to keep in mind that your family and friends love you. If they're pointing out to you that you are behaving negatively (something no one tends to see in themselves), it's because they love you and want to help you. So, don't get defensive. Be very open-minded and look for the signs yourself. The biggest sign is <u>no happy thoughts.</u>

* Aaron C. (Prostate cancer, Skin cancer)

Health is important to have. I was lucky that my cancer was caught early you know. I had a police friend of mine who died of prostate cancer, and he was younger than me. He didn't catch it in time. When he found out, his cancer was at stage IV, and he died within a year. Also, he had a 14-year old daughter he left behind. So, I think only of how devastating it would be for my children and how I can't be selfish or just think about myself in that regard.

I'm not afraid of surgery; never have been. Actually, it's like taking a great nap, you know. Some people are deathly afraid of hospitals. I'm not. I was never afraid of having surgery because I knew that the doctor I chose would be a good doctor, and he was definitely the best the hospital had.

I remember that there were a few things that were uncomfortable during treatment, but it was just a few, in the grand scheme of things. You've gotta look at it this way.

* Amor T. (Breast cancer, Ovarian cancer)

When I completed treatment and no longer had to return to the Cancer Center to get my port flushes, I felt sad. I also felt alone. The staff there, especially my doctor and oncology nurses there, were like family to me. I felt like I was also leaving behind my survivor sisters and brothers who shared my experience at the Cancer Center. We had created a "fun" group and with my last medical visit there, I didn't know when I would see them again. Well, as life would have it, I did see them many more times after, whether coincidentally or planned. It taught me again that we create our own opportunities and don't have to fall "victim" to our circumstances.

My new "normal" started when I changed my diet and lifestyle. I focus now on being thankful for EVERYTHING, even challenging situations (like being stuck in traffic when I'm late) because such situations enable me to see what I CAN do, i.e. take a deep breath, relax, think good thoughts and learn to manage my time better versus what I can't do, i.e. make traffic move with my frustrations. My stressful days are over for two reasons: (1) I am no longer working in a regular job in a toxic environment; I dictate my own hours in writing this book, and (2) I have finally found happiness, peace, stability, balance and true love in my life with Bill. Moving forward, I see more fun, fulfilling, learning life adventures.

As of this writing, I am in complete remission, meaning there is no evidence of cancer in body. I am fully aware, however, of the possibility of recurrence because it has happened to others. Nevertheless, I am not discouraged. Currently, there is an estimated 16.5 million cancer survivors in the United States and that number is projected to increase to 20.3 million by 2026. I believe there's a very strong possibility that with my focus on healthy living and proper nutrition together with the amazing advancements in western medicine working with proven complementary medicine, I will be one of the 20.3 million survivors in 2026. In the meantime, I will continue to work on being the best me I can possibly be and spread love and peace wherever I go.

* Cindy L. (Kidney cancer)

I'm part of midlife communities now. My friend Michelle and I started a Facebook group called "**Midlife at the Cabana.**" It's a perimenopause and menopause support group page where anyone who wants to stay awesome through midlife and beyond can join. It's a closed group site where members share their midlife experiences, have fun, and make friends. Those who want to join and add to the conversation just have to promise to be polite and respectful even if they do not agree with someone's position. No medical advice is given, and no promotion of products for sale is allowed. Search for us on Facebook: **Midlife at the Cabana - Perimenopause and Menopause Support**

I'm now living my life in certain increments, which is part of my new reality as a cancer survivor. I'm living in the now and living six months at a time, based on the scheduled follow-ups with my oncologist. Right now, I don't know what I'm facing or if new symptoms will arise or anything like that. My thoughts on these are off. That's kind of a new "normal' for me. I know over time that I'll learn to live with a certain amount of fear, and I'll also learn how to change my attitude towards it. I have to learn, or else I'll just go nuts.

I could choose to take anti-anxiety medications like Xanax or Ativan. But, they're very addicting and I would be doped up for the rest of my life if I chose to do that. But, I know that I definitely don't want to live like that; I want to enjoy life. So, I'm working hard to learn how to deal with my fears.

I told my doctor, "You know, I am a strong woman. I am one of the strongest women, mentally, that I know of, until cancer came and slapped me in the face." He told me, "You're still strong. However, having a strong personality or a strong character does not get somebody through this. Eventually, that strong personality or strong character is going to crumble." I realized the critical importance of getting a trained professional to help me cope and figure things out. Eventually, I learned to deal with my fears and anxieties; thanks to my psycho social treatment plan.

By the way, I know that, along with my new "normal", my family and friends who have been my support system are forced to live with me on a new "normal" too. I am so blessed and grateful to have them in my life.

ADVICE: Create that new "normal" of living with your fears and learn how to change your attitude towards them. Things are never going to go back to the way it was before your diagnosis. That's reality, and you can't change it. Besides, the people in your life have to decide if they can live with your new normal.

If you're having a hard time dealing with your new "normal," that's understandable. Nobody can get out of this experience unscathed. I suggest therapy for yourself and your caregivers if they too are having a hard time. There is family therapy. Hopefully, your treatment center offers this program.

Survivorship is individual for each person. A lot of us compare what life was before cancer and how it is after cancer. There are physical and mental limitations to consider and, along with them, worries on how to manage life with those limitations. The physical limitations tie in with the emotional because hey, I can't just go out and dump any sauce on whatever I'm eating now. That has been taken off of my food list. There are even certain whole food groups that I can't eat because my body is now functioning with only one kidney.

It's a scary thing.

I love bacon, Canadian ham, and sausage. Before my diagnosis, when I wanted a bacon sandwich, I just went and got one. But now, I can't. Before my diagnosis, I was able to lift a 50-pound bag of cement. Now, I can't. I can't even lift my 25-pound granddaughter. So that has a huge emotional impact. All I can do is sit on a rocking chair and have somebody put her on my lap.

"Things will get better": I keep telling myself that. My loved ones and my support system have been with me in this from early on. Although they've learned to live with my grunting or my other negative actions, I know that I need to cease the negativity. They also have to adjust and are going through their own sense of loss. What affects me, affects them too. Whatever I eat, they'll ultimately have to end up eating too. So, whatever I can't eat, they can't eat either. Think about it. We can't go out to some of our favorite restaurants, because I can't eat the food there. So, that has been taken away from them too. Fortunately, it's temporary and, together, we're learning to deal with it and just be thankful for what we have.

ADVICE: Yes, having cancer forces us to change a lot of things in life. You're not the same after treatment. You now have limitations that you didn't have before, and so you have to adjust. And, your loved ones and your support group have to adjust too. It can create a huge emotional impact for you and everyone involved. It's definitely not easy, but you can't give up. It's all temporary and, in time, you'll adjust and things will get better. You have to believe that, and you have to focus on that. Just learn to deal with it and be thankful for what you have, which is still a lot more than what many others have.

When it comes to support groups, there's a right time to join and a not-so-right time to join. After treatment, I found two support groups on Facebook and joined them. Next thing I knew, they were in my face all day, every day. I was just in the beginning stage of physical healing and I found myself getting so busy supporting other survivors on those sites that I forgot that I needed support too, so, I pulled myself out of those groups to focus on the things I needed to do for myself to heal.

ADVICE: Before you join a support group, think of how you want to participate or not participate. Think of how much time you would be willing to spend sharing with the group and how that would affect your daily activities. Think also of what you would be open to sharing and what kind of support you'd like to receive.

Since I was going through menopause, I joined a Facebook group called "Menopause Chicks." During one discussion, a woman talked about being dry and didn't know what to do. I immediately thought she should just get some lubrication. Since no one gave her any advice, I said, "I'm just being the elephant in the room here. We're talking about things like clitoral sensation and how it goes out the window. I'm just going to put that out there and be an open book." And by golly, 51 women got on the train and said, "Holy cow! Thank you for saying that!" Menopause Chicks is not a cancer support group although there are some cancer survivors in the group.

Since I'm a birth doula and women's issues, like menopause, diet, hormone replacement, diet and health are important to me, I decided to start my own website. I've since been working behind the scenes diligently to get it going. With that, I'm on a new path. I'm passionate about helping women through this phase in life, because quite frankly, there are so many people that sweep these important issues under the rug, something that also happens with issues cancer survivors face. We often hear, "You're going to be fine. Don't worry about it. When you return, everything will be like normal." Well, there isn't a "normal" like before. There is a "new normal."

* Rev. Linda S. (Pancreatic cancer 3x)

(Statement made before recently going into remission)

So, this is my life now. Five days a week for three consecutive weeks, I am at the clinic for lab work, chemo, and Neupogen shots. Then, I'm off from all of it for one week, but only if my labs allow for chemo. If not, the cycle stops for one week, and we begin again. I shared that to say that I find joy and contentment wherever I can and avoid negativity wherever I can. It is essential for my well-being. At least, I'm alive.

(Sharing given after PET scan resulted in NED "no evidence of disease")

Just met with my oncologist who reported that my PET/CT scan was normal. That means no suspicious activity was found in my body from my head to my thighs. Whew!!

My tumor markers remain quite low in the 100s and are fluctuating about 20 points from test to test, but that is still much better than the 3,191 they were a little over a year ago. It also means the cancer remains, so we continue to treat for complete curing AND healing. Whew! Thank you, God. Thank you family and friends for your continued prayers, blessings, good energy, mojos and everything else you have!

* Scott M. (Metastatic Colon cancer to the Prostate & Pancreas)

One way I've moved on is to share my story to give cancer patients hope and help them cope. At the Cancer Center, the nurses would sometimes ask me to introduce myself to a new patient who's there on day one. I would go up to them, introduce myself and just tell them my story. I don't ask them their story. I just say, "Hi, I'm Scott. I'm a stage IV colon cancer patient. I've been here six years, and I'm going into my seventh year." It surprises the new patients because I do not look sick. They see me, I'm healthy, and it gives them hope; it gives them faith. Some people are really, really bad off and having hope really, really helps them. And, I feel really good about myself for helping those people in that way.

Oftentimes, I counsel patients. If they're new, they'll ask me something like, "Well, what was that like for you?" I'll tell them my story; I don't hold back. I tell them exactly what happened, so people might be prepared if it were to happen to them.

I'm also doing pro bono Cancer Center advertisements for the hospital and the marketing department. Also, I enrolled in a fitness program that Stanford offered for twelve weeks free.

At the YMCA, they have the LIVESTRONG program where they have a staff person trained on some of the chemo side effects. They also have free Yoga for cancer patients. I did Restorative Yoga, which is a beginner type Yoga. Since all the patients in the program are cancer patients, you meet people and you share notes and you find some solace in the fact that you're not the only one going through this. And, it seems like once you have cancer, everybody around you has cancer or knows somebody who has cancer, which is true. It is a bond.

So, there's a lot ... there's almost too much out there. So, you find the support that you need and stick with that. You have a lot of options.

* Susan M. *(Ovarian cancer, Metastatic Pancreatic cancer to the Lungs)*

Through my HMO, Kaiser, I found the Roseville Wellness Center and began going there for meditation classes. I also started a yoga class here at "The Lodge" and I go twice a week. At the end of the class, we have a few minutes of meditation. I have learned to meditate at home and really enjoy the yoga, as it releases all negative thoughts and relaxes my stomach. If I have a bad stomach day and go to yoga, I am totally pain free when I leave. It has also helped my sciatica. In addition, I recently started going to the gym to walk on the treadmill three to four times a week. During summer, the heat where I live is in the 90s or 100s Fahrenheit, which makes walking outside difficult.

I attended my first meditation & mindfulness session recently at "The Wellness Within Center". It was great! A small group, but all so very friendly. I plan to continue the Tuesday morning classes, as it really helped me to relax and get more in touch with myself.

* Vida B.A. *(Breast cancer)*

Since I loved the head wraps I wore when I lost my hair to chemotherapy, I decided that I would design head wraps that are dressier. There are a lot of head wraps being sold online, but none like those I will be designing and selling. You see, women could wear my head wraps to dressy or formal occasions like weddings. I would also be an advocate for women with alopecia (hair loss) and would also donate some to cancer support organizations.

ADVICE: You can be creative in how you want to move forward. Talk with your family and friends. Ask for their input. Think about all the things you can enjoy and do differently. Create your new "normal" by enjoying your new lease on life, appreciating what you have and using your talents to share with others.

* Yesi L. *(Breast cancer: triple positive)*

I worked with a therapist and a psychologist. Fortunately, this therapy is covered by my insurance (United Healthcare). And the Cancer Center has a psychologist, which takes my insurance.

I listen to my body, and I listen to how I'm feeling. I acknowledge my feelings. When I do that, I am able to process them and then, let them go. They don't linger anymore, and they're not hurting me anymore. It definitely takes a lot of work.

ADVICE: Definitely, have a network of survivors you can reach out to. Network a lot and share experiences. I am definitely a lot better than I was before.

"Picking Up The Pieces" is a survivors' workshop that is offered by Cancer Care Point and Cancer Center. It is something that is optional. But, in my opinion, I feel that it should be mandatory immediately after you complete treatment. I believe that this survivors' workshop should be part of the treatment because it plays a significant role in the recovery process, which, in my opinion is the most difficult. The workshop can be a lifesaver and can definitely save you a lot of pain, especially in the emotional, psychological aspects of your life. It is also very important for caregivers to take as well because it helps you both understand one another. It also helps you understand your fears and struggles. Most of all, it helps you cope with your "New Normal".

CREATING YOUR OWN CANCER SURVIVOR NETWORK

---

* Aaron C. *(Prostate cancer, Skin cancer)*

I talked with just a couple of prostate cancer survivors over the phone. They were firefighters, and they gave me some good information.

* Amor T. (Breast cancer, Ovarian cancer)

After surviving breast cancer, I didn't think to reach out to other breast cancer survivors because I was too busy putting my cancer experience in the past and moving on with my life. My ovarian cancer journey three years later, however, presented a different set of circumstances, and I grew to appreciate life and slow it down enough to where I could relate to others also living with cancer. When the opportunity presents itself, I offer my assistance to help those going through active treatment or know of someone who is. I find fulfillment in being able to help others.

Many have asked me how I came to know all the cancer survivors featured in my book. Well, it really happened organically. The first cancer survivors I asked to be part of my book were my fellow Lions from the Foster City Lions Club: **Joan, Susan** and **Bob**. Then, I met **Glenn** at a Chemo Brain talk at the Cancer Center and he introduced me to **Scott** who was still going through treatment there. Scott told me about his good friend **Cindy L.** in Florida and I reached out to her. Early on, I had shared with my oncology nurses my dream of writing this book and one of them (ange RN Shelly) brought me and **Yesi** together. I contacted **Rachel** after our mutual friend, Veronica, introduced us to each other. When my mother-in-law Marty learned about my book, she told me about **Cindy R.** and her amazing story of survival. So, I reached out to her. In my bunco group, I learned that **Sondra** was also a survivor and asked her to share her experiences and wisdom. **Rev. Linda** was my former colleague at Mission Hospice & Home Care and I had been friends with **Hilda, Jacki, Rick** and **Aaron** for many years. When I learned that my former college classmates **Tet "Mesky"** and **Vida** had survived cancer, I asked them to share their cancer journeys too. And, last but certainly not the least, when my cousin Amy told me that her son, **JB**, at 21 years of age, had just survived a rare cancer, I was floored and knew that his story would be an inspiration for many, especially those from his generation. I think it's really awesome how we came together and I feel so blessed to have them in life.

I continue expanding my network, simply by reaching out and connecting, whether online or in my community. I truly believe that sharing is healing and it is food for the soul. I'm so blessed to be able to share with you all!.

* Cindy L. (Kidney cancer)

I have a good friend, Eric, whose son was my son Brennan's best friend. He had kidney cancer when he was very young and has never had a recurrence since. He's around 50 years old now. Eric also suffered two major heart attacks and, since he was very overweight then, he lost almost 200 pounds. When he learned that I was a cancer survivor, he said, "You're in a club that nobody wants to belong to. But, you're here." Eric is an inspiration to me.

Beth is someone I used to work with in New Mexico and we got reacquainted on Facebook about three years ago. I vaguely remembered that she had something with her kidney, but couldn't remember what it was because she never talked about it. When I shared my cancer diagnosis on Facebook, she told me that she was a survivor. And, for probably the past 30 years, Beth had been living with one kidney.

And then there's Greg who was diagnosed with kidney cancer 1998. When I first met him, he had just had a nephrectomy. I look up to Beth, Eric and Greg. They continuously inspire me, and I'm so grateful for their support.

> **ADVICE:** It really helps to connect with others who have survived cancer. Even though your individual experiences may differ, you'll still be able to relate to each other on many levels. Like my friend Eric said, "You're in a club that nobody wants to belong to. But, you're here."
>
> The biggest post-treatment obstacle for survivors is learning how to move on. No one can negate the fear of recurrence. It's a possibility we all have to live with. The cancer survivor support system is special and it is strong. Seek other survivors for advice and support. You'll find that there are many who want to help. As you get stronger in time, you'll be able to provide the support and advice needed by those going through the same anxieties and fears you experienced early in your survivorship.

* Jacki S. (Breast cancer)

After my lumpectomy, I did try to go to a cancer support group. I went twice and both times, I did not feel comfortable because I did not have the experience of being tired, of having awful side effects or of feeling depressed. When I went to the support group meetings, I felt so drained, because everybody there was depressed or sad. They had lymphedema and couldn't do anything. They were tired. They felt they didn't have any support. There was so much negativity there. I am a positive person, and I tried to put some positivity in there. But that went nowhere. I tried the support group a second time, but I did not feel any better, so I decided not to continue going to the support groups.

> **ADVICE:** My experience with cancer support groups just taught me that they weren't for me. It doesn't mean you will not benefit from them. They are there and, obviously, those who attend them feel like they're benefiting from the discussions. So, just know that they're there and available for you.

* Joan S. (Rectal cancer)

Find classes you can go to with people who have the same diagnosis, so you can learn what you're going to get into. I remember that was helpful. They met once a month, but it was on Tuesday evenings when I attend the Lions Club meetings, so I stopped going. It can be easy for some, but difficult for others. Try it and see for yourself if it will help you like it did me.

* Rachel S. (Breast cancer: triple negative)

I created my own cancer survivor network to a certain extent. I never went to any of the support groups for a couple of reasons: (1) because I didn't really have time; I felt I couldn't take my boys to the support group meetings with me and (2) I was too tired, and I didn't want to ask anybody to take me. I also had a third reason….and this might sound really bad, but…when I already have so much to take care of for myself, I didn't want to hear other peoples' stories. And, some of the people that I had talked to were very insistent that my experience was going to be the same as theirs. I got kind of tired of hearing things like: "You need to do this" or "You need to do that" or "This is what's going to happen". It's one thing to talk to somebody and hear their story. It's another thing to insist that your story is going to be the same as theirs because everybody's story is different. And so, I didn't go for those reasons.

I created my own cancer survivor network. I had a friend at work who went through a different type of cancer. She went through it about a year before I did, so I reached out to her, and we talked. Also, I had a friend in Florida, as well as a couple I was introduced to over the phone whom I'd call and we'd talk. My husband's HR manager also had cancer. I called her with questions also.

I actually have been in touch with a girl who recently got cancer; her cousin called out to me for help. Now, I talk with this girl almost every day. When we started, she asked me some questions. So, I told her, "Okay, I'm going to tell you a little bit about myself, and then I want to focus on you and how you're doing." I told her that because I believe that's what they really need. They don't need to hear everything that happened with me. They need to be comforted and they need to be able to get in touch with their welfare and situation. I can answer their questions if they really want to know about me. They don't need to know that I had bone pain for months and this is what I did. I'm not going to spill the details on them so, when I told her that the focus of our conversations was going to be her and how she's doing, she said "Okay!" and opened up a lot more.

> **ADVICE:** You are a cancer survivor and have choices in life. You can create your own cancer survivor network by reaching out to other cancer survivors. Do it your way; the way that makes the most sense to you, and never mind what other people think. Also, the word will get out that you survived this terrible disease and others new to cancer will then reach out to you for help. When that happens, you need to focus on the new cancer patient and how they are doing because it's not about you, it's about them. When you share yourself this way, you will feel good about yourself, and you will feel energized.

* Rick S. (CLL: Blood & Bone Marrow cancer)

There are cancer support groups where people who've gone through similar experiences with cancer understand each other and share together. I just didn't attend because I didn't want to dwell on my cancer. I have a tendency to dwell, so I just wanted to move on to other things.

The Leukemia Society is a good resource for CLL. They sent me a big folder that contained all the written pamphlets about leukemia.

* Sondra W. (Ovarian cancer 3x)

When I was going through treatment, my immune system was weak, and sometimes I had to be isolated, so, I didn't join any groups. However, any time I had a chance to talk to somebody while at the Cancer Center or the hospital, I did.

When I eventually got better and had more energy, I went to conferences and met people there. I shared and they shared, and that was really meaningful. I continue being on the lookout for classes or workshops offered by the hospital or other cancer organizations to not only network, but also to gain more insight and learn new ways of enjoying a healthier, cancer-free life. Now that I'm adjusting better during my second round of treatment, I have gone to two conferences and met people there. I am cautiously exploring activities that match my current energy level and taking the opportunity to network with other survivors. Sometimes, we'll choose to have a "NO CANCER DAY" when cancer is not in our conversation because we want to focus on only have enjoying ourselves without thinking about limitations.

> **ADVICE:** When you're going through treatment, talking with other patients can help you cope and even gain a better understanding of your experience. You don't have to join any groups. Just talking with anyone in the waiting room, like I did, can help you feel that you're not alone; there are actually people who can empathize with you and understand what you're going through.

* Scott M. (Metastatic Colon cancer to the Prostate & Pancreas)

I did network with other cancer survivors. I think that it's CRITICAL and I started with the Cancer Center's concierge. She had information on the support groups and things. Even talking with other cancer patients while I was getting my chemo infusions was important. There are a lot of support groups out there. Just put the word out. Even online support groups will help you out.

CURE is a magazine that's free for cancer patients. They have a website you can go into: www.curetoday.com. The magazine talks about all different types of cancers, what some of the latest research is, and stories about cancer survivors. They've got an online version. You can also subscribe to the print version if you prefer to read a magazine, like I do. I'm old school.

There's also the Cancer Club that's online that's HUGE! And you can actually join and just read other people's posts without ever posting anything.. It's a big blog and you can see what the topic is and what the questions are and what the responders all say. I've actually learned a tremendous amount from that website.

And then there's ColonTown, which is a HUGE national online community that's now starting to branch out. It's an invite-only, private website with different types of people. There's a "mayor" for each part of ColonTown, and we're starting local chapters here. ColonTown also has different sites. There's a spiritual site, a site that's all about test trials and where they're located, etc. Some people travel across the country to get involved with certain clinical trials and it's all around colorectal cancer. In our local club, we probably have 20 colon and colorectal cancer patients and we meet every three months. It's invite-only and private, so ileostomies, "the bags" and all that private stuff, patients or survivors of those cancers can talk about openly.

There are all sorts of resources out there. So again, just talk to other people. Ask them what did they use or what's worked for them. Or, you can check online too.

* Susan M. (Ovarian cancer, Metastatic Pancreatic cancer to the Lungs)

I joined RANN (Roseville Area Newcomers and Neighbors) a group of 500+ women. This group has women from Roseville, Lincoln, Auburn, Rocklin and Granite Bay. We have monthly luncheons with great speakers. There are many groups to join, i.e. golf, canasta, Mexican Train, cooking groups, poker, etc. I have met some wonderful women, many who also have had treatment for cancer.

Also, check with the hospital and your doctor's office to see what programs they offer. One hospital I stayed at had a support group and the other hospital had patients and family attend a workshop regarding the administration of chem. That hospital also offered a weekly support group.

~ 0 ~

OTHER INFORMATION YOU CAN USE

BASIC CANCER INFORMATION GUIDE

DEFINITION

Cancer is a name given to a collection of related diseases. In all types of cancer, some of the body's cells begin to divide without stopping and spread into surrounding tissues. Cancer can start almost anywhere in the body, which is made up of trillions of cells. Normally, human cells grow and divide to form new cells as the body needs them.

When cells grow old or become damaged, they die, and new cells take their place. When cancer develops, however, this orderly process breaks down. As cells become more and more abnormal, old or damaged cells survive when they should die, and new cells form when they are not needed. These extra cells can divide without stopping and may form growths called **tumors**. Many cancers form solid tumors, which are masses of tissue. Cancers of the blood, such as Leukemias, generally do not form solid tumors.

Cancerous tumors are **malignant**, which means they can spread into, or invade, nearby tissues. In addition, as these tumors grow, some cancer cells break off and travel to distant places in the body through the blood or lymph system and form new tumors far from the original tumor. Unlike malignant tumors, benign tumors do not spread into, or invade, nearby tissues. Benign tumors can sometimes be quite large, however. When removed, they usually don't grow back, whereas malignant tumors sometimes do grow back.

MAJOR TYPES OF CANCER

There are several types of cancer. Here is a list of what they are:

- **Carcinomas** are the most diagnosed cancer. They originate in the skin, lungs, breasts, pancrea, and other organs and glands.
- **Lymphomas** and **Multiple Myelomas** are cancers that begin in the lymphocytes, the cells of the immune system.
- **Leukemia** is a cancer that starts in blood-forming tissue, such as the bone marrow, and cause large numbers of abnormal blood cells to be produced and enter the blood.
- **Melanomas** are cancers that arise in the cells that make pigment in the skin.
- **Sarcomas** are cancers that begins in bone, cartilage, fat, muscle, blood vessels, or other soft or connective tissues of the body. They are uncommon.
- **Central Nervous System** cancers are cancers that begin in the tissues of the brain and spinal cord.

Understanding Cancer Stages and Grades

When solid cancerous tumors are found, they're diagnosed and assigned a grade and a stage. Oncologists use staging and grades to better understand the disease and select the best treatment.

Tumor grade is the same as cancer grade and indicates the rate of the cancer's growth and how likely it will spread. Cancer tumors are assigned a grade based on the appearance of their cells under a microscope. The more closely the cancer cells resemble normal cells, the lower the grade.

Cancer stage refers to the size of the tumor and if and how it has spread to other organs and tissues. Note that different types of cancer use the stage numbers in different ways. However, generally speaking, the higher the number, the more advanced the disease. Three criteria are used to staging solid tumors:

- T ... extent of the tumor
- N ... presence or absence of tumor cells in the lymph nodes
- M ... presence of absence of metastasis

Cancer Stages

Stage refers to the extent of your cancer, such as how large the tumor is, and if it has spread. Knowing your cancer stage allows your doctor to determine the best treatment for you.

- stage 0 ... indicates that the cancer is where it started (in situ) and hasn't spread
- stage I ... the cancer is small and hasn't spread anywhere else
- stage II ... the cancer has grown, but hasn't spread
- stage III ... the cancer is larger and may have spread to the surrounding tissues and/or the lymph nodes
- stage IV ... the cancer has spread from where it started to at least one other body organ; also known as "secondary" or "metastatic" cancer

Cancer Grades

The grade of a cancer depends on what the cells look like under a microscope. In general, a lower grade indicates a slower-growing cancer and a higher grade indicates a faster-growing one. The grading system that's usually used is as follows:

- grade 1 ... cancer cells look very similar to normal cells and are growing slowly
- grade 2 ... cancer cells don't look like normal cells and are growing more quickly than normal
- grade 3 ... cancer cells look very abnormal and are growing quickly
- GX ... means that doctors can't assess the grade. It is also called undetermined grade

General Types of Cancer Treatment

There are many types of cancer treatment. The types of treatment that you receive will depend on the type of cancer you have and how advanced it is. You may receive one type of treatment or a combination. Be sure to ask your doctor to what type or types of treatment you'll be receiving and why. Here are the more common cancer treatments used.

Brachytherapy
A type of radiation therapy in which sealed radioactive material is placed directly within or near the tumor site deliver a higher dose of internal radiation over a shorter period of time. Sometimes called internal radiation therapy.

Chemotherapy
A type of cancer treatment that uses drugs to kill cancer cells.

CyberKnife or CyberKnife Radiosurgery
A painless, noninvasive technology that offers delivery of high dose X-rays, focused precisely on a targeted region to treat tumors, brain and spine conditions, and cancers.

External radiation (external beam therapy)
A treatment that sends precise high levels of radiation directly to the cancer cells, using an external beam radiation therapy device.

Hormone Therapy
A treatment that slows or stops the growth of breast and prostate cancers that use hormones to grow.

Immunotherapy
A type of treatment that helps our immune system fight cancer.

Intensity Modulated Radiation Therapy (IMRT)
An advanced type of radiation technology that manipulates beams of radiation from any angle to conform to the shape of a tumor, thereby delivering radiation in a three-dimensional pattern that corresponds to the exact tumor location.

Photodynamic therapy (PDT)
Photodynamic therapy is a precise, patient-friendly way to treat some skin cancers and precancerous growths caused by sun damage, by injecting the bloodstream with a special, light-sensitive chemical.

Precision Medicine
Process that helps doctors select treatments that are most likely to help patients based on a genetic understanding of their disease.

Radiation therapy or Radiation Oncology
A type of cancer treatment that uses high doses of radiation to kill cancer cells and shrink tumors.
A treatment that uses special, high-energy radiation energy waves or particles to kill or shrink cancer cells and tumors.

Radiofrequency ablation (RFA)
A carefully controlled thermal heat treatment that uses high-energy radio waves to create very high heat in order to destroy cancer cells within certain areas.

Radiosurgery Radiation Treatment
A procedure utilizing highly accurate targeted radiation in large doses to effectively destroy a tumor or lesion.

Stem Cell Transplant
Procedure that restores blood-forming stem cells in those who have had their original stem cells destroyed by very high doses of chemotherapy or radiation therapy.

Stereotactic Ablative Body Radiotherapy (SABR)
A highly focused radiation treatment that, while using computerized imaging to precisely target a narrow X-ray beam, gives an intense dose of radiation concentrated on a tumor, while limiting the dose to the surrounding organs.

Surgery
When used to treat cancer, surgery is a procedure in which a surgeon removes cancer from your body.

Targeted Therapy
Cancer treatment that uses drugs or other substances to more precisely identify and attack changes in cancer cells that help them grow, divide and spread.

TrueBeam Linear Accelerator
An advanced image-guided radiation therapy system used to treat cancer with speed and accuracy while avoiding healthy tissues and organs.

CANCER AWARENESS RIBBON COLORS

Type of Cancer	Color	Type of Cancer	Color
All cancers	Lavender	Liver cancer	Green (Emerald)
Appendix cancer	Amber	Lung cancer	White
Bile Duct cancer	Green (Kelly)	Lymphoma	Lime
Bladder cancer	Purple/Yellow/Blue	Melanoma / Skin cancer	Black
Brain cancer	Grey	Mesothelioma	Pearl
Breast cancer (women)	Pink	Multiple Myeloma	Burgundy
Breast cancer (men)	Blue (light)	Non-Hodgkin's Lymphoma	Green (lime)
Carcinoid cancer	Zebra Stripe	Oral cancer	Burgundy/White
Cervical cancer	Teal/White	Osteosarcoma	Yellow
Childhood cancer	Gold	Ovarian cancer	Teal
Colon cancer	Blue (dark)	Pancreatic cancer	Purple
Endometrial cancer	Peach	Prostate cancer	Blue (light)
Esophageal cancer	Periwinkle	Rectal cancer	Blue
Ewing's Sarcoma	Yellow	Sarcoma/Bone cancer	Yellow
Gallbladder cancer	Green (Kelly)	Skin cancer	Orange
Head & Neck cancer	Burgundy/Ivory	Stomach cancer	Periwinkle
Hodgkin's Lymphoma	Violet	Testicular cancer	Orchid
Kidney cancer	Orange	Throat cancer	Burgundy/White
Laryngeal cancer	Burgundy / White	Thyroid cancer	Teal/Pink/Blue
Leiomyosarcoma	Purple	Uterine cancer	Peach
Leukemia	Orange	Honors Caregivers	Plum

AMERICAN CANCER ORGANIZATION WEBSITES

General Cancer Support

- American Cancer Society — https://www.cancer.org/
- Cancer CAREpoint — https://cancercarepoint.org/
- Cancer Horizons — https://www.cancerhorizons.com/
- Cancer.Net — https://www.cancer.net/
- CancerCare — https://www.cancercare.org/
- Cancer Treatment Centers of America — https://www.cancercenter.com/
- Cancer Support Community — https://www.cancersupportcommunity.org/
- Chemocare.com — http://www.chemocare.com/
- LiveStrong — https://www.livestrong.org/
- MayoClinic.org — https://www.mayoclinic.org/
- MDAnderson Cancer Center — https://www.mdanderson.org/
- National Cancer Institute — https://www.cancer.gov/
- Memorial Sloan Kettering Cancer Institute — https://www.mskcc.org
- WhatNext Cancer Support — https://www.whatnext.com/home

Financial Support

- American Cancer Society — https://www.cancer.org/
  - (800) 227-2345
- The Assistance Fund — https://tafcares.org/patients/
  - (855) 845-3663
- American Breast Cancer Foundation — http://www.abcf.org/
  - (410) 730-5105
- CancerCare — https://www.cancercare.org/
  - (800) 813-4673
- Cancer Financial Assistance Coalition — https://www.cancerfac.org/
- Cancer Support Community — https://www.cancersupportcommunity.org/
  - (888) 793-9355
- Good Days — https://www.mygooddays.org/
  - (877) 968-7233
- Healthwell Foundation — https://www.healthwellfoundation.org/
  - (800) 675-8416
- National Children's Cancer Society — https://www.thenccs.org/
  - (314) 241-1600
- National Foundation for Transplants — https://transplants.org/
  - (800) 489-3863
- Patient Access Network Foundation — https://panfoundation.org/index.php/en/
  - (866) 316-7263
- Patient Advocate Foundation Co-Pay Relief Program — https://panfoundation.org/index.php/en/
  - (866) 512-3861
- Patient Services, Inc. — https://www.patientservicesinc.org/
  - (800) 366-7741

Cancer-Specific Support

- **Breast Cancer**
  - Bay Area Cancer Connections   http://bcconnections.org/
  - Breast Cancer.org   http://www.breastcancer.org/
  - Living Beyond Breast Cancer   http://www.lbbc.org/
  - Susan G. Komen for the Cure   https://ww5.komen.org/
- **Colorectal Cancer**
  - Colorectal Cancer Alliance   https://www.ccalliance.org/
  - Colontown.org   https://colontown.org/
- **Kidney Cancer**
  - American Urological Association Foundation   http://www.urologyhealth.org/
- **Leukemia & Lymphoma**
  - Leukemia & Lymphoma Society   http://www.lls.org/
- **Lung Cancer**
  - American Lung Association   https://www.lung.org/
- **Ovarian Cancer**
  - Bay Area Cancer Connections   http://bcconnections.org/
  - National Ovarian Cancer Coalition (NOCC)   http://www.ovarian.org/
  - Ovarian Cancer National Alliance (OCNA)   https://ocrfa.org/
- **Pancreatic Cancer**
  - Pancreatic Cancer Action Network (PanCAN)   https://www.pancan.org/
- **Prostate Cancer**
  - Prostate Cancer Foundation   https://www.pcf.org/
  - Us TOO!   http://www.ustoo.org/
- **Sarcoma**
  - Sarcoma Alliance   https://sarcomaalliance.org/
  - Sarcoma Foundation of America   https://www.curesarcoma.org/
- **Skin Cancer**
  - American Melanoma Foundation   https://www.myamf.org/
  - The Skin Cancer Foundation   https://www.skincancer.org/

MISCELLANEOUS TIPS FROM SURVIVORS

* Aaron C. *(Prostate cancer. Skin cancer)*

I joined the Prostate Cancer Organization, but all they want is donations all the time. They didn't give me a whole lot of information. Most of it I found online, just doing my own research, and reading different articles about everything. There's a ton of information out there. Sources like the American Cancer Society or the Cure magazine didn't give me any additional information that I didn't find on my own.

Researching on my own was how I happened to find my doctors. I was searching other doctors online and found a guy who was a urologist in Arizona, who recommended the current doctor I use. He said, "Have you gone to so and so in Riverside?" I said, "No, I never knew he was out there." He goes, "Yeah, this guy's a great surgeon." So I contacted and interviewed this doctor in Riverside and he ended up being the doctor who trained the other doctors on Robotic Prostatectomies, like the one he performed on me.

* Amor T. *(Breast cancer. Ovarian cancer)*

Check out the Cancer Horizons website that has a ton of information about their resources, including free stuck, discounts and perks for cancer patients. https://www.cancerhorizons.com/free-stuff/cancer-freebies/

* Jacki S. (Breast cancer)

Something I'd like to share with everyone: Going into all my chemo treatments, I had a friend who is also one of the ice skaters I coach. She had other friends who also went through cancer and so she knew that to help out was a very positive thing for a cancer patient. So, she did something special for me. Before I went to each of my nine chemo sessions, she would hang a little gift bag containing five to seven fun pink things on my front door. They was every little pink thing you could think of, e.g.: A pink ribbon for my hair, a pink pen, a pink notebook, a pink pair of socks, a pink nail file, etc. So, before each chemo, I would open up my front door and there would be my pink goody bag! That wonderful and kind gesture definitely helped me feel better as a cancer patient and helped me cope with my chemo sessions.

I now continue my own support for breast cancer patients, by buying more pink clothes. I make donations too. I buy Estee Lauder cancer lipsticks (which donate to the cancer foundation). I look into stores while I'm shopping for pink things. And, for the month of October, which is breast cancer awareness month, I would get fun special things in the store. And so, that was a real fun special shopping time to buy pink. I would wear my pink clothes all month. And I would wear pink bracelets and pink necklaces and pink ribbons! I must say, the week before Halloween, I switch to my Halloween clothes. Still to this day, I wear pink all October. Also, I always look for the different companies that sell things to support breast cancer.

* Rachel S. (Triple Negative Breast cancer)

Handicap Placards

Before starting treatment, talk to your doctor and get a handicapped placard issued by the DMV. I would definitely take advantage of that.

PG&E Utility Bill Discount

You may be able to get a medical waiver to get lower utility rates. With PG&E, you have the doctor fill out a form and send it in, and PG&E will lower your energy rate. Mine are lowered for two years. When you go through chemo, you're going to go through hot flashes, you're going to go through cold spells ... you keep adjusting your energy to accommodate that.

* Sondra W. (Ovarian cancer 3x)

American Cancer Society is a great resource. They'll help you in different ways that you might not expect. For example, they'll help you with your wig or appearance-related effects of cancer with their "tlc" program. They'll also provide you with free transportation to and from your cancer-related medical appointments with their "Road to Recovery" program. Their "Personal Health Manager" is also another wonderful resource product that I've found really useful. They provide free to cancer patients.

Bay Area Cancer Connections is another great organization for breast and ovarian cancer patients in the San Francisco Bay Area. They have a lot of classes and speakers that address topics you may be interested in.

In November 2016, I attended their annual conference where they had a variety of really informative presentations, covering topics like recent clinical trials, living and working with cancer, optimizing everyday wellness, medical updates in the treatment and prevention of ovarian cancer, tips and tools to retain health sleep, cancer related cognitive changes, etc. They even gave me two wigs there. They were a wealth of assistance for me.

There's also **Cancer CAREPoint**, a non-profit organization that offers classes and provides a lot of free assistance to cancer patients too. They're wonderful, but I didn't use them as much, only because they're located a bit far for me. Still, for those for live closer, they definitely provide a lot of assistance there that will benefit cancer patients.

And then, of course, there's the **Living Strong, Living Well (LSLW)**, a 12-week, small-group strength and fitness training program specially designed for adult cancer survivors who have recently become de-conditions or chronically fatigued from their treatment and/or disease. This free program was offered at my hospital. The sessions are an hour-long and they trainers look at your entire situation to determine what exercises you'll be able to do.

* **Tet M.** (*colon cancer 3x*)

PLEASE, only follow reliable sites for information, such as Mayo Clinic, Canadian cancer Society, American cancer Society and Johns Hopkins Medicine. They are some of my go-to references. If you care about yourself, please stay away from blogs or sites that can easily scare you to death or provide wrong information. Remember that the internet is a double-edged sword. So, please use it wisely.

~ 0 ~

TIPS FOR THE CAREGIVER

Providing care for someone with cancer, be it your loved one, family member or friend is a HUGE gift. So, before anything else ... THANK YOU! Your giving of your time and energy helps them to cope with the sadness and the shock of their diagnosis, as well as, to maneuver through the maze of cancer treatment. It lets them feel they're valued and loved. Even though you may not quite know what to do, your making the choice to walk alongside your loved one, family member or friend is the first and most important step.

To be a caregiver doesn't mean only taking care of the cancer patient. It also means taking care of yourself. Being honest with yourself and the cancer patient from the get-go will ensure both your needs are met. Make your limits known as soon as you can ~ before they become a problem. This way, you and the cancer patient can better understand each other and adjust, as needed.

CAREGIVER FUNCTION EXAMPLES:

- Make sure the cancer patient eats and gets rest
- See that the cancer patient takes medicine as instructed
- Keep track of appointments
- Take care of insurance and billing issues, as necessary
- Drive the patient to/from appointments and take notes
- Act as a liaison with the medical team, speaking on behalf of the patient, if he/she is unable to
- Help the patient live as normal a life as possible
- Help feed, dress and bathe the patient

HOW TO LOVINGLY GUIDE THE CANCER PATIENT:

- **Keep the patient involved in planning their care.** This enables them to feel they still have a voice and some control over their life.
- **Let them make decisions.** This keeps their self-esteem intact and encourages them to be independent-thinking, If, in your opinion, they make poor choices, respectfully discuss it with them. (NOTE: If they decide to stop taking their medication or limit their activity, as instructed, then get help from the cancer care team.)
- **Agree on what the patient can safely do alone.** Let them do as much as they can.
- **Be gentle in your communications.** If you don't understand something they said or did, gently ask for help understanding what they said or did. And listen with an open mind. Never put them down, or worse, yell at them. Inject humor every once in awhile to lighten the air.
- **Solicit and heed feedback.** Ask your loved one how they see your caregiver-patient relationship working, so far. Heed whatever areas need to be adjusted.
- **Avoid applying pressure.** Instead, appeal to reason and find a way to meet in the middle when you don't agree on how to get certain things done.

- **Be patient**. Having cancer is painful, both physical and emotionally. Emotions run high and are more fragile whenever pain is experienced.
- **Simply be present.** Sometimes your loved one is angry, withdrawn, sad and quiet. Just try to be there for them and offer to listen. If they're not ready to talk, don't force them. They just need quiet time.

HOW TO TAKE CARE OF YOURSELF:

- Be sure to keep your own appointments, get enough sleep, exercise, eat healthy foods, and keep your normal routine, as much as possible.
- Don't try to do it all yourself! Reach out to others. Involve them in your life and in the things you must do for the cancer patient.
- Plan to do things you enjoy that cover the following activities:
  - Those that involve other people, e.g. lunch with a friend
  - Those that provide a sense of success, e.g. exercising or finishing a project
  - Those that make you feel good or relaxed, e.g. massage, watching a funny movie
- Keep a list of things other people can do to help. That way, when someone asks how they can help, you can give the list to them.
- Set aside some time during the day that is "cancer-free", i.e. focus on non-cancer related subject matters, e.g. world news, comedy show, social media, etc.
- Keep a journal of daily gratitude. Each night, before bed, no matter how tired or unmotivated you feel, simply write in one thing for which you are grateful.

~ 0 ~

HOW TO SUPPORT SOMEONE WITH CANCER

Many people struggle with what to say or do when they meet someone with cancer. They want to say the right thing, but are afraid they might say the wrong thing. Here are some Do's and Don'ts to help.

DOs	DON'Ts
• Do listen and be patient with them • Do pay attention to cues when you speak with them • Do pray for them • Simply be there for them - sometimes just being there is the best help of all. • Do encourage them to get a second opinion, if they're not happy with their doctor • Do send them a card or an email that will lift their spirits and make them laugh • Do give them a "Like" or a word of encouragement when they post something on Facebook or a social media site • Do offer to help them in specific ways, e.g. drive them to appointments, cook, take notes, pick up their kids, wash their dishes, do the laundry, research cancer organizations for them, etc. • Do offer to walk with them daily to keep their energy levels up. • (if applicable) Remember that their spouse and children need support too. Let them know. Let them talk or vent, if they need to. • Do be conscientious with your gift giving. Because chemo or other cancer treatment can cause nausea, please avoid anything with scents like perfumed candles, fragrant flowers, etc. Practical gifts are best, e.g. care package of healthy food, comfy slippers, blanket, etc.	• Don't offer advice unless asked specifically. • Don't tell them they'll be fine; you don't know that for a fact • Don't tell them you know what they're going through unless you've actually been through it • Don't' say you wish you can take the cancer away from them, because you can't; it's not reality. • Don't show them you're annoyed with their requests. • Don't tell them you're going to do something and then not do it. • Don't trivialize their concerns. Illness magnifies emotions and issues and, yes, sometimes unrealistically. • Don't complain about their requests or their situation. You wouldn't want others to do that to you if you were in their shoes. • Don't criticize them, even if you say it's constructive. It will come across as negative and does not benefit anyone. _____

~ o ~

GLOSSARY OF TERMS

(Most definitions were taken from the NCI Dictionary of Cancer Terms – National Cancer Institute www.cancer.gov)

	A
Abdominal Cavity	Area between abdominal wall and the spine. Organs of the abdominal cavity include the stomach, liver, gallbladder, spleen, pancreas, small intestine, kidneys, large intestine, and adrenal glands.
Abdominal Tap	A procedure to remove excess fluid from the abdominal cavity, which is the area between the abdominal wall and the spine. Excess fluid in the abdomen is called "ascites." Normally, there should be no ascites within the abdominal cavity
Abdominal Ultrasound	A procedure used to examine the organs in the abdomen. An ultrasound transducer (probe) is pressed firmly against the skin of the abdomen. High-energy sound waves fro, the transducer bounce off tissue and create echoes. The echoes are sent to a computer, which makes a picture called a sonogram. Also called "Transabdominal Ultrasound".
Abraxane	A drug used to treat breast cancer that has come back or spread to other parts of the body. It is also used with carboplatin to treat advanced non-small cell lung cancer in patients who are not able to have surgery or radiation therapy. It is also used with gemcitabine hydrochloride to treat pancreatic cancer that has spread to other parts of the body. It is being studied in the treatment of other types of cancer. Abraxane is a form of the anticancer drug paclitaxel and may cause fewer side effects than paclitaxel. It stops cancer cells from growing and dividing, and may kill them. It is a type of mitotic inhibitor and a type of anti-microtubule agent. Also called ABI-007, nanoparticle paclitaxel, paclitaxel albumin-stabilized nanoparticle formulation, and protein-bound paclitaxel.
Abscess	An enclosed collection of pus in tissues, organs, or confined spaces in the body. An abscess is a sign of infection and is usually swollen and inflamed.
Adenocarcinoma	Cancer that starts in glandular tissue, such as in the ducts or lobules of the breast or in the gland cells of the prostate.
Adhesiolysis	The term for the surgery that is performed to remove or divide adhesions so that normal anatomy and organ function can be restored and painful symptoms can be relieved. In some rare cases, adhesions form without visible or known tissue trauma.
Adhesions	Scar tissue that forms after surgery or injury. If the scar tissue tightens, it may bind together organs that are normally separate. This can sometimes cause problems, for instance, if there is partial or total blockage of the intestine.
Adjuvant Therapy	Treatment used in addition to the main treatment. It usually refers to hormone therapy, chemotherapy, radiation therapy, or immunotherapy added after surgery to increase the chances of curing the disease or keeping it in check.
Adriamycin	A brand name of doxorubicin hydrochloride, which is used to treat many types of cancer. This drug has been taken off the market and is no longer available.

Advanced Healthcare Directive	Legal document that tells the doctor and family what a person wants to future medical care if the person later becomes unable to make decisions for him or herself. This may include whether to start or when to stop life-sustaining treatments. Another type of advance directive lets you choose a person to make decisions for you if you become unable to do it for yourself.
Alopecia	The lack or loss of hair from areas of the body where hair is usually found. Alopecia can be a side effect of same cancer treatments.
Alpha Blocker	A drug that relaxes smooth muscle tissue. Alpha blockers are sometimes used to help men who have trouble passing urine because of benign prostatic hyperplasia (BPH) or other causes.
Alternative Therapy	An unproven therapy that is used instead of standard (proven) medical treatment. Some alternative therapies are known to cause harmful of even life-threatening side effects.
Amoxicillin	A drug used to treat some bacterial infections. Amoxicillin is a form of penicillin that is made in the laboratory. It kills certain types of bacteria. It is a type of antibiotic.
Anastrozole (Arimidex)	A drug used to treat certain types of breast cancer in postmenopausal women. It is also being studied in the treatment of other types of cancer. Anastrozole lowers the amount of estrogen made by the body. This may stop the growth of cancer cells that need estrogen to grow. Anastrozole is a type of nonsteroidal aromatase inhibitor. Also called Arimidex.
Anemia	A condition in which the number of red blood cells is below normal.
Anesthesia	A loss of feeling or awareness caused by drugs or other substances. Anesthesia keeps patients from feeling pain during surgery or other procedures. Local anesthesia is a loss of feeling in one small area of the body. Regional anesthesia is a loss of feeling in a part of the body, such as an arm or leg. General anesthesia is a loss of feeling and a complete loss of awareness that feels like a very deep sleep.
Anesthesiologist	A doctor who has special training in giving drugs or other agents to prevent or relieve pain during surgery or other procedures.
Angiogenesis	The formation of new blood vessels. Some cancer treatments work by blocking angiogenesis, which helps keep blood from reaching ("feeding") the tumor.
Angiography	A test in which a contrast dye is injected directly into a blood vessel that goes to the area that is being studied. A series of x-rays are then taken to who doctors the blood vessels around the tumor.
Antibacterial	A substance that kills bacteria or stops them from growing and causing disease.
Antibiotic	Drugs used to kill microorganisms (germs) that cause disease. Antibiotics may be made naturally by living organisms or they may be created in the lab. Since some cancer treatments can reduce the body's ability to fight infection, antibiotics may be used to treat or prevent these infections.
Antibody	A protein made by immune system cells and released into the blood. Antibodies defend the body against foreign agents, such as bacteria. These agents contain certain substances called antigens. Each antibody works against one certain antigen.
Antigen	Any substance that causes the body to make an immune response against that substance. Antigens include toxins, chemicals, bacteria, viruses, or other substances that come from outside the body. Body tissues and cells, including cancer cells, also have antigens on them that cause an immune response. They can also be used as markers in laboratory tests to identify those tissues or cells.
Antihistamine	A type of drug that blocks the action of histamines, which can cause fever, itching, sneezing, a runny nose, and watery eyes. Antihistamines are used to prevent fevers in patients receiving blood transfusions and to treat allergies, coughs, and colds.
Anti-inflammatory	Having to do with reducing inflammation.

Antioxidant	A substance that protects cells from the damage caused by free radicals (unstable molecules made by the process of oxidation during normal metabolism). Free radicals may play a part in cancer, heart disease, stroke, and other diseases of aging. Antioxidants include beta-carotene, lycopene, vitamins A, C, and E, and other natural and manufactured substances.
Anxiety	Feelings of fear, dread, and uneasiness that may occur as a reaction to stress. A person with anxiety may sweat, feel restless and tense, and have a rapid heartbeat. Extreme anxiety that happens often over time may be a sign of an anxiety disorder.
Arimidex (Anastrozole)	A drug used to treat certain types of breast cancer in postmenopausal women. It is also being studied in the treatment of other types of cancer. Arimidex lowers the amount of estrogen made by the body. This may stop the growth of cancer cells that need estrogen to grow. Arimidex is a type of nonsteroidal aromatase inhibitor. Also called Anastrozole.
Aromatase Inhibitor	A drug that prevents the formation of estradiol, a female hormone, by interfering with an aromatase enzyme. Aromatase inhibitors are used as a type of hormone therapy for postmenopausal women who have hormone-dependent breast cancer.
Arthralgia	Joint pain or physical discomfort where two or more bones meet to form a joint, ranging from mild to disabling.
Arthritis	A disease that causes inflammation and pain in the joints.
Ascites	Abnormal buildup of fluid in the abdomen that may cause swelling. In late-stage cancer, tumor cells may be found in the fluid in the abdomen. Ascites also occurs in patients with liver disease.
Aspiration	Removal of fluid or tissue through a needle. Also, the accidental breathing in of food or fluid into the lungs.
Asymptomatic	Not having any symptoms of a disease. Many cancers can develop and grow without causing symptoms, especially in the early stages. Screening tests such as mammograms and colonoscopies help find these early cancers before symptoms start, when the chances for cure are usually highest.
Atelectasis	Failure of the lung to expand (inflate) completely. This may be caused by a blocked airway, a tumor, general anesthesia, pneumonia or other lung infections, lung disease, or long-term bedrest with shallow breathing. Sometimes called a collapsed lung.
Augmentin	A drug used to treat bacterial infections. Adding the chemical clavulanate potassium to the antibiotic amoxicillin increases the amount of time the antibiotic stays active in the body. Augmentin is a type of combination antibiotic. Also called Amoxicillin-Clavulanate Potassium.
Autoimmune Disease	A condition in which the body recognizes its own tissues as foreign and directs an immune response against them.
Autologous	Use of the patient's own blood or tissue in a medical procedure; for example, using a woman's own tissue to rebuild her breast is called autologous tissue construction.
Avastin	A drug used alone or with other drugs to treat certain types of cervical, colorectal, lung, kidney, ovarian, fallopian tube, and primary peritoneal cancer, and glioblastoma (a type of brain cancer). It is also being studied in the treatment of other types of cancer. Avastin binds to a protein called vascular endothelial growth factor (VEGF). This may prevent the growth of new blood vessels that tumors need to grow. It is a type of anti-angiogenesis agent and a type of monoclonal antibody. Also called Bevacizumab.
Axillary	Pertaining to the armpit area, including the lymph nodes that are located there.
Axillary Dissection	Removal of the lymph nodes in the armpit (the axillary nodes). They are looked at under a microscope to see if they contain cancer.

Bacteria	A large group of single-cell microorganisms. Some cause infections and disease in animals and humans. The singular of bacteria is bacterium.
Basal Cell Carcinoma	Cancer that begins in the lower part of the epidermis (the outer layer of skin). It may appear as a small white or flesh-colored bump that grows slowly and may bleed. Basal cell carcinomas are usually found on areas of the body exposed to the sun. Basal cell carcinomas rarely metastasize (spread) to other parts of the body. They are the most common form of skin cancer. Also called Basal Cell Cancer.
Baseline	An initial measurement that is taken at an early time point to represent a beginning condition, and is used for comparison over time to look for changes. For example, the size of a tumor will be measured before treatment (baseline) and then afterwards to see if the treatment had an effect.
Benign	Not cancerous. Benign tumors may grow larger but do not spread to other parts of the body. Also called nonmalignant.
Bilateral	Affecting both the right and left sides of the body.
Biopsy	The removal of cells or tissues for examination by a pathologist. The pathologist may study the tissue under a microscope or perform other tests on the cells or tissue. There are many different types of biopsy procedures. The most common types include: (1) Incisional Biopsy, in which only a sample of tissue is removed; (2) Excisional Biopsy, in which an entire lump or suspicious area is removed; and (3) Needle Biopsy, in which a sample tissue or fluid is removed with a needle. When a wide needle is used, the procedure is called a Core Biopsy. When a thin needle is used, the procedure is called a Fine-Needle Aspiration Biopsy.
Bladder	A hollow organ in the pelvis with flexible, muscular walls. The bladder stores urine as it is made by the kidneys.
Blood Cancer	Cancer that begins in blood-forming tissue, such as the bone marrow, or in the cells of the immune system. Examples of blood cancer are leukemia, lymphoma, and multiple myeloma.
Blood Cell Count	A measure of the number of red blood cells, white blood cells, and platelets in the blood. The amount of hemoglobin (substance in the blood that carries oxygen) and the hematocrit (the amount of whole blood that is made up of red blood cells) are also measured. A blood cell count is used to help diagnose and monitor many conditions. Also called CBC, Complete Blood Count, and Full Blood Count.
Blood Draw	A procedure in which a needle is used to take blood from a vein, usually for laboratory testing. A blood draw may also be done to remove extra red blood cells from the blood, to treat certain blood disorders. Also called Phlebotomy and Venipuncture.
Blood Pressure	The force of circulating blood on the walls of the arteries. Blood pressure is taken using two measurements: systolic (measured when the heart beats, when blood pressure is at its highest) and diastolic (measured between heart beats, when blood pressure is at its lowest). Blood pressure is written with the systolic blood pressure first, followed by the diastolic blood pressure (for example 120/80).
Blood Sugar	Glucose (a type of sugar) found in the blood. Also called Glycemia.
Blood Test	A test done on a sample of blood to measure the amount of certain substances in the blood or to count different types of blood cells. Blood tests may be done to look for signs of disease or agents that cause disease, to check for antibodies or tumor markers, or to see how well treatments are working.
Blood Transfusion	A procedure in which whole blood or parts of blood are put into a patient's bloodstream through a vein. The blood may be donated by another person or it may have been taken from the patient and stored until needed. Also called Transfusion.

Bone Density	A measure of the amount of minerals (mostly calcium and phosphorous) contained in a certain volume of bone. Bone density measurements are used to diagnose Osteoporosis (a condition marked by decreased bone mass) to see how well Osteoporosis treatments are working, and to predict how likely the bones are to break. Low bone density can occur in patients treated for cancer. Also called BMD, bone mass and bone mineral density.
Bone Marrow	The soft, spongy tissue in the hollow middle of certain bones of the body. This is where new blood cells are made.
Bowel	The intestines, from the end of the stomach (pylorus) to the anus. The small bowel is the part of the intestine that goes from the bottom of the stomach to the large bowel. The large bowel goes from there to the anus, and is also called the colon.
Bowel Movement	Movement of feces (undigested food bacteria, mucus, and cells from the lining of the intestines) through the bowel and out the anus. Also called Defecation.
Bowel Obstruction	A partial or complete block of the small or large intestine that keeps food, liquid, gas, and stool from moving through the intestines in a normal way. Bowel obstructions may be caused by a twist in the intestines, hernias, inflammation scar tissue from surgery and certain types of cancer such as cancers of the stomach, colon, and ovary. They may also be caused by conditions that affect the muscles of the intestine, such as paralysis. Signs and symptoms may include pain and swelling in the abdomen, constipation, diarrhea, vomiting, and problems passing gas. Most bowel obstructions occur in the small intestine. Also called Intestinal obstruction.
BRCA1	A gene on chromosome 17 that normally helps to suppress cell growth. A person who inherits certain mutations (changes) in a BRCA1 gene has a higher risk of getting breast, ovarian, prostate, and other types of cancer.
BRCA2	A gene on chromosome 13 that normally helps to suppress cell growth. A person who inherits certain mutations (changes) in a BRCA2 gene has a higher risk of getting breast, ovarian, prostate, and other types of cancer.
Breast Cancer	Cancer that forms in tissues of the breast. The most common type of breast cancer is ductal carcinoma, which begins in the lining of the milk ducts (thin tubes that carry milk from the lobules of the breast to the nipple). Another type of breast cancer is lobular carcinoma, which begins in the lobules (milk glands) of the breast. Invasive breast cancer is breast cancer that has spread from where it began in the breast ducts or lobules to surrounding normal tissue. Breast cancer occurs in both men and women, although male breast cancer is rare.
Breast Carcinoma in Situ	There are 3 types of breast carcinoma in situ: ductal carcinoma in situ (DCIS), lobular carcinoma in situ (LCIS), and Paget disease of the nipple. DCIS is a noninvasive condition in which abnormal cells are found in the lining of a breast duct. The abnormal cells have not spread outside the duct to other tissues in the breast. In some cases, DCIS may become invasive cancer and spread to other tissues. At this time, there is no way to know which lesions could become invasive. LCIS is a condition in which abnormal cells are found in the lobules of the breast. This condition seldom becomes invasive cancer. However, having LCIS in one breast increases the risk of developing breast cancer in either breast. Paget disease of the nipple is a condition in which abnormal cells are found in the nipple only. Also called stage 0 breast carcinoma in situ.
Breast Density	A term used to describe the amount of dense tissue compared to the amount of fatty tissue in the breast on a mammogram. Dense breast tissue has more fibrous and glandular tissue than fat. There are different levels of breast density, ranging from little or no dense tissue to very dense tissue. The more density, the harder it may be to find tumors or other changes on a mammogram.
Breast Duct	A thin tube in the breast that carries milk from the breast lobules to the nipple. Also called milk duct.
Breast Implant	A silicone gel-filled or saline-filled sac placed under the chest muscle to restore breast shape.

| Amor Y. Traceski

Breast Reconstruction	Surgery to rebuild the shape of the breast after a mastectomy.
Breastbone	The long flat bone that forms the center front of the chest wall. The breastbone is attached to the collarbone and the first seven ribs. Also called sternum.
BUN	Nitrogen in the blood that comes from urea (a substance formed by the breakdown of protein in the liver). The kidneys filter urea out of the blood and into the urine. A high level of urea nitrogen in the blood may be a sign of a kidney problem. Also called blood urea nitrogen and urea nitrogen.

C

CA-125	A substance that may be found in high amounts in the blood of patients with certain types of cancer, including ovarian cancer. CA-125 levels may also help monitor how well cancer treatments are working or if cancer has come back. Also called cancer antigen 125.
Calcification	Deposits of calcium in the tissues. Calcification in the breast can be seen on a mammogram, but cannot be detected by touch. There are two types of breast calcification, macrocalcification and microcalcification. Macrocalcifications are large deposits and are usually not related to cancer. They are specks of calcium that may be found in an area of rapidly dividing cells. Many microcalcifications clustered together may be a sign of cancer.
Calcium	A mineral needed for healthy teeth, bones, and other body tissues. It is the most common mineral in the body. A deposit of calcium in body tissues, such as breast tissue, may be a sign of disease.
Calcium Carbonate	A form of the mineral calcium that is used to prevent or treat osteoporosis (a decrease in bone mass and density) and to treat heartburn and upset stomach. It is also being studied in the prevention of bone problems in people with cancer. It is a type of dietary supplement.
Cancer	A name given to a collection of related diseases. In all types of cancer, some of the body's cells begin to divide without stopping and spread into surrounding tissues. Cancer can start almost anywhere in the body, which is made up of trillions of cells.

Normally, human cells grow and divide to form new cells as the body needs them. When cells grow old or become damaged, they die, and new cells take their place. When cancer develops, however, this orderly process breaks down. As cells become more and more abnormal, old or damaged cells survive when they should die, and new cells form when they are not needed. These extra cells can divide without stopping and may form growths called tumors.

Many cancers form solid tumors, which are masses of tissue. Cancers of the blood, such as Leukemias, generally do not form solid tumors.

Cancerous tumors are malignant, which means they can spread into, or invade, nearby tissues. In addition, as these tumors grow, some cancer cells break off and travel to distant places in the body through the blood or lymph system and form new tumors far from the original tumor. Unlike malignant tumors, benign tumors do not spread into, or invade, nearby tissues. Benign tumors can sometimes be quite large, however. When removed, they usually don't grow back, whereas malignant tumors sometimes do. |
| Cancer Antigen 125 | A substance that may be found in high amounts in the blood of patients with certain types of cancer, including ovarian cancer. Cancer antigen 125 levels may also help monitor how well cancer treatments are working or if cancer has come back. Also called CA-125. |
| Capecitabine | A drug used to treat stage III colon cancer in patients who had surgery to remove the cancer. It is also used to treat metastatic breast cancer that has not improved after treatment with certain other anticancer drugs. Capecitabine is being studied in the treatment of other types of cancer. It is taken up by cancer cells and breaks down into 5-fluorouracil, a substance that kills tumor cells. Capecitabine is a type of antimetabolite. Also called Xeloda. |

CAPOX	An abbreviation for a chemotherapy combination used to treat advanced colorectal cancer. It is also being studied in the treatment of other types of cancer. It includes the drugs capecitabine and oxaliplatin. Also called CAPOX regimen.
Carboplatin	A drug that is used to treat advanced ovarian cancer that has never been treated or symptoms of ovarian cancer that has come back after treatment with other anticancer drugs. It is also used with other drugs to treat advanced, metastatic, or recurrent non-small cell lung cancer and is being studied in the treatment of other types of cancer. Carboplatin is a form of the anticancer drug cisplatin and causes fewer side effects in patients. It attaches to DNA in cells and may kill cancer cells. It is a type of platinum compound. Also called Paraplatin.
Carboplatin-Taxol Regimen	A chemotherapy combination used to treat endometrial, ovarian, and head and neck cancers, and non-small cell lung cancer that has spread. It includes the drugs carboplatin and paclitaxel (Taxol). Also called Carbo-Tax regimen, carboplatin-Taxol regimen, CaT regimen, and PC regimen.
Carcinogen	Any substance that causes cancer.
Carcinogenesis	The process by which normal cells are transformed into cancer cells.
Carcinoma	Cancer that begins in the skin or in tissues that line or cover internal organs.
Caregiver	A person who gives care to people who need help taking care of themselves. Examples include children, the elderly, or patients who have chronic illnesses or are disabled. Caregivers may be health professionals, family members, friends, social workers, or members of the clergy. They may give care at home or in a hospital or other health care setting.
CAT Scan (CT Scan)	A procedure that uses a computer linked to an x-ray machine to make a series of detailed pictures of areas inside the body. The pictures are taken from different angles and are used to create 3-dimensional (3-D) views of tissues and organs. A dye may be injected into a vein or swallowed to help the tissues and organs show up more clearly. A CAT scan may be used to help diagnose disease, plan treatment, or find out how well treatment is working. Also called computed tomography scan, computerized axial tomography scan, computerized tomography, and CT scan.
Catheter	A flexible tube used to deliver fluids into or withdraw fluids from the body.
CBC	A measure of the number of red blood cells, white blood cells, and platelets in the blood. The amount of hemoglobin (substance in the blood that carries oxygen) and the hematocrit (the amount of whole blood that is made up of red blood cells) are also measured. A CBC is used to help diagnose and monitor many conditions. Also called blood cell count, complete blood count, and full blood count.
CBC with Differential	A measure of the number of red blood cells, white blood cells, and platelets in the blood, including the different types of white blood cells (neutrophils, lymphocytes, monocytes, basophils, and eosinophils). The amount of hemoglobin (substance in the blood that carries oxygen) and the hematocrit (the amount of whole blood that is made up of red blood cells) are also measured. A CBC with differential is used to help diagnose and monitor many different conditions, including anemia and infection. Also called blood cell count with differential.
Cecum	A pouch that forms the first part of the large intestine. It connects the small intestine to the colon, which is part of the large intestine.
Cell	In biology, the smallest unit that can live on its own and that makes up all living organisms and the tissues of the body. A cell has three main parts: the cell membrane, the nucleus, and the cytoplasm. The cell membrane surrounds the cell and controls the substances that go into and out of the cell. The nucleus is a structure inside the cell that contains the nucleolus and most of the cell's DNA. It is also where most RNA is made. The cytoplasm is the fluid inside the cell. It contains other tiny cell parts that have specific functions, including the Golgi complex, the mitochondria, and the endoplasmic reticulum. The cytoplasm is where most chemical reactions take place and most proteins get made. The human body has more than 30 trillion cells.

Amor Y. Traceski

Cellulitis	Cellulitis is a common, yet potentially serious bacterial skin infection. The affected skin appears swollen and red and is typically painful and warm to the touch. Cellulitis usually affects the skin on the lower legs, but it can occur in the face, arms and other areas. Complications of cellulitis can be very serious. These can include extensive tissue damage and tissue death (gangrene). The infection can also spread to the blood, bones, lymph system, heart, or nervous system, which may lead to amputation, shock, or even death.
Cervix	The lower, narrow end of the uterus that forms a canal between the uterus and vagina.
Chemoembolization	A procedure in which the blood supply to a tumor is blocked after anticancer drugs are given in blood vessels near the tumor. Sometimes, the anticancer drugs are attached to small beads that are injected into an artery that feeds the tumor. The beads block blood flow to the tumor as they release the drug. This allows a higher amount of drug to reach the tumor for a longer period of time, which may kill more cancer cells. It also causes fewer side effects because very little of the drug reaches other parts of the body. Chemoembolization is used to treat liver cancer. Also called TACE and trans-arterial chemoembolization.
Chemotherapy	Treatment that uses drugs to stop the growth of cancer cells, either by killing the cells or by stopping them from dividing. Chemotherapy may be given by mouth, injection, or infusion, or on the skin, depending on the type and stage of the cancer being treated. It may be given alone or with other treatments, such as surgery, radiation therapy, or biologic therapy.
Chest Wall	Muscles, bones and joints that make up the area of the body between the neck and abdomen.
Chlorambucil-Prednisone Regimen	A chemotherapy combination used to treat chronic lymphocytic leukemia (CLL). It includes the drugs chlorambucil hydrochloride and prednisone. Also called chlorambucil-prednisone and CP.
Chronic Lymphocytic Leukemia (CLL)	An indolent (slow-growing) cancer in which too many immature lymphocytes (white blood cells) are found mostly in the blood and bone marrow. Sometimes, in later stages of the disease, cancer cells are found in the lymph nodes and the disease is called small lymphocytic lymphoma. Also called CLL.
Circulatory System	The system that contains the heart and the blood vessels and moves blood throughout the body. This system helps tissues get enough oxygen and nutrients, and it helps them get rid of waste products. The lymph system, which connects with the blood system, is often considered part of the circulatory system.
CLL or Chronic Lymphocytic Leukemia	An indolent (slow-growing) cancer in which too many immature lymphocytes (white blood cells) are found mostly in the blood and bone marrow. Sometimes, in later stages of the disease, cancer cells are found in the lymph nodes and the disease is called small lymphocytic lymphoma.
Colectomy	An operation to remove all or part of the colon. When only part of the colon is removed, it is called a partial colectomy. In an open colectomy, one long incision is made in the wall of the abdomen and doctors can see the colon directly. In a laparoscopic-assisted colectomy, several small incisions are made and a thin, lighted tube attached to a video camera is inserted through one opening to guide the surgery. Surgical instruments are inserted through the other openings to perform the surgery.
Colitis	Inflammation of the colon.
Colon	The longest part of the large intestine, which is a tube-like organ connected to the small intestine at one end and the anus at the other. The colon removes water and some nutrients and electrolytes from partially digested food. The remaining material, solid waste called stool, moves through the colon to the rectum and leaves the body through the anus.
Colon Cancer	Cancer that forms in the tissues of the colon (the longest part of the large intestine). Most colon cancers are adenocarcinomas (cancers that begin in cells that make and release mucus and other fluids).
Colonoscopy	Examination of the inside of the colon using a colonoscope inserted into the rectum. A colonoscope is a thin, tube-like instrument with a light and a lens for viewing. It may also have a tool to remove tissue to be checked under a microscope for signs of disease.

Colorectal Cancer	Cancer that develops in the colon (the longest part of the large intestine) and/or the rectum (the last several inches of the large intestine before the anus).
Colostomy	An opening into the colon from the outside of the body. A colostomy provides a new path for waste material to leave the body after part of the colon has been removed.
Colposcope	A lighted magnifying instrument used to check the cervix, vagina, and vulva for signs of disease.
Colposcopy	A procedure in which a lighted, magnifying instrument called a colposcope is used to examine the cervix, vagina, and vulva. During colposcopy, an instrument called a speculum is inserted into the vagina to widen it so that the cervix can be seen more easily. A vinegar solution may be used to make abnormal tissue easier to see with the colposcope. Tissue samples may be taken using a spoon-shaped instrument called a curette and checked under a microscope for signs of disease. Colposcopy may be used to check for cancers of the cervix, vagina, and vulva, and changes that may lead to cancer.
Combination Chemotherapy	Treatment using more than one anticancer drug.
Combination Therapy	Therapy that combines more than one method of treatment. Also called multimodality therapy and multimodality treatment.
Complementary & Alternative Medicine (CAM)	Forms of treatment that are used in addition to (complementary) or instead of (alternative) standard treatments. These practices generally are not considered standard medical approaches. Standard treatments go through a long and careful research process to prove they are safe and effective, but less is known about most types of complementary and alternative medicine. Complementary and alternative medicine may include dietary supplements, megadose vitamins, herbal preparations, special teas, acupuncture, massage therapy, magnet therapy, spiritual healing, and meditation. Also called CAM.
Complementary Medicine	Treatments that are used along with standard treatments, but are not considered standard. Standard treatments are based on the results of scientific research and are currently accepted and widely used. Less research has been done for most types of complementary medicine. Complementary medicine includes acupuncture, dietary supplements, massage therapy, hypnosis, and meditation. For example, acupuncture may be used with certain drugs to help lessen cancer pain or nausea and vomiting.
Complete Blood Count	A measure of the number of red blood cells, white blood cells, and platelets in the blood. The amount of hemoglobin (substance in the blood that carries oxygen) and the hematocrit (the amount of whole blood that is made up of red blood cells) are also measured. A complete blood count is used to help diagnose and monitor many conditions. Also called blood cell count, CBC, and full blood count.
Complete Hysterectomy	Surgery to remove the entire uterus, including the cervix. Also called total hysterectomy.
Complete Remission	The disappearance of all signs of cancer in response to treatment. This does not always mean the cancer has been cured. Also called complete response.
Compression	A pressing or squeezing together. In medicine, it can describe a structure, such as a tumor, that presses on another part of the body, such as a nerve. It can also describe the flattening of soft tissue, such as the breast, that occurs during a mammogram (x-ray of the breast).
Compression Garment	A tight-fitting, elastic garment, such as a sleeve or stocking. Compression garments are used in the treatment of lymphedema (swelling caused by a buildup of lymph fluid in tissue). They are also used to improve blood flow.
Computerized Axial Tomography Scan / CAT or CT scan	A procedure that uses a computer linked to an x-ray machine to make a series of detailed pictures of areas inside the body. The pictures are taken from different angles and are used to create 3-dimensional (3-D) views of tissues and organs. A dye may be injected into a vein or swallowed to help the tissues and organs show up more clearly. A computerized axial tomography scan may be used to help diagnose disease, plan treatment, or find out how well treatment is working. Also called CAT scan, computed tomography scan, computerized tomography, and CT scan.

Amor Y. Traceski

Cone Biopsy	procedure in which a cone-shaped piece of abnormal tissue is removed from the cervix. A scalpel, a laser knife, or a thin wire loop heated by an electric current may be used to remove the tissue. The tissue is then checked under a microscope for signs of disease. Cone biopsy may be used to check for cervical cancer or to treat certain cervical conditions. Types of cone biopsy are LEEP (loop electrosurgical excision procedure) and cold knife conization (cold knife cone biopsy). Also called conization.
Confusion	A mental state in which one is not thinking clearly.
Conization	A procedure in which a cone-shaped piece of abnormal tissue is removed from the cervix. A scalpel, a laser knife, or a thin wire loop heated by an electric current may be used to remove the tissue. The tissue is then checked under a microscope for signs of disease. Conization may be used to check for cervical cancer or to treat certain cervical conditions. Types of conization are LEEP (loop electrosurgical excision procedure) and cold knife conization (cold knife cone biopsy). Also called cone biopsy.
Constipation	A condition in which stool becomes hard, dry, and difficult to pass, and bowel movements don't happen very often. Other symptoms may include painful bowel movements, and feeling bloated, uncomfortable, and sluggish.
Contraindication	A symptom or medical condition that makes a particular treatment or procedure inadvisable because a person is likely to have a bad reaction. For example, having a bleeding disorder is a contraindication for taking aspirin because treatment with aspirin may cause excess bleeding.
Contrast Material	A dye or other substance that helps show abnormal areas inside the body. It is given by injection into a vein, by enema, or by mouth. Contrast material may be used with x-rays, CT scans, MRI, or other imaging tests.
Controlled Substance	A drug or other substance that is tightly controlled by the government because it may be abused or cause addiction. The control applies to the way the substance is made, used, handled, stored, and distributed. Controlled substances include opioids, stimulants, depressants, hallucinogens, and anabolic steroids. Controlled substances with known medical use, such as morphine, Valium, and Ritalin, are available only by prescription from a licensed medical professional. Other controlled substances, such as heroin and LSD, have no medical use and are illegal in the United States.
Conventional Medicine	A system in which medical doctors and other healthcare professionals (such as nurses, pharmacists, and therapists) treat symptoms and diseases using drugs, radiation, or surgery. Also called allopathic medicine, biomedicine, mainstream medicine, orthodox medicine, and Western medicine.
Conventional Treatment or Therapy	Treatment that is widely accepted and used by most healthcare professionals. It is different from alternative or complementary therapies, which are not as widely used. Examples of conventional treatment for cancer include chemotherapy, radiation therapy, and surgery.
Copay	The amount of money that a patient with health insurance pays for each healthcare service, such as a visit to the doctor, laboratory tests, prescription medicines, and hospital stays. The amount of the copay usually depends on the type of healthcare service. Also called copayment.
Core Biopsy	The removal of a tissue sample with a wide needle for examination under a microscope. Also called core needle biopsy.
Cortisone	A natural steroid hormone produced in the adrenal gland. It can also be made in the laboratory. Cortisone reduces swelling and can suppress immune responses.
Cramp	A sharp pain that occurs when a muscle suddenly contracts (tightens up). Cramps commonly occur in the abdomen and legs.
Creatinine	A substance that is made by the body and used to store energy. It is being studied in the treatment of weight loss related to cancer. It is derived from the amino acid arginine.

CT Scan or CAT Scan / Computerized Axial Tomography	A procedure that uses a computer linked to an x-ray machine to make a series of detailed pictures of areas inside the body. The pictures are taken from different angles and are used to create 3-dimensional (3-D) views of tissues and organs. A dye may be injected into a vein or swallowed to help the tissues and organs show up more clearly. A CT scan may be used to help diagnose disease, plan treatment, or find out how well treatment is working. Also called CAT scan, computed tomography scan and computerized axial tomography scan.
CT-Guided Biopsy	A biopsy procedure that uses a CT scan (a special type of x-ray linked to a computer) to find an abnormal area in the body and help guide the removal of a sample of tissue from that area. A needle is usually used to remove the sample, which is then checked under a microscope for signs of disease. A CT-guided biopsy may be done when the abnormal area is deep inside the body or when the doctor cannot feel a lump or mass.
Culture	The beliefs, values, and behaviors that are shared within a group, such as a religious group or a nation. Culture includes language, customs, and beliefs about roles and relationships. In medicine, culture also refers to the growth of microorganisms, such as bacteria and yeast, or human, plant, or animal cells or tissue in the laboratory.
Cure	To heal or restore health; a treatment to restore health.
Cyclosporine	A drug used to help reduce the risk of rejection of organ and bone marrow transplants by the body. It is also used in clinical trials to make cancer cells more sensitive to anticancer drugs.
Cymbalta	A drug used to treat depression and peripheral neuropathy (pain, numbness, tingling, burning, or weakness in the hands or feet) that can occur with diabetes. It is also being studied in the treatment of peripheral neuropathy caused by certain anticancer drugs. Cymbalta increases the amount of certain chemicals in the brain that help relieve depression and pain. It is a type of serotonin and norepinephrine reuptake inhibitor. Also called duloxetine hydrochloride.
Cyst	A closed, sac-like pocket of tissue that can form anywhere in the body. It may be filled with fluid, air, pus, or other material. Most cysts are benign (not cancer).
Cytotoxic Agent	A substance that kills cells, including cancer cells. These agents may stop cancer cells from dividing and growing and may cause tumors to shrink in size.
Cytotoxin	A substance that can kill cells.

D

Deductible	The amount of money that a patient with health insurance pays for healthcare services before the health insurance plan begins to pay. Healthcare services may include visits to the doctor, laboratory tests, prescription medicines, and hospital stays. Not all healthcare plans require a deductible. Usually, plans with higher deductibles have lower monthly premiums (payments).
Definitive Treatment	The treatment plan for a disease or disorder that has been chosen as the best one for a patient after all other choices have been considered.
Degenerative Disease	A disease in which the function or structure of the affected tissues or organs changes for the worse over time. Osteoarthritis, osteoporosis, and Alzheimer disease are examples.
Demerol	A drug used to treat moderate to severe pain. It binds to opioid receptors in the central nervous system. Demerol is a type of analgesic agent and a type of opioid. Also called meperidine hydrochloride.

Denosumab	A drug used to prevent or treat certain bone problems. Under the brand name Xgeva, it is used to prevent broken bones and other bone problems caused by solid tumors that have spread to bone. It is also used in certain patients to treat giant cell tumor of the bone that cannot be removed by surgery. Under the brand name Prolia, it is used to treat osteoporosis (a decrease in bone mass and density) in postmenopausal women who have a high risk of breaking bones. Denosumab is also being studied in the treatment of other conditions and types of cancer. It binds to a protein called RANKL, which keeps RANKL from binding to another protein called RANK on the surface of certain bone cells, including bone cancer cells. This may help keep bone from breaking down and cancer cells from growing. Also called AMG 162, Prolia, and Xgeva.
Department of Health and Human Services (DHHS)	The U.S. federal government agency responsible for protecting the public's health and providing important services, especially for people in need. The Department of Health and Human Services works with state and local governments throughout the country to do research and provide public health services, food and drug safety programs, health insurance programs, and many other services. There are several federal agencies that are a part of the Department of Health and Human Services. They include the Food and Drug Administration (FDA), the Centers for Disease Control and Prevention (CDC), the National Institutes of Health (NIH), and the Centers for Medicare and Medicaid Services (CMMS). Also called DHHS.
Device	An object that has a specific use. In medicine, wheelchairs, pumps, and artificial limbs are examples of devices.
DEXA Scan	An imaging test that measures bone density (the amount of bone mineral contained in a certain volume of bone) by passing x-rays with two different energy levels through the bone. It is used to diagnose osteoporosis (decrease in bone mass and density). Also called BMD scan, bone mineral density scan, DEXA, dual energy x-ray absorptiometric scan, dual x-ray absorptiometry, and DXA.
Dexamethasone	A drug used to reduce inflammation and lower the body's immune response. It is used with other drugs to treat leukemia, lymphoma, mycosis fungoides, and other types of cancer. Dexamethasone is also used to prevent or treat many other diseases and conditions. These include conditions related to cancer and its treatment, such as anemia, allergic reactions, swelling in the brain, and high levels of calcium in the blood. Dexamethasone is a type of corticosteroid.
Diabetes	Any of several diseases in which the kidneys make a large amount of urine. Diabetes usually refers to diabetes mellitus in which there is also a high level of glucose (a type of sugar) in the blood because the body does not make enough insulin or use it the way it should.
Diagnosis	The process of identifying a disease, condition, or injury from its signs and symptoms. A health history, physical exam, and tests, such as blood tests, imaging tests, and biopsies, may be used to help make a diagnosis.
Diaphragm	The thin muscle below the lungs and heart that separates the chest from the abdomen.
Diarrhea	Frequent and watery bowel movements.
Diazepam (Valium)	A drug used to treat mild to moderate anxiety and tension and to relax muscles. It is a type of benzodiazepine. Also called Valium.
DIEP Flap	A type of breast reconstruction in which blood vessels called deep inferior epigastric perforators (DIEP), and the skin and fat connected to them are removed from the lower abdomen and used for reconstruction. Muscle is left in place.
Digestion	The process of breaking down food into substances the body can use for energy, tissue growth, and repair.
Digestive System	The organs that take in food and turn it into products that the body can use to stay healthy. Waste products the body cannot use leave the body through bowel movements. The digestive system includes the salivary glands, mouth, esophagus, stomach, liver, pancreas, gallbladder, small and large intestines, and rectum.

Dilaudid	A drug used to treat moderate to severe pain. It may also be used to treat certain types of cough. Dilaudid is made from morphine and binds to opioid receptors in the central nervous system. It is a type of opioid and a type of analgesic agent. Also called Exalgo, hydromorphone hydrochloride, and Hydrostat IR.
Discharge	In medicine, a fluid that comes out of the body. Discharge can be normal or a sign of disease. Discharge also means release of a patient from care.
Disease Progression	Cancer that continues to grow or spread.
Disinfectant	Any substance or process that is used primarily on non-living objects to kill germs, such as viruses, bacteria, and other microorganisms that can cause infection and disease. Most disinfectants are harsh chemicals but sometimes heat or radiation may be used.
Diverticulitis	Inflammation of one or more pouches or sacs that bulge out from the wall of a hollow organ, such as the colon. Symptoms include muscle spasms and cramps in the abdomen.
Diverticulum	A small pouch or sac that bulges out from the wall of a hollow organ, such as the colon.
Docetaxel	A drug used to treat certain types of cancers of the breast, stomach, lung, prostate, and head and neck. It is being studied in the treatment of other types of cancer. Docetaxel kills cancer cells by stopping them from dividing. It is a type of taxane. Also called Taxotere.
Drug Interaction	A change in the way a drug acts in the body when taken with certain other drugs, herbals, or foods, or when taken with certain medical conditions. Drug interactions may cause the drug to be more or less effective, or cause effects on the body that are not expected.
Dry Orgasm	Sexual climax without the release of semen from the penis.
Duct	In medicine, a tube or vessel of the body through which fluids pass.
Ductal Carcinoma in Situ (DCIS)	The most common type of breast cancer. It begins in the lining of the milk ducts (thin tubes that carry milk from the lobules of the breast to the nipple). Ductal carcinoma may be either ductal carcinoma in situ (DCIS) or invasive ductal carcinoma. DCIS is a noninvasive condition in which abnormal cells are found in the lining of a breast duct and have not spread outside the duct to other tissues in the breast. In some cases, DCIS may become invasive cancer. In invasive ductal carcinoma, cancer has spread outside the breast duct to surrounding normal tissue. It also spreads through the blood and lymph systems to other parts of the body.
Ductal Carcinoma in Situ	A noninvasive condition in which abnormal cells are found in the lining of a breast duct. The abnormal cells have not spread outside the duct to other tissues in the breast. In some cases, ductal carcinoma in situ may become invasive cancer and spread to other tissues. At this time, there is no way to know which lesions could become invasive. Also called DCIS and intraductal carcinoma.
Duodenum	The first part of the small intestine. It connects to the stomach. The duodenum helps to further digest food coming from the stomach. It absorbs nutrients (vitamins, minerals, carbohydrates, fats, proteins) and water from food so they can be used by the body.
DVT (Deep Vein Thrombosis)	The formation of a blood clot in a deep vein of the leg or lower pelvis. Symptoms may include pain, swelling, warmth, and redness in the affected area. Also called deep vein thrombosis.
Dysfunction	A state of not functioning normally.
Dysplasia	Cells that look abnormal under a microscope but are not cancer.
Dyspnea	Difficult, painful breathing or shortness of breath.

Early Menopause	A condition in which the ovaries stop working and menstrual periods stop before age 40. Natural menopause usually occurs around age 50. A woman is said to be in menopause when she hasn't had a period for 12 months in a row. Early menopause can be caused by some cancer treatments, surgery to remove the ovaries, and certain diseases or genetic conditions. Also called premature menopause, premature ovarian failure, and primary ovarian insufficiency.
Early-Stage Breast Cancer	Breast cancer that has not spread beyond the breast or the axillary lymph nodes. This includes ductal carcinoma in situ and stage I, stage IIA, stage IIB, and stage IIIA breast cancers.
Early-Stage Cancer	A term used to describe cancer that is early in its growth, and may not have spread to other parts of the body. What is called early stage may differ between cancer types.
Edema	Swelling caused by excess fluid in body tissues.
Effusion	An abnormal collection of fluid in hollow spaces or between tissues of the body. For example, a pleural effusion is a collection of fluid between the two layers of membrane covering the lungs.
Embolism	A block in an artery caused by blood clots or other substances, such as fat globules, infected tissue, or cancer cells.
Embolization	A procedure that uses particles, such as tiny gelatin sponges or beads, to block a blood vessel. Embolization may be used to stop bleeding or to block the flow of blood to a tumor or abnormal area of tissue. It may be used to treat some types of liver cancer, kidney cancer, and neuroendocrine tumors. It may also be used to treat uterine fibroids, aneurysms, and other conditions. Types of embolization are arterial embolization, chemoembolization, and radioembolization.
Encapsulated	Confined to a specific, localized area and surrounded by a thin layer of tissue.
Endocervix	The inner part of the cervix that forms a canal that connects the vagina to the uterus. The endocervix is lined with cells that make mucus. During a pelvic exam, cells may be scraped from the endocervix. The cells are checked under a microscope for infection, inflammation, and cancer or changes that may become cancer.
Endocrine	Refers to tissue that makes and releases hormones that travel in the bloodstream and control the actions of other cells or organs. Some examples of endocrine tissues are the pituitary, thyroid, and adrenal glands.
Endocrine System	A system of glands and cells that make hormones that are released directly into the blood and travel to tissues and organs all over the body. The endocrine system controls growth, sexual development, sleep, hunger, and the way the body uses food.
Endocrine Therapy	Treatment that adds, blocks, or removes hormones. For certain conditions (such as diabetes or menopause), hormones are given to adjust low hormone levels. To slow or stop the growth of certain cancers (such as prostate and breast cancer), synthetic hormones or other drugs may be given to block the body's natural hormones. Sometimes surgery is needed to remove the gland that makes a certain hormone. Also called hormonal therapy, hormone therapy, and hormone treatment.
Endometrial	Having to do with the endometrium (the layer of tissue that lines the uterus).
Endometriosis	A benign condition in which tissue that looks like endometrial tissue grows in abnormal places in the abdomen.
Endorphin	One of several substances made in the body that can relieve pain and give a feeling of well-being. Endorphins are peptides (small proteins) that bind to opioid receptors in the central nervous system. An endorphin is a type of neurotransmitter.

Endoscope	A thin, tube-like instrument used to look at tissues inside the body. An endoscope has a light and a lens for viewing and may have a tool to remove tissue.
Endoscopy	A procedure that uses an endoscope to examine the inside of the body. An endoscope is a thin, tube-like instrument with a light and a lens for viewing. It may also have a tool to remove tissue to be checked under a microscope for signs of disease.
Enema	The injection of a liquid through the anus into the large bowel.
Epiglottis	The flap that covers the trachea during swallowing so that food does not enter the lungs.
Epinephrine	A hormone and neurotransmitter. Also called adrenaline.
Epithelium	A thin layer of tissue that covers organs, glands, and other structures within the body.
Erbitux	A drug used to treat certain types of head and neck cancer, and a certain type of colorectal cancer that has spread to other parts of the body. It is also being studied in the treatment of other types of cancer. Erbitux binds to a protein called epidermal growth factor receptor (EGFR), which is on the surface of some types of cancer cells. This may stop cancer cells from growing. Erbitux is a type of monoclonal antibody. Also called cetuximab.
Estrogen	A type of hormone made by the body that helps develop and maintain female sex characteristics and the growth of long bones. Estrogens can also be made in the laboratory. They may be used as a type of birth control and to treat symptoms of menopause, menstrual disorders, osteoporosis, and other conditions.
Estrogen Blocker	A substance that keeps cells from making or using estrogen (a hormone that plays a role in female sex characteristics, the menstrual cycle, and pregnancy). Estrogen blockers may stop some cancer cells from growing and are used to prevent and treat breast cancer. They are also being studied in the treatment of other types of cancer. An estrogen blocker is a type of hormone antagonist. Also called antiestrogen.
Estrogen Receptor	A protein found inside the cells of the female reproductive tissue, some other types of tissue, and some cancer cells. The hormone estrogen will bind to the receptors inside the cells and may cause the cells to grow. Also called ER.
Estrogen Receptor Negative	Describes cells that do not have a protein to which the hormone estrogen will bind. Cancer cells that are estrogen receptor negative do not need estrogen to grow, and usually do not stop growing when treated with hormones that block estrogen from binding. Also called ER-.
Estrogen Receptor Positive	Describes cells that have a receptor protein that binds the hormone estrogen. Cancer cells that are estrogen receptor positive may need estrogen to grow, and may stop growing or die when treated with substances that block the binding and actions of estrogen. Also called ER+.
Estrogen Replacement Therapy	Treatment with the hormone estrogen to increase the amount of estrogen in the body. It is given to women who have gone through menopause or to women who have early menopause caused by cancer treatment or by having their ovaries removed by surgery. Estrogen replacement therapy may help relieve symptoms of menopause, such as hot flashes, night sweats, vaginal dryness, and sleep problems. It may also help protect against osteoporosis (thinning of the bones) and lower the risk of breast cancer in postmenopausal women. Also called ERT.
Excision	Removal by surgery.
Explanation of Benefits	A summary of the costs of a medical treatment or other healthcare service that an insurance company may send to a patient after the patient has received the service. An explanation of benefits usually includes the date the patient received the service, how much the service cost, how much the health insurance plan paid, and how much the patient may need to pay the healthcare provider. Also called EOB.
Exploratory Surgery	Surgery to look inside the body to help make a diagnosis.

Extremely Dense Breast Tissue	A term used to describe breast tissue that is made up of almost all dense fibrous tissue and glandular tissue. On a mammogram, the dense areas of the breast make it harder to find tumors or other changes. Women who have extremely dense breast tissue have a higher risk of breast cancer than those who have little or no dense breast tissue. Extremely dense breast tissue is one of four categories used to describe a level of breast density seen on a mammogram. About 10% of women have this type of breast tissue.
F	
False-Negative Test Result	A test result that indicates that a person does not have a specific disease or condition when the person actually does have the disease or condition.
False-Positive Test Result	A test result that indicates that a person has a specific disease or condition when the person actually does not have the disease or condition.
Familial Cancer	Cancer that occurs in families more often than would be expected by chance. These cancers often occur at an early age, and may indicate the presence of a gene mutation that increases the risk of cancer. They may also be a sign of shared environmental or lifestyle factors.
Family History	A record of the relationships among family members along with their medical histories. This includes current and past illnesses. A family history may show a pattern of certain diseases in a family. Also called family medical history.
Fat Necrosis	Fat necrosis is a condition that occurs when a person experiences an injury to an area of fatty tissue, like the breast. Typically, when a person experiences damage to the breast tissue, the damaged cells die, and the body replaces them with scar tissue. However, sometimes the fat cells die, and they release their oily contents. As a result, a firm lump can form and resemble a cancerous cyst. Doctors call this lump an oil cyst. Damage to the fatty tissue can occur following a breast biopsy, radiotherapy, breast reconstruction, breast reduction or other breast surgery. Fat necrosis is harmless and, in most cases, the body will break it down over time (this could take a few months and even years). Surgery is usually avoided if possible because it can sometimes cause further fat necrosis. However, an operation to remove the fat necrosis may be recommended if: • the biopsy hasn't given enough information to confirm a diagnosis of fat necrosis • the fat necrosis is uncomfortable or tender • the lump or lumpy area doesn't go away by itself, or gets bigger
FDA (Food & Drug Administration)	An agency in the U.S. federal government whose mission is to protect public health by making sure that food, cosmetics, and nutritional supplements are safe to use and truthfully labeled. The FDA also makes sure that drugs, medical devices, and equipment are safe and effective, and that blood for transfusions and transplant tissue are safe. Also called Food and Drug Administration.
Fever	An increase in body temperature above normal (98.6 degrees F), usually caused by disease.
Fiber	In food, fiber is the part of fruits, vegetables, legumes, and whole grains that cannot be digested. The fiber in food may help prevent cancer. In the body, fiber refers to tissue made of long threadlike cells, such as muscle fiber or nerve fiber.
Fibroid	A benign smooth-muscle tumor, usually in the uterus or gastrointestinal tract. Also called leiomyoma.
Fibrosis	The growth of fibrous tissue.
Fiducial Marker	A medical device or small object placed in or on the body to mark an area for radiation treatment or surgery. For example, tiny gold seeds may be put into the prostate to mark a tumor before radiation therapy. This allows the doctor to give higher doses of radiation to the tumor with less harm to nearby healthy tissue.

Fine-Needle Aspiration (FNA) Biopsy	The removal of tissue or fluid with a thin needle for examination under a microscope. Also called FNA biopsy.
Flomax	A drug used to treat urinary problems caused by an enlarged prostate. Flomax relaxes the muscles of the prostate and bladder, which helps the flow of urine. It is a type of alpha blocker. Also called tamsulosin and tamsulosin hydrochloride.
Focal	In terms of cancer, limited to a specific area.
Follow-up	Monitoring a person's health over time after treatment. This includes keeping track of the health of people who participate in a clinical study or clinical trial for a period of time, both during the study and after the study ends.
Foreign	In medicine, foreign describes something that comes from outside the body. A foreign substance in the body's tissues, such as a bacterium or virus, may be recognized by the immune system as not belonging to the body. This causes an immune response. Other foreign substances in the body, such as artificial joints, are designed to not cause an immune response.
Frankincense	Frankincense, also known as olibanum, is made from the resin of the Boswellia tree. It typically grows in the dry, mountainous regions of India, Africa and the Middle East. It has a woody, spicy smell and can be inhaled, absorbed through the skin, steeped into a tea or taken as a supplement. Used in Ayurvedic medicine for hundreds of years, frankincense appears to offer certain health benefits, from improved arthritis and digestion to reduced asthma and better oral health. It may even help fight certain types of cancer.
Full Blood Count	A measure of the number of red blood cells, white blood cells, and platelets in the blood. The amount of hemoglobin (substance in the blood that carries oxygen) and the hematocrit (the amount of whole blood that is made up of red blood cells) are also measured. A full blood count is used to help diagnose and monitor many conditions. Also called CBC, and complete blood count.
G	
Gabapentin	A substance that is being studied as a treatment for relieving hot flashes in women with breast cancer. It belongs to the family of drugs called anticonvulsants.
Gallbladder	The pear-shaped organ found below the liver. Bile is concentrated and stored in the gallbladder.
Gemzar	A drug used to treat pancreatic cancer that is advanced or has spread. It is also used with other drugs to treat breast cancer that has spread, advanced ovarian cancer, and non-small cell lung cancer that is advanced or has spread. It is also being studied in the treatment of other types of cancer. Gemzar blocks the cell from making DNA and may kill cancer cells. Also called gemcitabine hydrochloride.
Gene	The functional and physical unit of heredity passed from parent to offspring. Genes are pieces of DNA, and most genes contain the information for making a specific protein.
General Anesthesia	A temporary loss of feeling and a complete loss of awareness that feels like a very deep sleep. It is caused by special drugs or other substances called anesthetics. General anesthesia keeps patients from feeling pain during surgery or other procedures.
Genetic	Having to do with genes. Most genes are sequences of DNA that contain information for making specific RNA molecules or proteins that perform important functions in a cell. The information in genes is passed down from parent to child. Sometimes, certain changes in genes can affect a person's risk of disease, such as cancer. These changes may be inherited or they may occur with age or exposure to environmental factors, such as diet, exercise, drugs, and chemicals.
Genetic Analysis	The study of a sample of DNA to look for mutations (changes) that may increase risk of disease or affect the way a person responds to treatment.

Genetic Counseling	A communication process between a specially trained health professional and a person concerned about the genetic risk of disease. The person's family and personal medical history may be discussed, and counseling may lead to genetic testing.
Genetic Predisposition	An inherited increase in the risk of developing a disease. Also called genetic susceptibility.
Genetic Testing	The process of analyzing cells or tissues to look for genetic changes that may be a sign of a disease or condition, such as cancer. These changes may be a sign that a person has an increased risk of developing a specific disease or condition. Genetic testing may also be done on tumor tissue to help diagnose cancer, plan treatment, or find out how well treatment is working.
Genetics	The study of genes and heredity. Heredity is the passing of genetic information and traits (such as eye color and an increased chance of getting a certain disease) from parents to offspring.
Germ	A bacterium, virus, or other microorganism that can cause infection and disease.
Gland	An organ that makes one or more substances, such as hormones, digestive juices, sweat, tears, saliva, or milk. Endocrine glands release the substances directly into the bloodstream. Exocrine glands release the substances into a duct or opening to the inside or outside of the body.
Glucose	A type of sugar; the chief source of energy for living organisms.
Glutamine	An amino acid used in nutrition therapy. It is also being studied for the treatment of diarrhea caused by radiation therapy to the pelvis.
Gold Seed Fiducial Markers	Tiny, gold seeds, about the size of a grain of rice, that are put in and/or around a tumor to show exactly where it is in the body. Doctors are then able to target the tumor directly and give higher doses of radiation with less harm to nearby healthy tissue. Also called gold fiducial marker seeds, gold fiducial markers, and gold seeds.
Grading	A system for classifying cancer cells in terms of how abnormal they appear when examined under a microscope. The objective of a grading system is to provide information about the probable growth rate of the tumor and its tendency to spread. The systems used to grade tumors vary with each type of cancer. Grading plays a role in treatment decisions.
Granocyte	Brand name for the medication lenograstim, which is a granulocyte colony-stimulating factor that helps stimulate the immune system. It is used when white blood cell counts get too low (neutropenia) to boost the number of white blood cells and prevent infection.
Gurney	a wheeled stretcher used for transporting hospital patients.
Guided Imagery	A technique in which a person focuses on positive images in his or her mind. It can help people reach a relaxed, focused state and help reduce stress and give a sense of well-being. Also called imagery.
Gynecologic	Having to do with the female reproductive tract (including the cervix, endometrium, fallopian tubes, ovaries, uterus, and vagina).
Gynecologic Oncologist	A doctor who has special training in diagnosing and treating cancers of the female reproductive organs.
Gynecologist	A doctor who has special training in diagnosing and treating female reproductive organ diseases.

H

Hand-Foot Syndrome	A condition marked by pain, swelling, numbness, tingling, or redness of the hands or feet. It sometimes occurs as a side effect of certain anticancer drugs. Also called palmar-plantar erythrodysesthesia.

Health Insurance Portability and Accountability Act (HIPAA)	A 1996 U.S. law that allows workers and their families to keep their health insurance when they change or lose their jobs. The law also includes standards for setting up secure electronic health records and to protect the privacy of a person's health information and to keep it from being misused. Also called HIPAA and Kassebaum Kennedy Act.
Health Insurance Premium	The amount of money that a patient pays monthly to a health insurance company for healthcare coverage. Coverage may include visits to the doctor, laboratory tests, prescription medicines, and hospital stays.
Healthcare Provider	A licensed person or organization that provides healthcare services.
Heart Rate	In medicine, the number of times the heart beats within a certain time period, usually a minute. The heart rate can be felt at the wrist, side of the neck, back of the knees, top of the foot, groin, and other places in the body where an artery is close to the skin. The resting heart rate is normally between 60 and 100 beats a minute in a healthy adult who is at rest. Measuring the heart rate gives important information about a person's health. Also called pulse.
Hemoglobin	A protein inside red blood cells that carries oxygen from the lungs to tissues and organs in the body and carries carbon dioxide back to the lungs. Testing for the amount of hemoglobin in the blood is usually part of a complete blood cell (CBC) test. It is used to check for conditions such as anemia, dehydration, and malnutrition.
Hemorrhage	In medicine, loss of blood from damaged blood vessels. A hemorrhage may be internal or external, and usually involves a lot of bleeding in a short time.
Hemorrhoid	An enlarged or swollen blood vessel, usually located near the anus or the rectum.
Heparin	A substance that slows the formation of blood clots. Heparin is made by the liver, lungs, and other tissues in the body and can also made in the laboratory. Heparin may be injected into muscle or blood to prevent or break up blood clots. It is a type of anticoagulant.
Hepatic Arterial Infusion	A procedure to deliver chemotherapy directly to the liver. Catheters are put into an artery in the groin that leads directly to the liver, and drugs are given through the catheters.
Hepatic Artery	The major blood vessel that carries blood to the liver.
Hepatic Portal Vein	A blood vessel that carries blood to the liver from the intestines, spleen, pancreas, and gallbladder. Also called portal vein.
Hepatocyte	A liver cell.
HER1	The protein found on the surface of some cells and to which epidermal growth factor binds, causing the cells to divide. It is found at abnormally high levels on the surface of many types of cancer cells, so these cells may divide excessively in the presence of epidermal growth factor. Also called EGFR, epidermal growth factor receptor, and ErbB1.
HER2 Negative	Describes cancer cells that do not have a large amount of a protein called HER2 on their surface. In normal cells, HER2 helps to control cell growth. Cancer cells that are HER2 negative may grow more slowly and are less likely to recur (come back) or spread to other parts of the body than cancer cells that have a large amount of HER2 on their surface. Checking for the amount of HER2 on some types of cancer cells may help plan treatment. These cancers include breast, bladder, ovarian, pancreatic, and stomach cancers. Also called human epidermal growth factor receptor 2 negative.
HER2 Positive	Describes cancer cells that have too much of a protein called HER2 on their surface. In normal cells, HER2 helps to control cell growth. When it is made in larger than normal amounts by cancer cells, the cells may grow more quickly and be more likely to spread to other parts of the body. Checking to see if a cancer is HER2 positive may help plan treatment, which may include drugs that kill HER2 positive cancer cells. Cancers that may be HER2 positive include breast, bladder, pancreatic, ovarian, and stomach cancers. Also called c-erbB-2 positive and human epidermal growth factor receptor 2 positive.

HER2/Neu	A protein involved in normal cell growth. It is found on some types of cancer cells, including breast and ovarian. Cancer cells removed from the body may be tested for the presence of HER2/neu to help decide the best type of treatment. HER2/neu is a type of receptor tyrosine kinase. Also called c-erbB-2, human EGF receptor 2, and human epidermal growth factor receptor 2.
Herceptin	A drug used to treat breast cancer that is HER2-positive (expresses the human epidermal growth factor receptor 2). It is also used with other drugs to treat HER2-positive stomach cancer that has not already been treated and has spread to other parts of the body. It is being studied in the treatment of other types of cancer. Herceptin binds to HER2 on the surface of HER2-positive cancer cells, and may kill them. It is a type of monoclonal antibody. Also called trastuzumab.
Hereditary	In medicine, describes the passing of genetic information from parent to child through the genes in sperm and egg cells. Also called inherited.
Hereditary Mutation	A gene change in a body's reproductive cell (egg or sperm) that becomes incorporated into the DNA of every cell in the body of the offspring. Hereditary mutations are passed on from parents to offspring. Also called germline mutation.
Hernia	A gene change in a body's reproductive cell (egg or sperm) that becomes incorporated into the DNA of every cell in the body of the offspring. Hereditary mutations are passed on from parents to offspring. Also called germline mutation.
Heterogeneously Dense Breast Tissue	A term used to describe breast tissue that is made up of mostly dense fibrous tissue and glandular tissue and also has some fatty tissue. On a mammogram, the dense areas of the breast make it harder to find tumors or other changes. Heterogeneously dense breast tissue is one of four categories used to describe a level of breast density seen on a mammogram. About 40% of women have this type of breast tissue.
High Blood Pressure	A blood pressure of 140/90 or higher. High blood pressure usually has no symptoms. It can harm the arteries and cause an increase in the risk of stroke, heart attack, kidney failure, and blindness. Also called hypertension.
High Blood Sugar	Higher than normal amount of glucose (a type of sugar) in the blood. High blood sugar can be a sign of diabetes or other conditions. Also called hyperglycemia.
High Grade	A term used to describe cells and tissue that look abnormal under a microscope. High-grade cancer cells tend to grow and spread more quickly than low-grade cancer cells. Cancer grade may be used to help plan treatment and determine prognosis. High-grade cancers usually have a worse prognosis than low-grade cancers and may need treatment right away or treatment that is more aggressive (intensive).
High-Dose Chemotherapy	An intensive drug treatment to kill cancer cells, but that also destroys the bone marrow and can cause other severe side effects. High-dose chemotherapy is usually followed by bone marrow or stem cell transplantation to rebuild the bone marrow.
High-Dose Radiation	An amount of radiation that is greater than that given in typical radiation therapy. High-dose radiation is precisely directed at the tumor to avoid damaging healthy tissue, and may kill more cancer cells in fewer treatments. Also called HDR.
High-Grade Lymphoma	A type of lymphoma that grows and spreads quickly and has severe symptoms. Also called aggressive lymphoma and intermediate-grade lymphoma.
High-Grade Squamous Intraepithelial Lesion	A growth on the surface of the cervix with moderately or severely abnormal cells. High-grade squamous intraepithelial lesions are usually caused by certain types of human papillomavirus (HPV) and are found when a Pap test is done. If not treated, these abnormal cells may become cancer and spread to nearby normal tissue. A high-grade squamous intraepithelial lesion is sometimes called moderate or severe dysplasia. Also called HSIL.
High-Risk Cancer	Cancer that is likely to recur (come back), or spread.

Hives	Itchy, raised red areas on the skin. Hives are caused by a reaction to certain foods, drugs, infections, or emotional stress. Also called urticaria.
Hormone	One of many substances made by glands in the body. Hormones circulate in the bloodstream and control the actions of certain cells or organs. Some hormones can also be made in the laboratory.
Hormone Receptor Negative	Describes cells that do not have a group of proteins that bind to a specific hormone. For example, some breast cancer cells do not have receptors for the hormones estrogen or progesterone. These cells are hormone receptor negative and they do not need estrogen or progesterone to grow. This can affect how the cancer is treated. Knowing if the cancer is hormone receptor negative may help plan treatment.
Hormone Receptor Positive	Describes cells that have a group of proteins that bind to a specific hormone. For example, some breast cancer cells have receptors for the hormones estrogen or progesterone. These cells are hormone receptor positive and they need estrogen or progesterone to grow. This can affect how the cancer is treated. Knowing if the cancer is hormone receptor positive may help plan treatment.
Hormone Replacement Therapy	Treatment with hormones to replace natural hormones when the body does not make enough. For example, hormone replacement therapy may be given when the thyroid gland does not make enough thyroid hormone or when the pituitary gland does not make enough growth hormone. Or, it may be given to women after menopause to replace the hormones estrogen and progesterone that are no longer made by the body. Also called HRT.
Hormone Therapy or Treatment	Treatment that adds, blocks, or removes hormones. For certain conditions (such as diabetes or menopause), hormones are given to adjust low hormone levels. To slow or stop the growth of certain cancers (such as prostate and breast cancer), synthetic hormones or other drugs may be given to block the body's natural hormones. Sometimes surgery is needed to remove the gland that makes a certain hormone. Also called endocrine therapy, hormonal therapy, and hormone treatment.
Hot Flash	A sudden, temporary onset of body warmth, flushing, and sweating (often associated with menopause).
Hyperbaric Oxygen	Oxygen that is given at a pressure that is higher than the pressure of the atmosphere at sea level. In medicine, breathing hyperbaric oxygen increases the amount of oxygen in the body. It is used in treating certain kinds of wounds, injuries, and infections. It is also used to treat carbon monoxide poisoning and other conditions in which the tissues are not getting enough oxygen. It is being studied in the treatment of some types of cancer. Hyperbaric oxygen may increase the amount of oxygen in cancer cells, which may make them easier to kill with radiation therapy and chemotherapy. It is a type of radiosensitizing agent and a type of chemosensitizing agent.
Hypersensitivity	An exaggerated response by the immune system to a drug or other substance.
Hypertension	A blood pressure of 140/90 or higher. Hypertension usually has no symptoms. It can harm the arteries and cause an increase in the risk of stroke, heart attack, kidney failure, and blindness. Also called high blood pressure.
Hyperthermia	Abnormally high body temperature. This may be caused as part of treatment, by an infection, or by exposure to heat.
Hyperthermia Therapy	A type of treatment in which body tissue is exposed to high temperatures to damage and kill cancer cells or to make cancer cells more sensitive to the effects of radiation and certain anticancer drugs.
Hyperthyroidism	Too much thyroid hormone. Symptoms include weight loss, chest pain, cramps, diarrhea, and nervousness. Also called overactive thyroid.
Hypothyroidism	Too little thyroid hormone. Symptoms include weight gain, constipation, dry skin, and sensitivity to the cold. Also called underactive thyroid.

Hysterectomy	Surgery to remove the uterus and, sometimes, the cervix. When the uterus and the cervix are removed, it is called a total hysterectomy. When only the uterus is removed, it is called a partial hysterectomy.

I

Ibrance	A cancer medicine that interferes with the growth and spread of cancer cells in the body. It is used to treat advanced or metastatic breast cancer in women and men. Also known as Palbociclib.
Idelalisib	A drug used with rituximab to treat chronic lymphocytic leukemia (CLL) that has come back. It is also used to treat follicular B-cell non-Hodgkin lymphoma (NHL) and small lymphocytic lymphoma (SLL) that have come back after treatment with other anticancer therapy. It is also being studied in the treatment of other types of cancer. Idelalisib blocks certain proteins, which may help keep cancer cells from growing and may kill them. It is a type of kinase inhibitor. Also called Zydelig.
Ileostomy	An opening into the ileum, part of the small intestine, from the outside of the body. An ileostomy provides a new path for waste material to leave the body after part of the intestine has been removed.
Ileum	The last part of the small intestine. It connects to the cecum (first part of the large intestine). The ileum helps to further digest food coming from the stomach and other parts of the small intestine. It absorbs nutrients (vitamins, minerals, carbohydrates, fats, proteins) and water from food to be used by the body.
Imaging Procedure or Test	A type of test that makes detailed pictures of areas inside the body. Imaging procedures use different forms of energy, such as x-rays (high-energy radiation), ultrasound (high-energy sound waves), radio waves, and radioactive substances. They may be used to help diagnose disease, plan treatment, or find out how well treatment is working. Examples of imaging procedures are computed tomography (CT), ultrasonography, magnetic resonance imaging (MRI), and nuclear medicine tests.
Immune Response	The activity of the immune system against foreign substances (antigens).
Immune System	A complex network of cells, tissues, organs, and the substances they make that helps the body fight infections and other diseases. The immune system includes white blood cells and organs and tissues of the lymph system, such as the thymus, spleen, tonsils, lymph nodes, lymph vessels, and bone marrow.
Immunodeficiency	The decreased ability of the body to fight infections and other diseases.
Immunostimulant	A substance that increases the ability of the immune system to fight infection and disease.
Immunosuppression	Suppression of the body's immune system and its ability to fight infections and other diseases. Immunosuppression may be deliberately induced with drugs, as in preparation for bone marrow or other organ transplantation, to prevent rejection of the donor tissue. It may also result from certain diseases such as AIDS or lymphoma or from anticancer drugs.
Immunotherapy	A type of biological therapy that uses substances to stimulate or suppress the immune system to help the body fight cancer, infection, and other diseases. Some types of immunotherapy only target certain cells of the immune system. Others affect the immune system in a general way. Types of immunotherapy include cytokines, vaccines, bacillus Calmette-Guerin (BCG), and some monoclonal antibodies.
Impairment	A loss of part or all of a physical or mental ability, such as the ability to see, walk, or learn.
Implant	A substance or object that is put in the body as a prosthesis, or for treatment or diagnosis.
Implant Displacement Views	A procedure used to do a mammogram (x-ray of the breasts) in women with breast implants. The implant is pushed back against the chest wall and the breast tissue is pulled forward and around it so the tissue can be seen in the mammogram. Also called Eklund displacement views and Eklund views.
In Situ	In its original place. For example, in carcinoma in situ, abnormal cells are found only in the place where they first formed. They have not spread.

Incision	A cut made in the body to perform surgery.
Incisional Biopsy	A surgical procedure in which a portion of a lump or suspicious area is removed for diagnosis. The tissue is then examined under a microscope to check for signs of disease.
Incontinence	Inability to control the flow of urine from the bladder (urinary incontinence) or the escape of stool from the rectum (fecal incontinence).
Incontinence Pads	An incontinence pad is a small, impermeable multi-layered sheet with high absorbency that is used as a precaution against urinary incontinence. It is generally made of cotton, if washable or paper, if disposable. Incontinence pads are usually placed in an undergarment or on a bed or chair under a person. They can come as panty-liners, inserts, pads or even available as replacement underwear.
Induction Therapy	The first treatment given for a disease. It is often part of a standard set of treatments, such as surgery followed by chemotherapy and radiation. When used by itself, induction therapy is the one accepted as the best treatment. If it doesn't cure the disease or it causes severe side effects, other treatment may be added or used instead. Also called first-line therapy, primary therapy, and primary treatment.
Infection	The invasion and growth of germs in the body. The germs may be bacteria, viruses, yeast, fungi, or other microorganisms. Infections can begin anywhere in the body and may spread all through it. An infection can cause fever and other health problems, depending on where it occurs in the body. When the body's immune system is strong, it can often fight the germs and cure an infection. Some cancer treatments can weaken the immune system, which may lead to infection.
Inflammatory	Having to do with inflammation (redness, swelling, pain, and a feeling of heat that helps protect tissues affected by injury or disease).
Infusion	A method of putting fluids, including drugs, into the bloodstream. Also called intravenous infusion.
Injection	Use of a syringe and needle to push fluids or drugs into the body; often called a "shot."
Insomnia	Difficulty in going to sleep or getting enough sleep.
Insulin	A hormone made by the islet cells of the pancreas. Insulin controls the amount of sugar in the blood by moving it into the cells, where it can be used by the body for energy.
Integrative Medicine	A type of medical care that combines conventional (standard) medical treatment with complementary and alternative (CAM) therapies that have been shown to be safe and to work. CAM therapies treat the mind, body, and spirit.
Internal Radiation Therapy	A type of radiation therapy in which radioactive material sealed in needles, seeds, wires, or catheters is placed directly into or near a tumor. Also called brachytherapy, implant radiation therapy, and radiation brachytherapy.
Internal Scars / Abdominal Adhesions	Tough tissue bands that form between the abdominal tissues and neighboring organs. They develop after surgery and make normally slippery internal tissues and organs stick together.
Interstitial Radiation Therapy	A type of internal radiation therapy in which radioactive material sealed in needles, seeds, wires, or catheters is placed directly into a tumor or body tissue.
Intestine	The long, tube-shaped organ in the abdomen that completes the process of digestion. The intestine has two parts, the small intestine and the large intestine. Also called bowel.
Intravenous or Intravenous Infusion	Into or within a vein. Intravenous usually refers to a way of giving a drug or other substance through a needle or tube inserted into a vein. Also called IV.

Invasive Breast Cancer or Infiltrating Breast Cancer	Cancer that has spread from where it began in the breast to surrounding normal tissue. The most common type of invasive breast cancer is invasive ductal carcinoma, which begins in the lining of the milk ducts (thin tubes that carry milk from the lobules of the breast to the nipple). Another type is invasive lobular carcinoma, which begins in the lobules (milk glands) of the breast. Invasive breast cancer can spread through the blood and lymph systems to other parts of the body.
Invasive Cancer	Cancer that has spread beyond the layer of tissue in which it developed and is growing into surrounding, healthy tissues. Also called infiltrating cancer.
Invasive Procedure	A medical procedure that invades (enters) the body, usually by cutting or puncturing the skin or by inserting instruments into the body.
Ionomycin	An antibiotic drug used to treat infection.
Irinotecan	The active ingredient in a drug used alone or with other drugs to treat colon cancer or rectal cancer that has spread to other parts of the body or has come back after treatment with fluorouracil. It is also being studied in the treatment of other types of cancer. Irinotecan blocks certain enzymes needed for cell division and DNA repair, and it may kill cancer cells. It is a type of topoisomerase inhibitor.
Irreversible Toxicity	Side effects that are caused by toxic substances or something harmful to the body and do not go away.
Irrigation	In medicine, washing out an organ (such as the stomach or colon), a body cavity, or a wound by flushing it with a fluid. Also called lavage.
IV	Into or within a vein. IV usually refers to a way of giving a drug or other substance through a needle or tube inserted into a vein. Also called intravenous.

J	
Jejunostomy	Surgery to create an opening into the jejunum (part of the small intestine) from the outside of the body. A jejunostomy allows a feeding tube to be put into the small intestine.
Jejunum	The middle part of the small intestine. It is between the duodenum (first part of the small intestine) and the ileum (last part of the small intestine). The jejunum helps to further digest food coming from the stomach. It absorbs nutrients (vitamins, minerals, carbohydrates, fats, proteins) and water from food so they can be used by the body.
Joint	In medicine, the place where two or more bones are connected. Examples include the shoulder, elbow, knee, and jaw.
J-Pouch Colorectal Anastomosis	A surgical procedure in which the colon is attached to the anus after the rectum has been removed. A 2-4 inch section of the colon is formed into a J-shaped pouch in order to replace the function of the rectum and store stool until it can be eliminated. This procedure is similar to the side-to-end coloanal anastomosis but a larger pouch is formed.

K	
Keloid	A thick, irregular scar caused by excessive tissue growth at the site of an incision or wound.
Kidney	One of a pair of organs in the abdomen. The kidneys remove waste and extra water from the blood (as urine) and help keep chemicals (such as sodium, potassium, and calcium) balanced in the body. The kidneys also make hormones that help control blood pressure and stimulate bone marrow to make red blood cells.

Kidney Cancer	Cancer that forms in tissues of the kidneys. The most common type of kidney cancer in adults is renal cell carcinoma. It forms in the lining of very small tubes in the kidney that filter the blood and remove waste products. Transitional cell cancer of the renal pelvis is kidney cancer that forms in the center of the kidney where urine collects. Wilms tumor is a type of kidney cancer that usually develops in children under the age of 5.
Kidney Failure	A condition in which the kidneys stop working and are not able to remove waste and extra water from the blood or keep body chemicals in balance. Acute or severe kidney failure happens suddenly (for example, after an injury) and may be treated and cured. Chronic kidney failure develops over many years, may be caused by conditions like high blood pressure or diabetes, and cannot be cured. Chronic kidney failure may lead to total and long-lasting kidney failure, called end-stage renal disease (ESRD). A person in ESRD needs dialysis (the process of cleaning the blood by passing it through a membrane or filter) or a kidney transplant. Also called renal failure.
Kidney Function	A term used to describe how well the kidneys work. The kidneys remove waste and extra water from the blood (as urine) and help keep chemicals (such as sodium, potassium, and calcium) balanced in the body. They also make hormones that help control blood pressure and stimulate bone marrow to make red blood cells. Also called renal function.
Killer T-Cell	A type of immune cell that can kill certain cells, including foreign cells, cancer cells, and cells infected with a virus. Killer T cells can be separated from other blood cells, grown in the laboratory, and then given to a patient to kill cancer cells. A killer T cell is a type of white blood cell and a type of lymphocyte. Also called cytotoxic T cell or lymphocyte.

L

Laparoscope	A thin, tube-like instrument used to look at tissues and organs inside the abdomen. A laparoscope has a light and a lens for viewing and may have a tool to remove tissue.
Laparoscopy	A procedure that uses a laparoscope, inserted through the abdominal wall, to examine the inside of the abdomen. A laparoscope is a thin, tube-like instrument with a light and a lens for viewing. It may also have a tool to remove tissue to be checked under a microscope for signs of disease.
Large Intestine	The long, tube-like organ that is connected to the small intestine at one end and the anus at the other. The large intestine has four parts: cecum, colon, rectum, and anal canal. Partly digested food moves through the cecum into the colon, where water and some nutrients and electrolytes are removed. The remaining material, solid waste called stool, moves through the colon, is stored in the rectum, and leaves the body through the anal canal and anus.
Laser Surgery	A surgical procedure that uses the cutting power of a laser beam to make bloodless cuts in tissue or to remove a surface lesion such as a tumor.
Latent	Describes a condition that is present but not active or causing symptoms.
Late-Stage Cancer	A term used to describe cancer that is far along in its growth, and has spread to the lymph nodes or other places in the body.
Lavage	In medicine, washing out an organ (such as the stomach or colon), a body cavity, or a wound by flushing it with a fluid. Also called irrigation.
Laxative	A substance that promotes bowel movements.
Lesion	An area of abnormal tissue. A lesion may be benign (not cancer) or malignant (cancer).
Leukemia	Cancer that starts in blood-forming tissue, such as the bone marrow, and causes large numbers of abnormal blood cells to be produced and enter the bloodstream.

Leukopenia	A decrease in the number of white blood cells (leukocytes) found in the blood, which places individuals at increased risk of infection.
Lidocaine	A substance used to relieve pain by blocking signals at the nerve endings in skin. It can also be given intravenously to stop heart arrhythmias. It is a type of local anesthetic and antiarrhythmic.
Lisinopril	A drug used to treat high blood pressure and certain heart conditions. It is also being studied in the prevention and treatment of side effects caused by some anticancer drugs. It blocks certain enzymes that cause blood vessels to constrict (narrow). It is a type of angiotensin-converting enzyme (ACE) inhibitor. Also called Prinivil and Zestril.
Liver	A large organ located in the upper abdomen. The liver cleanses the blood and aids in digestion by secreting bile.
Local Anesthesia	A temporary loss of feeling in one small area of the body caused by special drugs called anesthetics. The patient stays awake but has no feeling in the area of the body treated with the anesthetic. Local anesthetics may be injected or put on the skin to lessen pain during medical, surgical, or dental procedures. Some are available over-the-counter (without a doctor's order) and may help lessen local pain, irritation, and itching caused by conditions such as cold sores, sunburn, poison ivy, and minor cuts.
Local Therapy	Treatment that is directed to a specific organ or limited area of the body, such as the breast or an abnormal growth on the skin. Examples of local therapy used in cancer are surgery, radiation therapy, cryotherapy, laser therapy, and topical therapy (medicine in a lotion or cream that is applied to the skin).
Localized	In medicine, describes disease that is limited to a certain part of the body. For example, localized cancer is usually found only in the tissue or organ where it began, and has not spread to nearby lymph nodes or to other parts of the body. Some localized cancers can be completely removed by surgery.
Long-Term Side Effect	A problem that is caused by a disease or treatment of a disease and may continue for months or years. Long-term side effects of cancer treatment include heart, lung, kidney, or gastrointestinal tract problems; pain, numbness, tingling, loss of feeling, or heat or cold sensitivity in the hands or feet; fatigue; hearing loss; cataracts; and dry eyes or dry mouth.
Loop Electrosurgical Excision Procedure (LEEP)	A technique that uses electric current passed through a thin wire loop to remove abnormal tissue. Also called LEEP and loop excision.
Lorazepam	A drug that is used to treat anxiety and certain seizure disorders (such as epilepsy), and to prevent nausea and vomiting caused by chemotherapy. It belongs to the families of drugs called antiemetics and benzodiazepines.
Lovastatin	A drug used to lower the amount of cholesterol in the blood. It is also being studied in the prevention and treatment of some types of cancer. Lovastatin is a type of HMG-CoA reductase inhibitor (statin). Also called Mevacor.
Low Grade	A term used to describe cells and tissue that look almost normal under a microscope. Low-grade cancer cells look more like normal cells and tend to grow and spread more slowly than high-grade cancer cells.
Lower GI Series	X-rays of the colon and rectum that are taken after a person is given a barium enema.
Low-Grade Squamous Intraepithelial Lesion	Slightly abnormal cells are found on the surface of the cervix. Low-grade squamous intraepithelial lesion is caused by certain types of human papillomavirus (HPV) and is a common abnormal finding on a Pap test. It usually goes away on its own without treatment but sometimes the abnormal cells become cancer and spread to nearby normal tissue. Low-grade squamous intraepithelial lesion is sometimes called mild dysplasia. Also called LSIL.

Lumpectomy	An operation to remove the cancer and some normal tissue around it, but not the breast itself. Some lymph nodes under the arm may be removed for biopsy. Part of the chest wall lining may also be removed if the cancer is near it. Also called breast-conserving surgery, breast-sparing surgery, partial mastectomy, quadrantectomy, and segmental mastectomy.
Lung	One of a pair of organs in the chest that supplies the body with oxygen, and removes carbon dioxide from the body.
Lung Function	A term used to describe how well the lungs work in helping a person breathe. During breathing, oxygen is taken into the lungs, where it passes into the blood and travels to the body's tissues. Carbon dioxide, a waste product made by the body's tissues, is carried to the lungs, where it is breathed out. There are different tests to measure lung function. Also called pulmonary function.
Lymph / Lymphatic Fluid	The clear fluid that travels through the lymphatic system and carries cells that help fight infections and other diseases. Also called lymphatic fluid.
Lymph Node / Lymph Gland	A small bean-shaped structure that is part of the body's immune system. Lymph nodes filter substances that travel through the lymphatic fluid, and they contain lymphocytes (white blood cells) that help the body fight infection and disease. There are hundreds of lymph nodes found throughout the body. They are connected to one another by lymph vessels. Clusters of lymph nodes are found in the neck, axilla (underarm), chest, abdomen, and groin. For example, there are about 20-40 lymph nodes in the axilla. Also called lymph gland.
Lymph Node Dissection	A surgical procedure in which the lymph nodes are removed and a sample of tissue is checked under a microscope for signs of cancer. For a regional lymph node dissection, some of the lymph nodes in the tumor area are removed; for a radical lymph node dissection, most or all of the lymph nodes in the tumor area are removed. Also called lymphadenectomy.
Lymphadenectomy	A surgical procedure in which the lymph nodes are removed and a sample of tissue is checked under a microscope for signs of cancer. For a regional lymphadenectomy, some of the lymph nodes in the tumor area are removed; for a radical lymphadenectomy, most or all of the lymph nodes in the tumor area are removed. Also called lymph node dissection.
Lymphadenopathy	Disease or swelling of the lymph nodes.
Lymphatic System	The tissues and organs that produce, store, and carry white blood cells that fight infections and other diseases. This system includes the bone marrow, spleen, thymus, lymph nodes, and lymphatic vessels (a network of thin tubes that carry lymph and white blood cells). Lymphatic vessels branch, like blood vessels, into all the tissues of the body.
Lymphedema	A condition in which extra lymph fluid builds up in tissues and causes swelling. It may occur in an arm or leg if lymph vessels are blocked, damaged, or removed by surgery.
Lymphocyte	A type of immune cell that is made in the bone marrow and is found in the blood and in lymph tissue. The two main types of lymphocytes are B lymphocytes and T lymphocytes. B lymphocytes make antibodies, and T lymphocytes help kill tumor cells and help control immune responses. A lymphocyte is a type of white blood cell.
Lymphocytic Leukemia	A type of cancer in which the bone marrow makes too many lymphocytes (white blood cells).
Lymphoma	Cancer that begins in cells of the immune system. There are two basic categories of lymphomas. One kind is Hodgkin lymphoma, which is marked by the presence of a type of cell called the Reed-Sternberg cell. The other category is non-Hodgkin lymphomas, which includes a large, diverse group of cancers of immune system cells. Non-Hodgkin lymphomas can be further divided into cancers that have an indolent (slow-growing) course and those that have an aggressive (fast-growing) course. These subtypes behave and respond to treatment differently.

Lynch Syndrome	An inherited disorder in which affected individuals have a higher-than-normal chance of developing colorectal cancer and certain other types of cancer, often before the age of 50. Also called hereditary nonpolyposis colon cancer and HNPCC.
Lyrica	A drug used to treat nerve pain caused by diabetes or herpes zoster infection and certain types of seizures. It is being studied in the prevention and treatment of nerve pain in the hands and feet of cancer patients given chemotherapy. Lyrica is a type of anticonvulsant. Also called pregabalin.
Lysis of Adhesions	A surgery to cut bands of tissue that form between organs. These bands are called adhesions or internal scar tissues. They are often caused by scar tissue that formed after an earlier surgery. Adhesions can connect organs and tissues to each other. This can cause severe pain and stop organs from working well.

M

Magnetic Resonance Imaging (MRI)	A procedure in which radio waves and a powerful magnet linked to a computer are used to create detailed pictures of areas inside the body. These pictures can show the difference between normal and diseased tissue. Magnetic resonance imaging makes better images of organs and soft tissue than other scanning techniques, such as computed tomography (CT) or x-ray. Magnetic resonance imaging is especially useful for imaging the brain, the spine, the soft tissue of joints, and the inside of bones. Also called MRI, NMRI, and nuclear magnetic resonance imaging.
Maintenance Therapy	Treatment that is given to help keep cancer from coming back after it has disappeared following the initial therapy. It may include treatment with drugs, vaccines, or antibodies that kill cancer cells, and it may be given for a long time.
Malignant	Term used to describe tumors that can spread into, or invade, nearby tissues.
Mammogram	An x-ray of the breast.
Margin	The edge or border of the tissue removed in cancer surgery. The margin is described as negative or clean when the pathologist finds no cancer cells at the edge of the tissue, suggesting that all of the cancer has been removed. The margin is described as positive or involved when the pathologist finds cancer cells at the edge of the tissue, suggesting that all of the cancer has not been removed.
Marijuana	The dried leaves and flowering tops of the Cannabis sativa or Cannabis indica plant. Marijuana contains active chemicals called cannabinoids that cause drug-like effects all through the body, including the central nervous system and the immune system. Marijuana may help treat the symptoms of cancer or the side effects of cancer treatment, such as nausea and vomiting, pain, and cachexia (loss of body weight and muscle mass). Also called Cannabis.
Marker	A diagnostic indication that disease may develop.
Mass	In medicine, a lump in the body. It may be caused by the abnormal growth of cells, a cyst, hormonal changes, or an immune reaction. A mass may be benign (not cancer) or malignant (cancer).
Mastectomy	Surgery to remove part or all of the breast. There are different types of mastectomy that differ in the amount of tissue and lymph nodes removed.
Mediastinum	A membranous partition between two body cavities or two parts of an organ, especially that between the lungs.
Medicaid	A health insurance program for people who cannot afford regular medical care. The program is run by U.S. federal, state, and local governments. People who receive Medicaid may have to pay a small amount for the services they get.

Medi-Cal or California Medical Assistance Program	California's Medicaid program serving low-income individuals, including families, seniors, persons with disabilities, children in foster care, pregnant women, and childless adults with incomes below 138% of federal poverty level. Benefits include ambulatory patient services, emergency services, hospitalization, maternity and newborn care, mental health and substance use disorder treatment, dental (Denti-Cal), vision, and long-term care and supports.
Medical Oncologist	A doctor who has special training in diagnosing and treating cancer in adults using chemotherapy, hormonal therapy, biological therapy, and targeted therapy. A medical oncologist often is the main health care provider for someone who has cancer and gives supportive care, including coordination of treatment given by other specialists.
Medicare	A U.S. federal health insurance program for people aged 65 years or older and people with certain disabilities. Medicare pays for hospital stays, medical services, and some prescription drugs but people who receive Medicare must pay part of their healthcare costs.
Medicare Part D	A type of insurance that helps people with Medicare pay for prescription drugs. People with Medicare Part D have to pay an additional premium and part of their prescription drug costs, including deductibles and copayments. Medicare Part D is offered by private insurance companies approved by Medicare. It is a type of supplemental health insurance. Also called Medicare Prescription Drug Coverage.
Medication	A legal drug that is used to prevent, treat, or relieve symptoms of a disease or abnormal condition.
Mediport, Medi-Port, Port or Port-a-Cath	A device used to draw blood and give treatments, including intravenous fluids, drugs, or blood transfusions. The port is placed under the skin, usually in the chest. It is attached to a catheter (a thin, flexible tube) that is guided (threaded) into a large vein above the right side of the heart called the superior vena cava.
Meditation	A mind-body practice in which a person focuses his or her attention on something, such as an object, word, phrase, or breathing, in order to minimize distracting or stressful thoughts or feelings. Meditation may help relax the body and mind and improve overall health and well-being. It may be used to help relieve stress, pain, anxiety, and depression and to help with symptoms related to disease, such as cancer and AIDS. It is a type of complementary and alternative medicine (CAM).
Melanoma	A form of cancer that begins in melanocytes (cells that make the pigment melanin). It may begin in a mole (skin melanoma), but can also begin in other pigmented tissues, such as in the eye or in the intestines.
Melanoma in Situ	Abnormal melanocytes (cells that make melanin, the pigment that gives skin its natural color) are found in the epidermis (outer layer of the skin). These abnormal melanocytes may become cancer and spread into nearby normal tissue. Also called stage 0 melanoma.
Menopause	The time of life when a woman's ovaries stop producing hormones and menstrual periods stop. Natural menopause usually occurs around age 50. A woman is said to be in menopause when she hasn't had a period for 12 months in a row. Symptoms of menopause include hot flashes, mood swings, night sweats, vaginal dryness, trouble concentrating, and infertility.
Metastasis	The spread of cancer cells from the place where they first formed to another part of the body. In metastasis, cancer cells break away from the original (primary) tumor, travel through the blood or lymph system, and form a new tumor in other organs or tissues of the body. The new, metastatic tumor is the same type of cancer as the primary tumor. For example, if breast cancer spreads to the lung, the cancer cells in the lung are breast cancer cells, not lung cancer cells. The plural form of metastasis is metastases (meh-TAS-tuh-SEEZ).
Metastasize	To spread from one part of the body to another. When cancer cells metastasize and form secondary tumors, the cells in the metastatic tumor are like those in the original (primary) tumor.
Methotrexate	A drug used to treat many types of cancer. It is also used to treat rheumatoid arthritis and severe psoriasis (a type of skin condition). Methotrexate stops cells from using folic acid to make DNA and may kill cancer cells. It may also lower the body's immune response. Methotrexate is a type of antimetabolite and a type of antifolate. Also called amethopterin, MTX, Rheumatrex, and Trexall.

Mohs Micrographic Surgery	A surgical procedure used to treat skin cancer. Individual layers of cancer tissue are removed and examined under a microscope one at a time until all cancer tissue has been removed. Also called Mohs surgery.
Molecularly Targeted Therapy	In cancer, a type of treatment that uses drugs or other substances to target specific molecules involved in the growth and spread of cancer cells. Blocking these molecules may kill cancer cells or may keep cancer cells from growing or spreading. Molecularly targeted therapy may cause less harm to normal cells and may have fewer side effects than other types of cancer treatment.
Monitor	In medicine, to regularly watch and check a person or condition to see if there is any change. Also refers to a device that records and/or displays patient data, such as for an electrocardiogram (EKG).
Mucositis	A complication of some cancer therapies in which the lining of the digestive system becomes inflamed. Often seen as sores in the mouth.
Mucus	A thick, slippery fluid made by the membranes that line certain organs of the body, including the nose, mouth, throat, and vagina.
Multidisciplinary	In medicine, a term used to describe a treatment planning approach or team that includes a number of doctors and other health care professionals who are experts in different specialties (disciplines). In cancer treatment, the primary disciplines are medical oncology (treatment with drugs), surgical oncology (treatment with surgery), and radiation oncology (treatment with radiation).
Multiple Myeloma	A type of cancer that begins in plasma cells (white blood cells that produce antibodies). Also called Kahler disease, myelomatosis, and plasma cell myeloma.
Musculoskeletal	Having to do with muscles, bones, tendons, ligaments, joints, and cartilage.
Mutation	Any change in the DNA sequence of a cell. Mutations may be caused by mistakes during cell division, or they may be caused by exposure to DNA-damaging agents in the environment. Mutations can be harmful, beneficial, or have no effect. If they occur in cells that make eggs or sperm, they can be inherited; if mutations occur in other types of cells, they are not inherited. Certain mutations may lead to cancer or other diseases.
Myalgia	Pain in a muscle or group of muscles.

N

Narcotic	A substance used to treat moderate to severe pain. Narcotics are like opiates such as morphine and codeine, but are not made from opium. They bind to opioid receptors in the central nervous system. Narcotics are now called opioids.
National Cancer Institute	A part of the National Institutes of Health of the United States Department of Health and Human Services, it is the Federal Government's principal agency for cancer research. The National Cancer Institute conducts, coordinates, and funds cancer research, training, health information dissemination, and other programs with respect to the cause, diagnosis, prevention, and treatment of cancer. Access the National Cancer Institute Web site at http://www.cancer.gov. Also called NCI.
National Institutes of Health	A federal agency in the U.S. that conducts biomedical research in its own laboratories; supports the research of non-Federal scientists in universities, medical schools, hospitals, and research institutions throughout the country and abroad; helps in the training of research investigators; and fosters communication of medical information. Access the National Institutes of Health Web site at http://www.nih.gov. Also called NIH.
Nausea	A feeling of sickness or discomfort in the stomach that may come with an urge to vomit. Nausea is a side effect of some types of cancer therapy.

Needle Biopsy	The removal of tissue or fluid with a needle for examination under a microscope. When a wide needle is used, the procedure is called a core biopsy. When a thin needle is used, the procedure is called a fine-needle aspiration biopsy.
Negative Test Result	A test result that shows the substance or condition the test is supposed to find is not present at all or is present, but in normal amounts. In genetics, a negative test result usually means that a person does not have a mutation (change) in the gene, chromosome, or protein that is being tested. More testing may be needed to make sure a negative test result is correct.
Nephrectomy	Surgery to remove a kidney or part of a kidney. In a partial nephrectomy, part of one kidney or a tumor is removed, but not an entire kidney. In a simple nephrectomy, one kidney is removed. In a radical nephrectomy, an entire kidney, nearby adrenal gland and lymph nodes, and other surrounding tissue are removed. In a bilateral nephrectomy, both kidneys are removed.
Neutropenia	When a person has a low level of neutrophils. Neutrophils are a type of white blood cell. All white blood cells help the body fight infection. Neutrophils fight infection by destroying harmful bacteria and fungi (yeast) that invade the body. Neutrophils are made in the bone marrow. Bone marrow is the spongy tissue found in larger bones such as the pelvis, vertebrae, and ribs.
Neutropenic Diet	A special diet for those with neutropenia, cancer and weakened immune systems that incorporates dietary changes to prevent consumption of harmful bacteria in foods and beverages. It emphasizes the avoidance of the following: raw vegetables and fruits except oranges and bananas; takeout food and fast foods; aged cheese (blue, Roquefort, and Brie); deli meats; raw nuts or nuts roasted in shell; well water; and yogurt. Its usefulness has never been scientifically proven. However, neutropenic diets remain in place in many institutions even though their usefulness is controversial.
Neulasta	A drug used to treat neutropenia (a condition in which there is a lower-than-normal number of white blood cells) caused by some types of chemotherapy. It is used to help prevent infection in patients with certain types of cancer. Neulasta helps the bone marrow make more white blood cells. It is a form of filgrastim and is able to stay in the body longer. Neulasta is a type of colony-stimulating factor. Also called filgrastim-SD/01, Fulphila, and pegfilgrastim.
Neuropathy	A nerve problem that causes pain, numbness, tingling, swelling, or muscle weakness in different parts of the body. It usually begins in the hands or feet and gets worse over time. Neuropathy may be caused by cancer or cancer treatment, such as chemotherapy. It may also be caused by physical injury, infection, toxic substances, or conditions such as diabetes, kidney failure, or malnutrition. Also called peripheral neuropathy.
Neutropenia	A condition in which there is a lower-than-normal number of neutrophils (a type of white blood cell) in the blood.
Node Negative	Cancer that has not spread to the lymph nodes.
Node Positive	Cancer that has not spread to the lymph nodes.
Nodule	A growth or lump that may be malignant (cancer) or benign (not cancer).
Noninvasive	In medicine, it describes a procedure that does not require inserting an instrument through the skin or into a body opening. In cancer, it describes disease that has not spread outside the tissue in which it began.
Nonsteroidal Anti-Inflammatory Drug (NSAID)	A drug that decreases fever, swelling, pain, and redness. Also called NSAID.

Amor Y. Traceski

Normal Range	In medicine, a set of values that a doctor uses to interpret a patient's test results. The normal range for a given test is based on the results that are seen in 95% of the healthy population. Sometimes patients whose test results are outside of the normal range may be healthy, and some patients whose test results are within the normal range may have a health problem. The normal range for a test may be different for different groups of people (for example, men and women). Also called reference interval, reference range, and reference values.
Nuclear Medicine	A branch of medicine that uses small amounts of radioactive substances to make pictures of areas inside the body and to treat disease. In cancer, the radioactive substance may be used with a special machine (such as a PET scanner) to find the cancer, to see how far it has spread, or to see how well a treatment is working. Radioactive substances may also be used to treat certain types of cancer, such as thyroid cancer and lymphoma.
Nutrition	The taking in and use of food and other nourishing material by the body. Nutrition is a 3-part process. First, food or drink is consumed. Second, the body breaks down the food or drink into nutrients. Third, the nutrients travel through the bloodstream to different parts of the body where they are used as "fuel" and for many other purposes. To give the body proper nutrition, a person has to eat and drink enough of the foods that contain key nutrients.

O

Observation	In medicine, watching a patient's condition but not giving treatment unless symptoms appear or change.
Obstruction	Blockage of a passageway.
Omentectomy	Surgery to remove part or all of the omentum.
Omentum	A fold of the peritoneum (the thin tissue that lines the abdomen) that surrounds the stomach and other organs in the abdomen.
Ondansetron Hydrochloride	A drug used to prevent nausea and vomiting caused by chemotherapy and radiation therapy. It is also used to prevent nausea and vomiting after surgery. Ondansetron hydrochloride blocks the action of the chemical serotonin, which binds to certain nerves and may trigger nausea and vomiting. Blocking serotonin may help lessen nausea and vomiting. It is a type of serotonin receptor antagonist and a type of antiemetic. Also called Zofran.
Oophorectomy	Surgery to remove one or both ovaries.
Opioid	A substance used to treat moderate to severe pain. Opioids are like opiates, such as morphine and codeine, but are not made from opium. Opioids bind to opioid receptors in the central nervous system. Opioids used to be called narcotics. An opioid is a type of alkaloid.
Opioid Growth Factor	A substance that relieves pain and is being studied in the treatment of some types of cancer. Opioid growth factors bind to cells in the body, including tumor cells, which have opioid growth factor receptors on the surface. This may help stop the growth of the tumor cells. It may also prevent the growth of blood vessels that tumors need to grow. An opioid growth factor is a type of biological response modifier and a type of antiangiogenesis agent. Also called OGF.
Organ	A part of the body that performs a specific function. For example, the heart is an organ.
Osteopenia	A condition in which there is a lower-than-normal bone mass or bone mineral density (the amount of bone mineral contained in a certain amount of bone). Osteopenia is a less severe form of bone loss than osteoporosis.
Osteoporosis	A condition in which there is a decrease in the amount and thickness of bone tissue. This causes the bones to become weak and break more easily. Osteoporosis may be caused by older age, hormone changes, taking certain medicines, and not eating enough foods with calcium and vitamin D. It may also be caused by certain types of cancer and cancer treatment. It is most common in white and Asian women.

Ostomy	An operation to create an opening (a stoma) from an area inside the body to the outside. Colostomy and urostomy are types of ostomies.
Outcome	A specific result or effect that can be measured. Examples of outcomes include decreased pain, reduced tumor size, and improvement of disease.
Out-of-Pocket Cost	In medicine, the amount of money a patient pays for medical expenses that are not covered by a health insurance plan. Out-of-pocket costs include deductibles, coinsurance, copayments, and costs for non-covered healthcare services.
Outpatient	A patient who visits a health care facility for diagnosis or treatment without spending the night. Sometimes called a day patient.
Ovarian	Having to do with the ovaries, the female reproductive glands in which the ova (eggs) are formed. The ovaries are located in the pelvis, one on each side of the uterus.
Ovarian Cancer	Cancer that forms in tissues of the ovary (one of a pair of female reproductive glands in which the ova, or eggs, are formed). Most ovarian cancers are either ovarian epithelial cancers (cancer that begins in the cells on the surface of the ovary) or malignant germ cell tumors (cancer that begins in egg cells). Fallopian tube cancer and primary peritoneal cancer are similar to ovarian epithelial cancer and are staged and treated the same way.
Ovary	One of a pair of female glands in which the eggs form and the female hormones estrogen and progesterone are made. These hormones play an important role in female traits, such as breast development, body shape, and body hair. They are also involved in the menstrual cycle, fertility, and pregnancy. There is one ovary on each side of the uterus.
Overdose	An amount of drug that is more than what should be taken at one time.
Oxaliplatin	A drug used with other drugs to treat stage III colon cancer that was removed by surgery and colorectal cancer that is advanced. It is also being studied in the treatment of other types of cancer. Oxaliplatin damages the cell's DNA and may kill cancer cells. It is a type of platinum compound. Also called Eloxatin.
Oxycodone Hydrochloride	A drug used to treat moderate to severe pain. It is made from morphine and binds to opioid receptors in the central nervous system. Oxycodone hydrochloride is a type of analgesic agent and a type of opiate.
Oxygen	A colorless, odorless gas. It is needed for animal and plant life. Oxygen that is breathed in enters the blood from the lungs and travels to the tissues.
P	
Paclitaxel	A drug used to treat AIDS-related Kaposi sarcoma, advanced ovarian cancer, and certain types of breast cancer. It is also used with cisplatin to treat non-small cell lung cancer in patients who cannot be treated with surgery or radiation therapy. It is also being studied in the treatment of other types of cancer. Paclitaxel blocks cell growth by stopping cell division and may kill cancer cells. It is a type of antimitotic agent. Also called Taxol.
Pain Threshold	The point at which a person becomes aware of pain.
Premalignant	Likely to become cancer
Palpation	Examination by pressing on the surface of the body to feel the organs or tissues underneath.
Pancreas	A glandular organ located in the abdomen. It makes pancreatic juices, which contain enzymes that aid in digestion, and it produces several hormones, including insulin. The pancreas is surrounded by the stomach, intestines, and other organs.

Pancreatectomy	Surgery to remove all or part of the pancreas. In a total pancreatectomy, part of the stomach, part of the small intestine, the common bile duct, gallbladder, spleen, and nearby lymph nodes also are removed.
Pancreatic Cancer	A disease in which malignant (cancer) cells are found in the tissues of the pancreas. Also called exocrine cancer.
Pancreatitis	Inflammation of the pancreas. Chronic pancreatitis may cause diabetes and problems with digestion. Pain is the primary symptom.
Pancreatoduodenectomy	A type of surgery used to treat pancreatic cancer. The head of the pancreas, the duodenum, a portion of the stomach, and other nearby tissues are removed. Also called Whipple procedure.
Pap Test / Pap Smear	A procedure in which a small brush or spatula is used to gently remove cells from the cervix so they can be checked under a microscope for cervical cancer or cell changes that may lead to cervical cancer. It may also help find other conditions, such as infections or inflammation and is sometimes done at the same time as a pelvic exam.
Paralysis	Loss of ability to move all or part of the body.
Parametrium	The fat and connective tissue that surrounds the uterus. The parametrium helps connect the uterus to other tissues in the pelvis.
Parotid Gland Cancer	Cancer that forms in a parotid gland, the largest of the salivary glands, which make saliva and release it into the mouth. There are 2 parotid glands, one in front of and just below each ear. Most salivary gland tumors begin in parotid glands.
Parotidectomy	Surgery to remove all or part of the parotid gland (a large salivary gland located in front of and just below the ear). In a radical parotidectomy, the entire gland is removed.
Pathology Report	The description of cells and tissues made by a pathologist based on microscopic evidence, and sometimes used to make a diagnosis of a disease.
Patient Advocate	A person who helps guide a patient through the healthcare system. This includes help going through the screening, diagnosis, treatment, and follow-up of a medical condition, such as cancer. A patient advocate helps patients communicate with their healthcare providers so they get the information they need to make decisions about their health care. Patient advocates may also help patients set up appointments for doctor visits and medical tests and get financial, legal, and social support. They may also work with insurance companies, employers, case managers, lawyers, and others who may have an effect on a patient's healthcare needs. Also called patient navigator.
Patient-Controlled Analgesia (PCA)	A method of pain relief in which the patient controls the amount of pain medicine that is used. When pain relief is needed, the person can receive a preset dose of pain medicine by pressing a button on a computerized pump that is connected to a small tube in the body. Also called PCA.
Pegfilgrastim	A drug used to treat neutropenia (a condition in which there is a lower-than-normal number of white blood cells) caused by some types of chemotherapy. It is used to help prevent infection in patients with certain types of cancer. Pegfilgrastim helps the bone marrow make more white blood cells. It is a form of filgrastim and is able to stay in the body longer. Pegfilgrastim is a type of colony-stimulating factor. Also called filgrastim-SD/01, Fulphila, and Neulasta.
Pelvic Exam / Internal Exam	A physical exam of the vagina, cervix, uterus, fallopian tubes, ovaries, and rectum. First, the area outside the vagina is checked for signs of disease. A speculum is then inserted into the vagina to widen it so the vagina and cervix can be checked for signs of disease. Cell samples may be taken for a Pap test, or to test for sexually transmitted diseases or other infections. The doctor or nurse then inserts one or two lubricated, gloved fingers of one hand into the vagina and presses on the lower abdomen with the other hand to feel for lumps and check the size, shape, and position of the uterus and ovaries. The rectum may also be checked for lumps or abnormal areas. Also called internal exam.

Pelvis	The area of the body below the abdomen that contains the hip bones, bladder, and rectum. In females, it also contains the vagina, cervix, uterus, fallopian tubes, and ovaries. In males, it also contains the prostate and seminal vesicles.
Penicillin	A drug that is used to treat infection. It belongs to the family of drugs called antibiotics.
Peripheral Neuropathy	A nerve problem that causes pain, numbness, tingling, swelling, or muscle weakness in different parts of the body. It usually begins in the hands or feet and gets worse over time. Peripheral neuropathy may be caused by cancer or cancer treatment, such as chemotherapy. It may also be caused by physical injury, infection, toxic substances, or conditions such as diabetes, kidney failure, or malnutrition. Also called neuropathy.
Peritoneal Cavity	The space within the abdomen that contains the intestines, the stomach, and the liver. It is bound by thin membranes.
Peritoneal Fluid	A liquid that is made in the abdominal cavity to lubricate the surface of the tissue that lines the abdominal wall and pelvic cavity and covers most of the organs in the abdomen.
Peritoneum	The tissue that lines the abdominal wall and covers most of the organs in the abdomen.
PET Scan	A procedure in which a small amount of radioactive glucose (sugar) is injected into a vein, and a scanner is used to make detailed, computerized pictures of areas inside the body where the glucose is taken up. Because cancer cells often take up more glucose than normal cells, the pictures can be used to find cancer cells in the body. Also called positron emission tomography scan.
Phlebotomy / Blood Draw / Venipuncture	A procedure in which a needle is used to take blood from a vein, usually for laboratory testing. Phlebotomy may also be done to remove extra red blood cells from the blood, to treat certain blood disorders. Also called blood draw and venipuncture.
Phlegm	A more than normal amount of thick mucus made by the cells lining the upper airways and lungs. A buildup of phlegm may be caused by infection, irritation, or chronic lung disease, and can cause discomfort in the chest and coughing.
Physical Therapy	The use of exercises and physical activities to help condition muscles and restore strength and movement. For example, physical therapy can be used to restore arm and shoulder movement and build back strength after breast cancer surgery.
PICC – Peripherally Inserted Central Catheter	A device used to draw blood and give treatments, including intravenous fluids, drugs, or blood transfusions. A thin, flexible tube is inserted into a vein in the upper arm and guided (threaded) into a large vein above the right side of the heart called the superior vena cava. A needle is inserted into a port outside the body to draw blood or give fluids. A PICC may stay in place for weeks or months and helps avoid the need for repeated needle sticks. Also called peripherally inserted central catheter.
Plaque	In medicine, a small, abnormal patch of tissue on a body part or an organ. Plaques may also be a build-up of substances from a fluid, such as cholesterol in the blood vessels.
Plasma	The clear, yellowish, fluid part of the blood that carries the blood cells. The proteins that form blood clots are in plasma.
Pleura	A thin layer of tissue that covers the lungs and lines the interior wall of the chest cavity. It protects and cushions the lungs. This tissue secretes a small amount of fluid that acts as a lubricant, allowing the lungs to move smoothly in the chest cavity while breathing.
Pleural Effusion	An abnormal collection of fluid between the thin layers of tissue (pleura) lining the lung and the wall of the chest cavity.
Polyp	A growth that protrudes from a mucous membrane.

Portal Vein	A blood vessel that carries blood to the liver from the intestines, spleen, pancreas, and gallbladder. Also called hepatic portal vein.
Positive Test Result	A test result that shows that a person has the disease, condition, or biomarker for which the test is being done. In genetics, a positive test result usually means that a person has a mutation (change) in the gene, chromosome, or protein that is being tested. More testing may be needed to make a diagnosis or to make sure a positive test result is correct.
Positron Emission Tomography Scan / (PET Scan)	A procedure in which a small amount of radioactive glucose (sugar) is injected into a vein, and a scanner is used to make detailed, computerized pictures of areas inside the body where the glucose is taken up. Because cancer cells often take up more glucose than normal cells, the pictures can be used to find cancer cells in the body.
Post-Menopausal	Having to do with the time after menopause. Menopause ("change of life") is the time in a woman's life when menstrual periods stop permanently.
Postoperative	After surgery.
Post-Traumatic Stress Disorder (PTSD)	An anxiety disorder that develops in reaction to physical injury or severe mental or emotional distress, such as military combat, violent assault, natural disaster, or other life-threatening events. Having cancer may also lead to post-traumatic stress disorder. Symptoms interfere with day-to-day living and include reliving the event in nightmares or flashbacks; avoiding people, places, and things connected to the event; feeling alone and losing interest in daily activities; and having trouble concentrating and sleeping.
Precancerous	A term used to describe a condition that may (or is likely to) become cancer. Also called premalignant.
Prednisone	A drug used to lessen inflammation and lower the body's immune response. It is used with other drugs to treat leukemia and lymphoma and other types of cancer. It is also used alone or with other drugs to prevent or treat many other conditions. These include conditions related to cancer, such as anemia (a low level of red blood cells), allergic reactions, and loss of appetite.
Prescription	A doctor's order for medicine or another intervention.
Prevention	In medicine, action taken to decrease the chance of getting a disease or condition. For example, cancer prevention includes avoiding risk factors (such as smoking, obesity, lack of exercise, and radiation exposure) and increasing protective factors (such as getting regular physical activity, staying at a healthy weight, and having a healthy diet).
Preventive Mastectomy	Surgery to reduce the risk of developing breast cancer by removing one or both breasts before disease develops. Also called prophylactic mastectomy.
Primary Cancer or Primary Tumor	A term used to describe the original, or first, tumor in the body. Cancer cells from a primary cancer may spread to other parts of the body and form new, or secondary, tumors. This is called metastasis. These secondary tumors are the same type of cancer as the primary cancer.
Primary Care	Health services that meet most basic health care needs over time. Primary care includes physical exams, treatment of common medical conditions, and preventive care such as immunizations and screenings. Primary care doctors are usually the first health professionals patients see for basic medical care. They may refer a patient to a specialist if needed.
Primary Care Doctor (PCP)	A doctor who manages a person's health care over time. A primary care doctor is able to give a wide range of care, including prevention and treatment, can discuss cancer treatment choices, and can refer a patient to a specialist.
Progesterone	A type of hormone made by the body that plays a role in the menstrual cycle and pregnancy. Progesterone can also be made in the laboratory. It may be used as a type of birth control and to treat menstrual disorders, infertility, symptoms of menopause, and other conditions.

Prognosis	The likely outcome or course of a disease; the chance of recovery or recurrence.
Progression	In medicine, the course of a disease, such as cancer, as it becomes worse or spreads in the body.
Prophylactic	In medicine, something that prevents or protects.
Prostate	A gland in the male reproductive system. The prostate surrounds the part of the urethra (the tube that empties the bladder) just below the bladder, and produces a fluid that forms part of the semen.
Prostate Cancer	Cancer that forms in tissues of the prostate (a gland in the male reproductive system found below the bladder and in front of the rectum). Prostate cancer usually occurs in older men.
Prostatectomy	Surgery to remove part or all of the prostate and some of the tissue around it. Nearby lymph nodes may also be removed. It may be done through an open prostatectomy, in which an incision (cut) is made in the wall of the lower abdomen or the perineum, or by using a laparoscope (a thin, tube-like instrument with a light and lens for viewing).
Prosthesis	A device, such as an artificial leg, that replaces a part of the body.
Pruritis	Itching. Severe itching may be a side effect of some cancer treatments and a symptom of some types of cancers.
Psoriasis	A chronic disease of the skin marked by red patches covered with white scales.
Psychotherapy	Treatment of mental, emotional, personality, and behavioral disorders using methods such as discussion, listening, and counseling. Also called talk therapy.
Public Health Insurance	A program run by U.S. federal, state, or local governments in which people have some or all of their healthcare costs paid for by the government. The two main types of public health insurance are Medicare and Medicaid. Medicare is a federal health insurance program for people aged 65 years or older and people with certain disabilities. Medicaid and MediCal are public health insurance programs for some individuals and families with a low income or disabilities.
Pulmonary	Having to do with the lungs.
Pulse / Heart Rate	In medicine, the number of times the heart beats within a certain time period, usually a minute. The pulse can be felt at the wrist, side of the neck, back of the knees, top of the foot, groin, and other places in the body where an artery is close to the skin. The resting pulse is normally between 60 and 100 beats a minute in a healthy adult who is at rest. Measuring the pulse gives important information about a person's health. Also called heart rate.
Purine	One of two chemical compounds that cells use to make the building blocks of DNA and RNA. Examples of purines are adenine and guanine. Purines are also found in meat and meat products. They are broken down by the body to form uric acid, which is passed in the urine. High levels of uric acid in the body may cause gout.

Q

Qi	In traditional Chinese medicine, vital energy or life force that keeps a person's spiritual, emotional, mental, and physical health in balance.
Qigong	A form of traditional Chinese mind/body exercise and meditation that uses slow and precise body movements with controlled breathing and mental focusing to improve balance, flexibility, muscle strength, and overall health.

Radiation	Energy released in the form of particle or electromagnetic waves. Common sources of radiation include radon gas, cosmic rays from outer space, medical x-rays, and energy given off by a radioisotope (unstable form of a chemical element that releases radiation as it breaks down and becomes more stable). Radiation can damage cells. It is used to diagnose and treat some types of cancer.
Radiation Brachytherapy	A type of radiation therapy in which radioactive material sealed in needles, seeds, wires, or catheters is placed directly into or near a tumor. Also called brachytherapy, implant radiation therapy, and internal radiation therapy.
Radiation Therapy	The use of high-energy radiation from x-rays, gamma rays, neutrons, protons, and other sources to kill cancer cells and shrink tumors. Radiation may come from a machine outside the body (external-beam radiation therapy), or it may come from radioactive material placed in the body near cancer cells (internal radiation therapy or brachytherapy). Systemic radiation therapy uses a radioactive substance, such as a radiolabeled monoclonal antibody, that travels in the blood to tissues throughout the body. Also called irradiation and radiotherapy.
Radical Hysterectomy	Surgery to remove the uterus, cervix, and part of the vagina. The ovaries, fallopian tubes, and nearby lymph nodes may also be removed.
Radical Mastectomy	Surgery for breast cancer in which the breast, chest muscles, and all of the lymph nodes under the arm are removed. For many years, this was the breast cancer operation used most often, but it is used rarely now. Doctors consider radical mastectomy only when the tumor has spread to the chest muscles. Also called Halsted radical mastectomy.
Radio Wave	A type of wave made when an electric field and a magnetic field are combined. Radio waves are being studied in the treatment of several types of cancer and other conditions. The radio waves are sent through needles inserted into tumor tissue and may kill cancer cells. Radio waves are also used in MRI to create detailed images of areas inside the body.
Radioactive	Giving off radiation.
Radioactive Glucose	A radioactive form of glucose (sugar) often used during a positive emission tomography (PET) scan, a type of imaging test. In PET, a small amount of radioactive glucose is injected into a vein, and a scanner makes a picture of where the glucose is being used in the body. Cancer cells show up brighter in the picture because they are more active and take up more glucose than normal cells do. When used with PET, radioactive glucose helps find cancer cells in the body.
Radioactive Seed	A small, radioactive pellet that is placed in or near a tumor. Cancer cells are killed by the energy given off as the radioactive material breaks down and becomes more stable.
Radioembolization	A type of radiation therapy used to treat liver cancer or cancer that has spread to the liver. A thin, flexible tube is used to inject tiny beads that hold the radioactive substance yttrium Y 90 into the main blood vessel that carries blood to the liver. The beads collect in the tumor and in blood vessels near the tumor, and the yttrium Y 90 gives off radiation. This destroys the blood vessels that the tumor needs to grow and kills the cancer cells. Radioembolization is a type of internal radiation therapy. Also called intra-arterial brachytherapy.
Radiofrequency Ablation (RFA)	A procedure that uses radio waves to heat and destroy abnormal cells. The radio waves travel through electrodes (small devices that carry electricity). Radiofrequency ablation may be used to treat cancer and other conditions.
Radiology	The use of radiation (such as x-rays) or other imaging technologies (such as ultrasound and magnetic resonance imaging) to diagnose or treat disease.
Radiosurgery	A type of external radiation therapy that uses special equipment to position the patient and precisely give a single large dose of radiation to a tumor. It is used to treat brain tumors and other brain disorders that cannot be treated by regular surgery. It is also being studied in the treatment of other types of cancer. Also called radiation surgery, stereotactic radiosurgery, and stereotaxic radiosurgery.

Radiotherapy	The use of high-energy radiation from x-rays, gamma rays, neutrons, protons, and other sources to kill cancer cells and shrink tumors. Radiation may come from a machine outside the body (external-beam radiation therapy), or it may come from radioactive material placed in the body near cancer cells (internal radiation therapy or brachytherapy). Systemic radiotherapy uses a radioactive substance, such as a radiolabeled monoclonal antibody, that travels in the blood to tissues throughout the body. Also called irradiation and radiation therapy.
Reconstructive Surgery	Surgery that is done to reshape or rebuild (reconstruct) a part of the body changed by previous surgery.
Recover	To become well and healthy again.
Rectal Cancer	Cancer that forms in the tissues of the rectum (the last several inches of the large intestine closest to the anus).
Rectum	The last several inches of the large intestine closest to the anus.
Recurrence	Cancer that has recurred (come back), usually after a period of time during which the cancer could not be detected. The cancer may come back to the same place as the original (primary) tumor or to another place in the body. Also called recurrent cancer.
Red Blood Cell	A type of blood cell that is made in the bone marrow and found in the blood. Red blood cells contain a protein called hemoglobin, which carries oxygen from the lungs to all parts of the body. Checking the number of red blood cells in the blood is usually part of a complete blood cell (CBC) test. It may be used to look for conditions such as anemia, dehydration, malnutrition, and leukemia. Also called erythrocyte and RBC.
Referral	In medicine, the act of a doctor in which a patient is sent to another doctor for additional healthcare services.
Reflux	The backward flow of liquid from the stomach into the esophagus.
Refractory	In medicine, describes a disease or condition that does not respond to treatment.
Regeneration	In biology, regrowth of damaged or destroyed tissue or body part.
Regimen	A treatment plan that specifies the dosage, the schedule, and the duration of treatment.
Regional	In oncology, describes the body area right around a tumor.
Regional Lymph Node	In oncology, a lymph node that drains lymph from the region around a tumor.
Reglan	A drug that increases the motility (movements and contractions) of the stomach and upper intestine. It is used to treat certain stomach problems and nausea and vomiting caused by chemotherapy. It is a type of antiemetic and a type of motility agent. Also called metoclopramide.
Regression	A decrease in the size of a tumor or in the extent of cancer in the body.
Rehabilitation	In medicine, a process to restore mental and/or physical abilities lost to injury or disease, in order to function in a normal or near-normal way.
Relapse	The return of a disease or the signs and symptoms of a disease after a period of improvement. Relapse also refers to returning to the use of an addictive substance or behavior, such as cigarette smoking.
Remission	A decrease in or disappearance of signs and symptoms of cancer. In partial remission, some, but not all, signs and symptoms of cancer have disappeared. In complete remission, all signs and symptoms of cancer have disappeared, although cancer still may be in the body.

Renal Artery	The main blood vessel that supplies blood to a kidney and its nearby adrenal gland and ureter. There is a renal artery for each kidney.
Renal Function	A term used to describe how well the kidneys work. The kidneys remove waste and extra water from the blood (as urine) and help keep chemicals (such as sodium, potassium, and calcium) balanced in the body. They also make hormones that help control blood pressure and stimulate bone marrow to make red blood cells. Also called kidney function.
Resection	Surgery to remove tissue or part or all of an organ.
Respiratory System	The organs that are involved in breathing. These include the nose, throat, larynx, trachea, bronchi, and lungs. Also called respiratory tract.
Respiratory Therapy	Exercises and treatments that help improve or restore lung function.
Respite Care	Temporary care given to a person who is unable to care for himself or herself so that the usual caregivers can have a break. Respite care may include in-home care, adult daycare, or nursing home care.
Response	In medicine, an improvement related to treatment.
Restless Legs Syndrome	A condition in which a person has a strong urge to move his or her legs in order to stop uncomfortable sensations. These include burning, itching, creeping, tugging, crawling, or pain. These feelings usually happen when a person is lying or sitting down, and are worse at night. They can also occur in other parts of the body. Also called RLS.
Retch	The action of the stomach and esophagus to try to vomit (eject some or all of the contents of the stomach). Retching that does not cause vomiting is called dry heaves.

	S
Sacrum	The large, triangle-shaped bone in the lower spine that forms part of the pelvis. It is made of 5 fused bones of the spine.
Saline	A solution of salt and water.
Saliva	The watery fluid in the mouth made by the salivary glands. Saliva moistens food to help digestion and it helps protect the mouth against infections.
Salivary Gland	A gland in the mouth that produces saliva.
Salivary Gland Cancer	A rare cancer that forms in tissues of a salivary gland (gland in the mouth that makes saliva). Most salivary gland cancers occur in older people.
Salpingo-Oophorectomy	Surgical removal of the fallopian tubes and ovaries.
Sarcoma	A type of cancer that begins in bone or in the soft tissues of the body, including cartilage, fat, muscle, blood vessels, fibrous tissue, or other connective or supportive tissue. Different types of sarcoma are based on where the cancer forms. For example, osteosarcoma forms in bone, liposarcoma forms in fat, and rhabdomyosarcoma forms in muscle. Treatment and prognosis depend on the type and grade of the cancer (how abnormal the cancer cells look under a microscope and how quickly the cancer is likely to grow and spread). Sarcoma occurs in both adults and children.
Scan	A type of test that makes detailed pictures of areas inside the body. A scan may also refer to the picture that gets made during the test. Scans may be used to help diagnose disease, plan treatment, or find out how well treatment is working. There are many different types of scans, including computed tomography (CT) scans, magnetic resonance imaging (MRI) scans, and nuclear medicine scans (such as bone scans and liver scans). CT scans are done with an x-ray machine linked to a computer. MRI scans are done with radio waves and a powerful magnet linked to a computer. Nuclear medicine scans are done with small amounts of radioactive substances that are injected into the body and a special machine that detects the radioactive substance.

Scanner	In medicine, an instrument that takes pictures of the inside of the body.
Scar Tissue	Fibrous tissue that forms when normal tissue is destroyed by disease, injury, or surgery. For example, scar tissue forms when a wound heals after a cut, sore, burn, or other skin condition, or when an incision (cut) is made into the skin during surgery. It may also form inside the body when certain conditions, such as cirrhosis, cause normal tissue to become fibrous tissue.
Screening	Checking for disease when there are no symptoms. Since screening may find diseases at an early stage, there may be a better chance of curing the disease. Examples of cancer screening tests are the mammogram (for breast cancer), colonoscopy (for colon cancer), and the Pap test and HPV tests (for cervical cancer). Screening can also include doing a genetic test to check for a person's risk of developing an inherited disease.
Second Opinion	In medicine, the opinion of a doctor other than the patient's current doctor. The second doctor reviews the patient's medical records and gives an opinion about the patient's health problem and how it should be treated. A second opinion may confirm or question the first doctor's diagnosis and treatment plan, give more information about the patient's disease or condition, and offer other treatment options.
Secondary Cancer	A term used to describe cancer that has spread (metastasized) from the place where it first started to another part of the body. Secondary cancers are the same type of cancer as the original (primary) cancer. For example, cancer cells may spread from the breast (primary cancer) to form new tumors in the lung (secondary cancer). The cancer cells in the lung are just like the ones in the breast. Also called secondary tumor.
Secrete	To form and release a substance. In the body, cells secrete substances, such as sweat that cools the body or hormones that act in other parts of the body.
Sentinel Lymph Node	The first lymph node to which cancer is likely to spread from the primary tumor. When cancer spreads, the cancer cells may appear first in the sentinel node before spreading to other lymph nodes.
Sentinel Lymph Node Biopsy	Removal and examination of the sentinel node(s) (the first lymph node(s) to which cancer cells are likely to spread from a primary tumor). To identify the sentinel lymph node(s), the surgeon injects a radioactive substance, blue dye, or both near the tumor. The surgeon then uses a probe to find the sentinel lymph node(s) containing the radioactive substance or looks for the lymph node(s) stained with dye. The surgeon then removes the sentinel node(s) to check for the presence of cancer cells.
Sepsis	The presence of bacteria or their toxins in the blood or tissues.
Sequential Treatment	One treatment after the other.
Serotonin	A hormone found in the brain, platelets, digestive tract, and pineal gland. It acts both as a neurotransmitter (a substance that nerves use to send messages to one another) and a vasoconstrictor (a substance that causes blood vessels to narrow). A lack of serotonin in the brain is thought to be a cause of depression. Also called 5-hydroxytryptamine.
Short-Term Side Effect	A problem that is caused by treatment of a disease but usually goes away after treatment ends. Short-term side effects of cancer treatment include nausea, vomiting, diarrhea, hair loss, fatigue, and mouth sores.
Side Effect	A problem that occurs when treatment affects healthy tissues or organs. Some common side effects of cancer treatment are nausea, vomiting, fatigue, pain, decreased blood cell counts, hair loss, and mouth sores.
Sigmoid Colon	The S-shaped section of the colon that connects to the rectum.
Sigmoidoscope	A thin, tube-like instrument used to examine the inside of the colon. A sigmoidoscope has a light and a lens for viewing and may have a tool to remove tissue.

Amor Y. Traceski

Sigmoidoscopy	Examination of the lower colon using a sigmoidoscope, inserted into the rectum. A sigmoidoscope is a thin, tube-like instrument with a light and a lens for viewing. It may also have a tool to remove tissue to be checked under a microscope for signs of disease. Also called proctosigmoidoscopy.
Sign	In medicine, a sign is something found during a physical exam or from a laboratory test that shows that a person may have a condition or disease. Some examples of signs are fever, swelling, skin rash, high blood pressure, and high blood glucose.
Signaling Pathway	Describes a group of molecules in a cell that work together to control one or more cell functions, such as cell division or cell death. After the first molecule in a pathway receives a signal, it activates another molecule. This process is repeated until the last molecule is activated and the cell function is carried out. Abnormal activation of signaling pathways can lead to cancer, and drugs are being developed to block these pathways. These drugs may help block cancer cell growth and kill cancer cells.
Silicone	A synthetic gel that is used as an outer coating on breast implants and as the inside filling of some implants.
Sinus	A cavity, space, or channel in the body. Examples include hollow spaces in the bones at the front of the skull, and channels for blood and lymph. Sinuses may also be found in the heart, brain, kidney, and other organs.
Skin Cancer	Cancer that forms in the tissues of the skin. There are several types of skin cancer. Skin cancer that forms in melanocytes (skin cells that make pigment) is called melanoma. Skin cancer that forms in the lower part of the epidermis (the outer layer of the skin) is called basal cell carcinoma. Skin cancer that forms in squamous cells (flat cells that form the surface of the skin) is called squamous cell carcinoma. Skin cancer that forms in neuroendocrine cells (cells that release hormones in response to signals from the nervous system) is called neuroendocrine carcinoma of the skin. Most skin cancers form in older people on parts of the body exposed to the sun or in people who have weakened immune systems.
Skin Vesicle	A fluid-filled sac in the outer layer of skin. It can be caused by rubbing, heat, or diseases of the skin. Also called blister.
Small Intestine	A long tube-like organ that connects the stomach and the large intestine. It is about 20 feet long and folds many times to fit inside the abdomen. The small intestine has three parts: the duodenum, jejunum, and ileum. It helps to further digest food coming from the stomach. It absorbs nutrients (vitamins, minerals, carbohydrates, fats, proteins) and water from food so they can be used by the body. The small intestine is part of the digestive system.
Social Service	A community resource that helps people in need. Services may include help getting to and from medical appointments, home delivery of medication and meals, in-home nursing care, help paying medical costs not covered by insurance, loaning medical equipment, and housekeeping help.
Social Support	A network of family, friends, neighbors, and community members that is available in times of need to give psychological, physical, and financial help.
Social Worker	A professional trained to talk with people and their families about emotional or physical needs, and to find them support services.
Soft Diet	A diet consisting of bland foods that are softened by cooking, mashing, pureeing, or blending.
Soft Tissue	Refers to muscle, fat, fibrous tissue, blood vessels, or other supporting tissue of the body.
Soft Tissue Sarcoma	A cancer that begins in the muscle, fat, fibrous tissue, blood vessels, or other supporting tissue of the body.
Solid Tumor	An abnormal mass of tissue that usually does not contain cysts or liquid areas. Solid tumors may be benign (not cancer), or malignant (cancer). Different types of solid tumors are named for the type of cells that form them. Examples of solid tumors are sarcomas, carcinomas, and lymphomas. Leukemias (cancers of the blood) generally do not form solid tumors.

Sonogram	A computer picture of areas inside the body created by high-energy sound waves. The sound waves are bounced off internal tissues or organs and make echoes. The echoes form a picture of the body tissues on a computer screen. A sonogram may be used to help diagnose disease, such as cancer. It may also be used during pregnancy to check the fetus (unborn baby) and during medical procedures, such as biopsies. Also called ultrasonogram.
Standard Operating Procedure (SOP)	Written instructions for doing a specific task in a certain way. In clinical trials, SOPs are set up to store records, collect data, screen and enroll subjects, and submit Institutional Review Board (IRB) applications and renewals. Also called Standard Operating Procedure.
Spasm	A sudden contraction of a muscle or group of muscles, such as a cramp.
Spastic Colon	A disorder of the intestines commonly marked by abdominal pain, bloating, and changes in a person's bowel habits. This may include diarrhea or constipation, or both, with one occurring after the other. Also called IBS, irritable bowel syndrome, irritable colon, and mucus colitis.
Speculum	An instrument used to widen an opening of the body to make it easier to look inside.
Spine	The bones, muscles, tendons, and other tissues that reach from the base of the skull to the tailbone. The spine encloses the spinal cord and the fluid surrounding the spinal cord. Also called backbone, spinal column, and vertebral column.
Spirituality	Having to do with deep, often religious, feelings and beliefs, including a person's sense of peace, purpose, connection to others, and beliefs about the meaning of life.
Spleen	An organ that is part of the lymphatic system. The spleen makes lymphocytes, filters the blood, stores blood cells, and destroys old blood cells. It is located on the left side of the abdomen near the stomach.
Splenectomy	An operation to remove the spleen.
Sputum	Mucus and other matter brought up from the lungs by coughing.
Squamous Cell Carcinoma	Cancer that begins in squamous cells. Squamous cells are thin, flat cells that look like fish scales, and are found in the tissue that forms the surface of the skin, the lining of the hollow organs of the body, and the lining of the respiratory and digestive tracts. Most cancers of the anus, cervix, head and neck, and vagina are squamous cell carcinomas. Also called epidermoid carcinoma.
Stage	The extent of a cancer in the body. Staging is usually based on the size of the tumor, whether lymph nodes contain cancer, and whether the cancer has spread from the original site to other parts of the body.
Staging	Performing exams and tests to learn the extent of the cancer within the body, especially whether the disease has spread from where it first formed to other parts of the body. It is important to know the stage of the disease in order to plan the best treatment.
Stamina	The energy and strength to endure physical activity, stress, or illness over time.
Standard of Care	Treatment that is accepted by medical experts as a proper treatment for a certain type of disease and that is widely used by healthcare professionals. Also called best practice, standard medical care, and standard therapy.
Standard Operating Procedure (SOP)	Written instructions for doing a specific task in a certain way. In clinical trials, Standard Operating Procedures are set up to store records, collect data, screen and enroll subjects, and submit Institutional Review Board (IRB) applications and renewals. Also called SOP.

Staph Infection	A staph infection is caused by a Staphylococcus (or "staph") bacteria. Actually, about 25% of people normally carry staph in the nose, mouth, genitals, or anal area, and don't have symptoms of an infection. The foot is also very prone to picking up bacteria from the floor. The infection often begins with a little cut, which gets infected with bacteria. This can look like honey-yellow crusting on the skin. These staph infections range from a simple boil to antibiotic-resistant infections to flesh-eating infections. The difference between all these is the strength of the infection, how deep it goes, how fast it spreads, and how treatable it is with antibiotics. The antibiotic-resistant infections are more common in North America, because of our overuse of antibiotics. One type of staph infection that involves skin is called cellulitis and affects the skin's deeper layers. It is treatable with antibiotics. Staph infections become more serious when they go deeper in the body, entering the bloodstream, joints, lungs, or heart. These are known as invasive staph infections.
Statin	Any of a group of drugs that lower the amount of cholesterol and certain fats in the blood. Statins inhibit a key enzyme that helps make cholesterol. Statin drugs are being studied in the prevention and treatment of cancer.
Stem Cell	A cell from which other types of cells develop. For example, blood cells develop from blood-forming stem cells.
Stereotactic Biopsy	A biopsy procedure that uses a computer and a 3-dimensional scanning device to find a tumor site and guide the removal of tissue for examination under a microscope.
Steroid	Any of a group of lipids (fats) that have a certain chemical structure. Steroids occur naturally in plants and animals or they may be made in the laboratory. Examples of steroids include sex hormones, cholesterol, bile acids, and some drugs.
Steroid Drug	A type of drug used to relieve swelling and inflammation. Some steroid drugs may also have antitumor effects.
Stoma	A surgically created opening from an area inside the body to the outside.
Stomach	An organ that is part of the digestive system. The stomach helps digest food by mixing it with digestive juices and churning it into a thin liquid.
Stool	The material in a bowel movement. Stool is made up of undigested food, bacteria, mucus, and cells from the lining of the intestines. Also called feces.
Stress	In medicine, the body's response to physical, mental, or emotional pressure. Stress causes chemical changes in the body that can raise blood pressure, heart rate, and blood sugar levels. It may also lead to feelings of frustration, anxiety, anger, or depression. Stress can be caused by normal life activities or by an event, such as trauma or illness. Long-term stress or high levels of stress may lead to mental and physical health problems.
Strontium	A metal often used in a radioactive form for imaging tests and in the treatment of cancer.
Sulfa Drug	A type of antibiotic used to treat infection. Also called sulfonamide.
Sun Protection Factor (SPF)	A scale for rating the level of sunburn protection in sunscreen products. The higher the sun protection factor, the more sunburn protection it gives. Sunscreens with a value of 2 through 11 give minimal protection against sunburns. Sunscreens with a value of 12 through 29 give moderate protection. Sun protection factors of 30 or higher give high protection against sunburn.
Superficial	Affecting cells on the surface. Not invasive.
Superior Vena Cava	The large vein that carries blood from the head, neck, arms, and chest to the heart.

Supplemental Health Insurance	An additional insurance plan that helps pay for healthcare costs that are not covered by a person's regular health insurance plan. These costs include copayments, coinsurance, and deductibles. There are many different types of supplemental health insurance, including vision, dental, hospital, accident, disability, long-term care, and Medicare supplemental plans. There are also supplemental health insurance plans for specific conditions, such as cancer, stroke, or kidney failure. Some types of supplemental health insurance may also be used to help pay for food, medicine, transportation, and other expenses related to an illness or injury.
Supplemental Nutrition	A substance or product that is added to a person's diet to make sure they get all the nutrients they need. It may include vitamins, minerals, protein, or fat, and may be given by mouth, by tube feeding, or into a vein.
Suppository	A form of medicine contained in a small piece of solid material, such as cocoa butter or glycerin, that melts at body temperature. A suppository is inserted into the rectum, vagina, or urethra and the medicine is absorbed into the bloodstream.
Surgery	A procedure to remove or repair a part of the body or to find out whether disease is present. An operation.
Surgical Biopsy	The removal of tissue by a surgeon for examination by a pathologist. The pathologist may study the tissue under a microscope.
Surveillance	In medicine, closely watching a patient's condition but not treating it unless there are changes in test results. Surveillance is also used to find early signs that a disease has come back. It may also be used for a person who has an increased risk of a disease, such as cancer. During surveillance, certain exams and tests are done on a regular schedule. In public health, surveillance may also refer to the ongoing collection of information about a disease, such as cancer, in a certain group of people. The information collected may include where the disease occurs in a population and whether it affects people of a certain gender, age, or ethnic group.
Survival Rate	The percentage of people in a study or treatment group who are still alive for a certain period of time after they were diagnosed with or started treatment for a disease, such as cancer. The survival rate is often stated as a five-year survival rate, which is the percentage of people in a study or treatment group who are alive five years after their diagnosis or the start of treatment. Also called overall survival rate.
Survivor	One who remains alive and continues to function during and after overcoming a serious hardship or life-threatening disease. In cancer, a person is considered to be a survivor from the time of diagnosis until the end of life.
Survivorship	In cancer, survivorship focuses on the health and life of a person with cancer post treatment until the end of life. It covers the physical, psychosocial, and economic issues of cancer, beyond the diagnosis and treatment phases. Survivorship includes issues related to the ability to get health care and follow-up treatment, late effects of treatment, second cancers, and quality of life. Family members, friends, and caregivers are also considered part of the survivorship experience.
Survivorship Care Plan	A detailed plan given to a patient after treatment ends, that contains a summary of the patient's treatment, along with recommendations for follow-up care. In cancer, the plan is based on the type of cancer and the treatment the patient received. A survivorship care plan may include schedules for physical exams and medical tests to see if the cancer has come back or spread to other parts of the body. Getting follow-up care also helps check for health problems that may occur months or years after treatment ends, including other types of cancer. A survivorship care plan may also include information to help meet the emotional, social, legal, and financial needs of the patient. It may include referrals to specialists and recommendations for a healthy lifestyle, such as changes in diet and exercise and quitting smoking. Also called follow-up care plan.
Symptom	A physical or mental problem that a person experiences that may indicate a disease or condition. Symptoms cannot be seen and do not show up on medical tests. Some examples of symptoms are headache, fatigue, nausea, and pain.

Symptom Management	Care given to improve the quality of life of patients who have a serious or life-threatening disease. The goal of symptom management is to prevent or treat as early as possible the symptoms of a disease, side effects caused by treatment of a disease, and psychological, social, and spiritual problems related to a disease or its treatment. Also called comfort care, palliative care, and supportive care.
Syndrome	A set of symptoms or conditions that occur together and suggest the presence of a certain disease or an increased chance of developing the disease.
Synovial Membrane	A layer of connective tissue that lines the cavities of joints, tendon sheaths, and bursae (fluid-filled sacs between tendons and bones). The synovial membrane makes synovial fluid, which has a lubricating function.
Synthetic	Having to do with substances that are man-made instead of taken from nature.
Syringe	A small hollow tube used for injecting or withdrawing liquids. It may be attached to a needle in order to withdraw fluid from the body or inject drugs into the body.
Systemic	Affecting the entire body.
Systemic Disease	Disease that affects the whole body.
Systemic Therapy	Treatment using substances that travel through the bloodstream, reaching and affecting cells all over the body.

T

T-Cell	A type of white blood cell. T cells are part of the immune system and develop from stem cells in the bone marrow. They help protect the body from infection and may help fight cancer. Also called T lymphocyte and thymocyte.
Tamoxifen	A drug used to treat certain types of breast cancer in women and men. It is also used to prevent breast cancer in women who have had ductal carcinoma in situ (abnormal cells in the ducts of the breast) and in women who are at a high risk of developing breast cancer. Tamoxifen is also being studied in the treatment of other types of cancer. It blocks the effects of the hormone estrogen in breast tissue, which may help keep breast cancer cells from growing. Tamoxifen is a type of selective estrogen receptor modulator (SERM). Also called tamoxifen citrate.
Targeted Therapy	A type of treatment that uses drugs or other substances to identify and attack specific types of cancer cells with less harm to normal cells. Some targeted therapies block the action of certain enzymes, proteins, or other molecules involved in the growth and spread of cancer cells. Other types of targeted therapies help the immune system kill cancer cells or deliver toxic substances directly to cancer cells and kill them. Targeted therapy may have fewer side effects than other types of cancer treatment. Most targeted therapies are either small molecule drugs or monoclonal antibodies.
Taxane	A type of drug that blocks cell growth by stopping mitosis (cell division). Taxanes interfere with microtubules (cellular structures that help move chromosomes during mitosis). They are used to treat cancer. A taxane is a type of mitotic inhibitor and a type of antimicrotubule agent.
Taxol	A drug used to treat AIDS-related Kaposi sarcoma, advanced ovarian cancer, and certain types of breast cancer. It is also used with cisplatin to treat non-small cell lung cancer in patients who cannot be treated with surgery or radiation therapy. It is also being studied in the treatment of other types of cancer. Taxol blocks cell growth by stopping cell division and may kill cancer cells. It is a type of antimitotic agent. Also called paclitaxel.
Tendon	Tough, fibrous, cord-like tissue that connects muscle to bone or another structure, such as an eyeball. Tendons help the bone or structure to move.

Tetracycline	A drug used to treat bacterial infections. It stops the growth of bacteria by keeping them from making proteins. Tetracycline also binds to new bone tissue and is being studied as a way to detect bone growth. Tetracycline is a type of antibiotic and a type of bone-labeling agent.
Therapeutic	Having to do with treating disease and helping healing take place.
Thoracentesis / Pleural Tap	Removal of fluid from the pleural cavity through a needle inserted between the ribs.
Thrombosis	The formation or presence of a thrombus (blood clot) inside a blood vessel.
Thrush	A condition in which Candida albicans, a type of yeast, grows out of control in moist skin areas of the body. It is usually a result of a weakened immune system, but can be a side effect of chemotherapy or treatment with antibiotics. Thrush usually affects the mouth (oral thrush); however, rarely, it spreads throughout the entire body. Also called candidiasis and candidosis.
Thyroid	A gland located beneath the larynx (voice box) that makes thyroid hormone and calcitonin. The thyroid helps regulate growth and metabolism. Also called thyroid gland.
Thyroid Stimulating Hormone (TSH)	A hormone produced by the pituitary gland. Thyroid-stimulating hormone stimulates the release of thyroid hormone from thyroglobulin. It also stimulates the growth of thyroid follicular cells. An abnormal thyroid-stimulating hormone level may mean that the thyroid hormonal regulation system is out of control, usually as a result of a benign condition (hyperthyroidism or hypothyroidism). Also called TSH.
Tibia	The larger of two bones between the knee and ankle. Also called shinbone.
Tissue	A group or layer of cells that work together to perform a specific function.
Tissue Fluid	Fluid found in the spaces around cells. It comes from substances that leak out of blood capillaries (the smallest type of blood vessel). It helps bring oxygen and nutrients to cells and to remove waste products from them. As new tissue fluid is made, it replaces older fluid, which drains towards lymph vessels. When it enters the lymph vessels, it is called lymph. Also called interstitial fluid.
Total Hysterectomy	Surgery to remove the entire uterus, including the cervix. Also called complete hysterectomy.
Total Mastectomy	Surgery to remove the whole breast. Some of the lymph nodes under the arm may also be removed. Also called simple mastectomy.
Total PSA	The total amount of prostate-specific antigen (PSA) in the blood. It includes the amount of free PSA and the amount of PSA attached to other proteins.
Toxemia	Disease caused by the spread of bacteria and their toxins in the bloodstream. Also called blood poisoning and septicemia.
Toxic	Having to do with poison or something harmful to the body. Toxic substances usually cause unwanted side effects
Toxin	A poison made by certain bacteria, plants, or animals, including insects.
Tracer	A substance (such as a radioisotope) used in imaging procedures.
Tranquilizer	A drug that calms and soothes, and reduces stress and tension. Tranquilizers are used to treat anxiety and insomnia.
Transdermal	Absorbed through the unbroken skin.

Transfusion	A procedure in which whole blood or parts of blood are put into a patient's bloodstream through a vein. The blood may be donated by another person or it may have been taken from the patient and stored until needed. Also called blood transfusion.
Transitional Care	Support given to patients when they move from one phase of disease or treatment to another, such as from hospital care to home care. It involves helping patients and families with medical, practical, and emotional needs as they adjust to different levels and goals of care.
Transurethral Resection of the Prostate (TURP)	Surgery to remove tissue from the prostate using an instrument inserted through the urethra. Also called TURP.
Trauma	Injury to the body, or an event that causes long-lasting mental or emotional damage.
Treatment Cycle	A period of treatment followed by a period of rest (no treatment) that is repeated on a regular schedule. For example, treatment given for one week followed by three weeks of rest is one treatment cycle. When this cycle is repeated multiple times on a regular schedule, it makes up a course of treatment. Also called cycle of treatment.
Treatment Plan	A detailed plan with information about a patient's disease, the goal of treatment, the treatment options for the disease and possible side effects, and the expected length of treatment. A treatment plan may also include information about how much the treatment is likely to cost and about regular follow-up care after treatment ends.
Treatment Schedule	A step-by-step plan of the treatment that a patient is going to receive. A treatment schedule includes the type of treatment that will be given (such as chemotherapy or radiation therapy), how it will be given (such as by mouth or by infusion into a vein), and how often it will be given (such as once a day or once a week). It also includes the amount of time between courses of treatment and the total length of time of treatment.
Treatment Summary	A detailed summary of a patient's disease, the type of treatment the patient received, and any side effects or other problems caused by treatment. It usually includes results of laboratory tests (such as pathology reports and biomarker tests) and imaging tests (such as x-rays, CT scans, and MRIs), and whether a patient took part in a clinical trial. A treatment summary may be used to help plan follow-up care after treatment for a disease, such as cancer.
Trigger	In medicine, a specific event that starts a process or that causes a particular outcome. For example, chemotherapy, painful treatments, or the smells, sounds, and sights that go with them may trigger anxiety and fear in a patient who has cancer. In allergies, exposure to mold, pollen or dust may trigger sneezing, watery eyes, and coughing.
Triple Negative Breast Cancer	Describes breast cancer cells that do not have estrogen receptors, progesterone receptors, or large amounts of HER2/neu protein. Also called ER-negative PR-negative HER2/neu-negative breast cancer.
Tube-feeding	A way of giving medicines and liquids, including liquid foods, through a small tube placed through the nose or mouth into the stomach or small intestine. Sometimes the tube is placed into the stomach or small intestine through an incision (cut) made on the outside of the abdomen. Tube-feeding may be added to what a person is able to eat and drink, or it may be the only source of nutrition. It is a type of enteral nutrition. Also called gavage.
Tumor	An abnormal mass of tissue that results when cells divide more than they should or do not die when they should. Tumors may be benign (not cancer), or malignant (cancer). Also called neoplasm.
Tumor Board Review	A treatment planning approach in which a number of doctors who are experts in different specialties (disciplines) review and discuss the medical condition and treatment options of a patient. In cancer treatment, a tumor board review may include that of a medical oncologist (who provides cancer treatment with drugs), a surgical oncologist (who provides cancer treatment with surgery), and a radiation oncologist (who provides cancer treatment with radiation). Also called multidisciplinary opinion.
Tumor Burden / Tumor Load	Refers to the number of cancer cells, the size of a tumor, or the amount of cancer in the body. Also called tumor load.

Tumor Debulking	Surgical removal of as much of a tumor as possible. Tumor debulking may increase the chance that chemotherapy or radiation therapy will kill all the tumor cells. It may also be done to relieve symptoms or help the patient live longer. Also called debulking.
Tumor Grade	A description of a tumor based on how abnormal the cancer cells and tissue look under a microscope and how quickly the cancer cells are likely to grow and spread. Low-grade cancer cells look more like normal cells and tend to grow and spread more slowly than high-grade cancer cells. Grading systems are different for each type of cancer. They are used to help plan treatment and determine prognosis. Also called grade and histologic grade.
Tumor Marker	A substance found in tissue or blood or other body fluids that may be a sign of cancer or certain benign (noncancer) conditions. Most tumor markers are made by both normal cells and cancer cells, but they are made in larger amounts by cancer cells. A tumor marker may help to diagnose cancer, plan treatment, or find out how well treatment is working or if cancer has come back. Examples of tumor markers include CA-125 (in ovarian cancer), CA 15-3 (in breast cancer), CEA (in colon cancer), and PSA (in prostate cancer).
Tumor Marker Test	A test that measures the amount of substances called tumor markers in tissue, blood, urine, or other body fluids. Most tumor markers are made by both normal cells and cancer cells, but they are made in higher amounts by cancer cells. A high level of a tumor marker may be a sign of cancer or certain benign (noncancerous) conditions. A tumor marker test is usually done with other tests, such as biopsies, to help diagnose some types of cancer. It may also be used to help plan treatment or find out how well treatment is working or if cancer has come back.
Tumor Volume	The size of a cancer measured by the amount of space taken up by the tumor. For example, the tumor volume of prostate cancer is the percentage of the prostate taken up by the tumor.
Tumor-Derived	Taken from an individual's own tumor tissue; may be used in the development of a vaccine that enhances the body's ability to build an immune response to the tumor.
TURP	Surgery to remove tissue from the prostate using an instrument inserted through the urethra. Also called transurethral resection of the prostate.

U

Ulcer	A break on the skin, in the lining of an organ, or on the surface of a tissue. An ulcer forms when the surface cells become inflamed, die, and are shed. Ulcers may be linked to cancer and other diseases.
Ulceration	The formation of a break on the skin or on the surface of an organ. An ulcer forms when the surface cells die and are cast off. Ulcers may be associated with cancer and other diseases.
Ulcerative Colitis	Chronic inflammation of the colon that produces ulcers in its lining. This condition is marked by abdominal pain, cramps, and loose discharges of pus, blood, and mucus from the bowel.
Ultrasound	A procedure that uses high-energy sound waves to look at tissues and organs inside the body. The sound waves make echoes that form pictures of the tissues and organs on a computer screen (sonogram). Ultrasound may be used to help diagnose diseases, such as cancer. It may also be used during pregnancy to check the fetus (unborn baby) and during medical procedures, such as biopsies. Also called ultrasonography.
Ultrasound Transducer	A device that produces sound waves that bounce off body tissues and make echoes. The transducer also receives the echoes and sends them to a computer that uses them to create a picture called a sonogram. Transducers (probes) come in different shapes and sizes for use in making pictures of different parts of the body. The transducer may be passed over the surface of the body or inserted into an opening such as the rectum or vagina.
Ultrasound Guided Biopsy	A biopsy procedure that uses an ultrasound imaging device to find an abnormal area of tissue and guide its removal for examination under a microscope.

Undifferentiated	A term used to describe cells or tissues that do not have specialized ("mature") structures or functions. Undifferentiated cancer cells often grow and spread quickly.
Unilateral	Having to do with one side of the body.
Upper Extremity	The part of the body that includes the arm, wrist, and hand.
Upper Gastrointestinal (GI) Series	A series of x-ray pictures of the esophagus, stomach, and duodenum (the first part of the small intestine). The x-ray pictures are taken after the patient drinks a liquid containing barium sulfate (a form of the silver-white metallic element barium). The barium sulfate coats and outlines the inner walls of the upper gastrointestinal tract so that they can be seen on the x-ray pictures. Also called upper GI series.
Ureter	The tube that carries urine from the kidney to the bladder.
Urethra	The tube through which urine leaves the body. It empties urine from the bladder.
Urinalysis	A test that determines the content of the urine
Urinary	Having to do with urine or the organs of the body that produce and get rid of urine.
Urinary Tract	The organs of the body that produce and discharge urine. These include the kidneys, ureters, bladder, and urethra.
Urine	Fluid containing water and waste products. Urine is made by the kidneys, stored in the bladder, and leaves the body through the urethra.
Urticaria	Itchy, raised red areas on the skin. Urticaria are caused by a reaction to certain foods, drugs, infections, or emotional stress. Also called hives.
Uterus	The hollow, pear-shaped organ in a woman's pelvis. The uterus is where a fetus (unborn baby) develops and grows. Also called womb.

V

Vaginal Atrophy	A condition in which the tissues lining the inside of the vagina (birth canal) become thin, dry, and inflamed. This is caused by a decrease in the amount of estrogen (a female hormone) made by the body. Symptoms of vaginal atrophy include vaginal dryness, itching, and burning, and pain during sexual intercourse. Other symptoms include a burning feeling while urinating, feeling a need to urinate often or right away, and being unable to control the flow of urine. Vaginal atrophy most commonly occurs in women who have gone through menopause naturally or who have early menopause caused by certain types of cancer treatment (such as radiation therapy to the pelvis or chemotherapy) or by having their ovaries removed by surgery. Also called atrophic vaginitis.
Vaginal Cuff	The vaginal cuff is the upper portion of the vagina that opens up into the peritoneum and is sutured shut after the removal of the cervix and uterus during a hysterectomy. The vaginal cuff is created by suturing together the edges of the surgical site where the cervix was attached to the vagina
Value-Based Pricing	A system of setting the cost for a healthcare service in which healthcare providers are paid based on the quality of care they provide rather than the number of healthcare services they give or the number of patients they treat. Value-based pricing may give patients access to better treatments for lower costs. This may help reduce financial stress or hardship on patients receiving medical care.
Varubi	A drug used with other drugs to prevent nausea and vomiting caused by chemotherapy. Varubi blocks the action of chemicals in the central nervous system (CNS) that may trigger nausea and vomiting. It is a type of antiemetic. Also called rolapitant hydrochloride.
Vein	A blood vessel that carries blood to the heart from tissues and organs in the body.

Venipuncture	A procedure in which a needle is used to take blood from a vein, usually for laboratory testing. Venipuncture may also be done to remove extra red blood cells from the blood, to treat certain blood disorders. Also called blood draw and phlebotomy.
Venous Catheter	A thin, flexible tube that is inserted into a large vein, usually in the arm, chest, or leg. It is used to give intravenous fluids, blood transfusions, and chemotherapy and other drugs, and for taking blood samples. It avoids the need for repeated needle sticks.
Ventilator	In medicine, a machine used to help a patient breathe. Also called respirator.
Vertebral Column	The bones, muscles, tendons, and other tissues that reach from the base of the skull to the tailbone. The vertebral column encloses the spinal cord and the fluid surrounding the spinal cord. Also called backbone, spinal column, and spine.
Vesicle	A small sac formed by a membrane and filled with liquid. Vesicles inside cells move substances into or out of the cell. Vesicles made in the laboratory can be used to carry drugs to cells in the body.
Viral	Having to do with a virus.
Virus	In medicine, a very simple microorganism that infects cells and may cause disease. Because viruses can multiply only inside infected cells, they are not considered to be alive.
Visceral	The soft internal organs of the body, including the lungs, the heart, and the organs of the digestive, excretory, and reproductive systems.
Vital	Necessary to maintain life. Breathing is a vital function.
Vitamin	A nutrient that the body needs in small amounts to function and stay healthy. Sources of vitamins are plant and animal food products and dietary supplements. Some vitamins are made in the human body from food products. Vitamins are either fat-soluble (can dissolve in fats and oils) or water-soluble (can dissolve in water). Excess fat-soluble vitamins are stored in the body's fatty tissue, but excess water-soluble vitamins are removed in the urine. Examples are vitamin A, vitamin C, and vitamin E.

W

Warfarin	A drug that prevents blood from clotting. It belongs to the family of drugs called anticoagulants (blood thinners).
Watchful Waiting	Closely watching a patient's condition but not giving treatment unless symptoms appear or change. Watchful waiting is sometimes used in conditions that progress slowly. It is also used when the risks of treatment are greater than the possible benefits. During watchful waiting, patients may be given certain tests and exams. Watchful waiting is sometimes used in prostate cancer. It is a type of expectant management.
WBC	A type of blood cell that is made in the bone marrow and found in the blood and lymph tissue. WBCs are part of the body's immune system. They help the body fight infection and other diseases. Types of WBCs are granulocytes (neutrophils, eosinophils, and basophils), monocytes, and lymphocytes (T cells and B cells). Checking the number of WBCs in the blood is usually part of a complete blood cell (CBC) test. It may be used to look for conditions such as infection, inflammation, allergies, and leukemia. Also called leukocyte and white blood cell.
Well-Differentiated	A term used to describe cells and tissue that have mature (specialized) structures and functions. In cancer, well-differentiated cancer cells look more like normal cells under a microscope and tend to grow and spread more slowly than poorly differentiated or undifferentiated cancer cells.
Whipple Procedure	A type of surgery used to treat pancreatic cancer. The head of the pancreas, the duodenum, a portion of the stomach, and other nearby tissues are removed. Also called pancreatoduodenectomy.

White Blood Cell (WBC)	A type of blood cell that is made in the bone marrow and found in the blood and lymph tissue. White blood cells are part of the body's immune system. They help the body fight infection and other diseases. Types of white blood cells are granulocytes (neutrophils, eosinophils, and basophils), monocytes, and lymphocytes (T cells and B cells). Checking the number of white blood cells in the blood is usually part of a complete blood cell (CBC) test. It may be used to look for conditions such as infection, inflammation, allergies, and leukemia. Also called leukocyte and WBC.
Whole Cell Vaccine	Vaccine made from whole tumor cells that have been changed in the laboratory.
Wide Local Excision	Surgery to cut out the cancer and some healthy tissue around it.
Wound	A break in the skin or other body tissues caused by injury or surgical incision (cut).

X

Xanax	A drug used to treat anxiety disorders and panic attacks. It is being studied in the treatment of nausea and vomiting caused by some cancer treatments. It is a type of benzodiazepine. Also called alprazolam.
XELOX	An abbreviation for a chemotherapy combination used to treat colorectal cancer that has spread. It is also being studied in the treatment of other types of cancer. It includes the drugs capecitabine (Xeloda) and oxaliplatin. Also called XELOX regimen.
Xerostomia	Dry mouth. It occurs when the body is not able to make enough saliva.
Xgeva	A drug used to prevent bone problems caused by multiple myeloma or by solid tumors that have spread to the bone. It is also used in certain patients to treat giant cell tumor of the bone that cannot be removed by surgery. Xgeva is also used to treat hypercalcemia that is caused by cancer and did not get better after treatment with bisphosphonates. Xgeva binds to a protein called RANKL, which keeps RANKL from binding to another protein called RANK on the surface of certain bone cells, including bone cancer cells. This may help keep bone from breaking down and cancer cells from growing. Xgeva may also prevent the loss of calcium from the bones. It contains the active ingredient denosumab. Xgeva is a type of monoclonal antibody.
X-Ray	A type of radiation used in the diagnosis and treatment of cancer and other diseases. In low doses, x-rays are used to diagnose diseases by making pictures of the inside of the body. In high doses, x-rays are used to treat cancer.

Y

Yeast	A type of microorganism that is found almost everywhere, including inside the body. There are many different types of yeast. Some types are used to make foods, such as bread, cheese, and alcoholic drinks. Small amounts of a certain type of yeast normally live on the skin and in some parts of the body, such as the mouth, throat, and vagina. Yeast are a type of fungus.
Yeast Infection	A condition in which too much yeast grows in certain areas of the body and causes symptoms and disease. Small amounts of yeast normally live on the skin and in other parts of the body, such as the mouth, throat, and vagina. Sometimes, too much yeast can grow in these areas and cause infection. Yeast infections may also occur in the blood and spread throughout the body, but this is rare. Certain conditions, such as a weakened immune system, diabetes, pregnancy, hormone changes, and stress, and use of certain medicines may increase the risk of yeast infection.
Yoga	An ancient system of practices used to balance the mind and body through exercise, meditation (focusing thoughts), and control of breathing and emotions. Yoga is being studied as a way to relieve stress and treat sleep problems in cancer patients.
Yttrium Y 90	A radioactive form of the rare metal yttrium that is used in radiation therapy to treat some types of tumors. Yttrium Y 90 can be linked to a molecule, such as a monoclonal antibody, to help it locate and bind to certain substances in the body, including cancer cells. The radiation may kill the cancer cells.

Zofran	A drug used to prevent nausea and vomiting caused by chemotherapy and radiation therapy. It is also used to prevent nausea and vomiting after surgery. Zofran blocks the action of the chemical serotonin, which binds to certain nerves and may trigger nausea and vomiting. Blocking serotonin may help lessen nausea and vomiting. It is a type of serotonin receptor antagonist and a type of antiemetic. Also called ondansetron hydrochloride.
Zoladex	A drug used to treat prostate cancer and to relieve the symptoms of advanced breast cancer. It is also used to treat problems with the endometrium (lining of the uterus). Zoladex keeps the body from making the hormones luteinizing hormone-releasing hormone (LHRH) and luteinizing hormone (LH). This causes the testicles to stop making testosterone (a male hormone) in men, and the ovaries to stop making estradiol (a form of the hormone estrogen) in women. Zoladex may stop the growth of cancer cells that need testosterone or estrogen to grow. It is a type of LHRH agonist. Also called goserelin acetate and ZDX.
Zoloft	A drug used to treat depression. It is a type of selective serotonin reuptake inhibitor (SSRI). Also called sertraline.

AFTERWORD

When Amor first told me that she wanted to help others deal with cancer by writing a book about her experiences, I thought it would be interesting.

When she later told me that she would include other cancer survivors in the book, I thought that it was a great idea. But then, after she completed treatment and got to work talking to other survivors and recruiting them, I thought, "Wow, she really wants to do this and it would help a lot of people going through cancer treatment!"

Early on, Amor knew how she wanted her book to read. "Been There Done That: Practical Tips & Wisdom from Cancer Survivors to Cancer Patients" was always meant to be like a central guidebook for cancer patients. There was so much information to gather, transcribe and organize, it was sometimes overwhelming for her.

There was a big learning curve and a lot of stumbling blocks for her to overcome when writing this book. But because Amor was so passionate about getting the information out to help cancer patients, their caregivers, and other cancer survivors, she persisted.

Looking back at the entire process, it was a real grind and there were definitely challenges. Amor worked long nights and countless hours trying to get everything just right. She showed as much strength and determination as she had in fighting both of her cancers.

With the completion of this book, I can easily see how the material and advice will help cancer patients and caregivers through the difficulties of having to cope with and live with cancer.

I know because, as Amor's partner and caregiver, I've been there and done that too.

—Bill Stone